W9-BMC-362

DIFFICULT CARDIOLOGY III

For Maggie

DIFFICULT CARDIOLOGY III

Edited by

Graham Jackson FRCP FESC FACC
Consultant Cardiologist
Guy's Hospital
London, UK

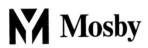 **Mosby**

St. Louis Baltimore Boston Carlsbad Chicago Naples New York Philadelphia Portland
London Madrid Mexico City Singapore Sydney Tokyo Toronto Wiesbaden

MARTIN DUNITZ

© Martin Dunitz Ltd 1997

First published in the United Kingdom in 1997 by
Martin Dunitz Ltd
The Livery House
7–9 Pratt Street
London NW1 0AE

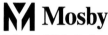 **Mosby**
Dedicated to Publishing Excellence

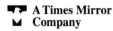 **A Times Mirror
Company**

Distributed in the U.S.A. and Canada by
Mosby–Year Book   Times Mirror Professional Publishing Ltd.
11830 Westline Industrial Drive   130 Flaska Drive
St. Louis, Missouri 63146   Markham, Ontario L6G 1B8

All rights reserved. No part of this publication may be
reproduced, stored in a retrieval system, or transmitted, in
any form or by any means, electronic, mechanical,
photocopying, recording or otherwise, without the prior
permission of the publisher.

A CIP catalogue record for this book is available from the
British Library

ISBN 1-85317-406-8

Composition by Keyword Typesetting Services Ltd
Printed and bound in Great Britain by
Biddles Ltd, Guildford and King's Lynn

CONTENTS

List of Contributors

AA Jennifer Adgey MD FRCP
Professor of Cardiology, Regional Medical
Cardiology Center, Royal Victoria Hospital,
Grosvenor Road, Belfast BT12 6BA,
Northern Ireland

Jacques D Barth MD PhD
Associate Professor of Preventive Medicine
and Cardiology, Atherosclerosis Research
Unit, University of Southern California, Los
Angeles, CA 90033, USA

D Gareth Beevers MD FRCP
Professor of Medicine, Department of
Medicine, City Hospital NHS Trust, Dudley
Road, Birmingham B18 7QH, UK

Andrew J Buda MD
Robert Morgandanes Professor, Section of
Cardiology, Department of Medicine, Tulane
University Medical Center, 1430 Tulane
Avenue, New Orleans, LA 70112, USA

**A John Camm MD QHP FRCP FESC
FACC**
Chairman, Department of Cardiological
Sciences, St George's Hospital Medical
School, Cranmer Terrace,
London SW17 0RE, UK

Stephen Campbell BSc MD FRCP
Consultant Cardiologist, Northern General
Hospital Trust NHS, Herries Road, Sheffield
S5 7AU, UK

**Douglas Chamberlain CBE KSG MD DSc
(Hon) FRCP FRCA FESC FACC**
Honorary Consultant Cardiologist, 25
Woodland Drive, Hove, East Sussex
BN3 6DH, UK

**John GF Cleland MD FRCP (UK) RESC
FACC**
British Heart Foundation Senior Research
Fellow, MRC Clinical Research Initiative in
Heart Failure and Honorary Consultant
Cardiologist, Western Infirmary, Glasgow
G11 6NT, UK

Richard Cooke BA (Law) MD MRCP (UK)
Consultant Cardiologist, Guys and St
Thomas NHS Trust, St Guy's Hospital,
Thomas Street, London, SE1 9RT, UK

Samer R Dibs MD
Clinical Assistant Professor, Section of
Cardiology, Department of Medicine, Tulane
University Medical Center, 1430 Tulane
Avenue, New Orleans, LA 70112, USA

Clare M Dollery BSc MRCP
MRC Clinical Training Fellow, The Hatter
Institute, Department of Academic and
Clinical Cardiology, University College
Hospital, Grafton Way, London WC1E 6DB,
UK

Leisa J Freeman MRCP
Associate Specialist in Cardiology, Walnut
Tree Farm, Benacre, Wrentham, Beccles,
Suffolk NR34 7L, UK

Jaswinder S Gill MD MRCP FACC
Consultant Cardiologist, Department of
Cardiological Sciences, St Guy's Hospital,
Thomas Street, London SE1 9RT, UK

Graham Jackson FRCP FESC FACC
Consultant Cardiologist, Department of
Cardiology, St Guy's Hospital, Thomas Street,
London SE1 9RT, UK

Frances L Johnson MD
Director, Cardiac Transplantation Services,
Veterans Affairs Palo Alto Heath Care
System, 38801 Miranda Avenue, Palo Alto,
CA 9304 and Clinical Faculty, Division of
Cardiovascular Medicine, Stanford
University of Medicine, Falk Cardiovascular
Research Building, Stanford,
CA 94305-5246, USA

Paul W Johnston MB MRCP
Senior Registrar, Regional Medical
Cardiology Center, Royal Victoria Hospital,
Grosvenor Road, Belfast BT12 6BA,
Northern Ireland

**Gregory YH Lip MD MRCP FACA
FACC**
Senior Lecturer in Medicine and Consultant
Cardiologist, Department of Medicine, City
Hospital NHS Trust, Dudley Road,
Birmingham B18 7QH, UK

Michael Marber PHD MRCP
Senior Lecturer, Honorary Consultant,
UMDS, St Thomas's Hospital, Lambeth Place
Road, London
SE1 7EH, UK

**John JV McMurray BSc MD MB ChB
MRCP**
Consultant Cardiologist, Department of
Cardiology, Western Infirmary, Glasgow
G11 6NT, UK

**John PD Reckless MD MB BS FRCP
MRCS**
Honorary Senior Lecturer, School of
Postgraduate Medicine, University of Bath,
and Consultant Physician, Royal United
Hospital, Bath BA1 3NG, UK

Peter Richardson MD FRCP
Consultant Cardiologist, King's College
Hospital, Denmark Hill, London SE5 9RS,
UK

John S Schroeder MD
Professor of Medicine, Division of Medicine,
Division of Cardiovascular Medicine,
Stanford University of Medicine, Falk
Cardiovascular Research Building, Stanford,
CA 94305-5246, USA

**Neil Sulke BSc (Hons) DM MRCP (UK)
FACC**
Consultant Cardiologist, Department of
Cardiology, Hunt House, St Guy's Hospital,
Thomas Street, London SE1 9RT, UK

Kim H Tan MD MRCP
Senior Registrar, Department of Cardiology,
Hunt House, St Guy's Hospital, Thomas
Street, London SE1 9RT, UK

Johan EP Waktare MB ChB MRCP
Clinical Research Registrar, Department of
Cardiological Sciences, St George's Hospital
Medical School, Cranmer Terrace, London
SW17 0RE, UK

Howard Why MD MRCP
Consultant Cardiologist, Burton Hospital,
Belvedere Road, Burton-on-Trent, Staffs
DE13 0RB, UK

Preface

The 'Difficult' books have proved very successful and I am grateful for the reception that they
have received. Criticisms have been constructive
and acted upon, and the helpful suggestions for
further chapters have been taken into account,
with many included in this volume. I must
admit that I did not expect to be editing a
third volume just seven years after the first,
but I believe it confirms the need for unconven-
tional books to complement the standard texts.

The objective is as before: to take a subject
where opinion is divided, review the evidence
and then to try to be as practical as possible.
The 'If I had...' addition to the chapters seems to
be very popular, with readers telling me that it's
the first section they turn to (rather like the
obituaries I was told!). I have tried to vary the
chapters as much as possible in the hope of
providing a book of general interest which is
applicable to a wide audience. However, I freely
admit that I have included subjects where I
personally feel the need for clear guidelines
and understanding (e.g. gene therapy) and I
hope that others feel the same. As I have said
in the previous volumes, what is difficult for
some is clear to others but even when it is
clear, it is often helpful to have the opinions
of others to give a more balanced perspective,
particularly if they are presented in a fresh and
interesting way.

We do not appear to be 'running out of
steam' with this idea and suggestions for the
fourth volume will be warmly welcomed. For
now, I hope that you enjoy this volume and
find the personalized style a readable way of
reviewing and agreeing or disagreeing with the
authors. Where guidelines are not clear a dis-
agreement is inevitable but it should always be
constructive, for our goal is a common one: to
improve the care of our patients whether their
management is straightforward or 'difficult'.

GJ
July 1997

Acknowledgements

I am, as always grateful, to my secretary Helen Symeou for co-ordinating the chapters. I am also grateful to Alan Burgess and Ian Mellor of Martin Dunitz who chased (and bullied!) the authors and have done an excellent job in bringing out the book quickly and keeping the chapters up-to-date. I must also thank all the authors and their secretaries for their hard work and finally Martin Dunitz for continuing to support the concept.

1

Primary and secondary cardiovascular prevention: one disease, two different management strategies?

Jacques D Barth

Introduction

Cardiovascular disease remains a primary healthcare issue with respect to its effect on human suffering and its economic impact. During the last decades, cardiovascular mortality in industrialized nations has declined.[1] However, cohort studies show that, in general, the incidence and prevalence of cardiovascular diseases have increased. And in the cases where the incidence and prevalence of coronary disease have not increased,[2] the best findings report that it has merely stayed the same as in prior years.

Both primary and secondary prevention of cardiovascular diseases are important.[3,4] While primary prevention deals with preventing and/or delaying the onset of coronary disease, secondary prevention focuses on preventing sequelae of established atherosclerotic heart disease. Apparently the primary prevention approach is superior and a variety of approaches used to prevent disease development have shown encouraging results. Dealing with the cause of the underlying problem is also more appropriate than trying to limit disease once damage has been done.

Why the success of primary prevention approaches has not yet resulted in a clear uniform policy is unfortunate. Opponents of primary prevention point to the fact that no scientific study has shown a primary prevention approach to be irrefutably more effective than other forms of prevention. However, in most studies each risk factor was considered as a separate contributor and managed as such. The underlying cause of most cardiovascular diseases is atherosclerosis, and as such the cause of the disease is multifactorial with each factor intertwined with others. Atherosclerotic cardiovascular diseases are a complex problem involving lipid deposition, blood pressure, rheologic forces, carbohydrate intolerance and thrombogenic aspects. The risk associated with anyone is compounded by the presence of the others. The risk associated with hypertension, hyperlipidemia or diabetes varies widely depending on the presence and level of other associated risk factors.[5-7] For example, at a given level of total cholesterol, risk is greatly affected by the total/high-density lipoprotein (HDL) cholesterol ratio. Total cholesterol alone does not decide risk — the two-way traffic of cholesterol must be assessed to complete the picture. Epidemiologic research has identified other factors contributing to coronary disease that include atherogenic personal attributes (e.g. type A psychological behavior, notably hostility) and the living habits which promote them, compromised coronary circulation and host susceptibility to these risk factors. Living habits, such as cigarette smoking or lack of exercise, independently affect the risk associated with any of the atherogenic traits. An individual's lifestyle, obesity and diet affect atherogenic factors and must be considered when assessing risk and implementing preventive measures. Optimal risk predictors require combining a quantitative assessment of all risk factors into a composite estimate.

The more extensive the atherosclerosis the more likely it is to lead to a complication (e.g. myocardial infarction and stroke).[8] However, atherosclerosis development is a slow process in itself and different risk factors decide the rate of acceleration of the process. Superimposed events like a myocardial infarction occur when a base of atherosclerosis that to some large extent remains lipid dependent is present.[9,10] The prudent approach is to interfere with the development of atherosclerosis itself to prevent cardiovascular disease and myocardial infarction. Prevention is the goal and cardiovascular risk factors should be modified as early as possible. A variety of prevention approaches to lower cardiovascular risk factors have been studied. These range from behavioral modification and drug intervention trials to the implementation of clinical endpoints (a myocardial infarction incidence) and an investigation focused on disease progression assessment.

The most important question (which has not been adequately addressed by these studies) is: what approach works the best for most individuals? In trying to answer this question a strict separation between primary and secondary prevention is somewhat of an artificial and illogical distinction, as atherosclerosis is a continuous and naturally progressive process. It should be kept in mind that the difference for any individual between primary and secondary prevention can be less than 24 hours. The occurrence of any one event during a lifelong, slowly progressive disease will interfere with the evolution of the disease in only a marginal way. The fact that 25% of patients show 'sudden cardiac death' as first signs of coronary heart disease shows that disease complications may occur suddenly.[11]

Another fact that blurs the distinction between primary and secondary prevention even more is that diagnosis of myocardial infarction is not straightforward. About 15% of those who suffer from a myocardial infarction do not experience any cardiovascular symptoms before the infarction.[12,13] A priori, separating primary and secondary prevention seems artificial and futile when trying to prevent a very real disease.

Primary prevention not only means before disability but also the avoidance of the need for (expensive) treatment for risks factors. Truly to prevent coronary disease, special attention must be given to lower socioeconomic and minority groups since a decline in morbidity and mortality of cardiovascular disease in these populations has not (yet) occurred. In the African-American population, hypertension is common, while diabetes and obesity remain the nemesis in the Hispanic/Latino population. Morbidity and mortality resulting from coronary disease remain number one in the developed world and have also gained the number-one spot in many developing countries. A recent prediction for the prevalence of the disease in the year 2020 indicates that cardiovascular diseases will increase even further and will remain the number-one disease and healthcare cost in the total world population.[14]

This chapter will focus on primary cardiovascular prevention, which will be defined as to retard, reduce and possibly reverse the growth of atherosclerotic disease to delay or prevent ischemic damage to the heart, extremities and brain. This review will be limited to studies designed to prevent (further) progression of the underlying cardiovascular disease, and will not look at studies which focus on preventing cardiovascular events.

Primary (observational) prevention studies

The Framingham Study

In the Framingham observational study, the benefits of modifying cardiovascular risk factors along with weight loss were identified as important factors in primary prevention of cardiovascular disease. This study was the first to identify that an elevated HDL-cholesterol level was inversely correlated with cardiovascular risks. It confirmed that low-density lipoprotein (LDL) cholesterol was positively correlated with a cardiovascular incidence.[15]

A recent publication on the effects of weight reduction showed that when subpopulations were compared with those whose body mass index (BMI) or weight changed least, men and women who lost weight during a 10-year period were older, heavier and had higher blood pressures and cholesterol levels initially but had the smallest gains in blood pressure and cholesterol levels. However, rates of cigarette smoking were higher, and rates of smoking cessation were lower. During 20 years of further follow-up, death rates were highest in those whose BMI decreased and in those with the highest BMI at study entry. Relative risks for death from cardiovascular disease, coronary heart disease and all causes were significantly greater by 33–61% in men whose BMI decreased after adjusting for age and risk factors for cardiovascular disease. In women, weight loss and weight gain were associated with higher relative risks for cardiovascular disease and coronary heart disease. However, the 38% increase in a total mortality rate among women who lost weight was statistically significant after adjusting for age.[16]

In summary, weight loss as a primary prevention measure was associated with improvements in blood pressure and cholesterol levels but was also associated with continued cigarette smoking, prevalent and incident cardiovascular disease, diabetes mellitus, other diseases and higher death rates. Leanness and maintenance of stable weight were beneficial to the prevention of cardiovascular morbidity and death.

The Chicago Studies

The Chicago Studies consisted of a group of long-term (ranging from 12 to 25 years) studies with men which focused on finding relationships between major risk factors, and mortality resulting from coronary artery disease (CAD) and overall mortality. Included in the Chicago Studies are the People's Gas Study, the Western Electric Study the Chicago Heart Association Study and the Multiple Risk Factor Intervention Trial.[17,18] A brief description of these studies and the significance of their findings is outlined below.

People's Gas Study (PG)/Western Electric Study (WE)

This longitudinal study followed 1119 men aged 25–39 for 25 years and 1235 men aged 40–59 years to track cardiovascular disease morbidity and mortality (PG). The WE study was a 24-year longitudinal study following 1882 men aged 40–55. Baseline nutrient data (dietary cholesterol) were also independently related to these mortality risks. Combined risk factor impact was strong for men of all baseline ages. Thus, for WE men, favorable levels compared to observed levels of serum cholesterol, blood pressure, cigarette use and dietary cholesterol were estimated to result in a 24-year risk of CAD death 69% lower, all-cause death 42% lower and longevity 9 years greater.[19]

Chicago Heart Association (CHA)

The Chicago Heart Association followed five groups of men and women over a 15-year period. These groups comprised 7873 men aged 25–39, 8515 men aged 40–59, 1490 men aged 60–74, 7082 women aged 40–59 and 1243 women aged 60–74. The study focused on tracking morbidity and mortality after healthy recommendations were given.

For CHA middle-aged and older women, favorable baseline levels of serum cholesterol, blood pressure and cigarette use were estimated to yield a 15-year CAD risk lower by 60% and longevity greater by 5 years.

Multiple Risk Factor Intervention Trial (MRFIT)

This 12-year project screened 11 098 men considered to be very low risk for CAD and compared them with a further 350 564 men. With a high degree of consistency, multivariate analyses showed independent positive relationships of baseline serum cholesterol, blood pressure and cigarette use to risk of death from CAD and other causes of death. Over 12 years, low-risk men (serum cholesterol < 4.71 mmol/l, systolic/diastolic blood pressure < 120/< 80 mm Hg, nonsmokers, nondiabetic, no previous heart attack) compared to all others were observed to have lower death rates by 89% for CAD, 79% lower for stroke, 86% lower for other cardiovascular diseases, 30% lower for cancers, 21% lower for a variety of other causes and 53% for all causes. The longevity for low-risk men was estimated to be more than 9 years longer than for all others. These findings show great potential for prevention of the CAD epidemic and for increased longevity with health through more healthy lifestyles with consequently lower cardiovascular risk factor levels.[20,21]

The inter-relationships among education, smoking and noncardiovascular (non-CVD) mortality were examined in middle-aged white males in the different studies. In each study, college graduates had the lowest prevalence of current smokers (as reported at the time of the study) and the highest prevalence of former smokers. In PG and WE, the relative risks of non-CVD death for those who did not attend college compared to those who did were 1.50 and 1.38. Differences in baseline cigarette smoking account for only 23–29% of the increased risks. For smoking-related causes, the relative risk of death for those who did not attend/graduate from college was 1.95 in WE, 2.13 in PG and 2.34 in CHA. These findings suggest that education is related inversely to mortality primarily through smoking and smoking-related causes of death. As smoking is becoming a habit of the less educated, these findings further underscore the need to target the lower end of the socioeconomic scale with a variety of smoking-cessation and other prevention programs.

Cardiovascular risk intervention

We will now look at risk factor modification studies aimed at minimizing the major cardiovascular risk factors.[22,23] These studies indicate the importance of cardiovascular risk factors in the prevention of CAD. The American Heart Association and fellow organizations in other countries have identified four major (modifiable) cardiovascular risk factors:

(i) Elevated/high blood cholesterol levels.
(ii) Elevated blood pressure.
(iii) Cigarette smoking.
(iv) A sedentary lifestyle.

Many minor risk factors have also been identified. However, modifying the major factors is an important key when we discuss primary prevention.

Elevated blood cholesterol — lipid profiles

With the help of the research studies outlined below, the direct and positive relationship between an elevated serum (LDL) cholesterol and the progression of cardiovascular disease is rarely disputed. HDL cholesterol is positively correlated with the prevention of both the progression of coronary disease and the occurrence of clinical events. These studies played an important role in our current understanding of the relationship between lipid profiles and CAD.[24,25] The following studies that have focused on this relationship should be considered.

The Coronary Drug Project

The Coronary Drug Project observed the effects of different lipid-mitigating drugs on the subsequent recurrence of complications of atherosclerosis. Fifteen years after the start of the study the group that had received niacin showed a significantly greater decrease in mortality (11%) when compared to the placebo group. This was true although the group took niacin for a very short period. The mortality for the other intervention groups (e.g. a thyroid hormone) was 52% whereas the mortality rate was 58% for the group given niacin during the initial phase of the project.[26]

The West of Scotland Study

The West of Scotland Study used the HMG-CoA reductase inhibitor, pravastatin, to lower LDL cholesterol. Results indicated that with the use of pravastatin, clinical events could be significantly lower in asymptomatic individuals with a relatively high blood cholesterol level. A total of 6595 men aged 45–64 with a mean plasma cholesterol level of 7.04 mmol/l received either 40 mg of pravastatin or a placebo. The average follow-up period was 4.9 years. In the placebo group, 248 definite coronary events occurred whereas only 174 occurred in the pravastatin group (31% reduction, p < 0.001). No increase in deaths from noncardiovascular causes in the pravastatin group was found, and a 22% reduction of death from any cause was also found for participants in the pravastatin group (p = 0.051). The West of Scotland Study showed for the first time that an initial cardiovascular event could be prevented by using lipid-lowering drugs.[27]

The Scandinavian Simvastatin Survival Study (4S)

The Scandinavian Simvastatin Survival Study was designed to evaluate the effects of cholesterol reduction with the HMG-CoA reductase inhibitor, simvastatin, on mortality and morbidity in patients with established CAD. A total of 4444 patients with angina pectoris or previous myocardial infarction and serum cholesterol levels of 5.5–8.0 mmol/l while treated with a lipid-lowering diet were randomly assigned to double-blind treatment with either simvastatin or a placebo. Over the 5.4 years of follow-up, simvastatin produced changes in total cholesterol (−25%), LDL cholesterol (−35%), and HDL cholesterol (+8%), with few adverse effects. Of patients in the placebo group 256 (12%) died compared to 182 (8%) in the simvastatin group, a risk reduction of 30% (p = 0.0003) attributable to a 42% reduction in the risk of coronary death. Noncardiovascular causes accounted for 49 deaths in the placebo group and 46 deaths in the simvastatin group.[28]

Primary intervention studies using only behavioral modification to affect lipid levels have not yet been reported. Animal data, genetic conditions that contribute to high cholesterol levels, post-mortem observations and a lipid atherosclerosis hypothesis explain our current understanding of the direct positive relationship between elevated cholesterol and the progression of cardiovascular disease. Complications of disease like sudden death or a myocardial infarction are dramatic events. However, often a slowly progressing sledging and atherosclerotic build-up remains the real culprit. It has been estimated that by the age of 40, about 40% of all men will have coronary narrowing of at least 50%, without suffering from any cardiac complaints. Again, when we look at real-life situations such as these, the strict distinction between primary and secondary prevention is an arbitrary one.

While lowering the lipid risk factors will slow the progression of coronary disease, it will not necessarily reverse the damage that has already been caused. Two studies have examined the impact of lipid-lowering medication on the progression and regression of CAD using sequential computerized coronary angiographies as methods. The interim analysis shows that lipid lowering with drugs decelerates progression of disease and dramatically decreases the likelihood of a clinical event but the regression of the disease itself remains a relatively rare phenomenon.[29,30] When drug and behavior modification strategies designed to induce regression of disease are compared and assessed by repeated quantitative assessed coronary angiographies, behavioral modifications are as successful or even better at reversing the disease than lipid-lowering medications.[31] To decide the associations of total, LDL and high-density lipoprotein (HDL) cholesterol with mortality from CAD and cardiovascular disease, 2541 white men aged 40–69 were studied for an average of 10.1 years. Seventeen per cent had some manifestation of cardiovascular disease at a baseline, while the remaining 83% did not. Among the men who had cardiovascular disease at a baseline, those with 'high' blood cholesterol levels (above 6.19 mmol/l) had a risk of death from cardiovascular disease (including coron-

ary heart disease) that was 3.45 times higher than that for men with 'desirable' blood cholesterol levels (below 5.16 mmol/l). All three lipid levels were also significant predictors of death from coronary heart disease alone ($p < 0.005$). Total cholesterol and LDL cholesterol levels were also significant predictors of death from cardiovascular and coronary heart disease in men without pre-existing cardiovascular disease, although these men remained at a lower level of absolute risk of death. Thus, the 10-year risk of death from cardiovascular disease for a man with pre-existing cardiovascular disease increased from 3.8% to almost 19.6% when his total cholesterol level increased from a 'desirable' level to a 'high' one. The corresponding risk for a man who was free of cardiovascular disease at a baseline increased from 1.7% to 4.9% with similar changes in total cholesterol. These findings suggest that total, LDL- and HDL-cholesterol levels are useful and accurate predictors of mortality, especially in men with pre-existing cardiovascular disease.[32]

In another meta-analysis, 24 847 male participants, with a mean age of 47.5 were studied.[33,34] Follow-up periods totaled 119 000 person years, during which 1147 deaths occurred. Mortality from coronary heart disease tended to be lower in men receiving interventions to reduce cholesterol when compared with mortality in control subjects ($p = 0.06$); however, total mortality was *not* affected by treatment. Lipid-lowering drug intervention treatments were found to reduce mortality from coronary heart disease ($p = 0.04$) significantly, while the reduction of cholesterol levels had no effect on mortality from cancer. And, surprisingly, a significant increase in deaths not related to illness (deaths from accidents, suicide or violence) in the groups receiving treatment was found when compared to controls ($p = 0.004$). Clearly, the association between the reduction of cholesterol concentrations and deaths not related to illness warrants further investigation. Additionally, the failure of cholesterol-lowering programs to affect overall survival shows that close examination is needed to appraise the real benefits of reducing cholesterol concentrations for the general population.[35,36]

Kuopio Atherosclerosis Prevention Study

The Kuopio Atherosclerosis Prevention Study (KAPS) is a population-based trial in the primary prevention of carotid and femoral atherosclerosis. A total of 447 men aged 44–65 years (mean 57) were randomized to pravastatin (40 mg/d) or placebo for three years. Fewer than 10% of the subjects had prior myocardial infarction. The outcome was the rate of carotid atherosclerotic progression of the annual ultrasound examinations in the average of the maximum carotid intima-media thickness (IMT). In the common carotid artery there was a treatment effect of 66%, in pravastatin 0.010 mm/y and in the placebo 0.029 mm/y (p < 0.002) at the overall mean baseline IMT of 1.35 mm. The treatment effect was larger in subjects with higher baseline IMT values and in smokers. It may be implied that LDL cholesterol lowering by pravastatin in hypercholesterolemic men in a primary prevention setting suggests an even greater effect in smokers than in nonsmokers.[37]

Program on the Surgical Control of Hyperlipidemia

The program on the Surgical Control of Hyperlipidemia (POSCH) was a controlled study to assess the effects of partial ileal bypass as a lipid-lowering intervention, on coronary atherosclerosis change, mortality and morbidity. LDL-cholesterol decreased during 7 years' follow-up by 59% whereas HDL-cholesterol and triglyceride levels basically remained the same. HDL_{2c} was significantly lower (p < 0.01) in the control group (0.22 mmol/l).

Apolipoprotein B was significantly lower in the intervention group and Apo-AI significantly higher at 7 years. Regression of disease was significantly correlated to persistent lowering of LDL cholesterol.[38]

Helsinki Heart Study

The Helsinki Heart Study was a randomized double-blind 5-year primary prevention trial to test the efficacy of HDL-cholesterol raising and triglycerides/LDL-cholesterol lowering using gemfibrozil.[39] Gemfibrozil (1200 mg/d) was given to 2051 middle-aged men (40–55 years) and 2030 men received a placebo. Triglycerides fell by 43%, LDL by 10% and HDL-cholesterol rose initially by 10%. A 34% reduction (p < 0.02) in cardiac endpoints was observed in the gemfibrozil group after 5 years of intervention. Fifty-six cardiac endpoints were observed in the intervention group versus 84 in the placebo population. As the initial baseline cholesterol was a relatively high 7.0 mmol/l, extrapolation to the general population seems difficult.

Oslo Diet and Antismoking Trial

The 15-year results of this trial have been summarized and published. This primary prevention study enrolled more than 1200 patients which were randomized to intervention (a low-saturated fat intake and quit-smoking advice) and control groups. The doctor–patient interaction was limited to an infrequent review of cardiovascular risk factors. This resulted in a 10% decrease in total cholesterol, total fat intake decreases from 40 to 27%, polyunsaturated fat/saturated fat ratio increases from 0.3 to 0.7%, and a decrease in triglycerides of 28%. HDL-cholesterol increased by 5% in those patients who lost weight. The conclusion of the 15-year follow-up data was that this intervention lead to a 5% decrease of risk of coronary heart disease for every 1% total cholesterol

		Intervention (n = 604)	Control (n = 628)	p
5 years	CHD death	6	14	ns
	Total death	16	24	ns
8.5 years	CHD death	7	19	0.037
	Total death	19	31	0.055
15 years	CHD death	24	48	0.004
	Total death	58	82	0.027

Adapted from Hjermann et al. as published in Betteridge and Barth.[42]

Table 1.1
Oslo Diet and Antismoking Trial (15 years' data).

lowering. In addition, cardiovascular death decreased by 50% in the intervention group whereas total death decreased by 30%. This study is one of the first to show that mortality will decrease when heart-healthy advice is given and followed (Table 1.1).[40,41]

National Heart, Lung and Blood Institute (NHLBI) type II study

This early trial used sequential coronary angiograms to compare change in coronary morphology between placebo and cholestyramine-treated patients with LDL-cholesterol above the 90th percentile of the general population. Cholestyramine decreased LDL-cholesterol by 26% whereas a low-fat diet alone induced only a decrease of 5%.[43] Cholestyramine retarded progression by 50% in comparison with the placebo population. A significant correlation was found to the level of LDL-cholesterol decrease and deceleration of progression of atherosclerosis. Triglycerides increased in both groups by 25%. A population of 116 patients with known CAD and hyperlipidemia were followed for 5 years. No significant difference was found in total events and mortality. Angiographic change was significantly (p < 0.03) progressive in the placebo group. New lesion formation and regression were essentially not

different. However, in lesions initially >50% progression was significantly less in the intervention group. It may be concluded from this trial that a reduction of LDL-cholesterol due to diet and cholestyramine decelerates progression of coronary atherosclerosis. HDL-subfractions were associated with slowing of progression and regression of disease whereas reduction in small LDL lead to a deceleration of disease alone.

The Lipid Research Clinics Coronary Primary Prevention Trial (LRC-CPPT)

This study was designed to assess in a primary setting the efficacy of a low-fat diet with or without the bile acid sequestrant cholestyramine.[44] Morbidity and mortality were assessed in 3806 men aged 35–59 years with primary hypercholesterolemia. During the 7-year study, total-cholesterol and LDL-cholesterol were reduced by 8% and 12% respectively as compared to the placebo group. A 19% reduction of fatal and nonfatal myocardial infarction was achieved (p < 0.05). In the cholestyramine group angina and bypass surgery were significantly reduced (20%, p < 0.01; 21%, p < 0.001 respectively). Individuals with the greatest reduction in risk showed the greatest benefit. As a rule of thumb, a 2% reduction in coronary risk would be the result of every 1% total cholesterol lowering.

The Pravastatin Multinational Study

The effects of pravastatin in patients with serum total cholesterol levels from 5.2 to 7.8 mmol/l plus two additional atherosclerotic risk factors were studied for outcomes on clinical events. In 1062 patients serum LDL-cholesterol fell by 26% during the 26 weeks of double-blind study and HDL-cholesterol increased by 7%. During the 26 weeks there were significantly more serious effects in the placebo group than in the intervention group. This study may indicate that acute lipid lowering will have a fairly rapid effect on events decline. It is unlikely that coronary morphology has changed so dramatically in 6 months' time to explain the impact.

Blood pressure

The correlation between elevated blood pressure and the development of cardiovascular disease, especially stroke, has been found to be strong and positive. In the Framingham Study, death from coronary heart disease and sudden death were two to four times higher when left ventricular hypertrophy (LVH) had been established. Studies that assessed the effects of hypotensive drugs on progression of coronary disease and coronary events have been, to some extent, inconclusive.[45] The somewhat disapointing results may be explained to some extent by the fact that until fairly recently hypotensive drugs adversely disturbed the lipid profile and caused the LDL to increase and the HDL to decrease. This might have resulted in trading in one cardiovascular risk factor for another. Newer hypotensive drugs do have a lipoprotein-neutral content, which is advantageous.

Behavioral modification trials to lower elevated blood pressure[17,46,47] seem to demonstrate the expected benefit of blood pressure lowering. In a study that compared different nonpharmacological intervention modes in lowering elevated blood pressure, three lifestyle interventions (weight reduction, sodium restriction and stress management) were carried out in a total of 2182 men and women for a period of 18 months.[48] The study indicated that an average weight reduction of 3.9 kg resulted in a decrease in diastolic blood pressure of 2.3 mmHg (p < 0.01) and a decrease in systolic blood pressure of 2.9 mmHg (p < 0.01). Sodium reduction resulted in a diastolic blood pressure decrease of 0.9 mmHg (p < 0.01) and a systolic decrease of 1.7 mmHg (p < 0.01). Stress management did not affect blood pressure. Supplements of calcium, potassium, magnesium or fish oils did not result in a significant decrease in blood pressure values. The effects of prolonged differences in diastolic blood pressure (DBP) on the risks of a stroke and CAD were estimated from 9 major prospective observational studies involving about 420 000 men and women who were followed up for intervals of 6–25 years. The results indicate that a prolonged difference of about 6 mmHg in DBP was associated with approximately 37% fewer strokes and 23% fewer CAD deaths and nonfatal myocardial infarctions. The effects of equivalent reductions in DBP produced by antihypertensive drug treatment but maintained for only a few years have been estimated in several overviews of randomized trials involving a total of 30 000–40 000 patients. The results of the overviews indicate that treatment reduced the risk of a stroke by about 40%, suggesting that most or all the long-term potential benefits for a stroke due to lower DBP were achieved within about 3 years of beginning treatment. The risks of nonfatal myocardial infarction and CAD death may have been reduced by about 10% among patients allocated to active treatment. Whatever the true effect of treatment on CAD, it would appear somewhat less than the difference in risk estimated from the observational studies for a prolonged difference in DBP of the same size. This apparent shortfall in benefit may reflect a long time-course for changes in DBP to have their full effects on CAD and possible adverse side-effects of the principal trial treatments, or both. A 5-year trial involving 201 men and women with high–normal blood pressure at a baseline demonstrated the ability to reduce the incidence of hypertension in participants randomized to a nutritional-hygienic interventional or control group. At follow-up, the incidence of hypertension was 8.8% among 102 intervention group participants versus 19.2% among 99 control group members. Mean trial blood pressure also was lower in the intervention compared with the control group (−1.2 and −1.9 mmHg, respectively, for diastolic blood pressure at worksite and office visits and −1.3 and −2.0 mmHg, respectively, for systolic blood pressure at the two sites). Net weight loss in the intervention group averaged 2.7 kg during the trial; sodium intake was reduced by 25% and reported alcohol intake decreased by 30%. The majority of intervention participants also reported an increase in physical activity. Effect on blood pressure was related particularly to the degree of weight loss. Results indicate that even a moderate reduction in risk factor for hypertension among hypertension-prone individuals contributes to the primary prevention of the disease.

A randomized controlled trial demonstrated the ability of nutritional intervention in place of antihypertensive drugs to maintain blood pressure at normal levels for 4 years in 39% of severely hypertensive patients whose blood pressure was previously well controlled by pharmacologic treatment. However, average blood pressures during the trial for patients in the intervention group were higher than those for a comparison group that continued to receive drug therapy throughout the study. Holter monitoring, echocardiography and electrocardiography done at 4 years to determine whether blood pressure differences between groups were associated with differences in cardiac status did not indicate any differences in cardiac status favorable to one group compared with the other. Further investigation in larger samples is needed to assess any long-term differences in cardiac status based on such 'alternative' therapies.[49]

Physical activity

The major cardiovascular risk factor in industrialized societies is a sedentary lifestyle that, if corrected could have the greatest impact on the prevention of cardiovascular disease.[50–54] Physical activity is inversely and causally related to the incidence of coronary heart disease (Figure 1.1) as derived from the NHANES study. In a secondary cardiovascular prevention setting, it has been shown that exercise in combination with diet may prevent progression of disease and clinical events. No study has been

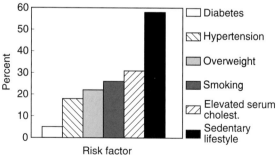

Figure 1.1
The relationship between the benefit of a modifiable cardiovascular risk factor and its prevalence.

shown to indicate prospectively the beneficial effects of exercise alone in a primary prevention setting. On the other hand, long-term follow-up studies have indicated that people who exercise do live longer and have fewer cardiovascular side-effects. It has been calculated that the relative risk of inactivity appears to be similar in magnitude to that of hypertension, hypercholesterolemia and smoking. Evidence for an independent role of increased physical activity in the primary prevention of coronary heart disease has grown in recent years. The relative risk of death from coronary heart disease, as derived from this meta-analysis, is 1.9 for sedentary compared with active occupations.[55] In the Honolulu Heart Study the association between physical activity and the 23-year incidence of coronary heart disease morbidity and mortality was assessed. This cohort study continues to follow 8006 Japanese-American men who were 45–68 years of age and living on Oahu, Hawaii, in 1965, for the development of coronary heart disease morbidity and mortality.[56] Exercise in the Framingham physical activity index was calculated by summing the product of average hours spent at each activity level and a weighting factor based on oxygen consumption. After age adjustment and using the lowest physical activity index tertile as a reference group, the relative risk for coronary heart disease incidence for the highest tertile of physical activity was 0.83. After adjusting for age, hypertension, smoking, alcohol intake, diabetes, cholesterol and BMI, the relative risk was 0.95. For coronary heart disease mortality, the age-adjusted relative risk was 0.74 and 0.85 after risk factor adjustment. These findings suggest that the impact of a physical activity index on coronary heart disease is mediated through its effects on hypertension, diabetes, cholesterol and BMI. These findings support the hypothesis that physical activity is inversely associated with coronary heart disease morbidity and mortality,

suggesting that physical activity interventions may have significant public health implications in the prevention of coronary heart disease.

In a recent statement by the US Surgeon General, primary attention was given to achieving group consensus concerning the recommended types and amounts of physical activity.[52] A concise 'public health message' was developed to express the recommendations of the experts. In summary, every US (and even UK?) adult should accumulate 30 minutes or more of moderate intensity physical activity, preferably on all days of the week.[49]

Cigarette smoking

Cigarette smoking seems to be the number-one contributor not just to cardiovascular disease and death but also as a major and still-growing risk factor and inducer of different types of disease.[57–59] The cumulative dose of cigarette smoking on the health of the original Framingham cohort (i.e. 5209 individuals aged 30–62 years at entry) after 34 years of follow-up was that a significant relationship was present between cigarette smoking and the incidence of lung cancer, stroke, transient ischemic attacks, intermittent claudication and total cardiovascular disease, and most especially the average annual death rate. Cigarette smoking was significantly related to coronary heart disease in men 45–64 years old, although not related in women or older men. The data confirm and extend the evidence of the detrimental influence of cigarette smoking on health.

The objective of the Multiple Risk Factor Intervention Trial (MRFIT) study was to investigate risk factors for death from different types of stroke among men. A total of 353 340 men were screened by 20 centers for the MRFIT in 1973–75. Vital status has been ascertained over an average of 12 years of follow-up. During this follow-up, 765 deaths from stroke were identified; 139 of these deaths were attributable to subarachnoid hemorrhage; 227 to intracranial hemorrhage; and 399 were classified as nonhemorrhagic stroke.[21] Blood pressure and cigarette smoking were strongly related to each type of stroke. Systolic blood pressure was a stronger predictor than diastolic blood pressure. With the exception of subarachnoid hemorrhage, death rates from each type of stroke increased with age and were higher for black men. The positive association of age and race with subarachnoid hemorrhage was much weaker than for the other types of strokes.

Other selected factors

Homocysteine

An elevated level of homocysteine is more common in patients with coronary artery disease or peripheral vascular disease. Increases in serum homocysteine may be related to vitamin B6 and/or vitamin B12 and folic acid.[60] A specific genetic trait, familial hyperhomocysteinemia, may be predisposing to premature coronary artery disease. The exact mechanism by which homocysteine induces an accelerated progression of atherosclerosis is yet unclear. An interrelationship between the above-mentioned vitamins, blood viscosity, fibrinogen and homocysteine levels implies a complex mechanism. The endothelial cell seems to play a role; so does probably an induction of smooth muscle cell proliferation. The level of homocysteine and premature development of coronary artery disease seems established. As homocysteine levels seem to be higher in women, an analysis in women with a 'normal' lipoprotein profile should be entertained. Treatment consists of the administration of folic acid 5 mg/day or vitamin B6 at 250 mg/day. Unfortunately, although this regimen lowers homocysteine levels, prospective studies using sequential

images of atherosclerosis or events are still lacking.

Elevated levels of homocysteine have been reported to be more prevalent in patients with CAD. The genetic contribution was assessed by homocysteine levels in 176 men with premature CAD (greater than 50% stenosis of a major epicardial coronary artery occurring before the age of 60 years) and in 255 controls free of cardiovascular disease. Homocysteine levels were higher in the CAD group compared with controls (13.9 versus 10.9 nmol/ml, $p < 0.001$); in addition, 28% of CAD patients had homocysteine levels above the 90th percentile of controls. Statistical analysis revealed that homocysteine levels were not related to the presence of hypertension, diabetes, smoking or plasma levels of lipoprotein cholesterol and apolipoproteins A-I and B. The families of 71 CAD patients were sampled and included 60 spouses and 239 first-degree relatives; 370 subjects were thus sampled. Spearman correlations between proband and spouses ($r = 0.264$, $p = 0.041$) and between mean values for parent and offspring ($r = 0.356$, $p = 0.002$) for homocysteine levels indicated that homocysteine levels are in part genetically determined. In 20 families (28.2%), the proband had homocysteine levels greater than the 90th percentile; familial segregation was observed in 10 of these kindreds. Therefore, 14% of CAD patients had familial hyperhomocysteinemia. In conclusion, the data suggest that plasma homocysteine is a risk factor for the development of CAD, independent of other cardiovascular risk factors, and that this elevation is in part genetically determined.[61]

Alcohol

It has been stated that alcohol may play some protective role in the development of cardiovascular disease. One or two glasses of red wine may increase HDL-cholesterol and result in an inverse relationship with atherosclerosis development (a.k.a. the French paradox). Suggestions about the nutrient intake that may explain this phenomenon have been made.[62,63] However, excess alcohol consumption has been associated with many other risk factors, e.g. hypertension. If both alcohol and lack of physical activity were assessed in the same population, ensuing coronary events could be explained by lack of exposure to physical activity.[64–66]

In a meta-analysis of 12 epidemiological, three case-control, and 10 separate prospective cohort studies, most epidemiological studies suggest that wine was more effective in reducing risk of mortality from heart disease than beer or spirits. Taken together, the three case control studies did not suggest that one type of drink was more cardioprotective than the others. Of the ten prospective cohort studies, four found a significant inverse association between risk of heart disease and moderate wine drinking, four found an association for beer and four for spirits. Results from observational studies, where alcohol consumption can be linked directly to an individual's risk of coronary heart disease, provide strong evidence that all alcoholic drinks are linked with lower risk. Thus a substantial portion of the benefit is from alcohol rather than other components of each type of drink. The 'French paradox' refers to the very low incidence of and mortality rates from ischemic heart disease in France, despite the fact saturated fat intakes, serum cholesterol, blood pressure and prevalence of smoking are no lower there than elsewhere.[63] To some extent this is due to under-reporting, but this is not the whole explanation. The relative immunity of the French to ischemic heart disease has been attributed to their high alcohol consumption and to their intake of antioxidant vitamins, both being supplied by wine.[67] The custom of drinking wine with the meal may confer protection against some of the adverse effects of the food.

Antioxidants

The relationship between vitamin C intake and mortality in the First National Health and Nutrition Examination Survey (NHANES I) Epidemiologic Follow-up Study cohort was assessed. This cohort is based on a representative sample of 11 348 noninstitutionalized US adults aged 25-74 years who were nutritionally examined during 1971–74 and followed up for mortality (1809 deaths) to 1984, a median of 10 years. An index of vitamin C intake has been formed from detailed dietary measurements and use of vitamin supplements.[68] The relation of the standardized mortality ratio (SMR) for all causes of death to increasing vitamin C intake is strongly inverse for males and weakly inverse for females. Among those with the highest vitamin C intake, males have an SMR of 0.65 for all causes, 0.78 for all cancers and 0.58 for all cardiovascular diseases; females have an SMR of 0.90 for all causes, 0.86 for all cancers and 0.75 for all cardiovascular diseases. Comparisons are made relative to all US whites, for whom the SMR is defined to be 1.00. There is no clear relation for individual cancer sites, except possibly an inverse relation for esophagus and stomach cancer among males. The relation with all causes of death among males remains after adjustment for age, sex and ten potentially confounding variables (including cigarette smoking, education, race and disease history). A recent study indicates that the antioxidants alpha tocopherol and beta carotene do not provide the prevention against cardiovascular disease that was expected.[69] Vasoreactivity and subsequently endothelial function were found to be disturbed. Vitamin E supplementation did not correct this finding on a short-term basis.[70]

Coffee

For many years, an association between coffee consumption and the risk of coronary heart disease has been suspected. Although based on small numbers of endpoints, a prospective study has suggested a particularly strong association between recent coffee drinking and the incidence of cardiovascular disease. The relationship of coffee consumption with the risk of myocardial infarction was assessed prospectively. The need for coronary artery bypass grafting or angioplasty and risk of a stroke in a cohort of 45 589 US men who were 40–75 years old in 1986 and who had no history of cardiovascular disease were analyzed. During two years of follow-up observation, 221 participants had a nonfatal myocardial infarction or died of coronary heart disease, 136 underwent coronary artery surgery or angioplasty and 54 had a stroke.[71] Total coffee consumption was not associated with an increased risk of coronary heart disease or stroke. The age-adjusted relative risk for all cardiovascular disease among participants who drank four or more cups of coffee per day was 1.04. Increasing levels of consumption of caffeinated coffee were not associated with higher risks of cardiovascular disease. Higher consumption of decaffeinated coffee, however, was associated with a marginally significant increase in the risk of coronary heart disease. Finally, no pattern of increased risk across the subgroups of participants with increasing intakes of caffeine from all sources was observed. Adjustment for major cardiovascular risk indicators, a dietary intake of fats and cholesterol intakes did not materially alter these associations. These findings do not support the hypothesis that coffee or caffeine consumption increases the risk of coronary heart disease or stroke.

Fish oils

Fish oil supplementation in individuals suffering from heterozygous familial hypercholesterolemia did not show a dramatic change in lipoprotein values. Therefore, the suggestions that n-3 fatty acid supplementation can be beneficial seems to be using a different pathway to prevent a cardiovascular event from occurring. Recent epidemiologic studies have shown that rates of cardiovascular disease are lower in populations such as the Greenland Eskimos than in those that do not eat seafood, even though the levels of dietary fat intake are often similar; (how may Eskimos are still adhering to that original diet?). Dietary fish oils are rich in eicosapentaenoic acid (EPA), a polyunsaturated fatty acid of the omega-3 series. EPA has been shown to prolong bleeding time and to decrease platelet aggregation and blood viscosity. EPA inhibits the production of prostaglandins from endogenous arachidonic acid, which is associated with the formation of thromboxane A2 and may also dampen cyclo-oxygenase and lipoxygenase metabolites involved in mediating endothelial cell proliferation. Dietary fish oils are now available in the form of EPA-enriched capsules. Short-term trials in humans have shown that EPA significantly reduces the levels of plasma triglycerides and may increase the levels of high-density lipoproteins; however, no consistent effect on serum cholesterol levels has been shown. The results of evaluations of EPA use in patients with renal disorders, mild hypertension, inflammatory disorders or hyperlipidemia have been promising.[72,73] On the basis of the epidemiologic and biologic evidence dietary fish oils warrant further study in extensive clinical trials. The original crosscultural comparisons between Greenland Eskimos and Danes and between Japan and western countries suggested that a high fish intake was associated with low mortality rates from coronary heart disease. More comprehensive crosscultural studies, e.g.

the Seven Countries Study, showed that the saturated fat content of the diet is more important than the amount of fish in explaining differences in coronary heart disease mortality between countries. Cohort studies carried out in cultures with a low level of fish consumption showed that persons who eat fish once or twice a week had lower mortality rates from coronary heart disease than persons who did not eat fish. The results of the epidemiological studies carried out so far suggest that a diet low in saturated fat in combination with a low level of fish consumption may be of importance for coronary heart disease prevention.[74]

Hormone replacement therapy

The results from the Postmenopausal Estrogen/ Progestin Intervention (PEPI) Trial indicate that estrogen substitution in postmenopausal women may prevent subsequent sequelae from occuring.[75] Although estrogen replacement therapy has been suggested,[76] no study has been published that indicates the benefits of prospective estrogens in preventing cardiovascular disease.

Type A behavior

A specific cardiovascular behavior has been associated with an increased risk of cardiovascular disease. This type A coronary-prone behavior has many aspects that are related to a feeling of time urgency, hostility, anger and psychological stress. This type of behavior is usually not recognized after the occurrence of a cardiovascular complication. No study has been published that indicates the benefits in a primary preventive setting of modifying type A behavior, although children seem more likely to be affected if their parents are considered type A personalities.[77,78] Hostility seems to contribute significantly to atherosclerosis development within type A behavior. Why most people contribute so much to the concept of stress as entity

to develop complications of atherosclerosis remains unclear.

Body fat distribution

A specific body fat distribution (abdominal obesity) is a separate and independent risk factor for cardiovascular disease. Even a small increase in weight is associated with an increase in risk. On the other hand no study has been published that indicates that a loss of excess weight will prevent cardiovascular complications or progression of disease. Whether this association is a direct or indirect one (insulin resistance?) is as yet not clear. Centralized obesity is associated with an increased likelihood for diabetes. Central obesity has been shown to be more prevalent in men and women who smoke. This may imply that in this population body fat distribution may be modified by behavioral factors.[79–81]

If trends in coronary heart disease that have occurred during the last decades are assessed, it becomes clear that in the white population and the more educated socioeconomic groups cardiovascular disease has dramatically declined. During the last decade the decline has been evening out. An explanation of this phenomenon may be found by realizing that the prevalence of obesity has increased significantly. Priorities in modifying cardiovascular risk factors as stated by patients should be taken into account in the management of the disease.[82]

Discussion

Given the fact that more than 250 cardiovascular risk factors have been recognized, a selection had to be made to indicate what may be the important factor in primary prevention of cardiovascular disease. A different relationship exists between the level of the risk factor and the contribution to cardiovascular risk (Figure 1.2) The relationship between smoking and risk

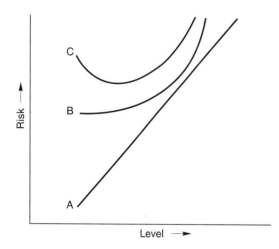

Figure 1.2
Relationship between the level of the risk factor and the contribution to risk. Line A depicts smoking, B blood cholesterol level, C blood pressure level.

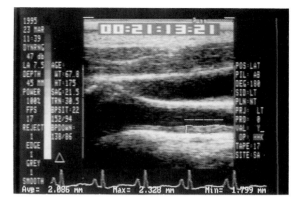

Figure 1.3
An example of a quantitative measurement of a thickened intima-media complex. A ruler of 1 cm depicts the measurement scope just below the carotid bifurcation in the far wall of the common carotid artery. A normal IMT average is up to 0.8 mm. This image is reproduced with permission of Prevention Concepts Inc. Santa Monica, CA.

seems linear whereas LDL-cholesterol has a more exponential risk contribution once the level is above the baseline value.

CAD is probably the most common example of a multifactorial disease that can be reduced in the incidence (if not prevented in some cases) by appropriate attention to and control of risk factors.[83] This conclusion is supported by large epidemiologic studies, confirmed by randomized intervention trials in which a putative risk factor is attacked with a specific therapy and put into context by the results of multiple risk factor intervention trials. The job of the physician is to take the pieces of scientific data regarding CAD and extrapolate them, if appropriate, to individual patients, who presumably will benefit from all the hard work their predecessors in clinical trials went through to prove that the intervention was successful. No agreement exists in the medical community to answer the question: what is the best way to assess the effect of risk factor modification? To prevent a

stroke or a myocardial infarct from occurring seems to be a different approach from assessing the disease itself using newer sonographic techniques like quantitative intima-media thickness (QIMT) of the carotid artery or brachial vasoreactivity assessment (Figure 1.3).

A possible way of dealing with the distinction between primary and secondary prevention may be related to an apparent lack of noninvasive low-cost tracking methods to detect and manage disease before a complication becomes apparent — as stated by Brown and Goldstein in a recent editorial in *Science*.[84] The acceptance by the research community of QIMT as surrogate for very early disease assessment should be expanded to include the general population.[85–89] The relationship between the different vascular beds and different age ranges indicates that the carotid artery seems to be a reliable surrogate (Figure 1.4). The advantage of knowing the extent of disease seems obvious. However, this issue seems far from settled.

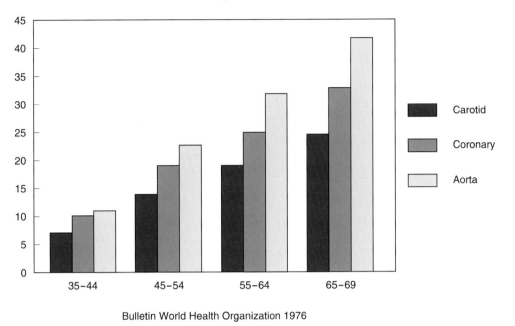

% Raised lesion coverage basal membrane

Bulletin World Health Organization 1976

Figure 1.4
Pathological findings in different vascular beds in different age ranges.

It has been proposed by Superko and Krauss that if aggressive lipoprotein lowering may induce regression, reduce clinical events and slow progression of coronary artery disease, the underlying mechanism must be different.[90] To extrapolate a reduction in clinical events to differences in pro/regression seems tricky. Trials using sequential angiography confirm the relative lack of pertinent relationship between the study of disease prevention and the occurrence of clinical events.[91] This actions remain unclear. Hypotheses about a more vulnerable cap on the atherosclerotic plaque would more likely result in a rupture and ensue in an occlusion of the vessel, resulting in ischemia or death of the distally located tissue. One needs to infer from this hypothesis that a soft cap may be the result of progression of disease.[92] This would be an unlikely phenomenon, as progression of the disease

may be accompanied by calcification and fibrous cap development. Therefore to use the results of some trial of lipid-lowering agents and to use clinical events and angiographic progression/regression of disease almost interchangeably seems fundamentally unscientific. The fact that atherosclerosis appears not to be an inert mass but a metabolic active substrate should be taken into account.

Given all this, and the previous focus on the management of the disease, several guidelines have emerged to prevent or retard the development of atherosclerosis. The recommendations seem simple but are sometimes difficult to follow.[93] The biggest breakthrough would be attained by encouraging people to exercise. This does not need to be to the extent that fitness clubs may want us to take it, but very simple measures can be quite effective:[94]

- Do not take the elevator to go up or down two floors;
- Park the car in a safe place but not too close to work. Walking, besides expending energy makes one feel psychologically better. Therefore, to measure the effects of exercise only by Metts seems to be only a small fraction of the benefit of exercising.

Diet has become a word most of us despise, but the reality is that most of us living in industrialized societies eat too many calories, consume an unbalanced diet and are unhappy with our body weight. A first step is, obviously, to know what you are eating. The second step would be to eat only half what is on your plate and to exercise. Find a partner so that you can support each other. When the urge to eat or indulge yourself appears, occupy your mind with something completely different.

Dietary assessment plays a crucial role in our ability to detect relationships between dietary exposure and disease causation. Nutritional problems are at the root of major mass diseases that are impediments to national and international health goals. This is as true for chronic undernutrition and famine as for many of the chronic diseases afflicting middle-aged and elderly people in industrialized and developing countries. High-quality dietary assessment provides a sound scientific foundation for the primary prevention of mass diseases, whereas inadequate assessment can produce false negative results and lead to apparent inconsistencies between crosspopulation and within-population findings for a particular disease.

The critical role of dietary assessment in the elucidation of disease causation is discussed with regard to high blood pressure, heart disease, breast cancer and several other major chronic diseases. Improved approaches to dietary assessment need to be made more widely known, not only between research scientists and health practitioners but also among policy-makers who require high-quality, dietary data for establishing nutrition goals and making policy decisions. For decades, dietary cholesterol has been recognized as the 'materia peccans' (Anitschkow) for the induction of atherosclerosis in animals. In rabbits, chickens and monkeys, the long-term feeding of small amounts of cholesterol leads to atherosclerosis despite little or no rise in serum total cholesterol, indicating an independent contribution of dietary cholesterol to atherogenesis over and above its influence on serum cholesterol, possibly through effects on serum cholesterol fractions (e.g. increased low-density lipoprotein cholesterol and decreased high-density lipoprotein cholesterol). In humans, ingestion of dietary cholesterol raises serum cholesterol, largely through its effect on low-density lipoprotein cholesterol. Over the range of intake in typical American diets, this effect is substantial, e.g. with 300 mg of cholesterol intake per 1000 kcal, rather than 100, serum cholesterol is on average about 6–7% higher, equivalent to a 12–14% greater risk of CAD. In international studies based on Food and Agriculture Organization and World Health Organization data, mean per capita dietary cholesterol levels are consistently related to CAD mortality rates. In addition, since 1981, four prospective within-population studies have shown that the dietary cholesterol intake of individuals is significantly related to their long-term CAD risk, independent of and in addition to serum cholesterol, blood pressure and cigarette use. On average, a 200 mg/1000 kcal higher intake of cholesterol at a baseline was associated with a 30% higher CAD rate. Conversely, lower intakes of cholesterol were associated with significantly lower risks of CAD, and of all causes of mortality as well. For example, in 19 years of follow-up in the Chicago Western Electric Study, a 200 mg/1000 kcal habitual lower cholesterol intake was associated with a 37% lower risk of death from any cause, equivalent to a life expectancy longer by 3.4 years.

When a physician advises a patient to modify unhealthy behaviors, the physician may be tempted to prescribe a target for change by selecting the single 'risk factor' that poses a threat to health. Since risk factor intervention efforts are less successful unless the target of the intervention is negotiated with the patient, these data should be of clinical importance in devising plans for behavioral change. The prevalence of these risk factors was markedly different from the Framingham Offspring Study population, used here as a comparison group. In the patients with CAD, only 3% had no risk factor (other than male sex), compared with 31% in the Framingham Offspring Study subjects. Most patients with CAD (97%) had greater than or equal to one additional risk factor. When the patients with CAD were divided by age groups (40–49 years, n = 109; 50–59, n = 191), no significant differences were observed in the prevalence of risk factors between the younger and older patients. The relevance of systemic hypertension (41 *vs.* 19%, $p < 0.001$), diabetes mellitus (12 *vs.* 1.1%, $p < 0.001$), cigarette smoking (67 *vs.* 28%, $p < 0.001$) and HDL cholesterol less than 0.90 mmol/l (63 *vs.* 19%, $p < 0.001$) was markedly higher in the patients with CAD than in Framingham Offspring Study subjects, whereas the prevalence of LDL cholesterol greater than or equal to 4.15 mmol/l was not significantly different between patients with CAD and Framingham Offspring Study subjects (26 *vs.* 26%). It is clear that risk factor modification does work. Different guidelines from both the European and American Heart Associations will help interested healthcare professionals to implement the science.[47,57,93,95,96]

In addition to the above-mentioned aspects, recent research indicates that it may even be more cost effective to start management early, given the fact that one deals with the same disease.[97,98] The Oslo diet study has indicated that not only will morbidity decrease in primary prevention but also mortality (Table 1.1). The pros and cons of primary cardiovascular prevention are listed in Table 1.2. Table 1.3 indicates the positive results of lowering cardiovascular events in a primary preventive setting.

In summary, if secondary prevention is obvious by modifying cardiovascular risk factors, similar criteria should be used to prevent the initial disease from developing. Low-cost noninvasive detecting and tracking devices (e.g. QIMT testing) are currently available to assist the patient and physician to ascertain the effects of the intervention after a period of only 12 months. The use of QIMT in early atherosclerosis assessment and tracking may help locate and identify people at risk of devel-

Pro	Contra
Dealing with the underlying problem	No definite scientific proof
Improvement of life's enjoyment	Facilitation realistic?
Preventing other diseases	Inducing other diseases

Table 1.2
Primary prevention approach.

	Duration	n	% change in lipid			CV events	p
			TC	LDL c	HDL c	Reduction	
CDP-niacin	7 years	3908	−10	NA	NA	14	<0.05
LRP-CPPT	7–10 years	3806	−8	−12	+4	19	<0.05
Helsinki Heart	5 years	4081	−10	−11	+12	33	<0.02
POSCH	10 years	838	−23	−38	+4	35	<0.001
4S	5.5 years	4444	−25	−35	+8	34	<0.0001
WOS	5.5 years	6595	−12	−16	+3	31	<0.001
KAPS	3 years	447	−18	−28	+4	21	<0.05

Table 1.3
Primary prevention intervention studies.

oping atherosclerosis and its complications. Therefore NOT to (re)focus on primary prevention when one disease is the culprit seems almost unethical.

If I had . . .

If I had a major cardiovascular risk factor without any signs or symptoms of heart disease, I would value my quality of life more. I would loose the extra 15 lbs that I carry and would exercise more diligently. I would schedule my 'health time' as I would my time to get to my office promptly. I would avoid the excuses that I make to eat too many unhealthy food products. I would abandon the feeling that I deserve high fat or high calorie products. Generally, I feel that I am doing pretty well by exercising and eating healthy meals; I have never smoked and must admit that I dislike to be around people who do smoke. I try to be a health-conscious model for my patients.

References

1 Higgins M, Thom T, Trends in CHD in the United States, *Int J Epidemiol* (1989)**19**:(**Suppl 1**):S58–S66.

2 Stamler J, Assessing diets to improve world health: nutritional research on disease causation in populations, *Am J Clin Nutr* (1994)**59**:146S–156S.

3 Bittner V, Primary and secondary prevention of ischemic heart disease, *Current Opin Cardiol* (1994)**9**:417–27.

4 Rossouw JE, Lewis B, Rifkind BM, The value of lowering cholesterol after myocardial infarction, *N Engl J Med* (1990)**323**:1112–19.

5 Jones PH, Gotto AM, Extending the benefit of lipid-regulating therapy to primary prevention, *Am J Cardiol* (1995)**76**:118C–121C.

6 Rich-Edwards JW, Manson JE, Hennekens CH, Buring JE, Medical progress: the primary prevention of coronary heart disease in women, *New Engl J Med* (1995)**332**:1758–66.

7 Manson JE, Tosteson H, Ridker PM et al, The primary prevention of myocardial infarction, *N Engl J Med* (1992)**326**:1406–16.

8 Cabin HS, Roberts WC, Relation of serum total cholesterol and triglyceride levels to the amount and extent of coronary arterial narrowing by atherosclerotic plaque in coronary heart disease, *Am J Med* (1982)**73**:227–34.

9 LaRosa JC, Hunninghake D, Bush D et al, The cholesterol facts: a summary of the evidence relating dietary fats, serum cholesterol and coronary heart disease: a joint statement by the American Heart Association and the National Heart, Lung, and Blood Institute, *Circulation* (1990)**81**:1721–33.

10 Barth JD, Arntzenius AC, Progression and regression of atherosclerosis. What roles for LDL-cholesterol and HDL-cholesterol: a perspective, *Eur Heart J* (1991)**12**:952–7.

11 Anderson KM, Wilson PWF, Odell PM, Kannel WB, An updated coronary risk profile: a statement for health professionals, *Circulation* (1991)**83**:356–62.

12 Kannel WB, Abbott RD, Incidence and prognosis of unrecognized myocardial infarction. An update on the Framingham Study, *N Engl J Med* (1984)**311**:1144–7.

13 Kannel WB, Abbott RD, Incidence and prognosis of unrecognized myocardial infarction, *N Engl J Med* (1984)**311**:1144–7.

14 Murray CH, Lopez A, *The global burden of disease: a comprehensive assessment of mortality and disability from diseases, injuries, and risk factors in 1990 and projected to 2020* (Harvard Medical School/WHO/World Bank: 1996).

15 Castelli WP, Garrison RJ, Wilson PW, Abbott RD, Kalousdian S, Kannel WB, Incidence of coronary heart disease and lipoprotein cholesterol levels. The Framingham Study, *J Am Med Assoc* (1986)**256**:2835–8.

16 Higgins M, D'Agostino R, Kannel W, Cobb J, Pinsky J, Benefits and adverse effects of weight loss. Observations from the Framingham Study, *Ann Intern Med* (1993)**119**:758–63.

17 Stamler R, Stamler J, Gosch FC et al, Primary prevention of hypertension by nutritional-hygienic means. Final report of a randomized, controlled trial, *J Am Med Assoc* (1989)**262**:1801–7.

18 Stamler J, Dyer AR, Shekelle RB, Neaton J, Stamler R, Relationship of baseline major risk factors to coronary and all-cause mortality, and to longevity: findings from long-term follow-up of Chicago cohorts, *Cardiology* (1993)**82**:191–222.

19 Clay CM, Dyer AR, Liu K et al, Education, smoking and non-cardiovascular mortality: findings in three Chicago epidemiological studies, *Int J Epidemiol* (1988)**17**:341–7.

20 Multiple Risk Factor Intervention Trial Research Group, Multiple Risk Factor Intervention Trial: risk factor changes and mortality results, *J Am Med Assoc* (1982)**248**:1465–77.

21 Neaton JD, Wentworth DN, Cutler J, Stamler J, Kuller L, Risk factors for death from different

types of stroke. Multiple Risk Factor Intervention Trial Research Group, *Ann Epidemiol* (1993)**3**:493–9.

22 Stamler J, Primary prevention of coronary heart disease. The last 20 years, *Am J Cardiol* (1981)**47**:722–35.

23 Cooper ES, Prevention: the key to progress, *Circulation* (1993)**87**:1430–3.

24 Stamler J, Shekele R, Dietary cholesterol and human coronary heart disease, *Arch Path Lab Med* (1988)**112**:1032–40.

25 Pekkanen J, Linn S, Heiss G et al, Ten-year mortality from cardiovascular disease in relation to cholesterol level among men with and without pre-existing cardiovascular disease, *N Engl J Med* (1990)**322**:1700–7.

26 Canner PL, Berge KG, Wenger NK et al, Fifteen year mortality in the Coronary Drug Project patients: long-term benefit with niacin, *JACC* (1986)**8**:1245–55.

27 Shepherd J, Cobbe SM, Ford I et al, Prevention of coronary heart disease with pravastatin in men with hypercholesterolemia, *N Engl J Med* (1995)**333**:1301–7.

28 Scandinavian Simvastatin Survival Group, Randomized trial of cholesterol lowering in 4444 patients with coronary heart disease: the Scandinavian Simvastatin Survival Study (4S), *Lancet* (1994)**344**:1383–9.

29 Blankenhorn DH, Selzer RH, Crawford DW et al, Beneficial effects of colestipol-niacin therapy on carotid atherosclerosis: two and four year reduction of intima-media thickness measured by ultrasound, *Circulation* (1993)**88**:20–9.

30 Mack WJ, Krauss RM, Hodis H, Lipoprotein subclasses in the Monitored Atherosclerosis Regression Study (MARS), *Arterioscl Thromb Vasc Biol* (1996)**16**:697–704.

31 Barth JD, Pixel or death experience from clinical trials assessing lipid lowering therapy, *Can J Cardiol* (1995)**11**:9C–14C.

32 Muldoon MF, Manuck SB, Matthews KA, Lowering cholesterol concentrations and mortality: a quantitative review of primary prevention trials, *Br Med J* (1990)**301**:309–14.

33 Muldoon MF, Manuck SB, Matthews KA, Lowering cholesterol concentrations and mortality: quantitative review of primary prevention trials, *Br Med J* (1990)**301**:309–14.

34 Kuller L, Borhani N, Furberg C et al, Prevalence of subclinical atherosclerosis and cardiovascular disease with associations in the cardiovascular health study, *Am J Epidemiol* (1994)**139**:1164–79.

35 Iribarren C, Reed DM, Burchfiel CM, Dwyer JH, Serum total cholesterol and mortality, *J Am Med Assoc* (1995)**273**:1926–32.

36 Sniderman AD, Ghezzo RH, Meta-analysis of the clinical outcomes of recent quantitative angiographic trials to lower plasma LDL in patients with CAD, *Can J Cardiol* (1994)**10**:10B–16B.

37 Salonen R, Nyyssonen K, Porkkala E et al, Kuopio Atherosclerosis Prevention Study (KAPS). A population-based primary preventive trial of the effect of LDL lowering on atherosclerotic progression in carotid and femoral arteries, *Circulation* (1995)**92**:1758–64.

38 Buchwald H, Matts JP, Fitch LL et al, for the Program on the Surgical Control of Hyperlipidemia (POSCH) group, Changes in sequential coronary arteriograms and subsequent coronary events, *J Am Med Assoc* (1992)**268**:1429–33.

39 Frick MH, Elo O, Haapa K et al, Helsinki Heart Study: primary prevention trial with gemfibrozil in middle aged men with dyslipidemia, *N Engl J Med* (1987)**317**:1237–45.

40 Hjermann I, Holme I, Gelve BK, Leren P, Effect of diet and smoking intervention on the incidence of coronary heart disease, *Lancet* (1981)**ii**:1303–10.

41 Kannel WB, Abbott RD, A prognostic comparison of asymptomatic left ventricular hypertrophy and unrecognized myocardial infarction: the Framingham Study, *Am Heart J* (1986)**111**:391–7.

42 Betteridge DJ, Barth JD, Summary of Cholesterol Consensus: a trans-Atlantic perspective, *Int J Cardiol* (1992)**37**:S3–S11.

43 Brensike JF, Levy RI, Kelsey SF et al, Effects of cholestyramine on progression of coronary arteriosclerosis: results of the NHLBI Type II Coronary Intervention Study, *Circulation* (1984)**69**:313–24.

44 Lipid Research Clinic Program, The LRC-CPPT results. I. Reduction in incidence of coronary heart disease, *J Am Med Assoc* (1984)**251**:351–74.

45 Pravastatin Multinational Study Group for Cardiac Risk Patients, Effects of pravastatin in patients with serum total cholesterol levels from 5.2 to 7.8 mmol/l (200–300 mg/dl) plus two additional atherosclerotic risk factors, *Am J Cardiol* (1993)**72**:1031–7.

46 Stamler J, Lifestyles, major risk factors, proof and public policy, *Circulation* (1978)**58**:3–18.

47 AHA Prevention Conference III, Behavior change and compliance: keys to improving cardiovascular health, *Circulation* (1993)**88**: 1376–407.

48 Trials of Hypertension Prevention Collaborative Research Group, The effects of non-pharmacologic interventions on blood pressure of persons with high normal levels: results of the Trials of Hypertension Prevention, Phase I, *J Am Med Assoc* (1992)**267**:1213–20.

49 Tyroler HA, Heyen S, Bartel A et al, Blood pressure and cholesterol as coronary heart disease risk factors, *Arch Intern Med* (1971)**128**: 907–14.

50 Fletcher GO, Lair SO, Blumenthal J et al., A statement on exercise, benefits and recommendations for physical activity programs for all Americans, *Circulation* (1992)**86**:340–4.

51 Kannel WB, Sorlie P, Some health benefits of physical activity: the Framingham study, *Arch Intern Med* (1979)**139**:857–61.

52 *Physical activity and health. A report of the Surgeon General* (US Department of Health and Human Services: Washington, DC, 1996).

53 Powell KE, Thompson PD, Caspersen CJ, Kendrick JS, Physical activity and the incidence of coronary heart disease, *Ann Rev Public Health* (1987)**8**:253–87.

54 Scragg R, Stewart A, Jackson R, Beaglehole, R, Alcohol and exercise in myocardial infarction and sudden coronary death in men and women, *Am J Epidemiol* (1987)**126**:77–85.

55 Pate RR, Pratt M, Blair SN et al, Physical activity and public health. A recommendation from the Centers for Disease Control and Prevention and the American College of Sports Medicine, *J Am Med Assoc* (1995)**273**:402–7.

56 Rodriguez BL, Curb JD, Burchfiel CM et al, Physical activity and 23-year incidence of coronary heart disease morbidity and mortality among middle-aged men. The Honolulu Heart Program, *Circulation* (1994)**89**:2540–4.

57 Rockville Department of Health and Human Services, *Reducing the health consequences of smoking: 25 years of progress. A report of the Surgeon General 1989* (Rockville Department of Health and Human Services, DHHS publication (CDC)89-8411:1989).

58 Freund KM, Belanger AJ, D'Agostino RB, Kannel WB, The health risks of smoking. The Framingham Study: 34 years of follow-up, *Ann Epidemiol* (1993)**3**:417–24.

59 Barrett-Connor E, Khaw KT, Cigarette smoking and increased central adiposity, *Ann Intern Med* (1989)**111**:783–7.

60 Verhoef P, Stampfer MJ, Buring JE et al, Homocysteine metabolism and risk of myocardial infarction: relation with vitamins B6, B12 and folate, *Am J Epidemiol* (1996)**143**:845–59.

61 Genest JJ Jr, McNamara JR, Upson B et al, Prevalence of familial hyperhomocyst(e)inemia in men with premature coronary artery disease, *Arterio Thromb* (1991)**11**:1129–36.

62 de Lorgeril M, Salen P, Martin J-L et al, Effect of a Mediterranean type of diet on the rate of cardiovascular complication in patients with coronary artery disease: insights into the cardioprotective effect of certain nutriments, *JACC* (1996)**28**:1103–9.

63 Burr ML, Explaining the French paradox, *J Royal Soc Health* (1995)**115**:217–19.

64 Gordon T, Kannel WB, Drinking habits and cardiovascular disease: the Framingham Study, *Am Heart J* (1983)**105**:667–73.

65 Steinberg D, Pearson TA, Kuller LH, Alcohol and atherosclerosis, *Ann Intern Med* (1991)**114**:967–76.

66 Klatsky AL, Armstrong MA, Friedman GD, Alcohol and mortality, *Ann Intern Med* (1992)**117**:646–54.

67 Rimm BE, Klatsky A, Grobbee D, Stampfer MJ, Review of moderate alcohol consumption and reduced risk of coronary heart disease: is the effect due to beer, wine, or spirits? *Br Med J* (1996)**312**:731–6.

68 Enstrom JE, Kanim LE, Klein MA, Vitamin C intake and mortality among a sample of the United States population, *Epidemiology* (1992)**3**:194–202.

69 The alpha Tocopherol, beta Carotene Cancer Prevention Study Group, The effect of vitamin E and beta carotene on the incidence of lung

cancer and other cancers in male smokers, *N Engl J Med* (1994)**330**:1029–35.

70   Elliott, TG, Barth JD, Mancini GB, Effects of vitamin E on endothelial function in men after myocardial infarction, *Am J Cardiol* (1995)**76**: 1188–90.

71   Grobbee DE, Rimm BE, Giovannucci E, Colditz G, Stampfer M, Willett W, Coffee, caffeine, and cardiovascular disease in men, *N Engl J Med* (1990)**323**:1026–32.

72   Kromhout D, N-3 fatty acids and coronary heart disease: epidemiology from Eskimos to western populations, *J Intern Med* (1989)**225**: 47–51.

73   Holub BJ, Dietary fish oils containing eicosa-pentaenoic acid and the prevention of athero-sclerosis and thrombosis, *Can Med Ass J* (1988)**139**:377–81.

74   Burr ML, Fehily AM, Gilbert JF et al, Effects of changes in fat, fish, and fibre intakes on death and myocardial infarction: diet and reinfarction trial (DART), *Lancet* (1989)**ii**:757–61.

75   The Writing Group for the PEPI Trial, Effects of estrogen or estrogen/progestin regimen on heart disease risk factors in postmenopausal women: the postmenopausal Estrogen/Proges-tin Intervention (PEPI) Trial, *J Am Med Assoc* (1995)**273**:199–208.

76   Stampfer MJ, Colditz GA, Estrogen replace-ment therapy and coronary heart disease: quan-titative assessment of epidemiologic evidence, *Prev Med* (1991)**20**:47–63.

77   Dembroski TM, MacDougal JM, Williams RB, Components of type A hostility and anger in relationship to angiographic findings, *Psycho-som Med* (1985)**47**:219–33.

78   Raikkeonen K, Predictive associations between type A behavior of parents and their children: a 6-year follow-up, *J Genetic Psychol* (1993)**154**:315–28.

79   American Heart Association, Guidelines for weight management programs for healthy adults, *Heart Disease and Stroke* (1994)**3**:221–8.

80   Bjorntorp P, Regional patterns of fat distribu-tion, *Ann Intern Med* (1985)**103**:994–5.

81   Reichley KB, Mueller WH, Hanis DL et al, Centralized obesity and cardiovascular disease risk in Mexican-Americans, *Am J Epidemiol* (1987)**125**:373–86.

82   Levenkron JC, Greenland P, Patient priorities for behavioral change: selecting from multiple coronary disease risk factors, *J Gen Internal Med* (1988)**3**:224–9.

83   Elliott WJ, Cardiovascular risk factors. Which ones can and should be remedied? *Postgrad Med* (1994)**96**:49–50,53–4,58.

84   Brown MS, Goldstein JL, Heart attacks: gone with the century? *Science* (1996)**272**:629 (edi-torial).

85   Hodis HN, Mack WJ, Barth JD, Carotid intima-media thickness as a surrogate end point for coronary artery disease, *Circulation* (1996) **94**:2311–12.

86   Adams MR, Nakagone H, Juergens CP et al, Intima-media thickness of the common carotid artery: a useful screening test prior to coronary angiography, *Circulation* (1994)**90** [2(1)23]: A0111.

87   Blankenhorn DH, Hodis HN, Arterial imaging and atherosclerosis reversal, *Arterioscler Thromb* (1994)**14**:177–92.

88   Salonen JT, Salonen R, Ultrasonographically assessed carotid morphology and the risk of coronary heart disease, *Arterioscler Thromb* (1991)**11**:1245–9.

89   Rauramaa R, Rankinen T, Tuomainen P, Vai-seanen S, Mercuri M, Inverse relationship between cardiorespiratory fitness and carotid atherosclerosis, *Atherosclerosis* (1995)**112**: 213–21.

90   Superko HR, Krauss RM, Coronary artery dis-ease regression. Convincing evidence for the benefit of aggressive lipoprotein management, *Circulation* (1994)**90**:1056–69.

91   Barth JD, Lipoproteins and the progression/regression of atherosclerosis, *Bailliere's Clin Epidem Metab* (1995)**4**:849–66.

92   Brown BG, Zhao XQ, Sacco DE, Albers JJ, Lipid lowering and plaque regression. New insights into prevention of plaque disruption and clinical events in coronary disease, *Circulation* (1993)**87**:1781–91.

93   National Cholesterol Education Program, Sec-ond report of the expert panel on detection, evaluation, and treatment of high blood choles-terol in adults (ATP II), *Circulation* (1994)**89**: 1333–445.

94   Berlin JA, Colditz GA, A meta-analysis of physical activity in the prevention of coronary heart disease, *Am J Epidemiol* (1990)**132**:612–28.

95   Krauss RM, Deckelbaum RJ, Ernst N et al, Dietary guidelines for healthy American adults. A statement for health professionals from the Nutrition Committee, American Heart Association, *Circulation* (1996)**94**:1795–800.

96   Recommendations of the European Atherosclerosis Society prepared by the International Task Force for Prevention of Coronary Heart Disease, Prevention of coronary heart disease: scientific background and new clinical guidelines, *Nutr Metab Cardiovasc Dis* (1992)**2**:113–56.

97   Sanford Schwartz J, The cost-effectiveness of cholesterol-lowering therapy: a guide for the perplexed, *JCOM* (1996) **3**:48–51.

98   Millar JA, Economic comparison of drug and lifestyle treatment of cardiovascular risk factors in high-risk patients, *Clin Exper Pharma Physio* (1995)**22**:217–19.

2

Diabetes and the heart

John PD Reckless

Introduction

Diabetes mellitus has a prevalence approaching 2% in the United Kingdom, but consumes over 8% of the UK National Health Service resources.[1] The largest proportion of this expenditure relates to the costs of managing macrovascular disease (MVD) found in diabetes. The incidence of both insulin dependent diabetes mellitus (IDDM) and noninsulin dependent diabetes mellitus (NIDDM), has been increasing, the latter partly because of increasing adiposity, reduced activity and longer life expectancy.

The introduction of insulin therapy in 1922 led to improved survival in younger diabetic patients, but MVD increasingly contributed to premature morbidity and mortality (Figure 2.1).[2] Coronary heart disease (CHD) is the major contributor to MVD and early death, as part of the spectrum of atherosclerosis and large vessel disease. End-organ damage also affects cerebral and peripheral vasculature.[3,4]

While there is an ongoing need to treat diabetes to avoid symptoms and acute complications (hypoglycaemia and ketoacidosis), and to treat and better prevent the specific microvascular complications of diabetes (neuropathy, nephropathy and retinopathy), substantial challenges exist still in prevention of MVD. Management and prevention of MVD has been rather an orphan in terms of interest, research and clinical effort compared with the immediate symptoms and microvascu-

lar complications of diabetes. More attention has been applied to IDDM patients or to insulin-requiring diabetic patients, even though they amount to 10% and 30% of the population respectively, while NIDDM has inappropriately been considered as 'mild' diabetes. The diabetes may remain 'mild' in terms of glycaemic symptoms or need for medication even after stroke, amputation, infarct, angina and cardiac failure have limited the patient.

The established risk factors for CHD and MVD — hypertension, hypercholesterolaemia and smoking — all apply to the diabetic population, and it is in their management that immediate opportunities lie. Beyond this, diabetes is itself a major independent risk factor for MVD, and a better understanding of the mechanisms underlying MVD will allow improved prevention.[5] The effects of these risk factors on cardiovascular mortality are shown in Figure 2.2.

Good diabetes control undoubtedly delays both the onset and the progression of microvascular disease-related retinopathy, nephropathy and neuropathy.[6] The DCCT trial did not show evidence of less MVD with improved glycaemic control because the study was not designed to examine MVD; the study population was of young IDDM patients whose MVD rates over 6 years were too low to allow statistical interpretation. The United Kingdom Prospective Diabetes Study[7] in NIDDM patients, which should report over the next 2 years, may provide some evidence here.

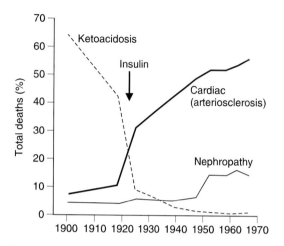

Figure 2.1
Changing patterns of mortality in diabetes over 60 years. Since the introduction of insulin, rates of death from acute complications have reduced considerably, but chronic, largely macrovascular, causes have become predominant. Data from Marble A, Insulin–clinical aspects: the first fifty years, Diabetes (1972)21:632–6.

Cessation of smoking, and indeed lack of initiation of the smoking habit, is of high priority in diabetes, because attention to correctable factors for MVD become more important as both disease frequency and disease prematurity rise.

Control of blood pressure has been demonstrated to be essential for protection against nephropathy and its progression, both in the general population and in people with diabetes.[8] With their mode of action, angiotensin converting enzyme (ACE) inhibitors appear to confer the additional benefit of protection against diabetic renal disease, over and above their hypotensive effects.[9,10]

In studies of lipid and lipoprotein levels as risk factors for CHD in the general population, high plasma and LDL cholesterol levels have received most attention, together with low levels of HDL. Little attention has been paid to triglyceride level, for while it is the most potent univariate risk factor for CHD, independent risk is lost or largely lost in multivariate analyses. Such statistical treatment may be flawed, as triglyceride is not independent of the other covariables. Alternative analyses, such as in the Procam study,[11] and a recent meta-analysis by Hokanson and Austin,[12] have drawn attention back to triglyceride.

Insufficient attention has been paid to lipid levels in diabetic patients in whom cholesterol and LDL cholesterol levels are normally similar to general population levels. In IDDM and insulin-treated diabetic patients HDL cholesterol levels are normal or high, and it is only in NIDDM that they are clearly low. The classical lipaemia of diabetes is hypertriglyceridaemia. In many patients poor diabetic control will contribute substantially to overproduction and impaired removal of triglyceride-rich lipoproteins. However, moderate hypertriglyceridaemia will often remain. It is becoming clear that the diabetic dyslipidaemia of moderately raised triglycerides and low HDL cholesterol levels are particularly atherogenic in this situation.[13,14] These abnormalities are associated with considerable, subtle, lipoprotein quality changes which will be considered later in more detail.

Therapeutic challenges exist in patient education, to encourage uptake of dietary, exercise and lifestyle changes across the diabetic population, and in prescribing practices of primary and secondary healthcare teams (in diabetology and other specialities), to encourage active and appropriate drug therapy for diabetes control, blood pressure control, and lipid modification. Once clinical CHD has been diagnosed, there has been some reluctance to offer interventional and therapeutic procedures to diabetic patients at rates commensurate with disease prevalence; this is only partly attributable to lesions that are less suitable for attention and to sicker patients.

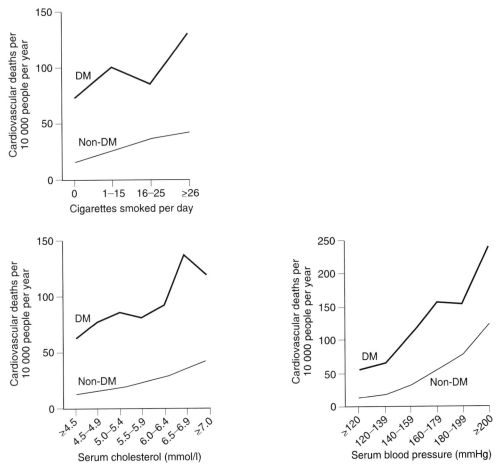

Figure 2.2
Deaths from cardiovascular disease over 12 years, and the effects of cigarette smoking, hypercholesterolaemia and hypertension in diabetic and nondiabetic men from the screenees of the multiple risk factor intervention trial. Data from Stamler et al.[5] DM, diabetes mellitus.

Mortality

Diabetic patients have increased mortality rates compared with the general population.[3,4] At any age of onset of diabetes, there is a reduction of about 30% in life expectancy (Figure 2.3).[3,4] One-third of a cohort of patients with IDDM at the Joslin clinic had died by age 55 years.[2]

Rates of CHD mortality in diabetes are increased about three-fold compared with the general population (Table 2.1).[3,4] Excess rates apply particularly to NIDDM, and (unlike the general population) to women with NIDDM.[15,16]

Morbidity

The Framingham study showed a three-fold increased incidence of CHD in the NIDDM subgroup compared with the nondiabetic age-

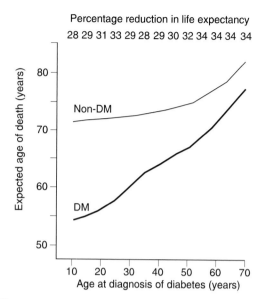

Percentage reduction in life expectancy
28 29 31 33 29 28 29 30 32 34 34 34 34

Figure 2.3
Life expectation by age at onset of diabetes, compared to nondiabetic controls. Percentage reduction in life expectancy is shown. Deaths within one week of first observation or hospital discharge are excluded. Data from the Joslin Clinic analysed by the Metropolitan Life Insurance Company; data from Marks and Krall.[4] DM, diabetes mellitus.

Cause of death	Death rate ratios for the diabetic to general population	
	Males	Females
Total vascular disease	2.4	3.4
Aged 15–44 years	12.2	19.5
Aged 45–74 years	2.2	3.2
Heart disease	2.0	3.2
Cerebrovascular disease	1.8	2.0
Renovascular	17.8	17.0

Table 2.1
*Relative mortality from vascular causes for diabetic patients of age 15–74 years first seen in the Joslin Clinic between 1950 and 1958 and traced to 1961. Data from Entmacher et al, Longevity of diabetic patients in recent years, Diabetes (1964) **13**:373–7, and from Marks and Krall.[4]*

and gender-matched population,[17] a shorter time to first or recurrent (nonfatal or fatal) CHD event,[18] and a high prevalence of overt and occult CHD at the time of diagnosis of NIDDM.[19,20] The high frequency of asymptomatic myocardial infarction found in electrocardiography has been suggested to be due to diabetic autonomic neuropathy.[21]

Atrioventricular and intraventricular conduction abnormalities associated with acute myocardial infarction are more common in diabetic subjects than in nondiabetic subjects.[22]

In the studies by Margolis et al.[20] and others,[23–26] diabetic women have a worse prognosis than those without diabetes and lose their premenopausal protection from CHD. It is of

interest to note that the prevalence of angina and myocardial infarction was increased in men and women at the time of diagnosis of NIDDM, and approached rates of those with established NIDDM.[27]

Cardiac failure is also markedly increased in diabetic subjects.[15] Echocardiography and radioisotope studies have demonstrated impaired systolic left ventricular function in systole and diastole[28] and may have some (but not an essential) relationship to diabetes duration and to the presence of specific diabetic complications (nephropathy and retinopathy). Various morphological changes have been observed more frequently in diabetes, for example perivascular and interstitial fibrosis. Separate from the excess of CHD, this suggests a specific diabetic heart muscle disease, perhaps akin to other diabetic microvascular complications. Furthermore, it has been suggested that left ventricular function may improve with better diabetic control.[29]

Risk factors

In the Multiple Risk Factor Intervention Trial[5] the 356 000 screenees were followed prospectively, highlighting the standard CHD risk factors of cigarette smoking, blood pressure, cholesterol and age. Independent of these, and of race and affluence, people with diabetes had three-times the CHD rate compared with people without diabetes.

This is reflected in the use of healthcare resources by the diabetic population for all purposes, which is four- to five-times the rate of the general population. In the USA, it was shown that 77% of all admissions and costs with diabetes complications were due to cardiovascular disease compared with 3%, 6% and 9% for retinopathy, nephropathy and neuropathy respectively.[30]

In countries such as Japan, where the rate of CHD in the general population is low, the diabetic subgroup also has a low rate, but it is still two- to four-fold greater than the nondiabetic population.[31] Rates of diabetes have been increasing in Japan,[31] as have prevalences of hyperlipidaemia and obesity,[32] while diabetes and impaired glucose tolerance have been shown to be associated with the incidence of stroke and CHD.[33]

The World Health Organization, through the St Vincent Declaration, has called for vigorous reduction in risk factors for CHD as part of required care of patients with diabetes.[34]

Smoking

MVD mortality is much increased in smokers compared with nonsmokers (see Figure 2.2),[5] although rates of cigarette smoking are not higher in those with diabetes. Smoking may elevate blood pressure acutely, and may limit hypotensive drug therapy efficacy. Direct effects of smoking affect arterial endothelium and are prothrombotic.

Specific studies of cigarette smoking in diabetic populations have not been widely performed, but Jarrett et al.[35] have suggested that smoking habits are not dissimilar in those with and without diabetes. Smoking has similar effects on increasing the relative CHD risk in both groups, although absolute CHD rates are higher in diabetic groups.[5,35]

The smoking habit should be discouraged, particularly in diabetic populations with higher MVD risks.

Hypertension

The causal relationship of blood pressure and MVD has been established in observational studies individually[5] and with meta-analysis.[36] In diabetes, hypertension has an increased prevalence, but also accelerates small and large vessel complications of diabetes; hypertension is rare in individuals surviving decades with diabetes. It has a multiplicative effect on MVD risk in diabetes,[17] and in impaired glucose tolerance.[37]

In diabetes plasma volume may increase, with a 10% increase in exchangeable sodium, and there is glomerular hyperfiltration with hyperglycaemia. Sodium and water retention may increase with progressive renal impairment, as blood pressure also rises. Those patients with established hypertension have a greater decline in renal function. Persistent proteinuria is the classical indicator of established diabetic renal disease, commencing as microalbuminuria, and progessing to intermittent and then persistent dipstick-positive proteinuria. In younger IDDM individuals, development of urinary albumin loss below levels of detection with dipsticks (microalbuminuria) is indicative of diabetic renal disease. This may also be true for older IDDM and NIDDM patients, but age and hypertension contribute to microalbuminuria without diabetes, making the finding less specific in these older diabetic groups.

About one-fifth of NIDDM patients and two-fifths of IDDM patients may develop evidence of nephropathy, up to two decades after onset of diabetes, but without necessarily progressing to end-stage renal disease requiring support.

Hyperglycaemia may accelerate development of diabetic renal disease, and good diabetic control may limit such development and help limit progression or early changes,[6] but once diabetic renal disease is established, blood pressure becomes the most important factor to control.[38]

Choice of hyptensive therapy is important, for the relatively lower efficacy of therapy in preventing CHD as opposed to cerebrovascular disease may relate to dyslipidaemic effects of beta blockers and thiazides.[39] Thiazides may also exacerbate NIDDM. Beta blockers may mask symptoms of, and recovery from hypoglycaemia in IDDM as well as worsening hypertriglyceridaemia.

Hyperlipidaemia

As in nondiabetic populations, MVD in IDDM and NIDDM patients is positively correlated with LDL cholesterol, and negatively with HDL cholesterol.[40–43] Concentrations of LDL cholesterol do not account for the excess CHD in diabetes, for in NIDDM versus nondiabetic groups the LDL cholesterol levels are similar or slightly lower.[44]

HDL cholesterol levels are normal in IDDM, but low in NIDDM. Relationships of HDL to vascular disease are inconsistent for IDDM patients, but clearly inversely related in those with NIDDM.

In the nondiabetic population, triglycerides are often the most important risk factor for CHD in univariate analysis.[12,45,46] The classical lipid abnormality of diabetes is hypertriglyceridaemia. Data are more limited for its relationship to CHD in diabetes.[13,14,40,47–49] However, triglycerides at entry into the Paris Prospective Study[14] were elevated in those men who died of CHD in the 11-year follow-up, compared with those who did not, after correction for hypertension, smoking, cholesterol and weight. A similar association between triglycerides and ECG ischaemia persisted after multivariate analysis in the WHO study.[13]

Insulin resistance syndrome

Many patients have coexistent hypertension, dyslipidaemia and diabetes mellitus or glucose intolerance, and hyperuricaemia or gout, high fibrinogen and high PAI-1 levels also occur (Table 2.2).[50] These abnormalities are associated with premature CHD and peripheral vascular disease.[51,52] The underlying metabolic abnormalities may be associated with insulin

---

- Hyperinsulinaemia
  Insulin resistance
- Central obesity android or abdominal, as opposed to buttocks and thigh (gynaecoid) obesity
- Hypertension
- High plasminogen activator inhibitor-1 levels

- Diabetes mellitus or IGT
- Hyperuricaemia or gout
- Mixed hyperlipidaemia and low HDL level (the atherogenic lipid profile)
- Premature macrovascular disease

Table 2.2
Features of the insulin resistance syndrome.

resistance, which may appear before other metabolic abnormalities are evident.[53]

Insulin resistance is associated with inadequately suppressed adipose tissue hormone-sensitive lipolysis resulting in increased nonesterified fatty acid flux to the liver as substrate for increased very low density lipoprotein (VLDL) triglyceride secretion.[54,55] Insulin resistance results in increased hepatic VLDL secretion,[56] but also impaired VLDL clearance from reduced lipoprotein lipase secretion and activity.

Features of the insulin resistance syndrome have been linked to birth weight, with subsequent risk of impaired glucose tolerance or NIDDM as an adult halving for each kilogram increase in birth weight.[57] Insulin resistance syndrome is also linked, with rates in adults falling from 30% in those of birth weight ≤ 2.5 kg to 6% in those of birth weight ≥ 4.3 kg.[58] Insulin resistance association with birth weight is independent of insulin resistance related to current adult body mass index or fat mass distribution.[59] Metabolic adaptation may occur in a fetus with impaired nutrition but may be permanently imprinted into adult biochemistry. How this change to fuel conservation occurs is not clear, and further investigation of underlying mechanisms is necessary to confirm this hypothesis, and to seek ways to obtain potential therapeutic benefits.

Triglyceride and HDL

Associated with overproduction and impaired clearance of VLDL, there is a longer residence time for VLDL. Impaired release of VLDL surface components and transfer to HDL may contribute to low HDL concentrations. Hepatic lipase activity increases with insulin resistance and is associated with conversion of HDL_2 to HDL_3 and lower total HDL,[60] which is in turn related to insulin resistance.[61]

Small dense LDL

Through the activity of cholesterol ester transfer proteins (CETP), there is an interchange of cholesterol ester from HDL and LDL to VLDL, with a reverse movement of triglyceride from triglyceride-rich lipoproteins to LDL and HDL. More exchange will occur with increased CETP activity, and also if there is longer VLDL plasma residence time. Triglyceride-enriched LDL and HDL particles become slightly smaller with hydrolysis of the triglyceride as they recycle past hepatic lipase for which they are good substrates. The smaller LDL particles (LDL_3) are poorer substrates for the LDL receptor than the more normal, larger, buoyant LDL_2. Although the change in size of LDL particles is quite small it is sufficient to allow conformational change in apoB-100, reducing apoB affinity for the LDL receptor in a manner that is probably independent of the triglyceride content.[62]

Slowly turning over LDL is linked to triglyceride levels, fasting and postprandially, and on and off triglyceride-lowering treatment.[63–65] Plasma triglyceride levels in the range of 1.5–3.5 mmol/L, which may not have attracted substantial clinical interest, are those in which small dense LDL_3 particles predominate. Treatment with fibric acid derivatives results not just in lowered plasma triglyceride levels, but also in substantial reduction in LDL_3.

A high concentration of small dense LDL_3 is associated with three- to seven-times the risk of CHD, independent of total LDL concentration,[66,67] and is also associated with low HDL cholesterol levels and moderate hypertriglyceridaemia. This pattern may be linked with insulin resistance, and has been termed the 'atherogenic lipid profile'.[68]

While most studies consider fasting plasma triglycerides, much of the time is spent in the postprandial state. These lipoprotein abnormalities are more obvious in the postprandial state, and exaggerated when fasting hypertriglyceridaemia is present.[69,70]

Glycaemic control and diabetic macrovascular disease

The microvascular complications (nephropathy, neuropathy and retinopathy) of diabetes are related to the duration of diabetes and its control.[71] While CHD and other macrovascular complications are considerably increased in diabetes, the relationship to good diabetic control is less distinct. Excess CHD was found not just in those with diabetes, but also in those with impaired glucose tolerance, and indeed in those with normal glucose tolerance but with blood glucose values in the top 5% of the normal distribution.[72–74]

Effects of therapy

Glucose

If glucose is important, one would expect tight glycaemic control to reverse or prevent diabetic complications. This has been demonstrated for microvascular complications in the Diabetes Control and Complications Trial,[6] in diabetic subjects with or without such complications at entry to the study. Macrovascular disease was decreased by 42% in this study, but the change was not significant as the study was in younger IDDM patients in whom prevalence rates of macrovascular disease were low.

There may be problems in establishing effects of glycaemic control in limiting CHD, because the threshold to develop excess CHD seems low (*see above*), and is lower than that for microvascular disease. Microvascular complications appear to require prevailing blood glucose levels of 11 mmol/L and above.[75,76] In patients with NIDDM, data are much more limited, and the results of the UKPDS are awaited.[7] Currently, initial efficacy results of different treatment regimens have been reported[77] but outcome data are not yet reported, and will need interpretation against a naturally deteriorating disease as pancreatic islet beta cell reserve fails.

Sulphonylureas

In studies of NIDDM cohorts, HDL cholesterol levels are low and tend to persist despite treatment. Patients treated with sulphonylureas may have lower HDL levels than NIDDM patients on other treatments,[78] but this may be a feature of the patient subgroups rather than a direct effect of the drug.

There was an unexpected increase in CHD events and mortality in the University Group Diabetes Program (UGDP) study,[79] a large interventional study of NIDDM treatments, implicating a first-generation sulphonylurea (tolbutamide). In UGDP CHD events were small in number, most occurred in a small number of centres, measures of long-term glycaemic control were not available, and the NIDDM was not severe. Even though there were these shortcomings, and the study has not been replicated, it should not be forgotten. Body weight increase and hyperinsulinaemia might offset the hypoglycaemic benefit,[77] but excess CHD did not occur in the insulin-treated group of UGDP.[79] Sulphonylurea treatment in the United Kingdom Prospective Diabetes Study Group[80] has not been shown to be harmful.

Biguanides

Metformin has moderate effect on triglycerides and perhaps on cholesterol in many, but not all studies. Triglyceride levels may improve, fasting or postprandially,[81,82,83] perhaps mostly in patients initially with hypertriglyceridaemia. HDL cholesterol is not substantially affected.

Metformin does not increase insulin secretion or cause weight increase or hypoglycaemia, but has extrapancreatic actions, probably increasing peripheral glucose utilization and suppressing hepatic gluconeogenesis. In the UKPDS study[80] metformin, sulphonylurea and insulin were equally effective, but outcomes for CHD and other cardiovascular mortality will not be known for about two years. This study will be important because, as with the sulphonylureas, doubts have been cast over another (no longer available) biguanide — phenformin — by the UGDP study,[79] where again excess CHD was found.

Insulin

On the one hand insulin has been implicated as an atherogenic factor,[84,85] while on the other, insulin treatment will improve glycaemic control, reduce hypertriglyceridaemia and is associated with higher levels of HDL cholesterol. Elevated plasma insulin is associated with CHD and precedes its development, but is normally accompanied by insulin resistance.[51] Insulin use has been linked to fatal coronary disease in the Pima Indians,[86] and to nonfatal CHD in other populations,[87] but diabetes severity was not controlled. However, intensive insulin treatment may correct increased cholesterol synthesis,[88] and reduce small dense LDL levels, and oxidation and glycation of lipoproteins.[89]

Where necessary, insulin should be used to improve glycaemic control. Certainly, IDDM patients using multiple insulin injections, continuous subcutaneous insulin infusions or,

shorter term, the artificial pancreas, demonstrate improved lipoprotein profiles.[90–92]

In the DCCT study[6] all the patients studied had IDDM only, and substantial effects on lipids and lipoproteins were not reported. Those patients receiving intensive treatment (compared with conventional treatment) showed a one-third reduction in the number of patients with LDL cholesterol > 4.14 mmol/L. However, this subgroup of patients is likely to have been only the top 10–15% of the LDL cholesterol distribution.

In NIDDM patients insulin treatment is appropriate where diabetic control is inadequate with other treatments, and may improve hypertriglyceridaemia. However, diabetic dyslipidaemia will very often persist, as will low HDL cholesterol levels.[78]

Hypotensive agents

The importance of blood pressure control is clearly established in diabetes, particularly if microalbuminuria develops. Indeed, the intervention levels of blood pressure should perhaps be a little lower than standard recommendations in young, microalbuminuric IDDM patients.

Standard thiazides and beta blockers may have specific relative contraindications in diabetes. The thiazides may be associated with an increase in impotence, in a patient group in which this is a particular issue. Similarly, in IDDM, beta blockers may mask the symptoms of hypoglycaemia and delay the rate of recovery from hypoglycaemia.[39] Both drug groups may be dyslipidaemic in susceptible individuals, and may aggravate diabetic dyslipidaemia.[39] While thiazide effects are dose-related, they may be present even at low doses. Where the use of these agents is not essential, alternatives should be considered as first-line treatment. If needed, for example beta blockers for angina, they should still be used.

ACE inhibitors and calcium antagonists are lipid neutral, and alpha blockers may be 'lipid-friendly'. ACE inhibitors may have a specific role in the protection of renal function in micro-albuminuric patients.

Lipids and lipoproteins

No major completed trials of primary or secondary prevention of CHD have included large numbers of IDDM or NIDDM patients, although such studies are now in progress. General population data have to be extrapolated to diabetes, but a causal role is suggested for diabetic dyslipidaemia, particularly with the increasing understanding of triglyceride-rich lipoprotein metabolism and small dense LDL.

In the Helsinki Heart Study gemfibrozil, which lowers triglycerides and elevates HDL (as well as reducing LDL moderately), was effective in reducing CHD rates.[93,94] Patients with high triglycerides and low HDL did as well or better than other subgroups, and while the number of diabetic patients within the group were small, their results were at least as good. The small number of diabetic patients within the Scandinavian Simvastatin Survial Study (4S)[95] had similar results to the whole patient group.

The 4S secondary prevention trial[95] showed reduction in total mortality of 30% (p = 0.003) and a reduction in CHD mortality of 42% (p < 0.00001). Also, in the West of Scotland primary prevention study (WOSCOPS)[96] CHD deaths and events were reduced by 31%, and total mortality by 22% (p = 0.051).

Fibrates

The fibrates may be the agents of choice in diabetes, particularly in NIDDM, where a mixed lipaemia is present. In some situations, with some fibrates, LDL cholesterol may rise rather than fall, reflecting more normal metabolism of triglyceride-rich lipoproteins through to LDL.[97–101] Excess small dense LDL_3 levels may be improved by fibrate treatment of mixed lipaemia, in people with NIDDM as well as IDDM.[69]

Statins

The hydroxymethylglutaryl Coenzyme-A reductase inhibitors (statins) are very potent reducers of plasma cholesterol and LDL cholesterol, with more modest effects on lowering triglycerides and raising HDL[95,96,102] and are very well tolerated. They have equivalent efficacy in diabetes for a given lipid profile compared with the non-diabetic population.

Resins

The resins — cholestyramine or colestipol — are very effective hypocholesterolaemic agents when well tolerated, but are less useful in mixed lipaemia, tending to increase triglyceride levels. They are therefore less often prescribed in diabetes.

Nicotinates

Nicotinic acid in pharmacological doses (1–3 g daily) inhibits lipolysis and can be very effective in reducing plasma triglyceride and VLDL triglyceride. However, it often has gastrointestinal side effects when taken in therapeutic doses, rarely may be hepatotoxic, and may worsen rather than improve glucose tolerance, perhaps because of rebound fattyacylaemia a few hours after ingestion. Acipimox (tetranicotinoyl-fructose) is better tolerated and longer acting, but less effective.[103]

Combination therapy

Combinations of drugs may be required for individuals at highest risk. Resin plus statin is an effective combination when hypercholesterolaemia is the prime abnormality. Statin plus fibrate is a logical combination, particularly when there is mixed lipaemia that is not controlled by diet and lifestyle changes and a single drug. This in currently used in specialist clinics for secondary prevention of coronary heart disease in some diabetic patients, but is outside data-sheet recommendations and product licences. The risk of the very rare, severe myositis seen with either group of drugs is increased during combination therapy with statin and fibrate, but it still uncommon.

If I had . . .

Primary prevention

If I diabetes it would concentrate my mind on the potential complications that might possibly come my way, both those microvascular and specific to diabetes and those macrovascular and not specific to diabetes but occurring with increased frequency. It would concentrate my mind on the data from the Joslin clinic in the 1960s, which suggested that life expectancy was reduced by about 30% at whatever age of onset of the diabetes. That the absolute reduction in life expectancy becomes less as one advances in age would not be a great consolation.

However, I would be optimistic that the prognosis may have improved over the last decades, and may continue to do so with further management advances. I would wish to extrapolate from the data that we do have. Passive inactivity on the basis that data are incomplete is not acceptable. Reasonable hypotheses exist, fully in keeping with other nondiabetic data, and while studies continue to test the hypotheses I would wish to act on best evidence at least until it is found deficient.[104]

My first efforts would be in correcting the metabolic abnormalities of my diabetes on the basis that diabetes duration multiplied by integrated metabolic defect is linked to risk of future CHD. I would be heartened by the results of the DCCT study,[6] which showed reduced risks of microvascular disease, and the hint of less macrovascular disease. I would have tightened up my variable diet, trying to reduce the indiscretions. I would increase efforts at regular physical exercise, aiming at 20–30 minutes of moderate breathlessness daily. I do not smoke, have normal blood pressure and a good lipid profile, but I would watch carefully for 'microhypertension' and would treat blood pressure at a lower threshold than I would without diabetes. I would recognize the amelioration of microalbuminuria and the slowing of the rate of renal function loss by active effective blood pressure control. Of the various agents I would note suggestions that ACE inhibitors may have a specific role in diabetic renal protection. I might avoid beta blockers without other reason than because of occasional loss of hypoglycaemia awareness in IDDM, and slower rate of recovery. I might avoid thiazides for their effects on potency, for their diabetogenic potential in NIDDM, and (as with beta blockers) for their dyslipidaemic potential even in lower dose. I would note the lipid-friendly possibilities of alpha blockers as an additional option.

My approach might vary with IDDM or NIDDM. NIDDM has a substantial CHD risk, worsened by central adiposity. I might not be able to avoid the latter fully if I had shown multiple elements of the insulin resistance syndrome, but would do my best. I would wish to have a cholesterol below 5 mmol/L and LDL cholesterol below 3.5 mmol/L. I would be much more concerned than many colleagues if I had moderate hypertriglyceridaemia (1.5–4.0 mmol/L) associated with a low HDL cholesterol (<1.1 mmol/L). The shift from buoyant LDL species to small dense LDL_3 occurs above a triglyceride value of 1.5 mmol/L. I would wait for the Israeli beza-fibrate study results with interest, and for another possible fibrate intervention study in Australasia. Correcting this classical diabetic dyslipidaemia may not be easy, but I would have a low threshold to initiate lipid lowering therapy, and would use fibrate of statin as most effective for me.

If it was my wife with the diabetes, and especially with NIDDM, I would be concerned because of the particularly increased macrovascular risk in IDDM and in NIDDM.

I would wish to have exercise testing at intervals, but recognizing that it may be less reliable than in nondiabetic patients, I would be prepared to have early coronary angiography. If I had microalbuminuria I would recognize my increased macrovascular risk and increase treatments where appropriate.

Secondary prevention

If I was unfortunate enough to have CHD already, I would be more aggressive in my management. I would wish to know about my left ventricular function, start ACE inhibition early, and control any trend to rising blood pressure. I would wish to know about my exercise reserve, and coronary artery anatomy with a view to treatment. Acutely, at the time of myocardial infarct or unstable angina, I would recognize my increased vulnerability.

I would lower my cholesterol to 4 mmol/L and my LDL cholesterol to less than 3 mmol/L with a statin. My triglycerides would be well below 1.5 mmol/L with fibrate treatment if needed, and hopefully with a consequent HDL cholesterol rise. That intervention data with fibrates are limited, and that patients with diabetes have mainly been excluded from big statin studies would not prevent my using them. I would be taking low-dose aspirin (75 mg daily), and would have been on this prior to my clinical CHD. If my macrovascular disease was cerebrovascular or peripheral vascular, I would still treat myself in the same way, although recognizing that data are less secure.

Although it is outside data-sheet recommendations, and without product licences, I would have a low threshold for the use of fibrate and statin in combination. Transaminase disturbance of significance is rare. Substantial asymptomatic CPK rise (up to 5–10-times normal) would not necessarily prevent treatment but is rarely seen, even with such combination therapy.

In both primary and secondary prevention I would be likely to move to insulin treatment if my glycaemic control was inadequate, and also if hypertriglyceridaemia persisted in NIDDM. I would wish to minimize my dosage by keeping thin and physically active and avoiding insulin resistance. I would be likely to use a four-times daily basal-bolus regimen, and would probably consider a rapid acting analogue insulin to match food absorption and to avoid the 30-minute injection-to-food requirement of soluble insulin.

All this said, I would recognize the persisting increased risk of vascular complications, and would watch treatment developments closely. Would it make me bring forward retirement? Perhaps, perhaps not!

References

1 Marks L, Counting the cost: the real impact of non-insulin-dependent diabetes. (King's Fund Policy Institute for the British Diabetic Association: London, 1996) 1–48.

2 Krowleski AS, Kosinski EJ, Warram JH et al, Magnitude and determinants of coronary heart disease in juvenile onset insulin dependent diabetes mellitus, *Am J Cardiol* (1987)**59**:750–5.

3 Reckless JPD, The epidemiology of coronary heart disease in diabetes mellitus. In: Taylor KG ed. *Diabetes and the heart* (Castle House Publications: Tunbridge Wells, 1987) 1–18.

4 Marks HH, Krall LP, Onset, course, prognosis and mortality in diabetes mellitus. In: Marble A, White P, Bradley RF, Krall LP, eds. *Joslin's diabetes mellitus* 11th ed. (Lea and Febiger: Philadelphia, 1971) 209–54.

5 Stamler J, Vaccaro O, Neaton JD, Wentworth D, for the Multiple Risk Factor Intervention Trial Research Group, Diabetes, other risk factors and 12 year cardiovascular mortality for men screened in the Multiple Risk Factor Intervention Trial, *Diabetes Care* (1993)**16**:434–44.

6 Diabetes Control and Complications Trial Group, Effect of intensive treatment of diabetes on the development and progression of long term complications in insulin dependent diabetes mellitus, *N Engl J Med* (1993)**329**:977–86.

7 United Kingdom Prospective Diabetes Study Group, The United Kingdom Prospective Diabetes Study (UKPDS): 8. Study design, progress and performance, *Diabetologia* (1991)**34**:877–90.

8 Mogensen CE, Longterm antihypertensive treatment inhibiting progression of diabetic retinopathy, *Br Med J* (1982)**285**:685–8.

9 Katz, R, Dunn T, Meyer S, Anderson S, Rennke HG, Brenner BM, Prevention of diabetic glomerulopathy by pharmacological amelioration of glomerular capillary hypertension, *J Clin Invest* (1986)**77**:1925–30.

10 Melbourne Diabetic Nephropathy Study Group, Comparison between perindopril and nifedipine in hypertensive and normotensive diabetic patients with microalbuminuria, *Br Med J* (1991)**302**:210–16.

11 Assmann G, Schulte H, The prospective cardiovascular Munster (PROCAM) study: prevalence of hyperlipidaemia in persons with hypertension and/or diabetes mellitus and the relationship to coronary heart disease, *Am Heart J* (1988)**116**:1713–24.

12 Hokanson JE, Austin MA, Triglyceride and coronary heart disease in men and women: meta-analysis of population based prospective studies, *Circulation* (1993)**88**:I–510.

13 West KM, Ahuja MMS, Bennett PH et al, The role of circulating glucose and triglyceride concentrations and their interactions with other risk factors as determinants of arterial disease in nine diabetic population samples from the World Health Organisation multinational study, *Diabetes Care* (1983)**6**:361–9.

14 Fontbonne A, Eschwege E, Cambien F et al, Hypertriglyceridaemia as a risk factor for coronary heart disease mortality in subjects with impaired glucose tolerance or diabetes, *Diabetologia* (1989)**32**:300–4.

15 Kannel WB, Role of diabetes in cardiac disease: conclusions from population studies. In: Zoneraich S, ed. *Diabetes and heart* (Charles C Thomas: Springfield, 1978) 97–122.

16 Reuanen A, Laakso M, Pyorala K, Cardiovascular and coronary heart disease mortality of diabetics and non-diabetics: impact of risk factors, *J Am Coll Cardiol* (1983)**1**:600 (abstr).

17 Kannel WB, McGee DI, Diabetes and glucose tolerance as risk factors for cardiovascular disease. The Framingham study, *Diabetes Care* (1979)**2**:120–6.

18 Abbott RD, Donahue RP, Kannel WB, Wilson PWF, The impact of diabetes on survival following myocardial infarction in men versus

women. The Framingham study, *J Am Med Assoc* (1988)**260**:3456–60.

19 Partamian JO, Bradley RF, Acute myocardial infarction in 258 cases of diabetes, *N Engl J Med* (1965)**273**:455–61.

20 Margolis JR, Kannel WB, Feinlieb M, Dawber TR, McNamara PM, Clinical features of unrecognized myocardial infarction: silent and symptomatic. Eighteen year follow up. The Framingham study. *Am J Cardiol* (1973)**32**:1–7.

21 Faerman I, Faccio E, Milei J et al, Autonomic neuropathy and painless myocardial infarction in diabetic patients. Histologic evidence of their relationship, *Diabetes* (1977)**26**:1147–58.

22 Czyzyk A, Krowleski AS, Szablowska S et al, Clinical course of myocardial infarction among diabetic patients, *Diabetes Care* (1980)**3**:526–9.

23 Barrett-Connor E, Wingard DL, Sex differential in ischaemic heart disease mortality in diabetics: a prospective population-based study, *Am J Epidemiol* (1983)**118**:489–96.

24 Heyden S, Heiss G, Bartel AG, Hames CG, Sex differences in coronary mortality among diabetics in Evans county, Georgia, *J Chronic Dis* (1980)**33**:265–73.

25 Smith JW, Marcus FI, Serokman R, Prognosis of patients with diabetes mellitus after myocardial infarction, *Am J Cardiol* (1984)**54**:718–21.

26 Molstad P, Nustad M, Acute myocardial infarction in diabetic patients, *Acta Med Scand* (1987)**222**:433–7.

27 Uusitupa M, Siitonen O, Aro A et al, Prevalence of coronary heart disease, left ventricular failure and hypertension in middle-aged, newly diagnosed type 2 (non-insulin-dependent) diabetic subjects, *Diabetologia* (1985)**28**:22–7.

28 Watson RDS, Waldron S, Heart disease and diabetes mellitus. In: Taylor KG, ed. *Diabetes and the heart* (Castle House Publications: Tunbridge Wells, 1987) 19–41.

29 Uusitupa M, Siitonen O, Aro A et al, Effect of correction of hyperglycaemia on left ventricular function in non-insulin-dependent (type 2) diabetics, *Acta Med Scand* (1983)**213**:363–8.

30 American Diabetes Association: Center for Economic Studies in Medicine, *Direct and indirect costs of diabetes in the United States in 1987* (American Diabetes Association: Alexandria, VA, 1988).

31 Ohmura T, Ueda K, Kiyohara Y et al, Prevalence of type 2 (non-insulin dependent) diabetes mellitus and impaired glucose tolerance in the Japanese general population: the Hisayama study, *Diabetologia* (1993)**36**:1198–203.

32 Fujishima M, Kiyohara Y, Ueda K, Hasuo Y, Kato I, Iwamoto M, Smoking as cardiovascular risk factor in low cholesterol population: the Hisayama study, *Clin Exp Hypertens* (1992)**A14**:99–108.

33 Fujishima M, Kiyohara Y, Kato I et al, Diabetes and cardiovascular disease in a prospective population survey in Japan, *Diabetes* (1996)**45**(**suppl 3**):S14–S16.

34 Krans HMJ et al, The St Vincent Declaration. *Diabetes care and research in Europe* (World Health Organization: Geneva, 1992).

35 Jarrett RJ, Keen H, Chakrabarti R, Diabetes, hyperglycaemia and arterial disease. In: Keen H, Jarrett J, eds. *Complications of diabetes* 2nd ed. (Edward Arnold: London, 1982) 179.

36 MacMahon S, Peto R, Cutler J et al, Blood pressure, stroke and coronary heart disease, Part 1. Prolonged differences in blood pressure: prospective observational studies corrected for the regression dilution bias, *Lancet* (1990)**335**:765–74.

37 Fuller JH, Shipley MJ, Rose G, Jarrett RJ, Keen H, Mortality from coronary heart disease and stroke in relation to degree of glycaemia: the Whitehall study, *Br Med J* (1983)**287**:867–70.

38 Parving HH, Andersen AR, Smidt UM, Svendsen PA, Early aggressive anti-hypertensive treatment reduces rate of decline in kidney function in diabetic nephropathy, *Lancet* (1983)**i**:1175–9.

39 Weidmann P, Ferrier C, Saxenhofer H et al, Serum lipoproteins during treatment with anti-hypertensive drugs, *Drugs* (1988)**35**(**suppl 6**):118–34.

40 Ronnemaa T, Laakso M, Kallio V, Pyorala K, Marniemi J, Puuka P, Serum lipids, lipoproteins and apolipoproteins and the excessive occurrence of coronary heart disease in non insulin dependent diabetic patients, *Am J Empidemiol* (1989)**130**:632–45.

41 Reckless JPD, Betteridge DJ, Wu P, Payne B, Galton DJ, High density and low density lipoproteins and prevalence of vascular disease in diabetes mellitus, *Br Med J* (1978)**i**:883–6.

42 Maser RE, Wolfson SK Jr, Ellis D et al, Cardiovascular disease and arterial calcification in insulin dependent diabetes mellitus: interrelation and risk factor profile, *Atheroscler Thromb* (1991)**11**:958–65.

43 Seviour PW, Teal TK, Richmond W, Elkeles RS, Serum lipids, lipoproteins and macrovascular disease in non-insulin dependent diabetics: a possible new approach to prevention, *Diabetic Med* (1988)**5**:166–71.

44 Reckless JPD, *Diabetes and lipids* (Martin Dunitz: London, 1994) 25.

45 Austin MA, Plasma triglyceride and coronary heart disease, *Arterioscler Thromb* (1992)**11**: 2–14.

46 Carlson LA, Bottiger LE, Ahfeldt PE, Risk factors for myocardial infarction in the Stockholm Prospective Study: a 14-year follow up focussing on the role of plasma triglycerides and cholesterol, *Acta Med Scand* (1979)**206**:351–60.

47 Santen RJ, Willis PW, Fajans SS, Atherosclerosis in diabetes mellitus: correlations with lipid levels, adiposity and serum insulin level, *Arch Intern Med* (1972)**130**: 833–43.

48 Nanka H, Five year incidence of major macrovascular complications in diabetes mellitus, *Horm Metab Res* (1985)**15**(suppl):15–19.

49 Laakso M, Ronnemaa T, Pyorala K, Kallio V, Puukka P, Penttila I, Atherosclerotic vascular disease and its risk factors in non-insulin dependent diabetic and non-diabetic subjects in Finland, *Diabetes Care* (1988)**11**:449–63.

50 Genest J, Cohn JS, Clustering of cardiovascular risk factors: targeting high risk individuals, *Am J Cardiol* (1995)**76**(suppl):8A–20A.

51 Reaven GM, Role of insulin resistance in human disease, *Diabetes* (1988)**37**:1595–607.

52 Laakso M, Insulin resistance and coronary heart disease, *Curr Opin Lipidol* (1996)**7**: 217–26.

53 Haffner SM, Valdez RA, Hazuda HP, Mitchell BD, Morales PA, Stern MP, Prospective analysis of the insulin resistance syndrome (syndrome X), *Diabetes* (1992)**41**:715–22.

54 McKeigue PM, Laws A, Chen YD, Marmot MG, Reaven GM, Relation of plasma triglyceride and apo B levels to insulin-mediated suppression of non-esterified fatty acids, *Arterioscler Thromb* (1993)**13**:1187–92.

55 Wiggins D, Gibbons GF, The lipolysis/esterfication cycle of hepatic triacylglycerol. It role in the secretion of very low density lipoprotein and its response to hormones and sulphonylureas, *Biochem J* (1992)**284**:457–62.

56 Kissebah AH, Adams PW, Wynn V, Interrelationships between insulin secretion and plasma free fatty acid and triglyceride kinetics in maturity onset diabetes and the effect of phenylethylbiguanide (phenformin), *Diabetologia* (1974)**10**:119–30.

57 Hales CN, Barker DJP, Clark PMS et al, Foetal and infant growth and impaired glucose tolerance at age 64, *Br Med J* (1991)**303**: 1019–22.

58 Barker DJP, Hales CN, Fall CHD, Osmond C, Phipps K, Clark PMS, Type 2 (non-insulin dependent) diabetes mellitus, hypertension and hyperlipidaemia (syndrome X): relation to reduced fetal growth, *Diabetologia* (1993)**36**: 62–7.

59 Lithell HO, McKeigue PM, Berglund L, Mohsen R, Lithell U-B, Leon DA, Relation of size at birth to non-insulin dependent diabetes and insulin concentrations in men age 50–60 years, *Br Med J* (1996)**312**:406–10.

60 Baynes C, Henderson AD, Anyaoku V et al, The role of insulin insensitivity and hepatic lipase in the dyslipidaemia of type 2 diabetes, *Diab Med* (1991)**8**:560–6.

61 Laakso M, Sarlund H, Mykkanen L, Insulin resistance is associated with lipid and lipoprotein abnormalities in subjects with varying degrees of glucose tolerance, *Arteriosclerosis* (1990)**10**:223–31.

62 Galeano NF, Milne R, Marcel YL et al, Apoprotein B structure and receptor recognition of trigylceride rich low density lipoprotein (LDL) is modified in small LDL but not in triglyceride-rich LDL of normal size, *J Biol Chem* (1994)**269**:511–19.

63 Caslake MJ, Packard CJ, Series JJ, Yip B, Dagen MM, Shepherd J, Plasma triglyceride and low density lipoprotein metabolism, *Eur J Clin Invest* (1992)**22**:96–104.

64 Caslake MJ, Packard CJ, Gaw A et al, Fenofibrate and LDL metabolic heterogeneity in hypercholesterolaemia, *Arterioscler Thromb* (1993)**13**:702–11.

65 Gaw A, Packard CJ, Caslake MJ et al, Effects of ciprofibrate on LDL metabolism in man, *Atherosclerosis* (1994)**108**:137–48.

66 Austin MA, Breslow JL, Hennekens CH, Buring JE, Willett WC, Krauss RM, Low density lipoprotein subclass patterns and risk of myocardial infarction, *J Am Med Assoc* (1988)**260**:1917–21.

67 Griffin BA, Freeman DJ, Tait GW et al, Role of plasma triglyceride in the regulation of plasma low density lipoprotein (LDL) subfractions: relative contribution of small, dense LDL to coronary heart disease risk, *Atherosclerosis* (1994)**106**:241–53.

68 Austin MA, King MC, Vranizan KM, Krauss RM, Atherogenic lipoprotein phenotype. A proposed genetic marker for coronary heart disease, *Circulation* (1990)**82**:495–506.

69 Harris C, Stirling C, Lloyd J, Reckless JPD, Qualitative diabetic lipoprotein change: postprandial profile and bezafibrate therapy, *Atherosclerosis* (1995)**115**:S52.

70 Tan KCB, Cooper MB, Ling KLE et al, Fasting and postprandial determinants for the occurrence of small dense LDL species in non-insulin dependent patients with and without hypertriglyceridaemia: the involvement of insulin, insulin precursor species and insulin resistance, *Atherosclerosis* (1995)**113**:273–87.

71 Pirart J, Diabetes mellitus and its degenerative complications: a prospective study of 4400 patients observed between 1947 and 1973, *Diabetes Care* (1978)**1**:166–88, 252–63.

72 Fuller JH, Shipley MJ, Rose G et al, Mortality from coronary heart disease and stroke in relation to degree of glycaemia: the Whitehall study, *Br Med J* (1983)**287**:867–70.

73 Eschwege E, Ducimetiere P, Thibult N et al, Coronary heart disease mortality in relation with diabetes, blood glucose and plasma insulin levels. The Paris Prospective study, ten years later, *Horm Metab Res* (1985)**15**(suppl):41–5.

74 Pyorala K, Savolainen E, Kaukola S et al, Plasma insulin as coronary heart disease risk factor: relationship to other risk factors and predictive value during the $9\frac{1}{2}$ year follow up of the Helsinki Policeman Study population, *Acta Med Scand* (1985)**701**(suppl):38–52.

75 Kuusisto J, Mikkanen L, Pyorala K, Laasko M, NIDDM and its metabolic control predict coronary heart disease in elderly subjects, *Diabetes* (1994)**43**:960–7.

76 Krolewski AS, Laffel LMB, Krolewski M, Quinn M, Warren JH, Glycolylated hemoglobin and the risk of microalbuminuria in patients with insulin-dependent diabetes mellitus, *N Engl J Med* (1995)**332**:1251–5.

77 United Kingdom Prospective Diabetes Study Group, The United Kingdom Prospective Diabetes Study (UKPDS): 13. Relative efficacy of randomly allocated diet, sulphonylurea, insulin or metformin in patients with newly diagnosed non-insulin dependent diabetes followed for three years, *Br Med J* (1995)**310**:83–8.

78 Stern MP, Mitchell BD, Haffner SM, Hazuda HP, Does glycaemic control of type II diabetes suffice to control diabetic dyslipidaemia? A community perspective, *Diabetes Care* (1992)**15**:638–44.

79 Klimt CR, Knatterud GL, Meinert CL, Prout TE, The University Group Diabetes Program: a study of the effects of hypoglycaemic agents on vascular complications in patients with adult-onset diabetes. I. Design, methods and baseline characteristics. II. Mortality results, *Diabetes* (1970)**19**(suppl 2):747–830.

80 United Kingdom Prospective Diabetes Study Group, The United Kingdom Prospective Diabetes Study (UKPDS): 16. Overview of 6 years' therapy of type II diabetes: a progressive disease, *Diabetes* (1995)**44**:1249–58.

81 Wu M-S, Johnston P, Sheu WH-H et al, Effect of metformin on carbohydrate and lipoprotein metabolism in NIDDM patients, *Diabetes Care* (1990)**13**:1–8.

82 Jeppesen J, Zhou M-Y, Chen YD, Reaven GM, Effect of metformin on postprandial lipaemia in patients with fairly to poorly controlled NIDDM, *Diabetes Care* (1994)**17**:1093–9.

83 Grant PJ, The effects of metformin on cardiovascular risk factors, *Diab Metab Rev* (1995)**11**(suppl):S43–S50.

84 Stout RW, Insulin and atheroma: 20 year perspective, *Diabetes Care* (1990)**13**:631–55.

85 Stout RW, Hyperinsulinaemia and athero-sclerosis, *Diabetes* (1996)**45**(suppl 3):S45–S46.

86 Nelson RG, Sievers ML, Knowler WC et al, Low incidence of fatal coronary disease in Pima Indians despite high prevalence of non-insulin dependent diabetes, *Circulation* (1990)**81**:987–95.

87 Janka HU, Ziegler AG, Standl E, Mehnert H, Daily insulin dose as a predictor of macrovascular disease in insulin treated non-insulin dependent diabetics, *Diabetes Metab* (1987)**13**: 359–64.

88 Scoppola A, Testa G, Frontoni S et al, Effects of insulin on cholesterol synthesis in type II diabetes mellitus, *Diabetes Care* (1995)**18**:1362–9.

89 Brunzell JD, Chait A, Lipoprotein pathophysiology and treatment. In: Rifkin H, Porte D, eds. *Ellemberg and Rifkin's diabetes mellitus: theory and practice* (Elsevier: New York, 1990) 756–67.

90 Pietri AO, Dunn FL, Grundy SM, Raskin P, The effect of continuous subcutaneous insulin infusion on very low density lipoprotein triglyceride metabolism in type I diabetes mellitus, *Diabetes* (1983)**32**:75–81.

91 Dunn FL, Raskin P, Belheimer DW, Grundy SM, The effect of diabetic control on very low density lipoprotein-triglyceride metabolism in patients with type II diabetes mellitus and marked hypertriglyceridaemia, *Metabolism* (1984)**33**:117–23.

92 Dunn FL, Carroll PB, Beltz WF, Treatment with artificial B cell decreases very low density lipoprotein triglyceride synthesis in type I diabetes, *Diabetes* (1987)**36**:661–6.

93 Frick MH, Elo O, Haapa K et al, Helsinki heart study: primary prevention trial with gemfibrozil in middle-aged men with dyslipidaemia, *N Engl J Med* (1987)**317**:1237–45.

94 Manninen V, Elo MO, Frick MH et al, Lipid alterations and decline in the incidence of coronary heart disease in the Helsinki Heart Study, *J Am Med Assoc* (1988)**260**:641–51.

95 Scandinavian Simvastatin Survival Study Group. Randomised trial of cholesterol lowering in 4444 patients with coronary heart disease: the Scandinavian Simvastatin Survival Study (4S), *Lancet* (1994)**344**:1383–9.

96 Shepherd J, Cobbe SM, Ford J et al, Prevention of coronary heart disease with pravastatin in men with hypercholesterolaemia. West of Scotland Coronary Prevention Study Group, *N Engl J Med* (1995)**333**:1301–7.

97 Vinik AI, Colwell JA, and Hyperlipidaemia in Diabetes Investigators, Effects of gemfibrozil on triglyceride levels in patients with NIDDM, *Diabetes Care* (1993)**16**:37–44.

98 Lahdenpera S, Tilly-Kiesi M, Vuorinen-Markkola H, Kuusi T, Taskinen MR, Effects of gemfibrozil on low density lipoprotein particle size, density distribution and composition in patients with type II diabetes, *Diabetes Care* (1993)**16**:584–92.

99 Garg A, Grundy SM, Gemfibrozil alone and in combination with lovastatin for treatment of hypertriglyceridaemia in NIDDM, *Diabetes* (1989)**38**:364–72.

100 Jones IR, Swai A, Taylor R, Miller M, Laker MF, Alberti KGMM, Lowering of plasma glucose concentrations with bezafibrate in patients with moderately controlled NIDDM, *Diabetes Care* (1990)**13**:855–63.

101 Stewart MW, Dyer RG, Alberti KGMM, Laker MF, The effects of lipid lowering on metabolic control and lipoprotein composition in type 2 diabetic patients with mild hyperlipidaemia, *Diabetic Med* (1995)**12**:250–7.

102 Sacks FM, Pfeffer MA, Moye LA et al, The effect of pravastatin on coronary events after myocardial infarction in patients with average cholesterol levels, *N Engl J Med* (1996)**335**: 1001–9.

103 Fulcher GR, Jones IR, Alberti KGMM, Improvement in glucose tolerance by reduction of lipid concentrations in non-insulin dependent diabetes mellitus, *Diabetes News* (1988)**9**:4–6.

104 Durrington PN, Prevention of macrovascular disease: absolute proof or absolute risk, *Diabetic Med* (1995)**12**:561–2.

3

Hypertension in women

Gregory YH Lip and D Gareth Beevers

Introduction

Hypertension is a major risk factor for premature death and morbidity from heart attacks, stroke and heart failure, and it is a common cause of end-stage renal failure. Over the past three decades, the marked reduction in death rates for cardiovascular disease and stroke is partly attributable to control of hypertension. Pooled clinical trial results have demonstrated for example, that a reduction in diastolic blood pressure by 5–6 mmHg results in a 38% reduction in stroke and a 16% reduction in coronary heart disease (CHD).[1]

Although there are probably more women than men with hypertension, most of our knowledge on the value of treating hypertension has been extrapolated from men to women. However, careful analysis of the large clinical trials of antihypertensive therapy does suggest that there are gender differences in the benefits of treatment, especially in mild hypertension. Indeed, these results do not support the current guidelines for the treatment of hypertensive women. Central to an understanding of the management of hypertension in women is an awareness of the role of oestrogens in cardiovascular disease. Furthermore, hypertension in women is closely related to other associated factors such as oral contraceptive use, pregnancy and the menopause, with its rapid fall in oestrogenic activity. All these factors have to be carefully considered in any assessment of blood pressure in women. Concerns about the use of

hormone replacement therapy in hypertensive postmenopausal women have also been voiced.

Hypertension as a cardiovascular risk factor in women

Hypertension is a particularly important risk factor for cardiovascular disease and stroke in women. For example, coronary artery disease is in general twice as common in hypertensive patients when compared with the normotensive population;[1,2] and hypertensive women are approximately four times more likely to have heart disease (relative risk 3.5; 95% confidence interval 2.8–4.5) and three times more likely to have a stroke (relative risk 2.6; 95% confidence interval 1.8–3.5) compared with normotensive women.[3] More women than men have hypertension after the age of about 50 years, reflecting the longer survival of women and the higher prevalence of hypertension among the elderly.

If other cardiovascular risk factors are also present, the treatment of hypertension and good blood pressure control are essential since a combination of risk factors synergistically increases the cardiovascular risk 'load' for individual women. The factors that predispose to CHD are similar for men and women, but their effects vary quantitatively depending on gender.[4,5] In the Rochester Coronary Heart Disease Project it was estimated that elimination of hypertension as a risk factor would reduce coronary heart disease by 45%; this is in comparison with a 64% reduction by smoking cessation, and a 45% reduction by use of oestrogen hormone replacement therapy.[6] However, the relative protection that women have against CHD compared with men persists even when they have the known risk factors, as seen in a 15-year follow-up study of over 8000 women and 7000 men aged 45–64 years.[7] Thus, with equal degrees of smoking, hypertension, lower social class and higher body mass index, women have consistently lower CHD mortality rates than men.[7] However, women are generally under-represented in trials of risk and intervention, and data are usually extrapolated from men to women.[8]

Epidemiology of hypertension in women

It is well established that there is a rise in blood pressure with age. In general, systolic blood pressure increases progressively with age, whereas diastolic blood pressure rises until the age of 60 years and then decreases. Overall, men also have slightly higher blood pressures than women and a slightly greater prevalence of hypertension.[9]

However, hypertension is a common problem in women, especially with increasing age. Statistics from the United Kingdom for 1991-1992 indicate that 31% of women aged 55–64 years were hypertensive or were receiving antihypertensive therapy; this proportion rises to 52% of those aged 64–74 years and 65% of women aged over 75 years.[10]

During the first four or five decades, the incidence of hypertension is higher in men than in women. Mean systolic pressure is usually significantly higher in men, but diastolic blood pressures apparently do not differ as much.[11] Some differences in the national prevalences of

hypertension are available from the USA, Australia and Korea.[9] In the National Health and Nutrition Examination Surveys (NHANES) III from the USA, blood pressures, particularly systolic, were higher in men than in women until 70 years of age, following which systolic pressure in women exceeded that in men and continued to be higher throughout the rest of life. By contrast, diastolic pressure levelled off at about age 50 years and then declined.[12] In the National Heart Foundation of Australia Risk Factor Prevalence Survey of men and women aged 26–64 years, men had higher pressures at all ages except age 64 years, when the mean systolic and diastolic pressures were similar in both sexes.[13] The prevalence of hypertension in the latter study was greater in men than women, except in the 60–64 years age group, when the prevalence was essentially identical (57.4% for men and 57.1% for women). In the Korean national survey, blood pressures were slightly higher in men than in women until age 50 years, when values for the two sexes became equal and remained so with increasing age; the prevalence of hypertension was also practically identical after age 50 years.[14] Data from the NHANES II study suggest that the prevalence of isolated systolic hypertension was less in women than in men, with black men having the highest prevalence.[15]

Women have less hypertension before the menopause, possibly because of higher circulating levels of oestrogen and lower androgen levels, or from reduced blood volume and viscosity resulting from menstrual loss.[16] However, beyond the age of 50 years the prevalence of hypertension appears to increase at a faster rate in women.[16,17] This rise in blood pressure with age is influenced by racial origin, with black hypertensive patients having a greater increase than white patients.[18] For example, hypertension was found to be more prevalent in African Americans aged 65–74 years (60%)

compared with whites (44%) and in black women compared with black men.[19,20] There is a steady increase in the prevalence of hypertension within each decade, with blacks having about twice the prevalence of whites.[20]

Thus, after the menopause, more women, especially black women, develop hypertension compared with men. However, epidemiological evidence suggests that in general, women tolerate hypertension better, live longer and have fewer complications than men with similar blood pressure levels.

Mechanisms of hypertension in women

Decreased sex hormones and increased sodium sensitivity have been suggested as potential mechanisms in the development of postmenopausal hypertension.[21] In addition, there may be a greater degree of volume expansion with age, as indicated by higher levels of atrial natriuretic factor and lower plasma renin activity.[16,22] Younger hypertensive women have a higher resting heart rate, cardiac index and pulse pressure, but a lower total peripheral resistance than younger hypertensive men, but these haemodynamic patterns tend to be similar in men and women older than 45 years.[23] As in men, higher plasma insulin levels also predict the subsequent development of hypertension.[24]

All these factors may be related to a rise in body mass index following the menopause, which is seen in some but not all women. It is unclear which is the primary phenomenon, to explain why reduction of circulating oestrogens is associated with rising blood pressure and cardiovascular risk.

There is also increasing recognition of the role of haemorheological and haemostatic factors in the development of hypertension and its complications.[25] Indeed, while the arterial tree is exposed to increased pressure flow, paradoxi-

cally the complications of hypertension are mainly thrombotic rather than haemorrhagic. These abnormalities of haemorheological indices, coagulation factors, arteriolar endothelial function and platelets may contribute to thrombus formation (thrombogenesis) in hypertensive patients, thus creating a prothrombotic (or hypercoagulable) state. There is evidence, for example, that these prothrombotic and rheological indices are abnormal in hypertensive patients even before they sustain any vascular complications.[25]

Abnormalities of platelet activation and aggregation are also well recognized in hypertensive patients and are significantly altered by antihypertensive drugs.[26–28] Rheological, platelet and coagulation factor abnormalities may therefore have some prognostic value in hypertensive patients. Finally, endothelial dysfunction or damage may be present as a result of hypertension, but endothelial damage may actually promote hypertension.[29] Such endothelial dysfunction is intimately related to coagulation factors (such as von Willebrand factor) and the process of thrombogenesis and atherogenesis.[25,30]

Many studies have demonstrated adverse changes in haemorheological and haemostatic factors following the menopause, which are reversed by the use of oestrogen hormone replacement therapy.[31–34] For example, in the large PEPI study, there was a significant reduction in plasma fibrinogen levels following HRT use.[33] The recent MRC trial found no significant changes in haemostatic factors following HRT use.[34]

Hypertension and target-organ damage

If target-organ damage (that is, heart attacks or strokes) is present in hypertensive patients, this confers additional cardiovascular risk. However, 'subclinical' target-organ damage is also associated with increased mortality and morbidity. Examples of this 'subclinical' end-organ damage in hypertensive patients include the presence of left ventricular hypertrophy (LVH) and microalbuminuria.

The presence of LVH has considerable prognostic implications,[2] with an increased risk of sudden death, arrhythmias (including ventricular arrhythmias and atrial fibrillation) and hypertensive heart failure. In addition, there is a twelve-fold increase in the risk of stroke, a four-fold increase in the risk of acute myocardial infarction and a three-fold increase in intermittent claudication.[2] Although the ECG is the commonest and easiest way of screening for LVH, it is best defined by calculation of the left ventricular mass index (LVMI) on echocardiography, adjusting for height and gender. There are age-specific criteria for defining LVH, as recommended by the Cornell investigators (LVMI $>134 \, g/m^2$ in men and $>110 \, g/m^2$ in women), or as defined by the Framingham study (LVMI $>131 \, g/m^2$ in men and $>100 \, g/m^2$ in women).[35] The Framingham investigators have also argued for indexing ventricular mass by height to avoid underestimating LVH related to obesity.

After adjusting for confounding factors, the relative risk of a coronary event in men and women increased by 1.67 and 1.60 respectively for every $50 \, g/m^2$ increment in left ventricular mass per unit of height.[36] In the Framingham study, women with isolated systolic hypertension showed a pattern of concentric hypertrophy, while in men an eccentric pattern was found. Adjusting for age, body mass index and diastolic pressure, the relative odds of LVH in such subjects was 2.58 in men and 5.94 in women.[37] This suggests that there is a greater tendency for women to develop LVH with elevations of systolic pressure, and this

may be a gender-determined response that contributes to the reduction in the male:female ratio of CHD, from 2.8 at age 45–54 years to 1.5 at age 75–84 years.[9] Hypertensive patients with LVH also have an increased risk of heart failure, which can be related to both systolic and diastolic dysfunction.[2] In particular, left ventricular systolic function is reduced in about 15% of hypertensive patients, which is related to an increased risk of cardiac ischaemia, myocardial infarction and arrhythmias. However, heart failure in hypertensive individuals can occasionally be due to diastolic dysfunction, with a poorly relaxing, noncompliant left ventricle.[38]

Low-level (20–200 mg/24h) albuminuria ('microalbuminuria') is an additional independent predictor of cardiovascular risk at all ages, with the excretion rate increasing with age in men but not women.[39] Microalbuminuria has been correlated with raised blood pressure in hypertensive patients, and is predictive of morbidity and mortality from cardiovascular disease.[39,40] This association has two possible explanations:[39] microalbuminuria is associated with an excess of known cardiovascular risk factors (such as lipid abnormalities and diabetes) and in addition, it may be a marker of established cardiovascular disease. In hypertension, microalbuminuria has also been correlated with abnormal plasma levels of von Willebrand factor, an index of endothelial dysfunction.[40] In addition, patients with essential hypertension and microproteinuria have been shown to have higher blood pressures and a higher prevalence of echocardiographic and electrocardiographic LVH.[41]

Hypertension and pregnancy

Hypertension occurs in around 5% of all pregnancies. However, this covers a wide range of conditions which carry different implications for pregnancy outcome and require different management strategies. Raised blood pressure may be a marker of underlying maternal disease or it may be a consequence of the pregnancy itself. Importantly however, hypertension in pregnancy affects the fetus as well as the mother, and can result in fetal growth retardation and, if severe, can increase both maternal and fetal morbidity and mortality. If recognized early and managed appropriately, many of these complications can be reduced.

Hypertensive diseases in pregnancy, including pre-eclampsia, remain major causes of maternal and fetal mortality in the UK, with an overall mortality rate of around 2%.[42] Although maternal mortality due to hypertension has fallen markedly over the last three decades, eclampsia remains an important cause of a significant number of deaths.[43,44] For example, pre-eclampsia is responsible for one-sixth of all maternal deaths[45] and a doubling of perinatal mortality.[46] However, most long-term follow-up data do not indicate an increased likelihood for the development of hypertension in later life among women who had pre-eclampsia compared with women who remained normotensive during pregnancy.

Antihypertensive drugs are used in pregnant women with hypertension to protect the mother's circulation, mostly against the risk of stroke. They have little effect on the progression of pregnancy-induced hypertension and do not significantly reduce the development of pre-eclampsia. However, they help maintain the pregnancy longer to allow the fetus to become more mature. Diuretics are usually of little use, except for relief of painful oedema and left ventricular failure and they do not prevent pre-eclampsia or reduce perinatal mortality. A review of the use of thiazides in uncomplicated hypertension in pregnancy concluded that there was no evidence of an adverse effect, although the incidence of hypertension and oedema was reduced.[47]

Probably the most widely used antihypertensive drug in pregnancy is α-methyldopa. This can be used to achieve blood pressure control with no long-term adverse effects on mother or fetus.[48,49] Drug withdrawal occurs in 15% due to unwanted side-effects, including depression, lethargy, sedation and postural hypotension. However, there is no evidence that α-methyldopa is associated with the development of postnatal depression, although some anxieties must remain in this area.

Beta blockers are generally safe and effective antihypertensive drugs in pregnancy. There is no evidence of a teratogenic effect and the drugs are well tolerated by the mother. Together with α-methyldopa, beta blockers were considered first-line antihypertensive drugs in pregnancy. However, there is some evidence that certain beta blockers may have adverse effects if used in very early pregnancy, especially at less than 20 weeks' gestation.[50,51] Thus, the time of initiation of beta blocker therapy is an important consideration in intrauterine growth retardation. Frishman and Chesner[52] suggest the following guidelines on the use of beta blockers in pregnancy:

- avoid the use of beta blockers during the first trimester of pregnancy;
- use the lowest possible dose;
- if possible, beta blockers should be discontinued 2–3 days prior to delivery, to limit their effects on uterine contractility and to avoid neonatal complications from beta blockade;
- use of beta blockers with beta-1 selectivity, intrinsic sympathomimetic activity, or alpha blocking activity may be preferable as these agents are less likely to interfere with beta-2 mediated uterine relaxation and peripheral vasodilatation.

Hydralazine is a second-line antihypertensive drug that is widely used in patients with severe hypertension and pre-eclampsia, but only rarely in the first trimester of pregnancy. Although it crosses the placenta, the only problem with hydralazine use in late pregnancy is thrombocytopenia.[53] Other adverse effects, such as headache, nausea and vomiting may be difficult to distinguish from imminent eclampsia.

Calcium antagonists are not licensed for use in pregnancy, although drugs such as nifedipine have been shown to be effective as a second-line agent where beta blockade or α-methyldopa was unsuccessful in controlling moderate to severe hypertension.[54,55] Prazosin is safe in pregnancy, with no records of teratogenesis.[56] However, there are no reliable data on the use of the newer, long-acting alpha blockers, such as doxazosin or terazosin. Finally, the ACE inhibitors have been associated with spontaneous abortions and fetal abnormalities, mainly skull ossification defects and anuria; such drugs are therefore absolutely contraindicated in pregnancy.[57–59]

Hypertension and the oral contraceptive pill

There is a slight increase in blood pressure in most women taking the oral contraceptive pill, which adds to their relative risk for increased cardiovascular disease.[60] For example, over a 2-year period, there was a mean increase in systolic blood pressure of 7.7 mmHg in women taking oestrogen–progestogen oral contraceptives, compared with a mean change of −1.2 mmHg in women using other methods of contraception.[60] This small rise is enough to raise the blood pressure beyond 140/90 mmHg in approximately 5% of women during a 5-year period. However, in more than half, the blood pressure returns to normal when oral contra-

ceptive use is stopped.[61] In a few women, severe hypertension occurs, leading to malignant phase hypertension and renal damage.[62]

It is uncertain whether oral contraceptives cause hypertension de novo or whether they are simply exaggerating a tendency in women who already have a propensity to develop hypertension. The exact mechanism of oral contraceptive-induced hypertension is uncertain, but changes in circulatory haemodynamics, haemorheological abnormalities, the renin–angiotensin–aldosterone system, insulin sensitivity and erythrocyte cation transport have been identified. For example, body weight, plasma volume and cardiac output are significantly increased in previously healthy women after 2–3 months of oral contraceptive use.[63] There is also an increase in sodium retention with use of oral contraceptives containing oestrogens and progestogens, with a 100–200 mEq increase in total body exchangeable sodium after 3 weeks.[64] Furthermore, oestrogens increase renin substrate and total renin activity,[65,66] whilst oral contraceptives containing 30–40 mg ethinyl oestradiol induce insulin resistance, and progesterone-only pills prolong the half-life of insulin.[67]

Women with hypertension secondary to oral contraceptive use should be managed as follows:[16]

(i) prescribe the lowest dose of oestrogen and progestogen, giving no more than a 6-month supply at a time;
(ii) measure blood pressure at least every 6 months;
(iii) stop use of oral contraceptives if blood pressure rises markedly and suggest use of an alternative contraceptive;
(iv) if blood pressure does not return to normal within 3 months, the patient should be 'worked-up' and treated for hypertension;

(v) if no alternative form of contraception is possible and oral contraceptive use must be continued, antihypertensive treatment may be needed to control blood pressure.

Hypertension and the menopause

The menopause is accompanied by a rise in systolic and diastolic blood pressures. This rise is independent of age, resulting in a higher prevalence of hypertension in women who are post-menopausal compared with those in the premenopausal state.[68] An increase in body weight is also a determinent of the postmenopausal increase in blood pressure.[69] Some workers have suggested that the blood pressure rise with increasing age may be related to the decrease in production of endogeneous female hormones that accompanies the menopause.[70] However, the menopause is associated with enhanced stress-induced cardiovascular responses and elevated ambulatory blood pressures during the day.[71]

There have been concerns about whether menopausal women with hypertension can take hormone replacement therapy. This area is discussed in more detail below.

Hypertension and hormone replacement therapy

There continues to be considerable reluctance and confusion when prescribing HRT to post-menopausal women who also have hypertension. In a survey of HRT prescribing habits, many clinicians avoided its use, especially if blood pressure was labile or remained difficult to control.[72] Particular concerns are related to the belief that HRT use may increase blood pressure. In younger women, for example, the use of high-dose oestrogen-containing oral con-

traceptives may be associated with an increase in systolic and diastolic blood pressures.[73,74]

In postmenopausal women the situation is less clear. In normotensive postmenopausal women, the use of HRT does not raise blood pressure and may even lower it.[70,75–80] A large retrospective study of HRT in hypo-oestrogenic normotensive women showed a significant reduction in the new development of hypertension among patients treated with oestrogen.[81] The recent, large prospective PEPI study also did not find any rise in blood pressures following use of HRT.[33]

The effects of HRT in hypertensive post-menopausal women have been investigated less, with few studies addressing this issue in the literature. Although hypertension can occur with postmenopausal oestrogen HRT, the majority of data suggest that HRT does not alter blood pressure or its lability. In a small Danish study, 12 normotensive and 12 hypertensive women were prospectively started on HRT, with a fall in systolic blood pressure being demonstrated in the hypertensive group after 6 months.[82] Pfeffer et al.[78] retrospectively studied 35 women (aged 52–87 years) with documented hypertension, in whom a fall in systolic blood presure was demonstrated following oral oestrogen therapy. In an open prospective study of 75 hypertensive menopausal women, we found no change in mean blood pressure over a median follow-up of 18 months, despite a significant rise in mean weight.[83] In women with uncontrolled hypertension, in whom HRT was prospectively discontinued, we found no signficant fall in mean blood pressure, suggesting that there is no significant pressor effect of HRT on blood pressure.[84] By contrast, a survey of 468 middle-aged women by Markovitz et al.[85] found that HRT use resulted in a small increase in both systolic and diastolic blood pressures compared to baseline; the main predictors of blood pressure changes were body weight or body mass index, and psychosocial factors, such as anger and anxiety.

The clinical evidence therefore suggests that HRT can safely be prescribed to hypertensive women. In fact, the lack of a rise in blood pressure with HRT may reflect a number of antihypertensive effects of oestrogen replacement, including the following:[16]

- vasodilatation, perhaps due to increased endothelium-dependent relaxation;[86]
- effects on cation fluxes that reduce intracellular calcium;[87]
- improvements in baroreceptor reflex sensitivity;[88]
- reversal of the hyperinsulinaemia seen postmenopausally.[89]

However, only a large, prospective, randomized, placebo-controlled study can allay any final doubts, although whether such a study would be feasible or ethical remains debatable. To study the effects of HRT on blood pressure in 100 symptomatic hypertensive postmenopausal women (and HRT would have to be withheld in 50% of them in a placebo-controlled study), it would be necessary to screen about 1000 symptomatic postmenopausal women (and therefore even more postmenopausal women to find those who are actually symptomatic).[90]

In view of the lack of consensus in the prescribing habits of HRT, we would suggest the following guidelines:[72]

(i) All clinicians should measure blood pressure before starting HRT;
(ii) In a normotensive postmenopausal woman, blood pressure should be measured annually following the start of HRT. One exception may be the use of Premarin®, where a follow-up blood pressure measurement should be made at 3

months, in view of reports of a possible rare idiosyncratic rise in blood pressure;[64]
(iii) In hypertensive menopausal women, blood pressure should at least be measured initially and thereafter 6-monthly, although if it is labile or difficult to control, 3-monthly measurements should be done;
(iv) If a hypertensive woman on HRT demonstrates a rise in blood pressure, careful monitoring or observation and perhaps an alteration or increase of antihypertensive treatment should be given.

With these guidelines, we feel that most women with hypertension would be able to have the benefits of HRT.

Antihypertensive drug therapy in women

Current recommendations concerning the treatment of hypertension do not distinguish between women and men. In 1993, the British Hypertension Society (BHS) and the Joint National Committee on Detection, Evaluation and Treatment of High Blood Pressure (JNC V) in the USA introduced updated guidelines for the management of hypertension.[91,92] These suggested that the thiazide diuretics and beta blockers should still be used as first-line or initial drugs, as they are effective and long-term outcome data from clinical trials show that they prevent myocardial infarction and stroke.[93] By contrast, the newer antihypertensives such as the calcium antagonists, ACE inhibitors and alpha blockers, were classed as 'alternative' drugs, only to be used when diuretics and beta blockers are 'contraindicated, ineffective or when side effects occur'. These guidelines encompass both men and women, and there was no differentiation between the sexes with respect to prescribing and adverse effects of antihypertensive therapy.

It has been suggested that the antihypertensive requirements of women have not been specifically studied in large-scale clinical trials. Of the nine major hypertension studies,[94–102] three (the Veteran's administration trials, the Oslo study and the Multiple Risk Factor Intervention Trial) did not include women,[96–98] three studied only elderly patients,[94,101,102] and three are considered to have been too short in duration of follow-up with insufficient numbers of women. Elderly hypertensive patients are paradoxically less likely to be treated than younger hypertensives;[103] as women are over-represented amongst the elderly, they are accordingly likely to be treated less often.[104] The earliest available data on treatment of hypertensive women come from the Hypertension Detection and Follow-up Program Cooperative group (HDFP), which was a community-based multicentre trial involving 10 940 subjects (of whom 46% were women and 44% were black), with a 5-year follow-up period.[95,105] However, antihypertensive therapy is of benefit in reducing the incidence of CHD by 25% in women with isolated systolic hypertension, a condition to which women are more susceptible by virtue of age distribution.[102]

Some studies have also shown an unexplained gender and ethnic difference in outcome. For example, the MRC study of patients aged 35–64 years showed a significant difference between men and women, with a 15% reduction in all-cause mortality among men, compared with a 26% increase in mortality among women, although women constituted 48% of the study population.[100] However, this apparent increase in mortality was not statistically significant because of the unexpectedly low mortality in the untreated control group of women. Furthermore, subgroup analysis of the Hypertension Detection and Follow-up Program study, where women constituted

46% of the study population, found that white hypertensive women had an adverse effect from antihypertensive therapy with a 2.5% increase in mortality, although there was a 28% reduction in mortality among black women.[95,105] This is compared to small reductions in mortality among men (18% in black men and 15% in white men).

Thus, when all the trials are considered together, women appear to have less benefit than men from antihypertensive treatment. In view of their lower cardiovascular risk and possible lower benefit from therapy, some authorities have suggested a more conservative approach towards the treatment of hypertension in women.[106] However, black women appear to have an undoubted benefit from treatment in the various studies. In black women, the onset of hypertension may occur as much as 10 years earlier than in white women. Furthermore, black patients may have had less access to health care, especially in the USA, and the improved access to treatment afforded by participation in the various studies may explain the greater treatment benefit.

However, in routine clinical practice there are generally few gender differences that are considered during prescribing of the various antihypertensive drug classes. There is the possibility that diuretic agents may protect those who are susceptible to postmenopausal osteoporosis.[107] Women may also experience different side effects from antihypertensive agents. For example, they more frequently develop a cough from the ACE inhibitors,[108,109] but are less likely to have the loss of sexual function commonly seen in men taking thiazide diuretics. However, the latter may be due to the fact that the appropriate questions have rarely been asked of women involved in clinical trials. In the large randomized trials of antihypertensive therapy, there is little mention of sexual dysfunction in women. The recently published Trial of Antihypertensive Intervention and Management (TAIM) study of low-dose thiazide diuretic or atenolol compared with placebo found no significant sexual impairment in drug-treated patients compared with placebo-treated women.[110] In addition, a study of efficacy, safety and quality-of-life effects of captopril in over 30 000 patients (of which 53% were women) showed that both men and women who had captopril substituted for other medications had similar improvements in sexual function.[111] By contrast, women (and men) in the TOMHS study reported reduced sexual activity with thiazide diuretics, but improved function with the long-acting alpha-blocker, doxozosin.[112] Finally, as lipid metabolism differs in women, information on the effects of antihypertensive therapy (especially with diuretics) on lipid metabolism in women and on its relation to the development of CHD is inadequate.[19] Thus, antihypertensive agents which have little impact on lipid profiles in male patients may have very different, perhaps harmful, effects in women.

The main precautions for antihypertensive drug prescribing for women pertain to concomitant diseases states, hypertension in pregnancy and the elderly hypertensive. However, nonpharmacological approaches should always be considered, including weight loss and increased physical activity, and approaches such as calcium supplementation have been helpful in women.[113]

Although beta blockers and thiazides have established survival and outcome benefits in patients with hypertension (and postmyocardial infarction), many patients with cardiovascular disease have contraindications to beta blockers, such as asthma or peripheral vascular disease, or have concomitant metabolic problems, such as diabetes or hyperlipidaemia, which preclude the use of thiazide diuretics. Recently published studies have suggested that calcium antagonists

may increase mortality in hypertensive patients.[114–116] While the results of these studies have been subject to much criticism and debate[117–119] and more long-term data are awaited, it would seem sensible to avoid using large doses of short-acting calcium antagonists and to use only the long-acting preparations. Dihydropyridine calcium antagonists, such as nifedipine capsules, should also be avoided in patients with unstable angina and previous myocardial infarction, unless beta blockers are given concomitantly. Calcium antagonists with negative inotropism, such as verapamil or diltiazem, should be avoided in patients with poor left ventricular function. Despite the well established benefits of ACE inhibitors in heart failure[120] and regression of hypertensive left ventricular hypertrophy,[121,122] this class of drug and the calcium antagonists have not been subject to long-term controlled trials to demonstrate their efficacy in reducing morbidity and mortality specifically in hypertensive patients.

In summary, there are significant differences in treatment outcome between white women and men, as well as between black and white women. However, the extent, direction and mechanisms of these differences are unclear. Treatment for black women is clearly beneficial, suggesting that aggressive screening and case finding are important considerations; by contrast, the data regarding aggressive treatment of white hypertensive women are equivocal, with some concern that such treatment may actually be harmful.[19]

If I had...

What if I was a young woman with hypertension? I would ensure that the reversible risk factors are detected and if possible, corrected, before starting antihypertensive therapy. For example, I would like a routine blood screen for renal function and diabetes, and to have my serum lipids checked. I would like an ECG as a simple screen for left ventricular hypertrophy and a urine test for proteinuria or glycosuria. I would also stop smoking, reduce my salt intake and if obese, reduce my weight.

If my raised blood pressure was oral contraceptive pill-induced, I would stop the pill and consider alternative contraception. If my raised blood pressure was pregnancy-induced, I would ensure careful observation, management and follow-up in a special obstetric unit with experience in looking after mothers with such problems. I would make strenuous efforts to avoid excessive weight gain with a combination of a prudent diet and plenty of exercise. If no other risk factors were present, I would receive antihypertensive drugs only if my diastolic blood pressure was consistently in excess of 95 mmHg, a slightly higher threshold than if I was a man.

If I was postmenopausal and hypertensive, I would again consider the above nonpharmacological interventions. If I was already on HRT, I would not like to stop it just because I was found to be hypertensive, but would like to have my blood pressure monitored carefully. If I was a black hypertensive woman, I would like aggressive treatment with antihypertensive treatment. If I sustained any complications of hypertension such as heart failure, renal impairment or stroke, I would ensure I had optimal hypertension control in addition to treatment for the complications. If I had atrial fibrillation, I would request prophylactic anticoagulation once my blood pressure was well controlled. Above all, I would want careful counselling and efficient long-term follow-up using the principles of evidence-based medicine!

References

1 Collins R, MacMahon SW, Blood pressure, antihypertensive drug treatment and the risks of stroke and of coronary heart disease, *Br Med Bull* (1994)**50**:272–98.

2 Lip GYH, Gammage MD, Beevers DG, Hypertension and the heart, *Br Med Bull* (1994)**50**:299–321.

3 Fiebach NH, Hebert PR, Stampfer MJ et al, A prospective study of high blood pressure and cardiovascular disease in women, *Am J Epidemiol* (1989)**130**:646–54.

4 Rich-Edwards JW, Manson JE, Hennekens CH, Buring JE, The primary prevention of coronary heart disease in women, *N Engl J Med* (1995)**332**:1758–66.

5 Brezinka V, Padmos I, Coronary heart disease risk factors in women, *Eur Heart J* (1994)**15**:1571–84.

6 Beard CM, Kottke TE, Annegers JF, The Rochester Coronary Heart Disease Project. Effect of cigarette smoking, hypertension, diabetes and setroidal estrogen use on coronary heart disease among 40- to 59-year old women, 1960 through 1982, *Mayo Clin Proc* (1989)**64**:1471–80.

7 Isles CG, Hole DJ, Hawthorne VM, Lever AF, Relation between coronary risk and coronary mortality in women of the Renfrew and Paisley survey: comparison with men, *Lancet* (1992)**339**:702–6.

8 Khaw K-T, Where are the women in studies of coronary heart disease? *Br Med J* (1993)**306**:1145–6.

9 Dustan HP, Gender differences in hypertension, *J Hum Hypertens* (1997) in press.

10 Marmot M, Brunner EJ, CHD risk among women. Whitehall II and other studies. In: Sharp I, ed. *Coronary heart disease: are women special?* (National Forum for Coronary Heart Disease Prevention: London, 1994) 57–70.

11 Zachariah PK, Sheps SG, Bailey KR, Wiltgen CH, Moore AG, Age-related characteristics of ambulatory blood pressure load and mean blood pressure in normotensive subjects, *JAMA* (1991)**265**:1414–17.

12 Burt VL et al, Prevalence of hypertension in the adult US population: results from the third National Health and Nutrition Examination Survey, 1988–1991, *Hypertension* (1985)**25**:305–13.

13 MacMahon SW, Blacket RB, Macdonald GJ, Hall W, Obesity, alcohol consumption and blood pressure in Australian men and women: the National Heart Foundation of Australia Risk Factor Prevalences Study, *J Hypertens* (1984)**2**:85–91.

14 Kim JS, Jones DW, Kim SJ, Hing YP, Hypertension in Korea: a national survey, *Am J Prev Med* (1994)**10**:200–4.

15 Kruczmarski RJ, Fiegal KM, Campbell SM, Johnson CL, Increasing prevalence of overweight among US adults — the National Health and Nutrition Examination Survey, 1989-1991, *JAMA* (1994)**272**:205–11.

16 Kaplan NM, The treatment of hypertension in women, *Arch Intern Med* (1995)**155**:563–7.

17 von Eiff AW, Blood pressure and estrogens, *Front Hormone Res* (1975)**3**:177–84.

18 Akinkugbe OO, World epidemiology of hypertension in blacks. In: Dallas Hall W, Saunders E, Shulman NB, eds. *Hypertension in blacks: epidemiology, pathophysiology and treatment* (Year Book Publishers: Chicago, 1985) 3–16.

19 Anastos K, Charney P, Charon RA, Cohen E, Jones CY, Marte C et al, Hypertension in women: what is really known. The women's caucus, Working Group on Women's Health of the Society of General Internal Medicine, *Ann Intern Med* (1991)**115**:287–93.

20 Cornoni-Huntley J, LaCroix AZ, Havlick RJ, Race and sex differentials and the impact of hypertension in the United States. The National Health and Nutritional Survey I Epidemiologic Follow-up Study, *Arch Intern Med* (1989)**149**:780–8.

21 Tominaga T, Suzuki H, Ogata Y et al, The role of sex hormones and sodium intake in

postmenopausal women, *J Hum Hypertens* (1991)**5**:494–500.

22 de Simone G, Devereux RB, Roman MJ et al, Gender differences in left ventricular anatomy, blood viscosity and volume regulatory hormones in normal adults, *Am J Cardiol* (1991)**68**:1704–8.

23 Messerli FH, Garavaglia GE, Schmieder RE, Sundgaard-Riise K, Nunez BD, Amodeo C, Disparate cardiovascular findings in men and women with essential hypertension, *Ann Intern Med* (1987)**107**:158–61.

24 Lissner L, Bengtsson C, Lapidus L, Kristjanssosn K, Wedel H, Fasting insulin in relation to subsequent blood pressure changes and hypertension in women, *Hypertension* (1992)**20**:797–801.

25 Lip GYH, Beevers DG, Abnormalities of rheology and coagulation in hypertension, *J Hum Hypertens* (1994)**8**:693–702.

26 Islim IF, Beevers DG, Bareford D, The effect of antihypertensive drugs on in vivo platelet activity in essential hypertension, *J Hypertens* (1992)**10**:379–83.

27 Metha J, Metha P, Platelet function in hypertension and effect of therapy, *Am J Cardiol* (1981)**47**:331–4.

28 Nyrop M, Zweifler AJ, Platelet aggregation in hypertension and the effects of antihypertensive treatment, *J Hypertens* (1988)**6**:263–9.

29 Luscher TF, The endothelium: target or promoter of hypertension? *Hypertension* (1990) **15**:482–5.

30 Lip GYH, Blann AD, von Willebrand factor and its relevance to cardiovascular disorders, *Br Heart J* (1995)**74**:580–3.

31 Meilahn EN, Kuller LH, Matthews KA, Kiss JE, Hemostatic factors according to menopausal status and use of hormone replacement therapy, *Ann Epidemiol* (1992)**2**:445–55.

32 Kroon UB, Tengborn SL, The effects of transdermal estradiol and oral conjugated estrogens on haemostatic variables, *Thromb Haemostat* (1994)**71**:420–3.

33 The Writing Group for the PEPI Trial, Effects of estrogen or estrogen/progestin regimens on heart disease risk factors in postmenopausal women. The Postmenopausal Estrogen/Progestin Interventions (PEPI) Trial, *JAMA* (1995)**273**:199–208.

34 Medical Research Council's General Practice Research Framework, Randomised comparison of oestrogen versus oestrogen plus progestogen hormone replacement therapy in women with hysterectomy, *Br Med J* (1996)**312**:473–8.

35 Koren MJ, Devereux RB, Risk, recognition and reversal of left ventricular hypertrophy in hypertension, *Curr Opinion Cardiol* (1991)**6**: 710–15.

36 Levy D, Garrison RJ, Savage DD, Kannel WB, Castell WP, Prognostic implications of echocardiographically determined left ventricular mass in the Framingham Heart Study, *N Engl J Med* (1990)**322**:1561–6.

37 Krumholz HM, Larson M, Levy D, Sex differences in cardiac adaptation to isolated systolic hypertension, *Am J Cardiol* (1993)**72**:310–13.

38 Fouad-Tarazi FM, Left ventricular diastolic dysfunction in hypertension, *Curr Opinion Cardiol* (1994)**9**:551–60.

39 Winocour PH, Microalbuminuria, *Br Med J* (1992)**304**:1196–7.

40 Pedrinelli R, Giampietro O, Carmassi F et al, Microalbuminuria and endothelial dysfunction in essential hypertension, *Lancet* (1994)**344**: 14–18.

41 Schmieder R, Grube E, Ruddel H, Schlebusch H, Schulte W, [Significance of microproteinuria for early detection of hypertension-induced end-organ damage], *Klin Wochenschr* (1990)**68**:256–62 (in German).

42 Douglas KA, Redman CWG, Eclampsia in the United Kingdom, *Br Med J* (1994)**309**:1395–400.

43 Redman CWG, Eclampsia still kills, *Br Med J* (1988)**296**:1209–10.

44 Sachs BP, Brown DAJ, Driscoll SG et al, Maternal mortality in Massachusetts. Trends and prevention, *N Engl J Med* (1987)**316**: 667–72.

45 Kaunitz AM, Hughes JM, Grimes DA, Smith JC, Rochat RW, Kafrissen ME, Causes of maternal mortality in the United States, *Obstet Gynecol* (1985)**65**:605–12.

46 Taylor DJ, The epidemiology of hypertension during pregnancy. In: Rubin PC, ed. *Handbook of hypertension. Vol 10. Hypertension in pregnancy* (Elsevier Science: Amsterdam, 1988) 223–40.

47 Collins R, Yusof S, Peto R, Overview of randomised trials of diuretics in pregnancy, *Br Med J* (1985)**290**:17–23.

48 Redman CWG, Beilin L, Bonnar J, Ounsted MK, Fetal outcome in trial of antihypertensive treatment in pregnancy, *Lancet* (1976)**2**:753–6.

49 Cockburn J, Moar VA, Ounsted M, Redman CWG, Final report of study on hypertension during pregnancy: the effects of specific treatment on the growth and development of children, *Lancet* (1982)**1**:647–9.

50 Butters L, Kennedy S, Rubin PC, Atenolol in essential hypertension during pregnancy, *Br Med J* (1990)**301**:587–9.

51 Lip GYH, Churchill D, Zarifis J, Beevers M, Shaffer L, Beevers DG, Cardiovascular drug use in early pregnancy, *Br Heart J* (1995)(**suppl 3**):166 (abstr).

52 Frishman WH, Chesner M, Beta-adrenergic blockers in pregnancy, *Am Heart J* (1988)**115**:147.

53 Widerlov E, Karlman I, Storsater J, Hydralazine-induced neonatal thrombocytopenia, *N Engl J Med* (1980)**303**:1235.

54 Constantine G, Beevers DG, Reynolds AL, Luesley DM, Nifedipine as a second line antihypertensive drug in pregnancy, *Br J Obstet Gynaecol* (1987)**94**:1136–42.

55 Walters BNJ, Redman CWG, Treatment of severe pregnancy associated hypertension with the calcium antagonist nifedipine, *Br J Obstet Gynaecol* (1984)**91**:330–6.

56 Lubbe WF, Hodge JV, Combined alpha- and beta-adrenoceptor antagonism with prazosin and oxprenolol in control of severe hypertension in pregnancy, *NZ Med J* (1981)**691**:169–72.

57 Pryde PG, Sedman AB, Nugent CE, Barr M, Angiotensin converting enzyme inhibitor fetopathy, *J Am Soc Nephrol* (1993)**3**:1575–82.

58 Editorial, Are ACE inhibitors safe in pregnancy? *Lancet* (1989)**2**:482–3.

59 Hanssens M, Keirse MJNC, Vankelecom F, Van Assche FA, Fetal and neonatal effects of treatment with angiotensin-converting enzyme inhibitors in pregnancy, *Obstet Gynecol* (1991)**78**:128–35.

60 Weir RJ, Hypertension secondary to contraceptive agents. In: Amery A, Fagard R, Lijnen P, Staessen J, eds. *Hypertensive cardiovascular disease: pathophysiology and treatment* (Martinus Nijhoff Publishers: Boston, 1982) 612–28.

61 Weir JW, Oral contraceptives and hypertension, *Hypertension* (1988)**11**(**suppl 2**):11–15.

62 Lim KG, Isles CG, Hodsman GP, Lever AF, Robertson JWK, Malignant hypertension in women of childbearing age and its relation to the contraceptive pill, *Br Med J* (1987)**294**:1057–9.

63 Walters WAW, Lim YL, Haemodynamic changes in women taking oral contraceptives, *J Obstet Gynecol Br Commonwealth* (1970)**77**:1007–12.

64 Crane MG, Harris JJ, Winsor W, Hypertension, oral contraceptive agents and conjugated estrogens, *Ann Intern Med* (1971)**74**:13–21.

65 Gordon MS, Chin WW, Shupnik MA, Regulation of angiotensinogen gene expression by estrogen, *J Hypertens* (1992)**10**:361–6.

66 Derkx FHM, Stuenkel C, Schalekamp MPA, Visser W, Huisveld IH, Schalekamp MADH, Immunoreactive renin, prorenin and enzymatically active renin in plasma during pregnancy and in women taking oral contraceptives, *J Clin Endocrinol* (1986)**63**:1008–15.

67 Godsland IF, Walton C, Felton C, Proudler A, Patel A, Wynn V, Insulin resistance, secretion and metabolism in users of oral contraceptives, *J Clin Endocrinol Metab* (1992)**74**:64–70.

68 Staessen J, Bulpitt CJ, Fagard R, Lijnen P, Amery A, The influence of menopause on blood pressure, *J Hum Hypertens* (1989)**3**:427–33.

69 Grobbee DE, van Hemert AM, Vandenbroucke JP, Hofman A, Valkenburg HA, Importance of body weight in determining rise and level of blood pressure in postmenopausal women, *J Hypertens* (1988)**6**(**suppl 4**):S614–16.

70 Regensteiner JG, Hiatt WR, Byyny RL, Tickett CK, Woodard WD, Moore LG, Short-term effects of estrogen and progestin on blood pressure of normotensive postmenopausal women, *J Clin Pharmacol* (1991)**31**:543–8.

71 Owens JF, Stoney CM, Matthews KA, Menopausal status influences ambulatory blood pressure levels and blood pressure changes during mental stress, *Circulation* (1993)**88**:2794–802.

72 Lip GYH, Beevers M, Churchill D, Beevers DG, Do clinicians prescribe hormone replacement therapy to hypertensive women? *Br J Clin Prac* (1995)49:61–4.

73 Khaw K-T, Peart WS, Blood pressure and contraceptive use, *Br Med J* (1982)285:403–7.

74 Weir RJ, Briggs E, Mack A, Naismith L, Taylor L, Wilson E, Blood pressure in women taking oral contraceptives, *Br Med J* (1974)1:533–5.

75 Christiansen C, Christensen MS, Hagen C, Stocklund KE, Transbøl I, Effects of natural estrogen/gestagen and thiazide on coronary risk factors in normal postmenopausal women, *Acta Obstet Gynecol Scand* (1981)60:407–12.

76 Lind T, Cameron EC, Hunter WM et al, A prospective controlled trial of six forms of hormone replacement therapy given to postmenopausal women, *Br J Obstet Gynaecol* (1979)86(suppl 3):1–29.

77 Perry I, Beevers M, Beevers DG, Leusley D, Oestrogens and cardiovascular disease, *Br Med J* (1988)297:1127.

78 Pfeffer RI, Kurosaki TT, Charlton SK, Estrogen use and blood pressure in later life, *Am J Epidemiol* (1979)110:469–78.

79 von Eiff AW, Plotz EJ, Beck KJ, Czernik A, The effects of estrogens and progestins on blood pressure regulation of normotensive women, *Am J Obstet Gynaecol* (1971)4:31–47.

80 Barrett-Connor E, Wingard D, Criqui MH, Postmenopausal estrogen use and heart disease risk factors in the 1980s, *JAMA* (1989)261:2095–100.

81 Hammond CB, Jelovsek FR, Lee KL, Creasman WT, Parker RT, Effects of long-term estrogen replacement therapy. I. Metabolic effects, *Am J Obstet Gynecol* (1979)133:525–36.

82 Jespersen CM, Arnung K, Hagen C et al, Effects of natural oestrogen therapy on blood pressure and renin-angiotensin system in normotensive and hypertensive menopausal women, *J Hypertens* (1983)1:361–4.

83 Lip GYH, Beevers M, Churchill D, Beevers DG, Hormone replacement therapy and blood pressure in hypertensive women, *J Hum Hypertens* (1994)8:491–4.

84 Zarifis J, Lip GYH, Beevers DG, The effects of discontinuing hormone replacement therapy in postmenopausal patients with uncontrolled

hypertension, *Am J Hypertens* (1996)8:1241–2.

85 Markovitz JH, Matthews KA, Wing RR et al, Psychological, biological and health behaviour predictors of blood pressure changes in middle-aged women, *J Hypertens* (1991)9:399–406.

86 Williams JK, Adams MR, Herrington DM, Clarkson TB, Short-term administration of estrogen and vascular responses of atherosclerotic coronary arteries, *J Am Coll Cardiol* (1992)20:452–7.

87 Stonier C, Bennett J, Messenger EA, Aber GM, Oestradiol-induced hypotension in spontaneously hypertensive rats: putative role for intracellular cations, sodium-potassium flux and prostanoids, *Clin Sci* (1992)82:389–95.

88 Muneta S, Dazai T, Iwata T et al, Baroreceptor reflex impairment in climacteric and ovariectomized hypertensive women, *Hypertens Res* (1992)15:27–32.

89 Proudler AJ, Felton CV, Stevenson C, Aging and the response of plasma insulin, glucose and C-peptide concentrations to intravenous glucose in postmenopausal women, *Clin Sci* (1992)83:489–94.

90 Lip GYH, Beevers DG, Zarifis J, Hormone replacement therapy and cardiovascular risk: the cardiovascular physicians' viewpoint, *J Intern Med* (1995)238:389–99.

91 Sever P, Beevers G, Bulpitt C et al, Management guidelines in essential hypertension: report of the second working party of the British Hypertension Society, *Br Med J* (1993)306:983–7.

92 Joint National Committee on Detection, Evaluation and Treatment of High Blood Pressure, The Fifth Report of the Joint National Committee on Detection, Evaluation and Treatment of High Blood Pressure (JNC V), *Arch Intern Med* (1993)153:154–83.

93 Collins R, MacMahon S, Blood pressure, antihypertensive drug treatment and the risks of stroke and coronary heart disease, *Br Med Bull* (1994)50:272–98.

94 Amery A, Brixko R, Clement D et al, Mortality and morbidity results from the European Working Party on High Blood Pressure in the Elderly trial, *Lancet* (1985)1:1349–54.

95 Hypertension Detection and Follow-up Program Cooperative Group, Five year findings

of the Hypertension Detection and Follow-up Program: II. Mortality by race, sex and age, *JAMA* (1979)**242**:2572–7.

96 Veterans Administration Cooperative Study Group on Antihypertensive Agents, Effects of treatment on morbidity in hypertension. II. Results in patients with diastolic blood pressure averaging 90–114 mmHg, *JAMA* (1970)**213**:1145–82.

97 Helgeland A, Treatment of mild hypertension: a five year controlled drug trial. The Oslo Study, *Am J Med* (1980)**69**:725–32.

98 Multiple Risk factor Intervention Trial Research Group, Risk factor changes and mortality results, *JAMA* (1982)**248**:1465–77.

99 National Heart Foundation of Australia, The Australian therapeutic trial in mild hypertension, *Lancet* (1980)**1**:1261–7.

100 Medical Research Council Working Party, MRC trial in mild hypertension: principal results, *Br Med J* (1985)**291**:197–204.

101 Medical Research Council Working Party, MRC trial of treatment of hypertension in older adults: principal results, *Br Med J* (1992)**304**:405–12.

102 SHEP Cooperative Research Group, Prevention of stroke by antihypertensive drugs treatment in older persons with isolated systolic hypertension. Final results of the Systolic Hypertension in the Elderly Program (SHEP), *JAMA* (1991)**265**:3255–64.

103 Dickerson JE, Brown MJ, Influence of age on general practitioner's definition and treatment of hypertension, *Br Med J* (1995)**310**:574.

104 Ray WA, Schaffner W, Oates JA, Therapeutic choice in the treatment of hypertension, *Am J Med* (1986)**81**(suppl 6C):9–16.

105 Schnall P, Alderman MH, Kern R, An analysis of the HDFP trial. Evidence of adverse effects of antihypertensive therapy on white women with moderate and severe hypertension, *J Med* (1984)**84**:299–301.

106 Jackson R, Barham P, Bills J, McLennan L, MacMahon S, Maling T, Management of raised blood pressure in New Zealand: a discussion document, *Br Med J* (1993)**307**:107–10.

107 Felson DT, Sloutskis D, Anderson JJ, Anthony JM, Kiel DP, Thiazide diuretics and the risk of hip fracture: results from the Framingham study, *JAMA* (1991)**265**:370–3.

108 Israili ZH, Hall WD, Cough and angioneurotic edema associated with angiotensin-converting enzyme inhibitor therapy, *Ann Intern Med* (1992)**117**:234–42.

109 Anonymous, Cough caused by ACE inhibitors, *Drug Ther Bull* (1994)**32**:28.

110 Wassertheil-Smoller S, Blaufox MD, Oberman A, Davis BR et al, Effect of antihypertensives on sexual function and quality of life: the TAIM study, *Ann Intern Med* (1991)**114**:613–20.

111 Schoenberger JA, Testa M, Ross AD, Brennan WK, Bannon JA, Efficacy, safety and quality of life assessment of captopril antihypertensive therapy in clinical practice, *Arch Intern Med* (1990)**150**:301–6.

112 Liebson PR, Grandits GA, Dianzumba S et al, Comparison of five antihypertensive monotherapies and placebo for change in left ventricular mass in patients receiving nutritional-hygienic therapy in the Treatment of Mild Hypertension Study (TOMHS), *Circulation* (1995)**91**:698–706.

113 Johnson NE, Smith EL, Freudenheim JL, Effects on blood pressure on calcium supplementation of women, *Am J Clin Nutr* (1985)**42**:12–17.

114 Psaty BM, Heckbert SR, Koepsell TD et al, The risk of myocardial infarction associated with antihypertensive drug therapies, *JAMA* (1995)**274**:620–5.

115 Furberg CD, Psaty BM, Meyer JV, Nifedipine: dose-related increase in mortality in patients with coronary heart disease, *Circulation* (1995)**92**:1326–31.

116 Pahor M, Guralnik JM, Corti MC et al, Long-term survival and use of antihypertensive medications in older persons, *J Am Geriatr Soc* (1995)**43**:1191–7.

117 Opie LH, Messerli FH, Nifedipine and mortality. Grave defects in the dossier [editorial], *Circulation* (1995)**92**:1068–73.

118 Lip GYH, Beevers DG, Are calcium antagonists safe in hypertension [editorial]? *Postgrad Med J* (1996)**72**:193–4.

119 Beevers DG, Sleight P, Short acting dihydropyridine (vasodilating) calcium channel blockers for hypertension: is there a risk? *Br Med J* (1996)**312**:1143-5.

120 Dargie HJ, McMurray JJV, Diagnosis and management of heart failure, *Br Med J* (1994)**308**:321–8.

121 Cruickshank JM, Lewis J, Moore V, Dodd C, Reversibility of left ventricular hypertrophy by differing types of antihypertensive therapy, *J Hum Hypertens* (1992)**6**:85–90.

122 Dahlöf B, Pennert K, Hansson L, Reversal of left ventricular hypertrophy in hypertensive patients. A metaanalysis of 109 treatment studies, *Am J Hypertens* (1992)**5**:95–110.

4

Coronary artery disease and women

Graham Jackson

Introduction

Over the past few years coronary artery disease (CAD) in women has become a topic of increasing interest.[1,2] At times it has seemed as if a new specialty was being created. From the outset it is important to recognize that CAD respects no race, religion or sex — it is a true equal-opportunity disease and equal-opportunity killer. However, CAD does present in different ways and with different degrees of severity depending on race and sex. It is these differences that are clinically important for they affect not only how we detect CAD but also how we initially manage and subsequently optimize individual patient care. I would like to emphasize the 'individual' at this point because it is the individual who makes up and is often hidden by the statistics, and in any review it is easy to forget what CAD really means to people and their families. We need to remember that for some a 2% mortality is a 100% mortality and there is no place for statistical complacency when advising on individual therapeutic options.

Epidemiology

The Framingham Study, which began in 1948, is the source of most of our information on CAD in women.[3] As a generalization, the clinical presentation of CAD occurs 10 years later in women than in men. Up to 60 years of age, one in five men and one in 17 women have had a coronary event: over 60 years of age, the incidence is equal at one in four for both sexes. Thus the incidence of CAD in women increases with age, notably after the menopause, and the only practical difference in CAD onset between men and women is 'when' rather than 'if'. Furthermore, CAD *does* affect premenopausal women and they account for 25% of all CAD deaths in those under 65 years of age.[4,5]

In the UK, 80 000 women and 100 000 men die from the consequences of CAD each year. In the USA, of 500 000 heart attack deaths each year, over 230 000 are in women. In addition, 87 000 American women die each year from stroke. Cardiovascular disease claims more women's lives than cancer, trauma and diabetes combined; the total is two-fold greater than total deaths from all kinds of cancer, and four-fold greater in white women and six-fold greater in black women than the number of deaths from the much-feared breast cancer.

While death is a sharp endpoint, disability and quality of life remain as important. Cardiovascular diseases are now considered to be the principal cause of disability in women. It is estimated that one-third of women with CAD below 65 years of age are disabled as a result and this increases to half in those over 65 years. Across all age groups, two-thirds of the women who suffer stroke are rendered permanently disabled.[2,6]

The most recent Framingham report, which examined gender differences, was published in

1993.[7] The differences in presentation (Table 4.1) are made more interesting by the better prognosis for women presenting with angina. This is almost certainly explained by a lower incidence of CAD (60–70%) for women at angiography compared with men (>90%). Not surprisingly, after 10 years of follow-up, subsequent myocardial infarction was twice as likely to be a problem in women initially presenting with infarction (34.8%) compared with women initially presenting with angina (17.8%).

Once women have sustained a myocardial infarct they have a worse prognosis, probably reflecting their increased age at presentation.[8,9] They are also more likely to have an increased risk factor profile with, in particular, an increased incidence of hypertension (49% women versus 35% men) and diabetes.[10] In women systolic blood pressure is second to age as the most important predictor of CAD, while in men it is fourth behind age, cholesterol and smoking.[3,11] Consequently, a higher incidence of diastolic heart failure might be expected and this probably explains the paradox of higher ejection fractions but an increased incidence of heart failure in women post-MI.

As our population ages, so the proportion of older women is increasing. Thus the problem of cardiovascular disease in women is going to present increasing management demands.

Indeed, as older women already outnumber older men, cardiovascular disease is now a greater cause of death in women (46%) than men (40%) in relative terms.[2] Although the incidence of CAD in men is declining, the evidence is less convincing in women, with reports of either a slower decline or even an increase in incidence. Therefore we have a major problem on our hands, and one that is increasing in size. Looking at cost alone, CAD costs the UK National Health Service £500 million per year, while in the USA the annual cost is $117 billion, with over half this cost being attributable to CAD in women.

It is evident that we must act to prevent cardiovascular disease and its consequences in women and men. Furthermore, we need to minimize the consequences of CAD after it has developed by aggressive secondary prevention.[11]

We can do this only by educating ourselves about the importance of cardiovascular disease in women and getting the message across to women that the threat of cancer is greatly exceeded by the threat of heart disease and stroke.

	Women	Men
Angina	47	32
Unstable angina	7	6
Infarct	32	46
Death	14	16

Table 4.1
Gender differences in CAD presentation (%).

- Women present more frequently with angina rather than MI or sudden death.
- Angina in women has a better prognosis due to an increased incidence of normal coronary anatomy.
- Women presenting with infarction have a worse prognosis due to increased age and risk factors.
- 40% of all coronary events in women are fatal.
- 67% of all sudden deaths in women occur without any history of previous CAD.

Key points

Anatomical differences

The female heart has 10% less left ventricular mass than the male heart and, in contrast to the male heart, may dilate on exercise with either a slower rise in ejection fraction or even a fall.[6,12] Thus assessments of ejection fraction on exercise are not as valid a means of identifying CAD in women. Women also tend to have smaller coronary arteries, which may present technical difficulties at the time of coronary artery bypass grafting (CABG) and adversely influence long-term graft patency.[13]

Risk factors

Whilst most of the risk factors for CAD are equally important in women and men, the degree of effect differs between the sexes.[4] Risk factors can be considered to be shared by the sexes (general risk factors) or unique to the sex (hormonal factors). Of course a combination may occur, thereby increasing risk, but accummulative risk for each sex does not imply equal risk because of the important protective factor of age in women, at least up to 75 years of age. Therefore, in viewing risk factors we need to take into account absolute risk as well as relative risk, men being at greater absolute risk than women.[14]

In general, women are under-represented in trials of risk and intervention and the data are not always easy to interpret as they have often, and at times inappropriately, been extrapolated from men to women.[15]

General risk factors

Smoking

Cigarette smoking increases the CAD risk by up to four times in women who smoke more than 20 cigarettes per day. Women who smoke are 3.6-times more likely than nonsmokers to sustain an MI.[16] There is a dose–response effect with even light smokers (<5 per day) doubling their risk. The risk increases further in smokers who are also hypertensive, diabetic, oral contraceptive users or women with hypercholesterolaemia.[4]

There is no evidence that 'low-yield' cigarettes claiming reduced tar, nicotine and carbon monoxide levels are safer although they are often promoted with women as the specific target.[17]

Cigarette smoking appears to be increasing in young women, often as a means of controlling weight. Slim (often too slim) and 'glamorous' women feature in advertisements for smoking, and marketing strategies often focus on female independence, success and sexuality. A woman (or man) who stops smoking can gain 4–5 kg in weight, and an image-conscious environment encourages smoking as a way (the wrong way) to stay slim.[18]

Stopping smoking improves survival in women who are healthy and women recovering from an MI with an estimated 50–80% reduction in CAD risk after 3–5 years.[19]

Cholesterol

Hypercholesterolaemia has been researched mainly in middle-aged men, but the majority of observational studies including women have shown a positive relationship between elevated cholesterol levels and CAD in women.[4,5] Before the menopause, women have an increased level of high-density lipoprotein (HDL) cholesterol which predicts a decreased CAD risk. After the menopause, total cholesterol rises along with low-density lipoprotein (LDL) cholesterol. The switch from increased HDL to increased LDL with age and change in hormonal status partly explain the increased CAD risk for women as they get older.

It is evident that full lipid profiles are essential in management of CAD risk as a reduction in total cholesterol containing predominantly HDL would be counterproductive. After the menopause, the rising LDL and falling HDL cholesterol levels may be modified by hormone replacement therapy (HRT).[20]

Possible explanations for the adverse changes in cholesterol levels are a decrease in hepatic LDL receptors and increase in hepatic lipase activity, leading to increased levels of circulating LDL. Postmenopausal women also have increased levels of lipoprotein (a), which is thought to be atherogenic.[21]

Evaluating the effects of lowering cholesterol in women is made difficult by their small numbers in either primary or secondary prevention trials.[15] The most recent primary prevention trial (WOSCOPS) concentrated on 6595 high-risk Scottish men:[22] other primary prevention trials contain too few women to identify any benefit (if present) of lipid lowering in healthy women.

We have more data from secondary prevention trials. The Scandinavian Simvastatin Survival Study (4S) included 827 (10%) women.[23] There was no difference in deaths comparing placebo (n = 25) with simvastatin (n = 27) at 5-year follow-up but there was a 35% decrease in major coronary events (91 versus 59). A similar study of pravastatin which included 119 (23%) women reported a significant decrease in cardiovascular events.[24] The Cholesterol and Recurrent Events (CARE) trial is the most recent. This allocated 4159 patients with MI (3–20 months before randomization) to 40 mg pravastatin daily or placebo.[25] The trial follow-up was 5 years and pravastatin led to a 28% reduction in LDL cholesterol, 14% reduction in triglycerides and 5% rise in HDL cholesterol. Clinically, pravastatin reduced nonfatal MI and CAD deaths by 24% (p = 0.002); although total deaths were lower in the pravastatin-treated group (180 versus 196), overall mortality was not significantly reduced. Women in this study showed greater cardiovascular benefits than men, with a reduction in fatal and nonfatal coronary events of greater than 45% (p = 0.001). The major cardiovascular benefit was overshadowed initially by an apparently significantly greater occurrence of nonfatal breast cancer in Pravastatin-treated women (twelve versus one on placebo). Careful reassessment of the data has been reassuring, with clear differences between the women arising by chance at entry to the trial. This has been reinforced by a systematic evaluation of other large Pravastatin trials identifying no increased risk. However this emphasises once more the importance of evaluating women in adequate numbers in secondary and primary prevention trials.

No similar breast cancer findings were seen with simvastatin (4S) and none have been recorded with fluvastain or lovastatin although female numbers remain small.

Studies of regression and progression of atheroma that have included women have shown benefits from lipid-lowering therapy similar to those in men.[26]

Although limited by numbers, the data favour lipid-lowering in women with evidence of CAD. The CARE trial dealing with women who had average cholesterol levels (<6.2 mmol/l)—in short 'typical' patients—demonstrated a substantial cardiovascular benefit: if 1000 women were treated for 5 years, 248 events would be avoided. There is as yet no evidence that *overall* mortality in women will be reduced. Observational data suggest lowering LDL and increasing HDL in healthy women would be beneficial although the data are not definitive. Women seem to tolerate high blood cholesterol levels better than men, especially if they have no other risk factors for CAD.[27]

Hypertension

Hypertension is discussed separately and in more detail elsewhere in this book. Hypertension is strongly associated with CAD in women. Women with CAD are twice as likely to be hypertensive as men and the incidence of hypertension increases with age. In the Nurses Health Study, after adjusting for age and other risk factors, hypertension led to a 3.5-fold increase in CAD risk for those aged 30–65 years.[28] A meta-analysis that included 14 611 women showed that a 7.5 mmHg difference in usual DBP independently increased CAD risk by 29% in both women and men.[29] All studies show increased CAD risk in white women who are hypertensive and this risk is also present for Asian women. Black women have less risk of CAD but increased risk of stroke.

While the CAD benefits of treating severe hypertension are clear for men and women, the evidence for treating women with mild hypertension is conflicting.[30] However, the benefits in reducing stroke are more convincing. A mean decrease in DBP of 6 mmHg reduces fatal and nonfatal stroke by 42% compared with fatal and nonfatal CAD at 14%.[29] In those over 65 years of age, trials of systolic and diastolic hypertension and isolated systolic hypertension, to which women are more susceptible, have included a significant number of women. In this age group antihypertensive treatment has afforded women a 36% reduction in stroke and a 25% reduction in CAD events (both significant).[31]

There is no evidence of sex differences in response to therapy.

Diabetes

Diabetes increases the CAD risk in women three-fold, neutralizing any protective sex advantage.[4] Mortality rates for CAD are up to seven-times higher among diabetic compared with nondiabetic women, and are up to four-times higher for diabetic compared with non-diabetic men.[32]

While the degree of diabetic control has not yet been shown to reduce CAD risk, the negative effects of diabetes are increased by other risk factors such as smoking, hypertension and obesity. At present, the main CAD preventive strategy in diabetes focuses on reducing other risk factors for CAD, although of course glycaemic control slows other diabetic complications and needs vigorous attention.

Other factors

Obese women are up to four-times more likely to die from CAD than lean women.[33] Obesity is also associated with other CAD risk factors such as diabetes, hypertension and hyperlipidaemia, which makes the assessment and intepretation of obesity as an independent risk factor difficult. Mortality from CAD is more strongly related to the ratio of waist:hip circumference (>0.8) than to weight alone.[33] Avoiding obesity reduces mortality with an estimated four-fold reduction in CAD risk.

Weight control is difficult without regular physical activity. Unfortunately, there is little evidence that physical activity *per se* reduces CAD in women, again because of a lack of studies, but the relationship of activity to other risk factors and obesity suggests that advice on weight loss combined with exercise will be beneficial.[4]

Mild to moderate alcohol consumption appears to reduce CAD risk in women but this benefit may be largely confined to women already at increased risk.[34] An alcohol intake of one glass of wine per day reduced CAD risk by 40%, while complete abstinence possibly increased the risk. A moderate intake (up to 2 units/day) may be beneficial, providing weight gain is avoided. Excess alcohol increases the risk of death from cardiovascular disease and

- Women are half as likely as men to develop CAD.
- Risk factor trials seldom include women and overall the number of women evaluated is small.
- Sound (and harmless) advice includes avoiding smoking, avoiding obesity and taking regular physical exercise.
- Hypertension merits detailed evaluation and monitoring.
- Hyperlipidaemia should be sought and corrected when CAD has been detected. Good primary prevention data in healthy women are not available and decisions on therapy should reflect the presence of other risk factors, e.g. diabetes and hypertension as well as patient preference.

Key points

heavy alcohol intake is a major preventable cause of all deaths.[4]

Hormonal risk factors

Oral contraceptives

There is no evidence that low-dose contraceptives increase coronary risk in women who do not smoke. Past use of oral contraceptives does not affect coronary risk in nonsmoking women. The combination of oral contraceptive use and smoking with higher-dose oral contraceptives increased cardiovascular risk seven-fold, but data on smoking and low-dose contraceptives are lacking.[35]

Women taking third-generation combined oral contraceptives (for example, low-dose ethinyl oestradiol plus gestodene and desogestrel) are no more likely to sustain an MI than nonusers.[36] Reports suggest they are less likely than second-generation agents (for example, low-

dose ethinyl oestradiol plus an earlier progestogen) to have an MI but this reduced risk, which needs to be confirmed, may be offset by an increased risk of venous thromboembolism.[37] It may be that low-dose aspirin in combination with third-generation pills could maximize cardiovascular benefit while minimizing the venous threat, but this is theoretical.

Women using oral contraceptives must be strongly urged not to smoke. Oral contraceptives and hypertension are discussed in Chapter 3.

Menopause and HRT

It is difficult to separate the effects of the menopause from age.[38] However, there is no doubt that the incidence of CAD rises significantly after the menopause, whether it is naturally or surgically induced. Women with an early surgical menopause have a 2.2-times higher risk of CAD compared with premenopausal women of a similar age. This change occurs as abruptly as the surgery, while any changes after a natural menopause are gradual, reflecting the gradual change in hormonal status.[4]

Hormone replacement therapy (HRT), especially oral oestrogen, favourably alters the ratio of LDL to HDL cholesterol as well as improving endothelial function and reducing fibrinogen.[39,40] HRT could be seen as an effective way of ameliorating the potential increased CAD risk associated with the menopause (menopausal changes include raised LDL, lowered HDL, raised lipoprotein (a) and clotting factors).

Unfortunately, we lack prospective randomized trial data to support emphatically the use of HRT and the benefit has been offset by the increased risk of breast and uterine cancer.[41,42] Matters are compounded by the fact that all the long-term beneficial data are based on the use of oral oestrogen, and the increased risk of breast cancer is not reduced by the cardiovascularly unproven addition of progesterone to oestrogen. Observational studies, which are limited by the possibility that healthy, educated and nonsmoking women may self-select themselves for HRT, show a 50% reduction in CAD risk for past users of oestrogen and 70% for continuing users — figures that are difficult to ignore.[39]

The drawback of oestrogen alone (unopposed oestrogen) is the increased risk of endometrial cancer when the uterus is intact. Pooled data indicate a 2.3-fold higher relative risk but no increased mortality (less invasive cancer). Combination therapy is therefore advocated when the uterus is intact. The Postmenopausal Estrogen/Progestin Trial (PEPT) was established to look at the differences between oestrogen alone, combination therapy (3 regimens) and placebo.[43] This 3-year randomized trial of 875 women reported recently on findings in women with no evidence of CAD at trial onset. Oral oestrogen had the most favourable impact on HDL levels, whereas combinations had less favourable HDL changes, but they were still significantly better than placebo. All active treatments reduced LDL by about 20% and the fibrinogen rise on placebo was not seen on active therapy. There were no treatment changes in blood pressure, weight or insulin. One-third of women with an intact uterus allocated to treatment with unopposed oestrogen had to be withdrawn because of adenomatous or endometrial hyperplasia. The authors concluded that the maximum benefit is found with unopposed oestrogen but this should be confined to women who have had a hysterectomy. Combination therapy is essential when a uterus is present. PEPI did suggest that benefits were seen in addition to health consciousness as 'healthy women' were as frequently present on randomization to the placebo group.[44]

The HRT debate remains open in several areas and current trials are designed to clarify outstanding issues, for example: Do diabetic women benefit? Is stroke helped? How long should HRT be advised? Is it as effective by patch as orally? The problem is that we have at least 5 years to wait for the Hormone Estrogen/Progestin Replacement Study (HERS) and 9 years for the Women's Health Initiative (WHI) to report and we need a clinical management plan in the interim. I adopt the following guidelines listed in Table 4.2.

We need to consider women's attitudes to HRT.[45] In a study of Stanford graduates, women feared breast cancer far more than heart disease and, in spite of recent publicity,

- HRT is indicated for menopausal symptoms.
- HRT is indicated for osteoporosis.
- HRT should be offered to those with established CAD as secondary prevention.
- HRT should be offered to those at high risk of CAD.
- HRT should not be offered if there is a personal history of cancer or a strong family history of breast cancer. Mammograms should be performed to alleviate any doubts.
- Women at low risk of CAD should make an educated decision on HRT, there being no evidence to support its blanket use.
- Hypertension, diabetes and stroke are not contraindications.

Table 4.2
Guidelines for HRT.

did not see themselves as being vulnerable to CAD. Perhaps these fears reflect the view that CAD is a more treatable condition than cancer.

Clinical evaluation

Women present more often with angina and men more often with an MI.[46,47] Women with chest pain are more prone to having atypical features and we have already established that there is a lower prevalence of CAD in women with chest pain, which in turn explains the better prognosis for women with angina.[48]

Atypical chest pain (Table 4.3) is more common in women probably because of a higher prevalence of less common causes of ischaemia such as microvascular angina, syndrome X, and nonischaemic syndromes such as mitral valve prolapse which is notoriously associated with

atypical pains, most often after rather than during exercise.

Even when angina is considered 'definite' or 'typical', CAD is present in only 60% of women compared with 20–40% when the pain is 'atypical' or 'probable' for angina. Thus the more typical the pain, the more likely the presence of CAD, but with a high incidence of normal coronary arteries, and thereby a good prognosis, it becomes imperative to establish the cause of the chest pain because of the impact of the diagnosis on every aspect of a woman's life.[1]

Compared with men, women with stable angina have pain more frequently at rest, during sleep and mental stress and it is more likely to affect the neck and shoulders.[47] The presence of atypical features as well as typical features does not decrease the likelihood of CAD. Perhaps because women have others (for example, their family) as a priority, they play down or

Typical	Atypical
Tightness	Sharp (not severe)
Pressure	Knife-like
Weight	Stabbing
Constriction	'Like a stitch'
Ache	'Like a needle'
Dull	Pricking feeling
Squeezing feeling	Shooting
Soreness	Reproduced by pressure or position
Crushing	Can walk around with it
'Like a band'	Continuous: 'It's there all day'
Breathless (tightness)	Located in left chest, abdomen, back, or arm in absence of mid-chest pain
Retrosternal	Unrelated to exercise
Precipitated by exertion* or emotion	Not relieved by rest or nitroglycerin
Promptly relieved by rest or nitroglycerin*	Relieved by antacids
	Characterized by palpitations without chest pain

Table 4.3
Characteristics of typical and atypical angina pectoris. *Required for diagnosis of definite angina by the Coronary Artery Surgery Study.[49]

belittle their own symptoms, which in turn could explain their later presentation to some extent. A woman with a little breathlessness ('my weight doctor') who doesn't want to bother the doctor but mentions it in passing should not be dismissed.

It is important that we evaluate women with chest pain as thoroughly as possible. A woman with no risk factors and atypical pain will be very unlikely to have CAD whereas a woman with more typical pain and one or two major risk factors will be more likely to have CAD. Where there are doubts or where risk needs to be assessed, noninvasive testing should be employed. However, because of the lower prevalence of CAD in women, the value of noninvasive tests will be lower. Nevertheless, a normal test at a good workload almost certainly will rule out CAD.

Exercise testing

If a woman has typical pain and an abnormal resting ECG we need look no further, but it is unusual for the resting ECG to be normal or equivocal. Exercise testing will be more accurate in detecting CAD when the prevalence is high (low false-positive rate) but there will be a higher false-negative rate. Thus, women have a higher false-positive rate and lower false-negative rate because of the lower prevalence overall of CAD. We also need to take into account exercise capacity, which is less in women, so that a normal test at a lower workload (<6 minutes on a Standard Bruce Protocol) is inconclusive, whereas a normal test at a good workload rules out significant CAD. On average, an abnormal exercise test has a 76% sensitivity and 71% specificity in women compared with 95% and 93% for men.[46]

It is likely that any test that is noninvasive will be made more useful by stratifying risk at referral (Figure 4.1).[47] Several suggestions have been made but a practical low-, moderate- and high-risk grouping is simple and clinically relevant.

In this categorization, a normal exercise test in a low-risk or moderate-risk patient will rule

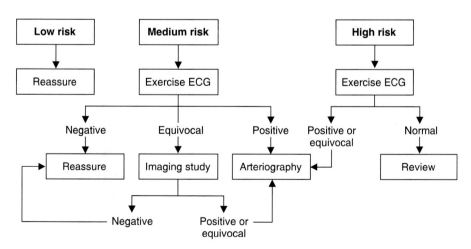

Figure 4.1
Low risk. *The estimated risk of CAD is less than 20%. The women are likely to be younger, have atypical pain and no risk factors of significance.* **Moderate risk**. *Risk is 20–80%. A mixture of typical and atypical pain. One major risk factor.* **High risk**. *>80% likelihood of CAD. Typical pain. Two major risk factors.*

out significant CAD. A positive test in a low-risk patient is likely to be false-positive so if anything, it should be avoided, whereas a positive or equivocal test in a moderate-risk or high-risk patient should lead on to further evaluation by imaging or coronary angiography.

Imaging

Few studies have looked specifically at the accuracy of imaging in women. Again, the accuracy will depend on the prevalence of CAD in the population. Breast attenuation is a problem in women and if the location of the breast varies between sequences, reversible ischaemia may be simulated. Taping the breast to the same location can simulate a fixed defect. Obesity may also pose problems with attenuation, which can occur with both planar and SPECT techniques.[50]

In the largest series (243) of women using exercise thallium-SPECT and a CAD diameter abnormality of >50%, the overall sensitivity was 71% and specificity 65%.[51] Sensitivity was 55% for women and 88% for men with single-vessel disease and 84% versus 93% for multivessel disease. It is difficult to argue a case for imaging above exercise testing other than in the moderate-risk group when, if the standard exercise test is equivocal, a normal perfusion study might obviate the need for angiography.

We do not know whether ^{99m}Tc-sestamibi SPECT or ^{82}Rb PET will improve the accuracy of imaging but adenosine SPECT thallium has been relatively disappointing (sensitivity: 82% in women; 95% in men).[52]

False-negatives imaging results do occur and may reflect submaximal exercise, a small female heart with small ischaemic areas to detect, less extensive CAD in younger women or less oestrogen-induced vasodilating effects postmenopause, reducing the difference between normally hyperaemic and less hyperaemic segments.

Stress echocardiography

Stress echocardiography appears to be of equivalent accuracy to nuclear studies.[53] Obesity and breast artifact are not major limitations. In one study of only 57 women who underwent angiography for typical and atypical pain, stress echocardiography had an overall sensitivity of 86% and specificity of 86%. Dipyridamole echocardiography had a 79% sensitivity and 93% specificity evaluated in 83 women and this compared with 72% sensitivity and 52% specificity for exercise testing alone.[54] Marwich et al. studied 161 women and recorded an 80% sensitivity and 81% specificity with this technique.[55]

Stress echocardiography appears to be more accurate and specific than exercise testing alone but the degree of difference does not justify the increased time and cost, except in moderate-risk cases where exercise testing alone is equivocal. It may have the edge over nuclear imaging but the scale of difference is far from impressive.

Coronary arteriography

When chest pain is problematic, the exercise test is abnormal or equivocal and the woman is considered high risk, the benefits of knowing the coronary anatomy in optimizing care outweigh the cost and minimal risk of cardiac catheterization.[56] We have to recognize that women are more likely to have normal coronary arteries but this should not deter us from thoroughly evaluating women's arteries when necessary. Trying to find a reason for not performing arteriography in the presence of an abnormal exercise test or imaging study is illogical — why do the tests if you are not prepared to follow them through?

Bias

The question of bias against women in the thorough evaluation of their condition is hotly debated.[1,57,58] It is difficult to distinguish any bias that may be due to sex from bias due to age and apparent bias may, in fact, be reflecting good clinical judgement in favour of women.[58,59] In the Survival and Ventricular Enlargement (SAVE) Study[60] women with the same degree of angina as men were less likely to undergo cardiac catheterization (15.4% versus 27.3%, p < 0.001) or CABG (5.9% versus 12.7%, p < 0.001) and the Yentl syndrome was born.[61] But this was 1991, and in 1994 another study discounted any sex bias in the referral for cardiac catheterization.[62] Furthermore, once angiography was performed there was no evidence of gender bias in referral for coronary artery revascularization procedures in 1995, whereas this might have been the case in 1991.[63]

Women estimate their own risk of CAD as being very low, with 73% of women estimating the risk to be less than 1% by the age of 70 years.[45] It is clear that CAD is just as much a woman's disease as a man's. I am constantly surprised by the lack of awareness of CAD as a woman's problem by women themselves and by healthcare professionals of either sex. Hiding behind hormones is no way to prevent CAD and it is no licence to ignore other risk factors.

Evaluating women with chest pain requires an awareness of the possibility of CAD in both physicians and women themselves. However, once this educational hurdle is overcome, the evidence from current practice is that any evaluation bias has been substantially reduced if not overcome.[1]

Treatment

Women have more severe disease, are older and more likely to be diabetic at presentation than men. Differences in therapy between the sexes must take into account these other variables. It appears that women experiencing infarction have similar rates of thrombolysis once they reach the coronary care unit.[64] This raises the question of whether age determines therapy and whether women, by sustaining infarcts at an older age, are placed at a disadvantage if age dictates entry to a coronary unit.[64] Thrombolysis is as effective in women as men, although women are at greater risk of haemorrhagic stroke and have a worse clinical outcome with more reinfarction and death.[63] Several studies have shown that women fare worse than men after an acute MI and that diabetic women are particularly at risk. In contrast, women have a more favourable outcome after the onset of angina, which is almost certainly due to the increased incidence of normal coronary arteries in women.

CABG rates do not appear to differ between men and women but the operative mortality tends to be higher in women (5.3% versus 2.5%,[66] 4.2% versus 2.1%[67]) especially in diabetics. Some of the increased operative risk may be related also to small vessel size.

Angioplasty is as successful in women as men. In one study of nearly 5000 patients (1224 women and 3726 men)[68] women were older, more likely to be diabetic, hypertensive, have had a previous infarction and have involvement of the left anterior descending artery. The angioplasty success rates were similar but women had a higher procedural mortality (1.1% versus 0.3%, p = 0.001). Corrected for body surface area, there was no increased risk. Event-free survival was better for women than men. Another study of 3557 patients (27%

women) found no periprocedural mortality related to sex alone.[69]

The prognostic benefits from beta blockers, ACE inhibitors and aspirin are applicable to women as well as men. However, some unwanted effects of these drugs are different (for example, cough caused by ACE inhibitors is more common in women), or can have different implications (such as impotence). Anxieties about tamoxifen are unfounded as it significantly reduces serum cholesterol in postmenopausal women with breast cancer[70] and this might explain the tamoxifen-related reduction in fatal myocardial infarction reported in Scotland.[71]

Women are less likely to attend rehabilitation programmes which offer valuable secondary prevention postinfarction, post-CABG or post-PTCA.[72] Women who do attend have high dropout rates. Post-MI women return to work less frequently and take longer to recover in general than men. This may reflect the lack of appropriate advice for women and begs the question of whether rehabilitation tailored to women's needs may be more successful.

Racial differences

Mortality rates and risk factors for CAD in black and white women showed no difference over a 30-year follow-up.[73] This contrasts with the evidence for increased risk in the Asian population,[74] perhaps due to the increased prevalence of insulin resistance.

Conclusions

CAD is an increasing problem in women. Education is essential to dispel the myth that it is a man's disease. Risk-factor modification is essential and attempts must be made to curtail the increase in teenage smoking. Women often have atypical chest pain which should be thoroughly evaluated. Women benefit as much as men from coronary care, thrombolysis, CABG and PTCA but are more likely to have advanced disease, be hypertensive, diabetic and be older at presentation and thereby have increased complications and mortality. Evidence of a sex rather than age bias remains but it is far less than 5 years ago. To experience the benefits of modern therapy more fully, women must present earlier in the disease process — it is unclear why they do not do so.

If my wife had...

If my wife had chest pain I would take it seriously, as she has a strong family history of premature death due to CAD on the male side. I would ask a colleague to assess her and would expect a careful history and examination to follow. I know that she is at low risk — a nonsmoker (lifelong), with normal blood pressure, and cholesterol <5.0 mmol/L but I am aware that she is menopausal. We have checked the above in view of her family history and she is already on HRT supervised by our very good GP.

If the chest pain history was suspicious I would expect an exercise ECG to be arranged. I would be reassured and I hope she would, by a normal result after at least 9 minutes of the Bruce protocol. If the exercise test was inconclusive or positive, I would hope she would be advised to undergo coronary arteriogaphy. I do not consider this a risky procedure in the right pair of hands but I would request it be performed at a tertiary centre with full back-up facilities. Complications do occur and I would take no chances.

While waiting for evaluation, I would advise her to begin aspirin at 75 mg/day, assess the response to GTN and commence atenolol 50 mg/day. Stopping therapy is as easy as starting it too late.

If normal coronary arteries were detected I would know we could buy some more CDs, as the prognosis is good. We would both improve our lifestyle, taking regular exercise and watching weight. Teamwork is needed. I would hope she could manage without drugs although I recognize that syndrome X could be a possibility and we all know how difficult that is to manage.

Significant CAD would worry me because I wouldn't have predicted it and I don't like it when all we know proves to be inaccurate. I would hope to be involved in any management decision and to help decide on the merits of the options available. If intervention was necessary I would confer with the colleagues I respect and of whose ability I am sure. I would encourage rehabilitation and a healthy lifestyle with less stress. I cannot pretend that I wouldn't worry because the CAD would have developed in a low-risk environment and I would have no handles to grip with regard to minimizing subsequent risk. I am also acutely aware of the fact that informed consent in our case would be very informed and that perhaps due to pressure, my own similar patients are less informed than they should be.

The positive side of detecting CAD would be the optimism that we could do something about it. Other illnesses are not as kind.

References

1 Jackson G, Coronary artery disease and women, *Br Med J* (1994)**309**:555–7.

2 Wenger NK, Speroff L, Packard B, Cardiovascular health and disease in women, *N Engl J Med* (1993)**329**:247–56.

3 Lerner DJ, Kannel WB, Patterns of coronary heart disease morbidity and mortality in the sexes: a 26 year follow-up of the Framingham population, *Am Heart J* (1986)**111**:383–90.

4 Rich-Edwards JW, Manson JE, Hennekens CH, Buring JE, The primary prevention of coronary heart disease in women, *N Engl J Med* (1995)**332**:1758–66.

5 Kitler ME, Coronary disease: are there gender differences? *Eur Heart J* (1994)**15**:409–17.

6 Wenger NK, Coronary heart disease in women: a 'new' problem. *Hosp Pract* (1992)**27**:59–74.

7 Murabito JM, Evans JC, Larson MG, Levy D, Prognosis after the onset of coronary heart disease. An investigation of differences in outcome between the sexes according to initial coronary disease presentation, *Circulation* (1993)**88**: 2548–55.

8 Becker RC, Terrin M, Ross R et al, for the TIMI investigators, Comparison of clinical outcomes for women and men after acute myocardial infarction, *Ann Intern Med* (1994)**120**: 638–45.

9 Jenkins JS, Flaker GC, Nolte B et al, Causes of higher in-hospital mortality in women than men after acute myocardial infarction, *Am J Cardiol* (1994)**73**:319–22.

10 Topol EJ, Califf RM, George BS et al, Insights derived from the Thrombolysis and Angioplasty in Myocardial Infarction (TAMI) trials, *J Am Coll Cardiol* (1988)**12**:24a–31a.

11 Brezinka V, Padmos I, Coronary heart disease risk factors in women, *Eur Heart J* (1994)**15**: 1571–84.

12 Higginbottom MB, Morris KG, Coleman RE, Cobb FR, Sex related differences in the normal cardiac response to upright exercise, *Circulation* (1984)**70**:357–66.

13 O'Connor NJ, Morton JR, Birkmeyer JD et al, Effect of coronary artery diameter in patients undergoing coronary bypass surgery, *Circulation* (1996)**93**:652–5.

14 Fetters JK, Peterson ED, Shaw LJ, Newby LK, Califf RM, Sex-specific differences in coronary artery disease risk factors, evaluation and treatment: have they been adequately evaluated? *Am Heart J* (1996)**131**:796–813.

15 Khaw KT, Where are the women in studies of coronary heart disease? *Br Med J* (1993)**306**: 1145–6.

16 Parish S, Collins R, Peto R et al, Cigarette smoking, tar yields, and non-fatal myocardial infarction: 14,000 cases and 32,000 controls in the United Kingdom, *Br Med J* (1995)**311**: 471–7.

17 Palmer JR, Rosenberg L, Shapiro S, 'Low yield' cigarettes and the risk of non-fatal myocardial infarction in women, *N Engl J Med* (1989)**320**: 1569–73.

18 Califano JA, The wrong way to stay slim, *N Engl J Med* (1995)**333**:1214–16.

19 Rosenberg L, Palmer JR, Shapiro S, Decline in the risk of myocardial infarction among women who stop smoking, *N Engl J Med* (1990)**322**: 213–17.

20 Walsh BW, Schiff I, Rosner B et al, Effects of post menopausal estrogen replacement on the concentrations and metabolism of plasma lipoproteins, *N Engl J Med* (1991)**325**:1196–204.

21 Soma MR, Osnago-Gadda I, Paoletti R et al, The lowering of lipoprotein (a) induced by estrogen and progesterone replacement therapy in post-menopausal women, *Arch Intern Med* (1993)**153**:1462–8.

22 Shepherd J, Cobbe SM, Ford I et al, Prevention of coronary heart disease with pravastatin in men with hypercholesterolaemia, *N Engl J Med* (1995)**333**:1301–7.

23 Scandinavian Simvastatin Survival Study Group, Randomised trial of cholesterol lowering in 4444 patients with coronary heart

disease: the Scandinavian Simvastatin Survival Study (4S), *Lancet* (1994)**344**:1383–9.

24 The Pravastatin Multinational Study Group for Cardiac Risk Patients, Effects of pravastatin in patients with serum total cholesterol levels from 5.2 to 7.8 mmol/liter (200–300 mg/dl) plus two additional atherosclerotic risk factors, *Am J Cardiol* (1993)**72**:1031–7.

25 Sacks FM, Pfeffer MA, Moye LA et al. The effect of Pravastatin on coronary events after myocardial infarction in patients with average cholesterol levels, *N Engl J Med* (1996) **335**:1001–9.

26 MAAS Investigators, Effect of simvastatin on coronary atheroma: the Multicentre Anti-Atheroma Study (MAAS), *Lancet* (1994)**344**:633–8.

27 Isles CG, Hole DJ, Hawthorne VM, Lever AF, Relation between coronary risk and coronary mortality in women of the Renfrew and Paisley survey: comparison with men, *Lancet* (1992)**339**:702–6.

28 Fiebach NH, Hebert PR, Stampfer MJ et al, A prospective study of high blood pressure and cardiovascular disease in women, *Am J Epidemiol* (1989)**130**:646–54.

29 Collins R, Peto R, MacMahon S et al, Blood pressure, stroke, and coronary heart disease. 2. Short-term reductions in blood pressure: overview of randomised drug trials in their epidemiological context, *Lancet* (1990)**335**:827–38.

30 Kaplan NM, The treatment of hypertension in women, *Arch Intern Med* (1995)**155**:563–7.

31 SHEP Cooperative Research Group, Prevention of stroke by antihypertensive drug treatment in older persons with isolated systolic hypertension, *JAMA* (1991)**265**:3255–64.

32 Manson JE, Colditz GA, Stampfer MJ et al, A prospective study of maturity-onset diabetes mellitus and risk of coronary heart disease and stroke in women, *Arch Intern Med* (1991)**151**:1141–7.

33 Manson JE, Willett WC, Stampfer MJ et al, Body weight and mortality among women, *N Engl J Med* (1995)**333**:677–85.

34 Fuchs CS, Stampfer MJ, Colditz GA et al, Alcohol consumption and mortality in women, *N Engl J Med* (1995)**332**:1245–50.

35 Hennekens CH, Evans D, Peto R, Oral contraceptive use, cigarette smoking and myocardial infarction, *Br J Fam Plann* (1979)**5**:66–7.

36 Lewis MA, Spitzer WO, Heinemann LAJ et al, Third generation oral contraceptives and risk of myocardial infarction: an international case-control study, *Br Med J* (1996)**312**:88–90.

37 Spitzer WO, Lewis MA, Heinemann LAJ et al, Third generation oral contraceptives and risk of venous thromboembolic disorders: an international case-control study, *Br Med J* (1996)**312**:83–8.

38 Gordon J, Kannel WB, Hjortland MC, McNamara PM, Menopause and coronary heart disease. The Framingham Study, *Ann Intern Med* (1978)**89**:157–61.

39 Stampfer MJ, Colditz GA, Willett WC et al, Postmenopausal estrogen therapy and cardiovascular disease: ten year follow-up from the Nurses' Health Study, *N Engl J Med* (1991)**325**:756–62.

40 Stevenson JC, Crook D, Godsland IF, Influence of age and menopause on serum lipids and lipoproteins in healthy women, *Atherosclerosis* (1993)**98**:83–90.

41 Colditz GA, Hankinson SE, Hunter DJ et al, The use of estrogens and progestins and the risk of breast cancer in postmenopausal women, *N Engl J Med* (1995)**332**:1589–93.

42 Davidson NE, Hormone-replacement therapy — breast versus heart versus bone, *N Engl J Med* (1995)**332**:1638–9.

43 The Writing Group for the PEPI Trial, Effects of estrogen or estrogen/progestin regimens on heart disease risk factors in postmenopausal women: the Postmenopausal Estrogen/Progestin Interventions Trial, *JAMA* (1994)**273**:199–208.

44 Healy B, PEPI in Perspective, *JAMA* (1995)**273**:240–1 (editorial).

45 Pilote L, Hlatky MA, Attitudes of women toward hormone therapy and prevention of heart disease, *Am Heart J* (1995)**129**:1237–8.

46 Sullivan AK, Holdright DR, Wright CA et al, Chest pain in women: clinical, investigative and prognostic features, *Br Med J* (1994)**308**:883–6.

47 Douglas PS, Ginsburg GS, The evaluation of chest pain in women, *N Engl J Med* (1996)**334**:1311–15.

48 Holdright DR, Fox KM, Characterisation and identification of women with angina pectoris, *Eur Heart J* (1996)17:510–17.

49 CASS principal investigators and their associates – Coronary Artery Surgery Study (CASS): a randomized trial of coronary artery bypass surgery survival data, *Circulation* (1983) **68**: 939–50.

50 De Puey EG, Garcia EV, Optimal specificity of thallium — 201 SPECT through recognition of imaging artifacts, *J Nucl Med* (1989)30:441–9.

51 Chae SC, Heo J, Iskandrian AS et al, Identification of extensive CAD in women by exercise single-photon emission computer tomographic (SPECT) thallium imaging, *J Am Coll Cardiol* (1993)21:1305–11.

52 Pancholy S, Gioia G, Russel J et al, Detection of CAD in women, *Circulation* (1995)**92**:1–13.

53 Saivada SG, Ryan T, Fineberg NS et al, Exercise echocardiographic detection of CAD in women, *J Am Coll Cardiol* (1989)14:1440–7.

54 Masini M, Picano E, Lattanzi F et al, High dose dipyridamole echocardiography test in women: correlation with exercise electrocardiography test and coronary arterography, *J Am Coll Cardiol* (1988)**12**:682–5.

55 Marwich TH, Anderson T, Williams MJ et al, Exercise echocardiography is an accurate and cost efficient technique for the detection of CAD in women, *J Am Coll Cardiol* (1995)**26**: 329–35.

56 De Bono D et al, Complications of diagnostic cardiac catheterisation: results from 34041 patients in the United Kingdom, confidential enquiry into cardiac catheter complications, *Br Heart J* (1993)70:297–300.

57 Laskey WK, Gender differences in the management of coronary artery disease: bias or good clinical judgement, *Ann Intern Med* (1992)**116**: 869–71.

58 Bickell NA, Pieper KS, Lee KL et al, Referral patterns for coronary artery disease treatment: gender bias or good clinical judgement, *Ann Intern Med* (1992)116:791–7.

59 Adams JN, Jamieson M, Rawles JM et al, Women and myocardial infarction: agism rather than sexism? *Br Heart J* (1995)73:87–91.

60 Steingort RM, Packer M, Hamm P et al, Sex differences in the management of coronary artery disease, *N Engl J Med* (1991)**325**:226–30.

61 Healy B, The Yentl syndrome, *N Engl J Med* (1991)**325**:274–6.

62 Mark DB, Shaw LK, Delong ER et al, Absence of sex bias in the referral of patients for cardiac catheterisation, *N Engl J Med* (1994)**330**: 1101–6.

63 Bell MR, Bergar PB, Holmes DR et al, Referral for coronary artery revascularisation procedures after diagnostic coronary angiography, *J Am Coll Cardiol* (1995)**25**:1650–5.

64 Lincoff AM, Califf RM, Ellis SG et al, Thrombolytic therapy for women with myocardial infarction: is there a gender gap? *J Am Coll Cardiol* (1993)**22**:1780–7.

65 Hannaford PC, Kay CR, Ferry S, Agism as explanation for sexism in provision of thrombolysis. *Br Med J* (1994) 309:573.

66 Barbir M, Lazem F, Ilsley C et al, Coronary artery surgery in women compared with men: analysis of coronary risk factors and in-hospital mortality in a single centre, *Br Heart J* (1994)71:408–12.

67 Davis KB, Chaitman B, Ryan T et al, Comparison of 15-year survival for men and women after initial medical or surgical treatment for coronary artery disease: a CASS registry study, *J Am Coll Cardiol* (1995)25:1000–9.

68 Arnold AM, Mick MJ, Piedmonte MR, Simpfendorfer C, Gender differences for coronary angioplasty, *Am J Cardiol* (1994)74:18–21.

69 Bell MR, Holmes DR, Berger PB et al, The changing in-hospital mortality of women undergoing percutaneous transluminal coronary angioplasty, *JAMA* (1993)269:2091–5.

70 Love RR, Wiebe DA, Newcomb PA et al, Effects of tamoxifen on cardiovascular risk factors in postmenopausal women, *Ann Intern Med* (1991)**115**:860–4.

71 McDonald CC, Stewart HJ et al, Fatal myocardial infarction in the Scottish adjuvant tamoxifen trial, *Br Med J* (1991)303:435–7.

72 McGee HM, Horgan JH, Cardiac rehabilitation programmes: are women less likely to attend? *Br Med J* (1992)305:283–4.

73 Keil JE, Sutherland SE, Knapp RG et al, Mortality rates and risk factors for coronary disease in black as compared with white men and women, *N Engl J Med* (1993)**329**:73–8.

74 Bhatnagar D, Anand IS, Durrington PN et al, Coronary risk factors in people from the Indian subcontinent in West London and their siblings in India, *Lancet* (1995)**345**:405–9.

5

Angina and concomitant disease

John JV McMurray

Introduction

While it is common to discuss the management of 'angina' as if this syndrome occurs in isolation, the reality is that many patients with angina have concomitant disease that alters the approach to treatment.

Angina with left ventricular dysfunction and heart failure

That this is true is seen nowhere more clearly than in patients with chronic heart failure (CHF). It is perhaps important to state at the outset that angina and heart failure frequently exist. Many of the large heart failure trials have done the disservice of giving the contrary impression by excluding patients on the basis of an exercise test limited by angina or ECG evidence of ischaemia. The truest reflection of reality is the SOLVD Registry, a huge database of patients with multisystem disease older than those who are usually randomized into clinical trials.[1–3] In the SOLVD Registry approximately 60% of patients with CHF also reported angina. This reflects the fact that most cases of heart failure are due to coronary heart disease and previous myocardial infarction. What are the therapeutic options? Medically, we can consider the standard antianginal classes, i.e. calcium channel antagonists, nitrates and beta blockers.

Calcium channel blockers

Though efficacious antianginal agents these drugs may aggravate the heart failure syndrome.[4,5] There is evidence that short-acting dihydropyridine calcium antagonists, such as nifedipine, lead to neuroendocrine activation, sodium and water retention, and clinical deterioration.[6–9] Diltiazem is known to increase the risk of developing hear failure in patients with impaired left ventricular function (Figure 5.1).[10] Verapamil, like the aforementioned calcium antagonists, is negatively inotropic though in one large postinfarction study did not appear to exacerbate heart failure.[11] Its safety in patients with frank CHF is not known.

A major breakthrough in this area, however, has been the demonstration that the very long-acting dihydropyridine, amlodipine, does not increase the risk of clinical deterioration or death. In the PRAISE trial amlodipine had an overall neutral effect on morbidity and mortality in patients with severe CHF (Figure 5.2).[12] Curiously, in a prespecified subgroup analysis, there was even a reduction in mortality in patients with 'nonischaemic' CHF receiving amlodipine.

If a calcium channel blocker must be used in a patient with angina and heart failure, amlodipine is the drug of choice.

Nitrates

Though often considered as an ideal treatment for patients with heart failure and angina it is

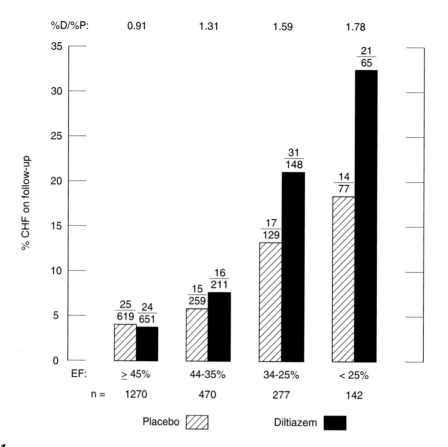

Figure 5.1
Percent of patients with new or worsened congestive heart failure (CHF) during long-term follow-up is shown for four groups defined solely by baseline ejection fraction (EF): ≥0.45, 0.44–0.35, 0.34–0.25, and <0.25. Paired bars demonstrate occurrence of late CHF in placebo- and diltiazem-treated subsets. Number of patients with CHF (numerator) and total number in each subset (denominator) are displayed above each bar. At top of figure, value for each group shows percent of patients with late CHF among those given diltiazem (D) divided by percent of patients with late CHF among those given placebo (P). Data are shown for 2159 patients with baseline measurement of EF. Diltiazem-associated increase in late CHF is progressively larger as baseline EF is reduced.

unlikely that nitrates are of anything other than limited benefit. It is commonly and incorrectly thought that nitrates are beneficial in heart failure *per se*; there is no evidence for this belief.[13] Nitrates are, however, undoubtedly efficacious antianginal agents. They are also, however, necessarily of limited value because of the problem of tolerance.[14]

It is now common to prescribe a long-acting formulation, usually first thing in the morning, to avoid daytime, exercise-induced angina. It must be realized, however, that such an approach (and such formulations) leave the patient without anti-ischaemic protection during the night and, perhaps most importantly, in the early-morning predose period. It is in this period that the risk of infarction, sudden death and other serious events is greatest.[15]

Nitrates do not, therefore, provide 24-hour anti-ischaemic protection.

Beta blockers

Beta blockers should normally be regarded as first-line antianginal therapy, especially in patients with previous myocardial infarction (i.e. most heart failure patients).[16–18] Although these drugs have been shown to improve prognosis after infarction, especially in patients with impaired left ventricular function, and to reduce the risk of sudden, presumed arrhythmic death, especially in patients with heart failure complicating infarction, beta blockers have been traditionally considered to be contraindicated in patients with CHF.

While conventional (large) doses of beta blockers, introduced abruptly, can lead to cata-strophic (even fatal) haemodynamic deterioration, there is considerable evidence that very small doses of these drugs, introduced cautiously and titrated up over weeks and months, may lead to an improvement in ventricular function and clinical status.[19–22] Paradoxically, this benefit seemed, initially, to be most marked or even confined to patients with nonischaemic dilated cardiomyopathy.[23]

More recently, however, carvedilol has been shown to be of benefit in patients with CHF, regardless of aetiology.[21,24,25] Carvedilol has also been shown to reduce mortality — a finding that is somewhat controversial and awaits confirmation (Figure 5.3). Depending on the results of further trials, such as BEST, CIBIS 2 and MERIT, it may be the beta blockers become the drug of choice for the patient with angina and CHF.[22]

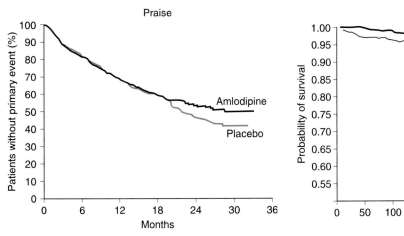

Figure 5.2
Kaplan–Meier plots of the time to the first primary event (death or cardiovascular morbidity) among 571 patients with chronic heart failure receiving amlodipine and 582 receiving placebo. As compared with the placebo group, the amlodipine group had a 9% lower risk of a primary event (95% confidence interval, 24% lower to 10% higher; p = 0.31).

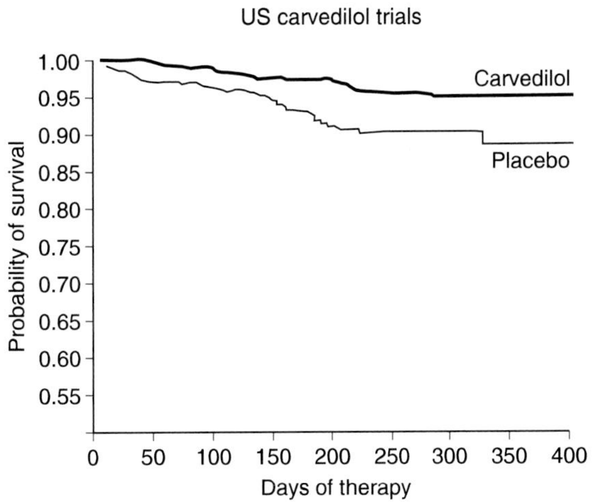

Figure 5.3
US carvedilol trials: a multicentre phase III clinical trial programme consisting of four concurrent randomized placebo controlled trials involving 1094 CHF patients with NYHA class II–IV symptoms and LVEFS of ⩽0.35. Mortality was reduced by 65% in the carvedilol groups (P = 0.0001).

ACE inhibitors

Studies of ACE inhibitors as antianginal agents have been disappointing.[26–28] While some have suggested angiotensin-converting enzyme a benefit, most have been neutral and at least one has suggested that ACE inhibition may aggravate angina.

Though the prevention arm of the Studies of Left Ventricular Dysfunction (SOLVD) and the Survival and Ventricular Enlargement (SAVE) study suggested that ACE inhibitors can reduce new acute coronary events in patients with coronary heart disease and impaired left ventricular function, this benefit has not been confirmed in the recent, prospective, Quinapril Ischaemic Events Trial (QUIET) where patients undergoing coronary angioplasty were randomized to receive placebo or the ACE inhibitor, quinapril.[28–31] In this trial patients had preserved left ventricular function. A number of much larger trials which will address this question are also underway (Figure 5.4).

Aspirin

Though generally regarded to be of therapeutic value in patients with coronary heart disease, concerns have been raised that asprin may at least partially antagonize the beneficial actions

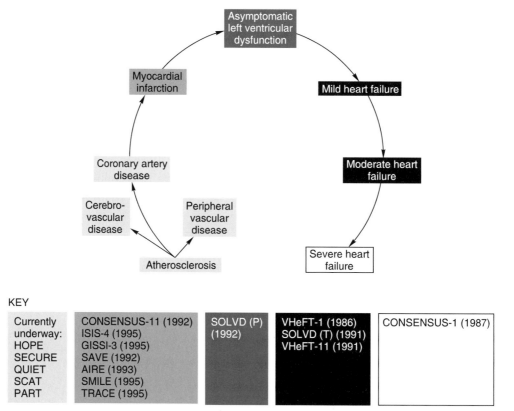

Figure 5.4
The expanding role of ACE inhibitors in cardiovascular disease: key published and ongoing trials.

of ACE inhibitors in patients with left ventricular dysfunction.[32] There is also evidence from the second Persantin and Apsirin Reinfarction Study (PARIS 2) that antiplatelet therapy may be of little benefit in patients with significant left ventricular dysfunction.[33]

Surgery

While many patients with angina and heart failure might not be considered for coronary artery bypass grafting (CABG) because of their advanced age and multisystem disease, it is still unfortunately the case that others are denied CABG because of the mistaken belief that poor left ventricular function and heart failure are contraindications to surgery.

Paradoxically, of course, it is precisely these patients who seem to have the most to gain prognostically (and, potentially, symptomatically) (Figure 5.5).[34,35] Indeed, patients with angina and heart failure are probably a greatly underinvestigated group. With the growing realization that ventricular dysfunction may be reversible if it is due to chronic low-flow ischaemia (so-called 'hibernating' myocardium), and that ischaemia may often manifest as breathlessness, it is likely that there is a subgroup of patients with CHF who stand to obtain not only an improvement in angina but also in ventricular function with CABG. There is also evidence that this is the case with left ventricular ejection faction increasing after surgery.[35] This author's approach is to consider cardiac catheterization in patients with angina and heart failure, with a view to revascularization for prognostic reasons if the patient is young enough and otherwise fit enough to undergo CABG. To reluctant surgeons, concerned about poor ventricular function, the author points out that painful myocardium (i.e. causing angina) must be viable myocardium. In the patient with medically refractory angina who really is not a candidate for CABG or angioplasty (see below), then transcutaneous laser myocardial revascularization may hold some promise.

Coronary angioplasty

Patients with medically refractory angina, who do not have a prognostic indication for surgery, can also be considered for percutaneous transluminal coronary angioplasty (PTCA). Though there are no good data from randomized controlled comparative trials, evidence from registries suggests that PTCA carries a considerably increased risk in patients with poor left ventricular function and that outcome may be inferior to that after surgery.[36] This author only considers PTCA, therefore, when CABG is not possible.

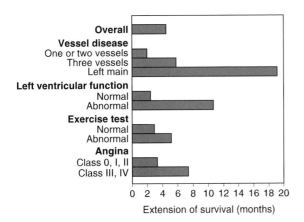

Figure 5.5
The prognostic benefits of CABG appear greatest in those who are most symptomatic.

Angina and hyperlipidaemia

Perhaps the most common accompaniment of angina is hyperlipidaemia. The recent 'statin' studies have removed any lingering doubt that effective reduction of cholesterol slows the progression of coronary atherosclerosis, may even lead to regression of atheroma and prevents new clinical events.[37–47] In keeping with this, cholesterol reduction improves endothelial function, increases myocardial bloodflow and reduces myocardial ischaemia. The most convincing evidence of a reduction in clinical events comes from the Scandanavian Simvastatin Survival Study (4S) where 19% of the 4444 randomized patients had a history of angina but not previous infarction.[37,42] This subgroup had a 26% reduction in the rate of major coronary events, a benefit that was statistically significant and proportionally similar to that seen in the main group of patients in 4S, i.e. survivors of myocardial infarction (Table 5.1).[42] This subgroup analysis of 4S is backed up by two other analyses.[38,43] Meta-analysis of the small statin studies, published or presented prior to 4S, showed a 44% reduction in overall mortality in patients receiving active treatment.[38] The majority of patients in these smaller

studies had angina rather than a previous infarction. Indeed, many had relatively mild or diffuse coronary atherosclerosis and were felt not to need further intervention or were deemed to be unsuitable for further intervention, i.e. the type of patient about whom cardiologists often despair with respect to therapeutic options! A separate meta-analysis, the Pravastatin Atherosclerosis Intervention Program, came to a similar conclusion.[43]

The average total cholesterol in most of these recent statin studies was approximately 6–6.5 mmol/l (Table 5.2). Clearly, however, the question arises as to the benefit or otherwise of lipid-lowering therapy in patients with total plasma cholesterol concentrations below, say, 5.5 mmol/l (the 4S treatment threshold). Epidemiologically there is still a direct relationship between population cholesterol concentration and coronary heart disease mortality at much lower cholesterol concentrations.[45] The

| Subgroup (n) | Patients with a major coronary event | | |
	Placebo	Simvastatin	Risk reduction
Aspirin (1637)	28	20	34
No aspirin (2807)	28	19	33
Beta blocker (2525)	28	20	36
No beta blocker (1919)	28	19	31
<60 years (2162)	28	18	39
≥60 years (2282)	28	21	29
Angina only (918)	18	14	26
Previous MI (3526)	31	21	35
Female (827)	22	15	35
Male (3617)	29	21	34

Table 5.1
Analysis of subgroups in the 4S study (%).

	4S n = 4444	CARE n = 4159	PMNSG n = 1062	MARS n = 247	CCAIT n = 331	PLAC-I n = 408	PLAC-II n = 151	MAAS n = 381	REGRESS n = 884
Mean age (yr)	58	59	55	58	53	57	62	55	60
Male (%)	81	86	76	91	81	77	85	88	100
Cholesterol (mmol/l)	6.74	5.4	6.75	5.99	6.46	5.97	6.05	6.44	~6.0
Angina (%)	21	20	40	41	66	–	–	68	–
Previous MI (%)	79	100	34	60	55	43	63	54	47
Treatment	Simvastatin	Pravastatin	Pravastatin	Lovastatin	Lovastatin	Pravastatin	Pravastatin	Simvastatin	Pravastatin

Table 5.2
Summary of recent secondary prevention studies using HMG CoA reductase inhibitors.

recent Cholesterol And Recurrent Events (CARE) study has, however, been interpreted as showing no benefit in reducing LDL cholesterol below 3.2. mmol/l.[46] A separate analysis, including CARE but also the post-CAGB trial, still, I feel, leaves this question open (Figure 5.6).[48,49] Indeed, I believe the totality of epidemiological, pathophysiological and clinical trial evidence to date supports a policy of aggressive cholesterol reduction in all patients with established coronary disease aiming for a total cholesterol of <5 mmol/l and LDL cholesterol of < 4 mmol/l.[44,48]

This policy is also applicable to patients undergoing coronary intervention for their angina. Though cholesterol reduction does not prevent restenosis following angioplasty it does have all the benefits already alluded to. The recent National Institutes of Health post-CABG trial, mentioned above, emphasizes the importance of vigorous cholesterol reduction after bypass surgery.[49] In this trial there were fewer graft occlusions and coronary events in patients randomized to 'aggressive' lipid-lowering therapy compared to 'standard' lipid-lowering therapy.

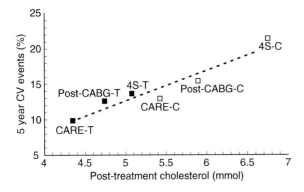

Figure 5.6
The events from different trials are plotted in relation to the cholesterol levels during the randomized period. Note the continuous relation across the entire range of cholesterol values depicted. The CV events included vary slightly between trials: CV death or MI in 4S; CV death or MI in CARE; CV death, MI, stroke, revascularization, or unexpected death in Post-CABG Trial. The total cholesterol level in the Post-CABG Trial is derived using the values for LDL, triglycerides, and HDL.

Angina and hypertension

The combined anti-ischaemic and antihypertensive actions of beta blockers make these agents, in this author's mind, the drugs of choice in patients with angina and high blood pressure. Indeed there is some evidence from clinical trials in angina (ASSIST) and hypertension that beta blockers may improve prognosis in both these conditions.[51–53] Conversely, there is controversial evidence that at least some calcium channel blockers may worsen prognosis both in patients with coronary heart disease and in patients with hypertension.[54–57]

This hazard, if real, is probably confined to the short-acting dihydropyridine calcium antagonists, at least in patients with coronary heart disease. In the patient who really cannot tolerate a beta blocker (usually only asthmatics) the second drug of choice is a rate-limiting calcium channel blocker. Here the preferred agent is probably verapamil as it does not seem to aggravate left ventricular dysfunction and, according to the DAVIT studies, may reduce coronary events in infarct survivors.[58,59] Also, in a reasonably large outcome study in angina, verapamil-treated patients did not fare worse than those treated with metoprolol.[60] The only possible exception to the above would be patients with angina, hypertension and significant left ventricular systolic dysfunction. Here amlodipine would probably be the drug of choice although cautious use of carvedilol might also be considered. This, of course, presumes that an ACE inhibitor has been given.[50]

The usual considerations apply to the use of PTCA and CABG in the patient with angina and hypertension. Similarly, the usual approaches to secondary prevention of coronary heart disease (aspirin, cholesterol reduction, etc.) and investigation for causes of secondary hypertension should also apply.

Angina and chronic obstructive airways disease/ asthma

Asthma is an absolute contraindication to use of a beta blocker and, in asthmatic patients, as in hypertensives, the first-line treatment of angina should be a rate-limiting calcium channel antagonist, such as verapamil or diltiazem. Nitrates can be added as second-line therapy. CABG is usually possible with modern anaesthetic techniques though PTCA probably has a greater role to play in these patients. In contrast with asthma, patients with chronic obstructive airways disease (COAD) usually do tolerate beta blockers quite well and it is often worth at least trying these drugs in the patient with refractory angina.

Angina and peripheral vascular disease

One of the greatest therapeutic myths is that beta blockers are contraindicated in patients with peripheral vascular disease (PVD). It is in fact rare for patients with PVD to complain of any clinical deterioration when given a beta blocker, and controlled clinical trials support this observation. Indeed, some calcium channel blockers, by inducing a 'steal' phenomenon, exacerbate claudication though this does not seem to be true of verapannil.[63] It is worth recalling that, in the Beta Blocker Heart Attack Trial (BHAT), the incidence of newly reported intermittent claudication was similar in the propranolol and placebo groups.[61] In patients with a history of intermittent claudication, fewer propranolol than placebo-treated patients had this complaint recorded as an adverse event. The Stockholm Metoprolol trial reported fewer leg amputations in the beta blocker group than the placebo group.[62]

The major challenge in patients with PVD usually arises when it comes to cardiac catheterization because of refractory symptoms or a positive stress test. Femoral access and aortic passage may be difficult or impossible. Brachial access will be easier but the subclavian and carotid arteries will often be diseased and the risk of cerebral embolism during the procedure is much greater than normal. Left main coronary artery stenosis and renal artery stenosis are much more common in these patients and must be anticipated by the catheterizer.

A not uncommon patient, at least in Glasgow, is one with poor left ventricular function, hypertension, severe angina and carotid-cerebrovascular disease; often the patient will have concomitant lung disease and diabetes. Such patients are a therapeutic minefield and detection of, and treatment of, renal artery stenosis can often be a critical component of successful management, i.e. by ameliorating hypertension and enabling use of an ACE inhibitor for poor LV function — manoeuvres that in themselves will often lessen angina or at least improve the patient's chances of being suitable for CABG or PTCA.

Angina and diabetes

Beta blockers

Another common therapeutic myth is that beta blockers should not be used in patients with diabetes. This arose from the observation that beta blockers, particularly those that are non-selective, may mask the symptoms and change the normal physiological responses to hypoglycaemia in insulin-treated diabetics. While this may be considered a relative contraindication in insulin-treated patients it should definitely not apply to noninsulin-treated patients. It is relevant to recall that in the postinfarction trials diabetic patients obtained a particularly large risk reduction with beta blockers.[18,64] It is this author's practice to use beta blockers as first-line antianginal therapy in insulin-treated diabetics unless they are prone to regular hypoglycaemic attacks.

Angioplasty

Recent results from the National Heart, Lung and Blood Institute (NHLBI)-sponsored BARI study have shown that PTCA is significantly less successful in the long-term control of symptoms.[65–67] In a 'clinical alert' the NHLBI has advised that diabetic patients on oral hypoglycaemic agents or insulin, who need multivessel coronary revascularization, undergo CABG rather than PTCA. This recommendation is based on an analysis of outcome among the 352 diabetics in BARI, which is a trial that randomized patients with significant stenoses of at least two major epicardial coronary vessels and severe or unstable angina. Five-year mortality in diabetics undergoing CABG was 19% compared to 35% among those randomized to PTCA (p= 0.03).

Angina, peptic ulceration and active oesophagitis

Asprin is undoubtedly associated with an increased risk of gastrointestinal haemorrhage (Table 5.3) especially at higher doses. There is good evidence that 75 mg (or less) may be a sufficient daily maintenance dose to achieve an antiplatelet effect in patients with coronary disease and that larger doses increase the risk of gastrointestinal bleeding.[68] Although 'dyspepsia' is common in the general population this symptom is probably not a sufficient reason to avoid aspirin therapy. The patient with barium or endoscopically proven ulceration is, however, a real problem. Fortunately, new antiplatelet therapies are becoming available which, unlike their predecessors, e.g. dipyridamole, do have therapeutic efficacy. The most promising prospect for routine, safe oral use is clopidogrel.[69] Unlike aspirin, this agent does not act via cyclo-oxygenase and, hence, does not inhibit the production of cytoprotective

Events per 1000 patient years of treatment		
Risk	Haematemesis	0.2–1.0
	Melaena	2.1–7.0
	All GI bleeding	2.5–7.7
	Peptic ulcer	0.5–3.3
	Hospital admission for peptic ulcer	3.5
Benefit	Any major vascular event (e.g. death, MI, CVA)	18

GI = gastrointestinal
MI = myocardial infarction
CVA = cerbrovascular accident

Adapted from Weil J et al *Br Med J* 1995; **310**: 827–30 and Roderick PK et al *Br J Clin Pharmac* 1993; **35**: 219–26.

Table 5.3
Risk/benefit from aspirin.

prostaglandin E2 in the gastrointestinal lining. Instead, clopidogrel inhibits ADP-dependent platelet aggregation. Clopidogrel was slightly more effective than aspirin in reducing vascular events in the recent CAPRIE study (Figure 5.7).[69]

Angina and atrial fibrillation

There is no doubt that warfarin therapy reduces the risk of thromoembolism and stroke in patients with atrial fibrillation, many of whom have associated coronary heart disease.[70,71] Warfarin is also superior to aspirin in this respect, especially in patients with structural heart disease.[70,71] Therefore, if a patient with angina also has left ventricular hypertrophy or left ventricular dysfunction and atrial fibrillation they should receive warfarin therapy, aiming to obtain an INR of 2.0–2.5. The unanswered question is whether or not both aspirin *and* warfarin are indicated. Both agents are of benefit postinfarction and have a different mechanism of action.[72,73] In some settings, e.g. in patients with prosthetic valves, the combination is better than monotherapy.[74] There is certainly an argument for considering low dose aspirin and warfarin in a patient with angina, atrial fibrillation and structural heart disease.

A beta blocker, alone or in combination with a rate-limiting calcium channel blocker, should provide sufficient rate control.[75] Digoxin is probably best avoided as there is a lingering concern that it increases myocardial electrical instability and the risk of sudden death.[76]

Angina and ventricular arrhythmias

Sudden death in the patient with angina usually occurs in the context of left ventricular systolic dysfunction. Beta blockers have been convincingly shown to reduce sudden cardiac death postinfarction and the same is probably true of ACE inhibitors.[77] By contrast, Class I antiarrhythmic drugs have been shown to increase mortality in this setting.[79–80] Amiodarone, however, may reduce sudden death but overall mortality was not reduced in EMIAT or CAMIAT.[80,82] Recently, MADIT has shown that an implantable defibrillator significantly reduces the risk of death in infarction survivors with impaired LV function and inducible ventricular arrhythmias that are not pharmacologically suppressible.[83] A significantly greater proportion of defibrillator patients (26%) received beta blockers compared to conventional therapy patients (8%), making the overall result of this trial somewhat difficult to interpret. In other words, the whole issue of how best to treat asymptomatic ventricular arrhythmias in the patient with coronary heart disease is very complex and there is probably not yet a consensus on management.

Angina and smoking

Many patients with coronary heart disease continue to smoke and this habit adversely affects their prognosis. There is now good evidence that nicotine replacement therapy approximately doubles the chance of smoking cessation and this therapy appears to be safe in patients with stable coronary heart disease. Patches seem to be more effective than gum, there is little value in extending treatment beyond eight weeks. Complete abstinence in the first two weeks of therapy is vital. Weaning is not necessary. Counselling adds little to the effectiveness of treatment.[84,85]

If I had...

I will probably have developed angina many months or even years after a myocardial infarction; it is hoped that, these days, early reversible ischaemia is detected and treated. Because my infarction was some time ago I may have been denied important new therapies and been burdened with ineffective or even hazardous ones, e.g. diltiazem or nifedipine.

I see three objectives of treatment, all of which are inter-related. I want symptom relief and improvement in prognosis — improvement related to retarding the pathophysiology of coronary disease and improvement related to modifying favourably the pathophysiology of left ventricular dysfunction.

I wish treatment with a beta blocker. I may well have been denied this because more than 60% of infarct survivors in the UK (and elsewhere) are. I suspect it is people like myself with poor left ventricular function who are most likely to be denied treatment but who have most to gain. I believe nonselective beta block-

ers are better, not necessarily as antianginals but as antiarrhythmics and, perhaps, in preventing reinfarction. I might choose carvedilol because, if my left ventricular dysfunction is significant, I feel I would tolerate it better, initially.

I also want to receive a statin, regardless of my plasma cholesterol concentration and I want to reduce my cholesterol (and triglycerides) as much as possible. I would aim for an LDL cholesterol of below 0.5 mmol/l. I might have to take atorvastatin to achieve these goals.

I expect to be treated with an ACE inhibitor. I believe bigger doses are better and would aim for 20 mg twice daily of enalapril, if I could tolerate it. My hope is that this would not only stabilize my left ventricular function (LV) but probably also reduce my risk of a new coronary event and, even, an arrhythmia as suggested by a recent analysis of the AIRE study and TRACE. I believe that the ACE inhibitor and statin will probably also act synergistically to improve my endothelial function.

I am concerned that the aspirin–ACE inhibitor interaction is real. I would either take a very low dose of aspirin or the equivalent of a low dose such as 75 mg of an enteric-coated preparation. Alternatively, I would consider taking clopidogrel, if I could obtain it (Figure 5.7).

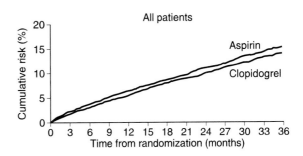

Figure 5.7
Cumulative incidence of stroke, MI, or vascular death (intention to treat analysis).

If my angina remained troublesome I would add amlodipine rather than a nitrate. I hope I would, however, be on the waiting list for a coronary angiogram! If I had angina and left ventricular systolic dysfunction I would expect to have a coronary angiogram. I am clearly at high risk of an adverse outcome and would, if at all possible, wish to be considered for coronary artery bypass grafting, if that were indicated. In other words if I have three-vessel disease or two-vessel disease, including a very proximal left anterior descending (LAD) lesion, I would ask for surgery. If I had single-vessel disease with a stenosis involving my proximal LAD I would still prefer an internal mammary graft to PTCA and probably to medical therapy. This is because the clinical trials comparing CABG to PTCA show surgical superiority with this type of lesion. If I had a stenosis involving just one of my other major coronary vessels I would want to think long and hard about what to do. While I would be happy to stick to medical therapy if my LV function was normal and my symptoms settled, I am not so sure if my LV function is impaired. My gut instinct tells me that improved perfusion of an area of myocardium that is both painful and mechanically dysfunctioning is probably a good thing.

References

1   Bangdiwala SI, Weiner DH, Bourassa MG et al, Studies of Left Ventricular Dysfunction (SOLVD) registry: rationale, design, methods and description of baseline characteristics, *Am J Cardiol* (1992)**70**:347–53.

2   Bourassa MG, Gurne O, Bangdiwala SI et al, Natural history and patterns of current practice in heart failure, *J Am Coll Cardiol* (1993)**22**: 14A–19A.

3   Young JB, Weiner DH, Yusuf S et al, Patterns of medication use in patients with heart failure: a report from the Registry of Studies of Left Ventricular Dysfunction (SOLVD), *Southern Med J* (1995)**88**:514–23.

4   Packer M, Kessler PD, Lee WH, Calcium-channel blockade in the management of severe chronic congestive heart failure: a bridge too far, *Circulation* (1987)**75**:V-56–V-64.

5   Packer M, Second generation calcium channel blockers in the treatment of chronic heart failure: are they any better than their predecessors? *J Am Coll Cardiol* (1989)**14**:1339–42.

6   Packer M, Lee WH, Medina N et al, Prognostic importance of the immediate hemodynamic response to nifedipine in patients with severe left ventricular dysfunction, *J Am Coll Cardiol* (1987)**10**:1303–11.

7   Packer M, Pathophysiological mechanisms underlying the adverse effects of calcium channel-blocking drugs in patients with chronic heart failure, *Circulation* (1989)**80**:IV-59–IV67.

8   Elkayam U, Amin J, Mehra A et al, A prospective, randomized, double-blind, crossover study to compare the efficacy and safety of chronic nifedipine therapy with that of isosorbide dinitrate and their combination in the treatment of chronic congestive heart failure, *Circulation* (1990)**82**:1954–61.

9   Barjon JN, Rouleau JL, Bichet D et al, Chronic renal and neurohumoral effects of the calcium entry blocker nisoldipine in patients with congestive heart failure, *J Am Coll Cardiol* (1987)**9**:622–30.

10 Goldstein, RE, Boccuzzi SJ, Cruess D et al, Diltiazem increases late-onset congestive heart failure in postinfarction patients with early reduction in ejection fraction, *Circulation* (1991)**83**:52–60.

11 Hansen JF, Effect of verapamil on mortality and major events after acute myocardial infarction (The Danish Verapamil Infarction Trial II — DAVIT II), *Am J Cardiol* (1990)**66**:779–85.

12 Packer M, O'Connor CM, Ghali JK et al, Effect of amlodipine on morbidity and mortality in severe chronic heart failure, *N Eng J Med* (1996)**335**:1107–14.

13 Packer M, Are nitrates effective in the treatment of chronic heart failure? Antagonist's viewpoint, *Am J Cardiol* (1990)**66**:458–61.

14 Elkayam U, Mehra A, Shotan A, Ostrzega E, Nitrate resistance and tolerance: potential limitations in the treatment of congestive heart failure, *Am J Cardiol* (1992)**70**:98B–104B.

15 Peters RW, Muller JE, Goldstein S et al, Propranolol and the morning increase in the frequency of sudden cardiac death (BHAT Study), *Am J Cardiol* (1989)**63**:1518–20.

16 Yusuf S, Peto R, Lewis J et al, Beta blockade during and after myocardial infarction: an overview of the randomized trials, *Prog Cardiovasc Dis* (1985)**27**:335–71.

17 Yusuf S, Anand S, Avezum A Jr et al, Treatment for acute myocardial infarction. Overview of randomized clinical trials, *Eur Heart J* (1996)**17**:16–29.

18 Boissel JP, Furberg CD, Friedman LM et al, The Beta-Blocker Pooling Project (BBPP): subgroup findings from randomized trials in post infarction patients, *Eur Heart J* (1988)**9**:8–16.

19 Waagstein F, Bristow MR, Swedberg K et al, Beneficial effects of metoprolol in idiopathic dilated cardiomyopathy, *Lancet* (1993)**342**: 1441–6.

20 Lechat P, Jaillon P, Fontaine ML et al, A randomized trial of beta-blockade in heart failure: the Cardiac Insufficiency Bisoprolol Study (CIBIS),*Circulation* (1994)**90**:1765–73.

21 Packer M, Bristow MR, Cohn JN et al, The effect of carvedilol on morbidity and mortality in patients with chronic heart failure, *N Engl J Med* (1996)**334**:1349–55.

22 Cleland JGF, Bristow MR, Erdmann E et al, Beta-blocking agents in heart failure. Should they be used and how? *Eur Heart J* (1996)**17**:1629–39.

23 Zarembski DG, Nolan PE Jr, Slack MK, Lui CY, Meta-analysis of the use of low-dose beta-adrenergic blocking therapy in idiopathic or ischemic dilated cardiomyopathy, *Am J Cardiol* (1996)**77**:1247–50.

24 Colucci WS, Packer M, Bristow MR et al, Carvedilol inhibits clinical progression in patients with mild symptoms of heart failure, *Circulation* (1996)**94**:2800–6.

25 Packer M, Colucci WS, Sackner-Bernstein JD et al, Double-blind, placebo-controlled study of the effects of carvedilol in patients with moderate to severe heart failure: the PRECISE Trial, *Circulation* (1996)**94**:2793–9.

26 Pepine CJ, Ongoing clinical trials of angiotensin-converting enzyme inhibitors for treatment of coronary artery disease in patients with preserved left ventricular function, *J Am Coll Cardiol* (1996)**27**:1048–52.

27 Young JB, ACE inhibitors and ischemic heart disease, *Coron Artery Dis* (1995)**6**:272–80.

28 Lonn EM, Yusuf S, Jha P et al, Emerging role of angiotensin-converting enzyme inhibitors in cardiac and vascular protection, *Circulation* (1994)**90**:2056–69.

29 Rutherford JD, Pfeffer MA, Moye LA et al, Effects of captopril on ischemic events after myocardial infarction: results of the survival and ventricular enlargement trial, *Circulation* (1994)**90**:1731–8.

30 Yusuf S, Pepine CJ, Garces C et al, Effect of enalapril on myocardial infarction and unstable angina in patients with low ejection fractions, *Lancet* (1992)**340**:1173–8.

31 Texter M, Lees RS, Pitt B et al, The QUinapril Ischemic Event Trial (QUIET) design and methods: evaluation of chronic ACE inhibitor therapy after coronary artery intervention, *Cardiovasc Drugs Ther* (1993)**7**:273–82.

32 Cleland JGF, Bulpitt CJ, Falk RH et al, Is aspirin safe for patients with heart failure? *Br Heart J* (1995)**74**:215–19.

33 Klimt CR, Knatterud GL, Stamler J, Meier P, Persantine-aspirin reinfarction study. Part II. Secondary coronary prevention with persantine and aspirin, *J Am Coll Cardiol* (1986)**7**:251–69.

34 Yusuf S, Zucker D, Peduzzi P et al, Effect of coronary artery bypass graft surgery on survival: overview of 10-year results from randomised trials by the Coronary Artery Bypass Graft Surgery Trialists Collaboration, *Lancet* (1994)**344**:563–70.

35 Elefteriades JA, Tolis G Jr, Levi E et al, Coronary artery bypass grafting in severe left ventricular dysfunction: excellent survival with improved ejection fraction and functional state, *J Am Coll Cardiol* (1993)**22**:1411–17.

36 Holmes DR Jr, Detre KM, Williams DO et al, Long-term outcome of patients with depressed left ventricular function undergoing percutaneous transluminal coronary angioplasty: the NHLBI PTCA Registry, *Circulation* (1993)**87**:21–9.

37 Pedersen TR, Randomised trial of cholesterol lowering in 4444 patients with coronary heart disease: the Scandinavian Simvastatin Survival Study (4S), *Lancet* (1994)**344**:1383–9.

38 McMurray J, Slattery J et al, Scandinavian simvastatin study (4S) (1), *Lancet* (1994)**344**:1765–6.

39 Sacks FM, Rouleau JL, Moye LA et al, Baseline characteristics in the cholestrol and recurrent events (CARE) trial of secondary prevention in patients with average serum cholesterol levels, *Am J Cardiol* (1995)**75**:621–3.

40 Pedersen TR, Kjekshus J, Berg K et al, Baseline serum cholesterol and treatment effect in the Scandinavian Simvastatin Survival Study (4S), *Lancet* (1995)**345**:1274–5.

41 Pfeffer MA, Sacks FM, Moye LA et al, Cholesterol and recurrent events: a secondary prevention trial for normolipidemic patients, *Am J Cardiol* (1995)**76**:98C–106C.

42 Kjekshus J, Pedersen TR, Reducing the risk of coronary events: evidence from the Scandinavian Simvastatin Survival Study (4S), *Am J Cardiol* (1995)**76**:64C–68C.

43 Byington RP, Jukema JW, Salonen JT et al, Reduction in cardiovascular events during pravastatin therapy: pooled analysis of clinical events of the pravastatin atherosclerosis inter-

vention program, *Circulation* (1995)**92**:2419–25.

44 Marchioli R, Marfisi RM, Carinci F, Tognoni G, Meta-analysis, clinical trials, and transferability of research results into practice: the case of cholesterol-lowering interventions in the secondary prevention of coronary heart disease, *Arch Intern Med* (1996)**156**:1158–72.

45 Chen Z, Peto R, Collins R et al, Serum cholesterol concentration and coronary heart disease in population with low cholesterol concentrations, *Br Med J* (1991)**303**:276–82.

46 Sacks RM, Pfeffer MA, Moye LA et al, The effect of pravastatin on coronary events after myocardial infarction in patients with average cholesterol levels, *N Engl J Med* (1996)**335**:1001–9.

47 Buchwald H, Campos CT, Boen JR et al, Gender-based mortality follow-up from the program on the surgical control of the hyperlipidemias (POSCH) and meta-analysis of lipid intervention trials: women in POSCH and other lipid trials, *Ann Surg* (1996)**224**:486–500.

48 Yusuf F, Anand S, Cost of prevention — the case of lipid-lowering, *Circulation* (1996)**93**:1774–6.

49 Campaeu L, Knatterud GLMK, Domanski M et al, Effect of aggressive lowering of low- density lipoprotein cholesterol levels and low-dose anticoagulation on obstructive changes in saphenous-vein coronary-artery bypass grafts, *N Engl J Med* (1997) **336**:153–62.

50 Kostis JB, The effect of enalapril on mortal and morbid events in patients with hypertension and left ventricular dysfunction, *Am J Hypertension* (1995)**8**:909–14.

51 Pepine CJ, Cohn PF, Deedwania PC et al, Effects of treatment on outcome in mildly symptomatic patients with ischemia during daily life: the atenolol silent ischemia study (ASIST), *Circulation* (1994)**90**:762–8.

52 Shinton RA, Beevers DG, A meta-analysis of mortality and coronary prevention in hypertensive patients treated with beta-receptor blockers, *J Hum Hypertension* (1990)**4**:31–4.

53 Wikstrand J, Warnold I, Tuomilehto J et al, Metoprolol versus thiazide diuretics in hypertension: morbidity results from the MAPHY study, *Hypertension* (1991)**17**:579–88.

54 Yusuf S, Calcium antagonists in coronary artery disease and hypertension: time for reevaluation? *Circulation* (1995)**92**:1079–82.

55 Furberg CD, Psaty BM, Meyer JV, Nifedipine. Dose related increase in mortality in patients with coronary heart disease, *Circulation* (1995)**92**:1326–31.

56 Furberg CD, Psaty BM, Corrections to the nifedipine meta-analysis (letter), *Circulation* (1996) **93**:1475–6.

57 Psaty BM, Heckbert SR, Koepsell TD et al, The risk of myocardial infarction associated with antihypertensive drug therapies, *J Am Med Assoc* (1995)**274**:620–5.

58 Yusuf S, Held P, Furberg C, Update of effects of calcium antagonists in myocardial infarction or angina in light of the second Danish verapamil infarction trial (DAVIT-II) and other recent studies, *Am J Cardiol* (1991)**67**:1295–7.

59 Yusuf S, Verapamil following uncomplicated myocardial infarction: promising, but not proven, *Am J Cardiol* (1996)**77**:421–2.

60 Rehnqvist N, Hjemdahl P, Billing E et al, Effects of metoprolol vs verapamil in patients with stable angina pectoris. The Angina Prognosis Study in Stockholm (APSIS), *Eur Heart J* (1996)**17**:76–81.

61 Bagger JP, Helligsoe P, Randsbaek F et al, Effect of verapamil in intermittent claudication – A randomized, double-blind, placebo-controlled, cross-over study after individual dose-response assessment, *Circulation* (1997) **95**:411–14.

62 Beta Blocker Heart Attack Trial Research Group, A randomised trial of propranolol in patients with acute myocardial infarction. II. Morbidity results, *J Am Med Assoc* (1983)**250**:2814–19.

63 Olsson G, Lubsen J, van Es GA, Rehnqvist N, Quality of life after myocardial infarction: effect of long term metoprolol on mortality and morbidity, *Br Med J* (1986)**292**:1491–3.

64 Kendall MJ, Lynch KP, Hjalmarson A, Kjekshus J, Beta-Blockers and sudden cardiac death, *Ann Intern Med* (1995)**123**:358–67.

65 Alderman EL, Andrews K, Bost J et al, Comparison of coronary bypass surgery with angioplasty in patients with multivessel disease: the Bypass Angioplasty Revascularization

Investigation (BARI) investigators, *N Engl J Med* (1996)**335**:217–25.

66 Kip KE, Faxon DP, Detre KM et al, Coronary angioplasty in diabetic patients: the National Heart, Lung, and Blood Institute percutaneous transluminal coronary angioplasty registry, *Circulation* (1996)**94**:1818–25.

67 St Claire DA Jr, King SB III, Effect of diabetes mellitus on outcome after percutaneous transluminal coronary angioplasty, *Coron Artery Dis* (1996)**7**:744–52.

68 JullMoller S, Edvardsson N, Jahnmatz B et al, Double-blind trial of aspirin in primary prevention of myocardial infarction in patients with stable chronic angina pectoris, *Lancet* (1992)**340**:1421–5.

69 Gent M, A randomised, blinded, trial of clopidogrel versus aspirin in patients at risk of ischaemic events (CAPRIE), *Lancet* (1996)**348**:1329–39.

70 Cleland JGF, Cowburn PJ, Falk RH, Should all patients with atrial fibrillation receive warfarin? Evidence from randomized clinical trials, *Eur Heart J* (1996)**17**:674–81.

71 Cowburn P, Cleland JGF, SPAF-III results, *Eur Heart J* (1996)**17**:1129.

72 Almony GT, Lefkovits J, Topol EJ, Antiplatelet and anticoagulant use after myocardial infarction, *Clin Cardiol* (1996)**19**:357–65.

73 Julian DG, Chamberlain DA, Pocock SJ et al, A comparison of aspirin and anticoagulation following thrombolysis for myocardial infarction (the AFTER study): a multicentre unblinded randomised clinical trial, *Br Med J* (1996)**313**:1429–31.

74 Turpie AGG, Gent M, Laupacis A et al, A comparison of aspirin with placebo in patients treated with warfarin after heart-valve replacement, *N Engl J Med* (1993)**329**:524–9.

75 Lewis RV, McMurray J, McDevitt DG, Effects of atenolol, verapamil, and xamoterol on heart rate and exercise tolerance in digitalised patients with chronic atrial fibrillation, *J Cardiovasc Pharmacol* (1989)**13**:1–6.

76 Leor J, Goldbourt U, Behar S, Is it safe to prescribe digoxin after acute myocardial infarction? Update on continued controversy, *Am Heart J* (1995)**130**:1322–3.

77 Kober L, TorpPedersen C, Carlsen JE et al, A clinical trial of the angiotensin-converting-enzyme inhibitor trandolapril in patients with left ventricular dysfunction after myocardial infarction, *N Engl J Med* (1995)**333**:1670–6.

78 Rogers WJ, Epstein AE, Arciniegas JG et al, Preliminary report: effect of encainide and flecainide on mortality in a randomized trial of arrhythmia suppression after myocardial infarction, *N Engl J Med* (1989)**321**:406–12.

79 Rogers WJ, Epstein AE, Arciniegas JG et al, Effect of the antiarrhythmic agent moricizine on survival after myocardial infarction, *N Engl J Med* (1992)**327**:227–33.

80 Epstein AE, Hallstrom AP, Rogers WJ et al, Mortality following ventricular arrhythmia suppression by encainide, flecainide, and moricizine after myocardial infarction: the original design concept of the Cardiac Arrhythmia Suppression Trial (CAST), *JAMA* (1993)**270**:2451–5.

81 Julian DG, Camm AJ, Frangin G et al, Randomised trial of effect of amiodarone on mortality in patients with left-ventricular dysfunction after recent myocardial infarction: EMIAT, *Lancet* (1997)**349**:667–74.

82 Cairns JA, Connolly SJ, Roberts R et al, Randomised trial of outcome after myocardial infarction in patients with frequent or repetitive ventricular premature depolarisations: CAMIAT, *Lancet* (1997)**349**:675–82.

83 Moss AJ, Hall WJ, Cannom DS et al, Improved survival with an implanted difibrillator in patients with coronary heart disease at high risk for ventricular arrhythmia, *N Engl J Med* (1996)**335**:1933-40.

84 Fiore MC, Jorenby DE, Baker TB et al, Tobacco dependence and the nicotine patch—clinical guidelines for effective use, *JAMA* (1997)**268**:2687–94.

85 Fiore MC, Smith SS, Jorenby DE et al, The effectiveness of the nicotine patch for smoking cessation–a metanalysis, *JAMA* (1994)**271**:1940–7.

6

To stent or not to stent?

Kim H Tan and Graham Jackson

Introduction

Since its inception in 1977, percutaneous trans-luminal coronary angioplasty has established itself as an efficacious procedure in the treatment of obstructive coronary artery disease.[1] However, despite marked advances in angioplasty technology, greater operator experience, and the use of adjunctive pharmacotherapy, deficiencies persist which have restricted its application. The two primary limitations of conventional balloon angioplasty are early abrupt vessel closure at the time of the procedure causing acute complications, and late restenosis that leads to recurrent ischaemia.[2–11] New interventional devices such as atherectomy and laser have been introduced in an effort to improve upon these deficiencies and expand the application of percutaneous revascularization. Although many of these devices have improved the acute results, most have not fulfilled their expectations in salvaging abrupt vessel occlusion and preventing late restenosis.[12–16] As a result, the initial enthusiasm has waned as experience has increased. However in contrast, the last few years has seen a dramatic increase in the utilization of stents, which have adopted a prominent and expanding role in today's practice of interventional cardiology.

Dotter and Judkins were the first to propose stenting as a technique for transluminal treatment of an arteriosclerotic obstruction,[17] and the first stents were implanted in human coronary arteries in 1986 by Sigwart et al.[18] Much of our current understanding and expectations from intracoronary stenting have been derived from early observational studies combined with recent well conducted and comprehensive randomized trials. Although preliminary data showed that intracoronary stenting proved its utility in overcoming the two major residual problems of conventional balloon angioplasty, initially they also highlighted the substantial risks associated with stenting which may be considered likely to outweigh the benefits. The perceived need for intensive anticoagulation therapy required prolonged hospitalization and resulted in bleeding problems (manifesting as a need for transfusions or major peripheral vascular complications occurring at the femoral puncture site). Early reports also demonstrated a 3.5–17% risk of acute or subacute thrombosis of the stent, depending on the stent design and indications for implantation, with resulting serious clinical sequelae.[19–33] Importantly, stent implantation was (and remains) expensive, and the long-term results remains unknown. These difficulties were the main reasons why major concerns were raised about the use of stent implantation in the early 1990s.

However, it is fair to say that the early stent technique was crude, and stents were frequently imprecisely and inadequately employed. Furthermore, there were marked inconsistencies in operator technique, equipment design, and adjunct pharmacotherapy. Over the last few years the pioneering work of some investigators has made great strides in overcoming some of the deficiencies and risks associated with intra-coronary stenting. This in turn has led to a relatively uncontrolled expansion of the indications for stenting, including clinical settings in which the evidence to support its use remains elusive, leading to a phenomenon currently termed as 'stent fever'.

This chapter aims to review the available evidence on the use of intracoronary stents in the various angiographic and/or clinical settings. The role of anticoagulation and antiplatelet therapy and intravascular ultrasound in guiding stent employment will also be discussed. A management strategy for each of the clinical settings, based on currently available evidence and risk–benefit analysis rather than on the technical feasibility of stenting, will then be proposed.

Indications for coronary stenting

The decision of whether or not to deploy a stent after an interventional procedure is based either on the angiographic findings or clinical status of the patient. The current indications for intracoronary stenting include:

- bail-out therapy of acute and threatened vessel closure,
- nonelective treatment of a suboptimal angiographic result after conventional balloon angioplasty,
- elective stenting of primary lesions in native coronary arteries, saphenous vein grafts, restenotic lesions, and total occlusions.

Before implanting a stent, the clinical indication, the angiographic parameters, and the structural design of the available stents must be taken into consideration. There are currently more than 10 stent designs commercially available (Table 6.1, Figure 6.1). Familiarity

with the technical properties of the various stent designs (in particular, the profile in the unexpanded state, trackability, longitudinal flexibility, mechanism of employment, and whether shortening occurs with deployment) holds the key to a successful intracoronary stent implantation.

Bail-out stenting

The ischaemic complications encountered during balloon mechanical barotrauma (death, myocardial infarction, and emergency coronary artery bypass surgery) arise frequently as a result of abrupt occlusion of the vessel being dilated, with a reported incidence ranging from 2% to 14%.[34–39] Although the proposed mechanisms responsible for abrupt vessel occlusion include subintimal haemorrhage, thrombus formation, arterial spasm, and acute elastic recoil, the inciting event is usually a complex dissection with occlusive intimal flap formation. Current treatment strategies for dealing with abrupt vessel occlusion include redilatation (prolonged inflations, larger balloons, or auto-

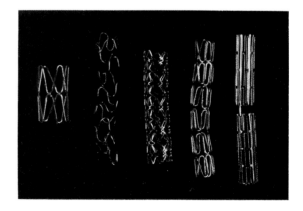

Figure 6.1
Examples of some of the commercially available coronary stents. From left to right: Microstent (6 mm), Wiktor, Nir, Microstent (18 mm), Palmaz-Schatz.

Coronary stent	Deployment	Design	Composition	Metallic SA	Radio-opacity
Gianturco-Roubin	Balloon-expandable	Clam shell flexible coil loop	Stainless steel	~ 10%	±
Palmaz-Schatz	Balloon-expandable	Slotted tube	Stainless steel	~ 20%	±
Multilink	Balloon-expandable	Zig-zag serial rings joined by multiple links	Stainless steel	7–15%	±
Wallstent	Self-expanding	Multiple wire braid	Colbalt-based alloy (Elgiloy)	~ 20%	++
Microstent	Balloon-expandable	Zig-zag axial struts, welded/ unwelded in series	Stainless steel	~ 8%	++
Freedom	Balloon-expandable	Single wire fish bone	Stainless steel	11–15%	++
Wiktor	Balloon-expandable	Single wire sinusoidal helicoid coil	Tantalum	~ 8%	+++
Cordis	Balloon-expandable	Single wire sinusoidal helicoid coil	Tantalum	~ 15%	++++
Nir	Balloon-expandable	Multicellular rectangular mesh	Stainless steel	14–19%	±
ACT One	Balloon-expandable	Slotted tube	Nitinol	~ 39%	++

Metallic SA = surface area of stent when expanded to noincal diameter.

Table 6.1
Structural designs of some of the commercially available coronary stents.

perfusion balloons), intracoronary vasodilators, or intracoronary thrombolytics.[40–43] The efficacy is limited and ischaemic complications persist in a substantial proportion of patients despite these manoeuvres.

By virtue of their scaffolding nature, stents are unmatched in their ability to seal a dissection and restore vessel patency. In the bail-out situation, the tough primary lesion has already been dilated when the stent is being implanted and the function of the stent is to restore the threatened vessel to near normal geometry by pushing plaque material and dissected intimal flaps aside. Hence, irrespective of their design, most of the commercially available stents have been used successfully for this purpose, although it is likely that those with a low metallic surface area may be more suited to the more thrombogenic substrate of bail-out stenting (Figure 6.2). These observational studies have suggested that implantation of the Wallstent, Gianturco-Roubin stent, Palmaz-Schatz stent, Microstent, and Wiktor stent may be of value in bail-out management and reduce the need for emergency bypass surgery.[44–49] Accordingly, bail-out stenting (stent-by) is now considered a definitive treatment and not just a bridge to surgery (stand-by). However, despite the gratifying acute results, long-term follow-up data are lacking. Currently in progress are multiple prospective randomized trials (for example, GRACE and TASC II) comparing the immediate and long-term efficacy of bail-out stenting with long balloon inflation or other interventional devices. The results of some of these trials should become available in the near future and preliminary results have been encouraging.[50,51]

Elective stenting

Restenosis, the phenomenon of renarrowing at the treatment site after conventional balloon angioplasty, occurs in 30–50% of patients within the first 6 months.[52–55] The exact pathophysiological mechanisms that lead to restenosis remain unclear, which means that they are likely to be multifactorial. In addition to the contribution of early elastic recoil, coronary spasm, platelet deposition, and neointimal hyperplasia, recent studies have shown that chronic geometric remodelling also plays an important role in the process of restenosis.[56] Despite the extensive theoretical benefits, the influence of pharmacological treatment on restenosis remains unproven.[57] Many new devices were introduced in an attempt to reduce the amount of intimal hyperplasia by producing a less reactive luminal surface and providing a larger post-treatment luminal diameter. However, apart from primary stent implantation, most of these devices have, until now, failed to reduce the problem of restenosis and provide better long-term outcome than conventional balloon angioplasty.[58–62]

Stents reduce restenosis by preventing early elastic recoil, resetting the vessel size of the stented segment, and resisting late geometric remodelling (Figures 6.3 and 6.4). The normalized rheology results in less turbulent blood flow across the stented segment. This should reduce the 'response to injury' cascade, which ultimately leads to smooth muscle cell proliferation and neointimal hyperplasia.[63,64] Since the primary objective of elective stenting is to reduce late restenosis, a stent design with extensive scaffolding and strong radial force should be used. This will prevent early encroachment on the lumen by intimal protrusion and recoil, and reduce late lumen renarrowing due to intimal hyperplasia through the interstrut intervals.

Despite the encouraging results of observational studies on the benefits of intracoronary stenting with multiple stent designs, to date only the Palmaz-Schatz tubular slotted design has been demonstrated by the rigours of comprehensive randomized trials to improve

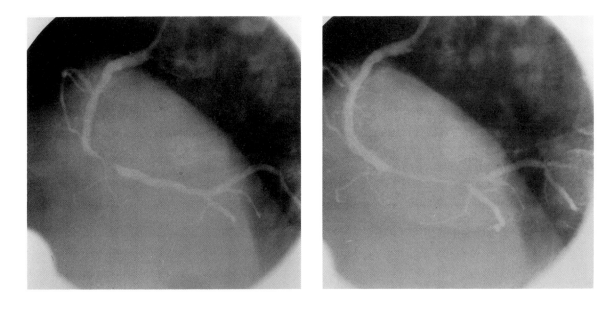

A   B

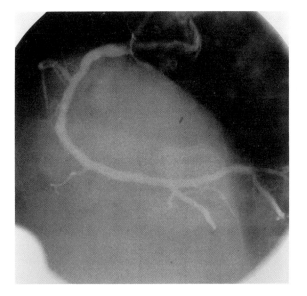

C

Figure 6.2
Bail-out stenting (LAO projection). (A) High-grade lesion in the right coronary artery. (B) Abrupt occlusion with extensive spiral dissection after balloon dilatation. (C) Final angiographic outcome after implantation of a single long Microstent.

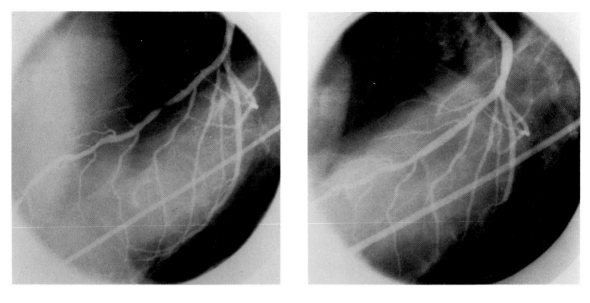

A

B

Figure 6.3
Elective stenting (LAO projection with cranial tilt). (A) Focal high-grade lesion in the mid-segment of the left anterior descending artery. (B) Final angiographic result after implantation of a single Multilink stent.

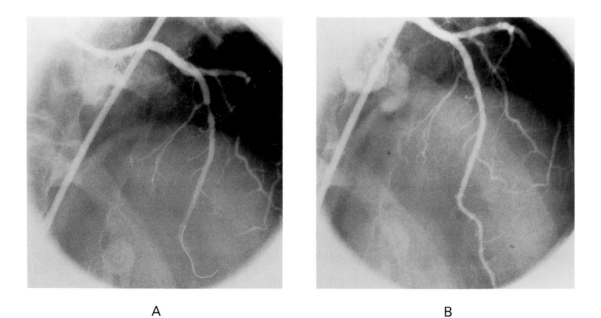

A

B

Figure 6.4
Elective stenting (RAO projection with cranial tilt). (A) Focal high-grade lesion in the mid-segment of the left anterior descending artery. (B) Final angiographic result after implantation of a single Palmaz-Schatz stent.

late angiographic and clinical outcome over conventional balloon angioplasty.[19,20] In fact, the STRESS and BENESTENT trials (see Table 6.2 for definitions of trial acronyms) have been instrumental in popularizing the recent enormous increase in stent utilization. These trials have shown that fewer patients with stents underwent repeat target vessel revascularization for ischaemia than patients treated with conventional balloon angioplasty, and the benefit was maintained up to at least 1 year after the procedure.[65] Multiple clinical trials are currently in progress to evaluate the efficacy of the various other stent designs in reducing restenosis (for example, WIDEST, START). Whereas these randomized studies will go a long way towards improving our ability to decide whether or not to implant a stent electively, many patients with complex coronary disease are not being included in the study populations, especially those with small vessel diameter, long lesions, ostial lesions, and bifur-

cational lesions. At present, the decision on whether or not to implant a stent in these patients will have to rely on clinical judgement in the absence of data from randomized trials.

Conditional stenting

The term conditional stenting refers to the nonelective use of stents in the treatment of a suboptimal result after conventional balloon angioplasty. This strategy is reasonable because dilatation with conventional balloon angioplasty is required in most patients before they undergo intracoronary stent placement. However, there is no universally accepted definition of a suboptimal angiographic result, and the final post-treatment luminal diameter that interventionists consider acceptable has changed over the years. Early definitions of angiographic success required a reduction in stenosis severity of only 10–20% of normal luminal diameter; this remains the definition used by

GRACE	Gianturco-Roubin stent in Acute Closure Evaluation
TASC II	Trial of Angioplasty and Stents in Canada
STRESS	STEnt REStenosis Study
BENESTENT	BElgian NEtherlands STENT study
WIDEST	WIktor in DEnovo STenosis study
START	STent versus Angioplasty Restenosis Trial
CAVEAT	Coronary Angioplasty Versus Excisional Atherectomy Trial
SAVED	Stent versus balloon Angioplasty for aortocoronary saphenous VEin bypass graft Disease
SPACTO	Stent versus PTCA After recanalization of Chronic Total coronary Occlusions
SICCO	Stenting In Chronic Coronary Occlusion trial
REST	REstenosis STent study
STENTIM	STENTing In acute Myocardial infarction
STAMI	STenting for Acute Myocardial Infarction
PAMI	Primary Angioplasty for Myocardial Infarction trial
MUSIC	Multicentre Ultrasound Stent In Coronary artery disease
MUST	MUlticentre Stents Ticlopidine study
TASTE	Ticlopidine Aspirin STent Evaluation

Table 6.2
Acronyms of clinical trials.

the National Heart, Lung, and Blood Institute.[66,67] The guidelines published by the American College of Cardiology/American Heart Association define angiographic success as a ≥20% change in luminal diameter, with the final diameter stenosis <50%.[68] Given the generally accepted doctrine 'the bigger, the better', operators are now striving for better acute angiographic results.[69,70] Data from the Thoraxcentre in The Netherlands have shown that 'stent-like' conventional balloon angioplasty results, defined as diameter stenosis of ≤30%, result in a clinical and angiographic long-term outcome equivalent to stenting.[71] Hence, it is now more commonly accepted that a residual stenosis after conventional balloon angioplasty of >30% is considered suboptimal. In this setting, as for elective stenting, the primary objective is to prevent early recoil and reduce late restenosis (Figure 6.5). Hence a stent proffering strong radial support with extensive scaffolding will be preferable. Several observational studies have reported on the feasibility and efficacy of this approach.[72,73] Furthermore, Kimura et al. have shown that, compared with a cohort of patients treated with conventional balloon angioplasty alone, patients receiving an intracoronary Palmaz-Schatz stent had no significant loss in diameter gain at 24-hour follow-up angiography and a lower incidence of restenosis at 6-month follow-up angiography.[74] Rodriguez et al. also reported that, compared with a control group, intracoronary Gianturco-Roubin stent implantation in patients who exhibit early loss in minimal luminal diameter detected at 24-hour angiography improves the long-term angiographic outcome and reduces the need for subsequent revascularization procedures.[75] However, despite the increasing enthusiasm among interventionists to treat these suboptimal results with stent implantation, this practice is not supported by any data from randomized

trials. Given that stents undoubtedly promote a more extensive intimal proliferative response than balloon angioplasty, we should await the results of randomized trials before drawing final conclusions on the merits of stent implantation in this clinical setting.

Stenting in saphenous vein grafts

Treatment options are limited for patients who have recurrent symptoms from saphenous vein graft disease after prior coronary artery bypass grafting. The three major mechanisms that play a role in saphenous vein graft occlusion are thrombosis, intimal hyperplasia, and atherosclerosis.[76] Despite improvements in myocardial protection and increased surgical experience, repeat operation is associated with higher mortality and morbidity, and provides less satisfactory symptom relief than is achieved with the primary operation.[77,78] Although conventional balloon angioplasty has been applied with encouraging acute results, periprocedural complications are not uncommon, and frequently occur as a result of distal particulate embolization of atheroma in the older saphenous vein grafts, which tend to contain diffuse, bulky, friable, and thrombotic lesions.[79–82] Moreover, the resenosis rate is strikingly high at 60–70%.[83,84] Many new devices have been introduced as alternatives to conventional balloon angioplasty, including extraction and directional atherectomy and excimer laser angioplasty.[85–90] Despite the encouraging results of earlier observational studies, only one randomized study has been completed. The CAVEAT II study has demonstrated that directional atherectomy has little advantage over conventional balloon angioplasty in focal low-risk saphenous vein graft lesions and the problems of distal particulate embolization and late restenosis remain unsolved.[91,92]

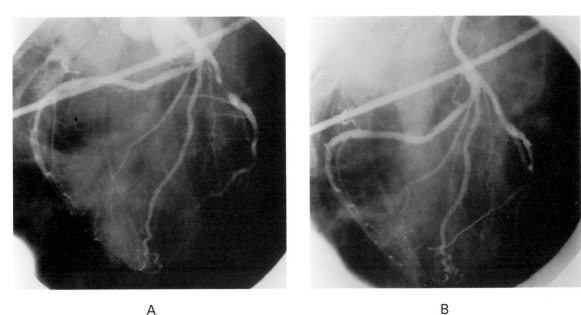

A   B

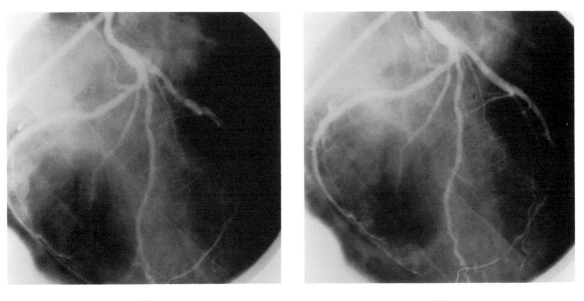

C   D

Figure 6.5
Conditional stenting (RAO projection with caudal tilt). (A) High-grade lesion in the proximal segment of the left anterior descending artery. (B) Good angiographic result immediately after balloon dilatation. (C) Elastic recoil occurring 5 minutes after balloon dilatation. (D) Final angiographic result after implantation of a single NIr stent.

The ability of stents to provide a more predictable angiographic outcome and reduce distal particulate embolization into the subtended coronary artery bed, is attributable to their latticework designs, which prevent plaque dislodgement and entrap the friable atheromatous debris (Figures 6.6 and 6.7). In addition, the enhanced resistance to radial compression may prevent external saphenous vein graft compression and geometric plaque remodelling, which may reduce late lumen loss. In this clinical setting, stents with extensive scaffolding, higher metallic surface area, and short interstrut distance, for example the Wallstent, should be chosen.[93] Observational studies have suggested that stent implantation results in a greater improvement in immediate angiographic results, lower embolization frequency, and more favourable long-term outcomes than conventional coronary angioplasty.[94–98] Preliminary results from the SAVED trial, comparing conventional balloon angioplasty with stent implantation of focal *de novo* saphenous vein graft stenoses, have shown that stenting was associated with a higher procedural success rate, a larger improvement in postprocedure minimal luminal diameter, and a trend towards fewer non-Q wave myocardial infarcts and greater net luminal gain at 6 months.[99] The final results are eagerly awaited to allow proper assessment of the full impact of stent placement for the treatment of saphenous vein graft lesions.

Stenting in chronic total occlusions

Chronic total occlusions are found in 10–20% of patients referred for coronary angioplasty.[67] Although the procedure is technically feasible, recanalization of a chronic total occlusion by

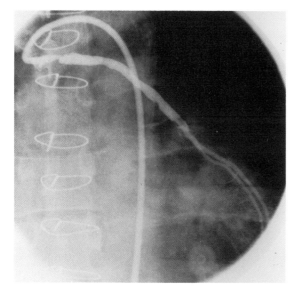
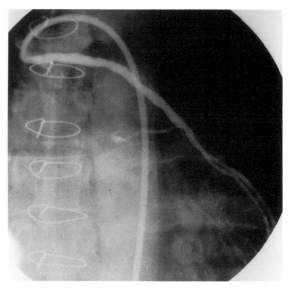

A   B

Figure 6.6
Stenting in saphenous vein grafts (PA projection with caudal tilt). (A) Proximal and distal lesions in a saphenous vein graft to the circumflex marginal artery. (B) Final angiographic result after implantation of two Multilink stents.

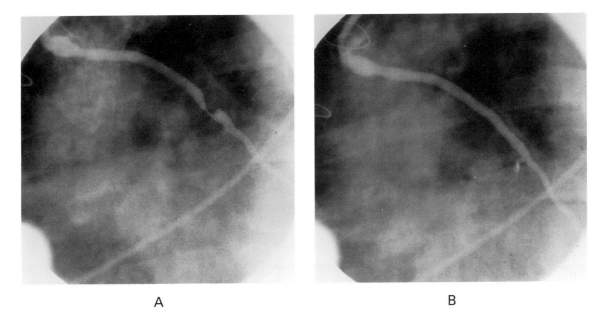

A   B

Figure 6.7
Stenting in saphenous vein grafts (LAO projection). (A) Lesion in the body of a saphenous vein graft to the circumflex marginal artery. (B) Final angiographic result after implantation of a single Palmaz-Schatz stent.

angioplasty is often considered to be a relative contraindication because of low initial success rates, high equipment costs, long periods of exposure to fluoroscopy, and disappointingly high rates of restenosis ranging from 40% to 77%.[100–104] Thus, many patients with chronic total occlusions are referred for coronary artery bypass surgery, even in the presence of single-vessel coronary artery disease. Given the complexity of the procedure, preventive therapy to reduce the likelihood of restenosis after successful recanalization is of particular importance in this subset of patients. The theoretical mechanisms by which stent implantation may lower the rate of restenosis are those that have already been discussed under the section on elective stenting. These include reducing the incidence of undetected abrupt closure, achieving a larger final minimal lumen diameter, limiting acute and chronic recoil, and resisting late geometric remodelling (Figure 6.8). After recanalization of chronic total occlusions, the vessel distal to the point of occlusion is often found to be extensively diseased, and the use of long stents or multiple stents is often necessary to reconstruct the entire vessel. To date, published results for stenting of chronically occluded vessels have been limited to observational series.[105] The results from these studies have suggested that stent implantation is associated with a beneficial long-term angiographic outcome. These favourable results have provided the impetus for randomized clinical trials, many of which are currently in progress (for example, SPACTO, SICCO). Preliminary data from the SICCO trial — a multicentre, randomized, controlled study — have shown that primary stenting in chronic coronary occlusions improves the long-term clinical and angiographic outcome.[106]

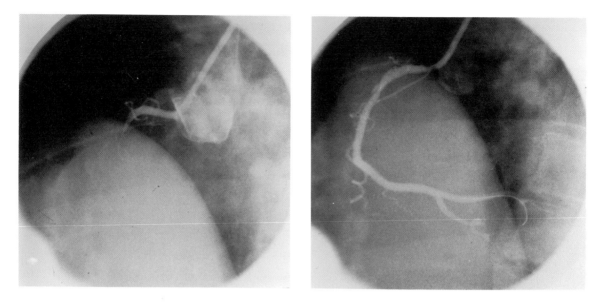

A   B

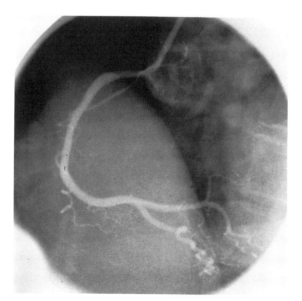

C

Figure 6.8
Stenting in chronic total occlusions (LAO projection). (A) Chronic total occlusion of a right coronary artery. (B) Occlusion recanalized with balloon angioplasty. (C) Final angiographic result after implantation of a single Microstent.

Stenting in recurrent (secondary) restenosis

With the expansion of the indications for percutaneous interventional procedures, the management of patients with recurrent restenosis has become a common but difficult clinical problem. Although treatment of restenosis with a repeat angioplasty has become routine clinical practice and is accepted as an integral part of the overall revascularization strategy, it is nevertheless associated with a significant incidence of further restenosis, ranging from 26% to 34%.[107–110] Since intracoronary stent implantation has been shown to improve late angiographic outcome in *de novo* lesions, it makes intuitive sense that stent implantation in this clinical setting should provide long-term clinical benefit. However, there is little information on the efficacy of stent implantation in this clinical setting and the limited observational data have shown disparate results.[111–113] Preliminary results of the REST study, a multicentre randomized trial comparing the implantation of a single Palmaz-Schatz stent with balloon angioplasty in patients with restenosis in native coronary arteries, have shown favourable acute and long-term angiographic outcomes with intracoronary stenting.[114] Results from other randomized trials that are ongoing should allow an informed assessment of the merits of stenting in restenotic lesions.

Stenting in acute coronary syndromes

After an acute myocardial infarction, early coronary artery recanalization reduces infarct size and improves survival. Recanalization can be achieved by either an intravenous thrombolytic agent or immediate coronary angioplasty, first introduced by Hartzler et al. in 1983.[115] Three recent prospective randomized studies have confirmed the greater effectiveness of immediate angioplasty in restoring patency and preventing reocclusion of the infarct-related artery compared with the best thrombolytic treatment.[116–118] Although conventional balloon angioplasty is usually successful, failure to achieve reperfusion is associated with a high mortality.[119–122] Furthermore, the incidence of reocclusion with conventional balloon angioplasty in acute coronary syndromes is greater than in the elective setting because of a greater risk of significant intimal dissection and the local environment is highly thrombogenic.[20,25,123] Although reocclusion is often asymptomatic, the survival benefit is negated.[120,122]

The use of intracoronary stents to maintain patency in acute myocardial infarction and unstable angina, especially if intracoronary thrombus is present, has been contraindicated because of the intense activation of the clotting mechanism and high incidence of subacute stent occlusion.[124] Although it seems logical to avoid the placement of thrombogenic stents into an artery that potentially contains fresh thrombus, recent registry studies from Neumann et al., Le May et al., STENTIM I French Registry, and the Stent Without Coumadin French Registry have shown that with the improvement of implantation techniques and the development of better antithrombotic strategies, not only can a high primary success in restoring vessel patency be achieved, but the thrombotic risk is also dramatically reduced.[125–128] Furthermore, the presence of angiographically visible intracoronary thrombus does not preclude a good outcome and is not predictive of reocclusion (Figure 6.9).[129] Although these results are encouraging, the precise indication for stenting as an adjunct to immediate coronary angioplasty in patients with acute coronary syndromes and the optimal antithrombotic

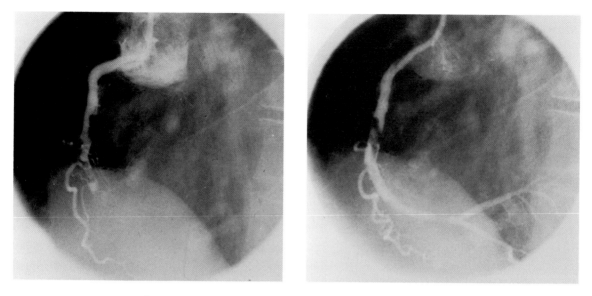

A   B

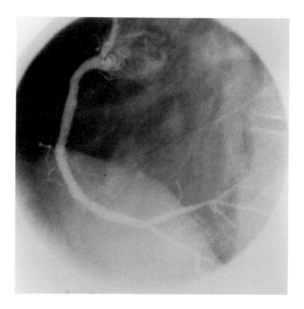

C

Figure 6.9
Stenting in acute coronary syndromes (LAO projection). (A) Occluded right coronary artery in a patient with unstable angina. (B) Angiographic appearance after balloon dilatation with evidence of extensive thrombus formation. (C) Final angiographic result after implantation of three Microstents.

strategy, remains to be determined by randomized trials (for example, PAMI III, STENTIM II, STAMI).

Anticoagulation regimen and intravascular ultrasound

Although the efficacy of stents in various clinical settings has been demonstrated, subacute stent thrombosis has emerged as a serious potential complication. Since coronary stents are metallic and thrombogenic, various anticoagulation regimens have been advocated, including the use of heparin, dextran, warfarin, aspirin, sulphinpyrazone, dipyridamole, and thrombolytics. Despite a stringent anticoagulation regimen, the incidence of subacute stent thrombosis remains significant, ranging from 3.5% to 17%, depending on the stent design and indications for implantation.[19–21,24,27–33] This aggressive anticoagulation regimen also resulted in a high incidence of bleeding complications, manifesting as major peripheral vascular complications or need for transfusions, and subsequently prolonged hospital stay.

Colombo et al. were the first to suggest that the key issue in prevention of subacute stent thrombosis is optimization of stent implantation and not perfect control of haemostasis.[130] The use of intravascular ultrasound has shown that more than 80% of stents may be underexpanded despite apparent angiographically successful implantation, even with automated quantitative analysis. Incomplete stent apposition, persistence of residual luminal narrowing due to incomplete or asymmetrical stent expansion, proximal or distal dissections not covered by the stent, poor inflow or outflow, small vessel diameter less than 3 mm, and presence of significant disease of the proximal and distal reference segment are factors that predispose to stent thrombosis. These investigators have shown that if the entire lesion is treated routinely using high-pressure dilatation and intravascular ultrasound to document optimal stent expansion and lesion coverage, then anticoagulation would be rendered superfluous. Hence, the post-stenting medication protocol has been modified accordingly, and the stringent anticoagulation regimen consisting of heparin, aspirin, and coumadin have been replaced by the combination of aspirin and/or ticlopidine. The improved stent implantation technique and the modified antithrombotic regimen have reduced the subacute stent thrombosis rate to less than 2% and virtually abolished the bleeding complications.[131,132] These registry data have been validated by the preliminary results from the MUSIC trial.[133] This is a multicentre, open, prospective, observational study to test the concept of using intravascular ultrasound-guided optimized stent expansion to obviate the need for systemic anticoagulation. The incidence of subacute stent thrombosis in this study was 0.6%.

However, intravascular ultrasound is a time-consuming and costly investigation which is not without risk.[134] Furthermore, the routine use of high-pressure inflation with a larger balloon during stent implantation may obviate the need for intravascular ultrasound guidance. This view is supported by the encouraging data from the Stent Without Coumadin French Registry, which reported on more than 1000 patients treated with aspirin and ticlopidine after stenting without using intravascular ultrasound guidance. The incidence of subacute stent thrombosis was less than 2%.[131] The MUST study — an open, prospective, multicentre, observational study — was designed to validate the concept of stenting with aspirin and ticlopidine as sole post-stenting treatment without intravascular ultrasound guidance.[135] Preliminary results have shown a subacute thrombosis rate of 1.2%. Similar conclusions have also been reached by the TASTE study.[136] Hence, the precise role of intravascular ultrasound in guiding stent implantation must be specifically addressed in a randomized trial before it can be advocated widely, especially in the current financial climate. Several randomized trials will soon report whether implantation guided by ultrasound is necessary and gives a better long-term outcome.

Research into novel methods of rendering the stent more thromboresistant are also in progress. A covalently heparin-bound Palmaz-Schatz stent will be studied in the BENESTENT II clinical trial and results from the pilot phase have shown a 0% subacute stent thrombosis rate with just aspirin and ticlopidine.[137] Other adjunct pharmacology that has shown promise includes improved antiplatelet agents (for example, monoclonal antibodies to glycoprotein IIb/IIIa) and antithrombins such as hirudin and Hirulog.[138,139]

Contraindications for stenting

Despite the multitude of clinical settings in which stenting is either indicated and/or beneficial, there are still some absolute or relative contraindications to stent implantation. In these situations, stents should be avoided if at all possible and an alternative management strategy should be sought, although this may not always be available. Contraindications include:

- any bleeding diathesis or active peptic ulcer disease which renders either antiplatelet or anticoagulation treatment a contraindication,
- inadequate guiding catheter support,
- small vessel diameter <2.5 mm,
- vessels with poor distal run-off, which increases the risk of stent thrombosis,

- extreme vessel tortuosity, which reduces the likelihood of successful stent delivery and implantation at the lesion site,
- large amount of thrombus at the lesion site, although the presence of thrombus *per se* need not deter stent implantation,
- undilatable or heavily calcified stenosis, which may require pretreatment with rotational atherectomy.

Conclusions

When Andreas Gruntzig introduced coronary balloon angioplasty in 1977, he could not have foreseen how quickly this technique would develop and become accepted as part of routine clinical practice. His pioneering work opened the era of interventional cardiology and since then, coronary balloon angioplasty has emerged as a major tool in the armamentarium for treating coronary artery disease. The growth of coronary balloon angioplasty has triggered the development of new coronary revascularization technologies, in an attempt to overcome some of the limitations of the original angioplasty technique. For new devices to become established, they must be able to demonstrate clear advantages over conventional balloon angioplasty, especially where the latter tends to do poorly (for example, with complex lesion morphology) or prove their clinical utility in overcoming some of the residual problems of conventional angioplasty (for example, abrupt vessel closure and restenosis). With many of these devices, the initial promise has not been fulfilled, and the expectations have been scaled back accordingly. The only exception is intracoronary stents, which have fulfilled their initial promise, and appear to have realized an increasing potential in ever-expanding clinical settings. Stents appear to be unmatched in their ability to:

- restore vessel patency in the event of an abrupt occlusion,
- improve acute lumen dimensions, long-term angiographic and clinical outcome,
- offer a more predictable early and late angiographic outcome in saphenous vein grafts.

Stents are also establishing a bigger role in the treatment of chronic total occlusions, acute coronary syndromes, and recurrent restenosis. Despite their apparent potential, maintaining an awareness of the many potential problems and deficiencies will hopefully facilitate meaningful progress in this vital field. Not least are the cost implications in a time of limited resources and financial constraints, especially as the in-hospital and 1-year cost analyses of stenting compared with conventional balloon angioplasty are currently discouraging (Figure 6.10).[140] Hopefully, further prospective cost analysis studies taking into account ongoing refinements in stent design, implantation techniques, and antithrombotic regimens, will clarify the economic impact of this proecudure. None the less, based on available data, coronary stent implantation has already become

established in interventional therapeutic cardiology. Future refinements should be directed at improving stent designs (optimal metal coverage ratios, greater size and length variability, improved flexibility, better delivery systems, and increased radio-opacity), extending the indications to more complex clinical settings (small vessels, longer lesions, unfavourable morphology, and multivessel coronary stenting), optimizing implantation strategies, and improving adjuvant therapies.

If I had . . .

If I had a coronary artery lesion that required coronary angioplasty, I would choose my interventional cardiologist very carefully! In particular, he or she should be performing a high volume of percutaneous interventional procedures on a regular basis and have proven experience in intracoronary stent implantation. His or her familiarity with the advantages and limitations of the various stent designs that are currently commercially available would also be essential.

Prior to the procedure, I would like my cardiologist to have formulated a procedural

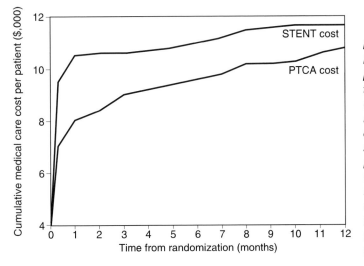

Figure 6.10

Plot of cumulative medical care costs in patients assigned to initial percutaneous transluminal coronary angioplasty (PTCA) or coronary stenting in the multicentre STRESS trial. Total 1-year cost is significantly higher with coronary stenting (US$11 656 versus US$10 865; p < 0.001). Reproduced and modified with permission from Cohen DJ et al, In-hospital and one-year economic outcomes after coronary stenting or balloon angioplasty. Results from a randomized clinical trial, Circulation (1995)**92**:2480–7.

strategy, to ensure the right equipment is available, and to ensure surgical stand-by is available — whilst the risks are low, I would like to avoid them. In addition, I would like him or her to be aware of any absolute contraindication to intracoronary stenting that I may have, such as vessel tortuosity, bleeding diathesis, and small vessel size. If there were no contraindications, I would like to be treated with aspirin and ticlopidine prior to the procedure.

If I had a threatened or abrupt occlusion complicating conventional balloon angioplasty, I would like my cardiologist to implant a stent immediately providing that there were no absolute contraindications. I would like him or her to choose a coil stent because of the low metallic surface area.

If I had a *de novo* lesion, and the conventional balloon angioplasty result was perfect with no evidence of dissection and a stent-like appearance angiographically, I would be happy not to have a stent. I am aware that this is a rare occurrence. If the angiographic results of the balloon angioplasty were anything but perfect, I would like my cardiologist to implant a stent electively, using a Palmaz-Schtaz tubular slotted stent if available, to improve my long-term angiographic outcome, especially if the lesion was located in a major epicardial vessel of 3 mm or greater in size. When the covalently heparin-coated stents are made available, I would be keen for him or her to use this instead.

If I had a saphenous vein graft lesion, I would definitely want to undergo elective stent implantation, if possible without any predilatation, or using an undersized balloon if necessary. I would like a stent with an extensive scaffolding and latticework design such as the Wallstent or the Palmaz-Schatz tubular slotted stent.

If I had a chronic total occlusion, a lesion with recurrent restenosis, or an acute coronary syndrome requiring percutaneous intervention, I would probably like a stent to be implanted after successful conventional balloon angioplasty, although I would like my cardiologist to weigh up the pros and cons of the situation, taking account of the clinical and angiographic indications and contraindications.

In all the above clinical settings, I would like my cardiologist to ensure that the stent has been fully deployed, the entire lesion is covered adequately, there is good inflow and outflow, and there is no residual luminal narrowing. If intravascular ultrasound was available, I would like him or her to use it to ensure the mentioned criteria are met. If not, I would like him or her to perform post-stenting high-pressure inflation with an oversized balloon.

After the procedure was successfully performed, I would like to have aspirin and ticlopidine as my sole post-stenting antithrombotic regimen. I would continue to take the ticlopidine for 4 weeks and the aspirin indefinitely. I would ensure that my full blood count was checked to identify ticlopidine-induced neutropenia.

Finally, I would ask myself how I got into this predicament in the first place and vigorously address my lifestyle and risk factors. No-one on the catheterization table wishes he'd spent more time in the office!

References

1 Grüntzig AR, Transluminal dilatation of coronary artery stenosis [letter], *Lancet* (1978)**1**:263.

2 Ellis SG, Roubin GS, King SB III et al, Angiographic and clinical predictors of acute closure after native vessel coronary angioplasty, *Circulation* (1988)**77**:372–9.

3 Detre KM, Holmes DR Jr, Holubkov R et al, and coinvestigators of the National Heart, Lung, and Blood Institute's Percutaneous Transluminal Coronary Angioplasty Registry, Incidence and consequences of periprocedural occlusion: the 1985–1986 National Heart, Lung, and Blood Institute Percutaneous Transluminal Coronary Angioplasty Registry, *Circulation* (1990)**82**:739–50.

4 de Feyter PJ, van den Brand M, Jaarman G, van Domburg R, Serruys PW, Suryapranata H, Acute coronary artery occlusion during and after percutaneous transluminal coronary angioplasty. Frequency, prediction, clinical course, management, and follow-up, *Circulation* (1991)**83**:927–36.

5 de Feyter PJ, de Jaegere PPT, Serruys PW, Incidence, predictors and management of acute coronary occlusion after coronary angioplasty, *Am Heart J* (1994)**127**:643–51.

6 Lincoff AM, Popma JJ, Ellis SG, Hacker JA, Topol EJ, Abrupt vessel closure complicating coronary angioplasty: clinical, angiographic and therapeutic profile, *J Am Coll Cardiol* (1992)**19**:926–35.

7 Nobuyoshi M, Kimura T, Nosaka H et al, Restenosis after successful percutaneous transluminal coronary angioplasty: serial angiographic follow-up of 229 patients, *J Am Coll Cardiol* (1988)**12**:616–23.

8 Serruys PW, Luijten HE, Beatt KJ et al, Incidence of restenosis after successful coronary angioplasty: a time related phenomenon. A quantitative angiographic study in 342 consecutive patients at 1, 2, 3 and 4 months, *Circulation* (1988)**77**:361–72.

9 Le Feuvre C, Bonan R, Cote G et al, Five- to ten-year outcome after multivessel percutaneous transluminal coronary angioplasty, *Am J Cardiol* (1993)**71**:1153–8.

10 Holmes DR, Vlietstra RE, Smith HC et al, Restenosis after percutaneous transluminal coronary angioplasty (PTCA): a report from the PTCA registry of the National Heart, Lung, and Blood Institute, *Am J Cardiol* (1984)**53**:77C-81C.

11 Hirshfeld JW, Schwartz JS, Jugo R et al, and the M-HEART investigators. Restenosis after coronary angioplasty: a multivariate statistical model to relate lesion and procedure variables to restenosis, *J Am Coll Cardiol* (1991)**18**:647–56.

12 Hinohara T, Robertson GC, Selmon MR et al, Restenosis after directional coronary atherectomy, *J Am Coll Cardiol* (1992)**20**:623–32.

13 Litvack F, Margolis J, Eigler N et al, Percutaneous excimer laser coronary angioplasty: results of the first 110 procedures, *J Am Coll Cardiol* (1990)**15(suppl A)**:25A (abstr).

14 Waller BF, 'Crackers, breakers, stretchers, drillers, scrapers, shavers, burners, welders and melters' — the future treatment of atherosclerotic coronary artery disease? A clinical-morphologic assessment, *J Am Coll Cardiol* (1989)**13**:969–87.

15 Adelman AG, Cohen EA, Kimball BP et al, A comparison of directional atherectomy with balloon angioplasty for lesions of the left anterior descending coronary artery, *N Engl J Med* (1993)**329**:228–33.

16 Topol EJ, Leya F, Pinkerton CA et al, for the CAVEAT Study Group, A comparison of directional atherectomy with coronary angioplasty in patients with coronary artery disease, *N Engl J Med* (1993)**329**:221–7.

17 Dotter CT, Judkins MP, Transluminal treatment of arteriosclerotic obstruction. Description of a new technique and a preliminary report of its application, *Circulation* (1964)**30**:654–70.

18 Sigwart U, Puel J, Mirkovitch V, Joffre F, Kappenberger L, Intravascular stents to prevent occlusion and restenosis after transluminal angioplasty, *N Engl J Med* (1987)**316**:701–6.

19 Serruys PW, de Jaegere P, Kiemeneji F et al, for the BENESTENT Study Group, A comparison of balloon-expandable-stent implantation with balloon angioplasty in patients with coronary artery disease, *N Engl J Med* (1994)**331**:489–95.

20 Fischman DL, Leon MB, Baim DS et al, for the Stent Restinosis Study Investigators, A randomized comparison of coronary-stent placement and balloon angioplasty in the treatment of coronary artery disease, *N Engl J Med* (1994)**331**:496–501.

21 Haude M, Erbel R, Issa H et al, Subacute thrombotic complications after intra-coronary implantation of Palmaz-Schatz stents, *Am Heart J* (1993)**126**:15–22.

22 Haude M, Erbel R, Straub U, Dietz U, Meyer J, Short and long term results after intra-coronary stenting in human coronary arteries: monocentre experience with the balloon-expandable Palmaz-Schatz stent, *Br Heart J* (1991)**66**:337–45.

23 Levine MJ, Leonard BM, Burke JA et al, Clinical and angiographic results of balloon-expandable intra-coronary stents in right coronary artery stenosis, *J Am Coll Cardiol* (1990)**16**:332–9.

24 Schatz RA, Baim DS, Leon MB et al, Clinical experience with the Palmaz-Schatz coronary stent. Initial results of a multicenter study, *Circulation* (1991)**83**:148–61.

25 Serruys PW, Strauss BH, Beatt KJ et al, Angiographic follow-up after placement of a self-expanding coronary-artery stent, *N Engl J Med* (1991)**324**:13–17.

26 Goy JJ, Sigwart U, Vogt P et al, Long-term follow-up of the first 56 patients treated with intra-coronary self-expanding stents (the Lausanne experience), *Am J Cardiol* (1991)**67**:569–72.

27 Herrmann HC, Buchbinder M, Clemen MW et al, Emergent use of balloon-expandable coronary artery stenting for failed percutaneous transluminal coronary angioplasty, *Circulation* (1992)**86**:812–19.

28 Kastrati A, Schömig A, Dietz R, Neumann FJ, Richardt G, Time course of restenosis during the first year after emergency coronary stenting, *Circulation* (1993)**87**:1498–1505.

29 Schömig A, Kastrati A, Dietz R et al, Emergency coronary stenting for dissection during percutaneous transluminal coronary angioplasty: angiographic follow-up after stenting and after repeat angioplasty of the stented segment, *J Am Coll Cardiol* (1994)**23**:1053–60.

30 Roubin GS, Cannon AD, Agrawal SK et al, Intracoronary stenting for acute and threatened closure complicating percutaneous transluminal coronary angioplasty, *Circulation* (1992)**85**:16–27.

31 Malosky SA, Hirshfeld JW Jr, Herrmann HC, Comparison of results of intra-coronary stenting in patients with unstable vs. stable angina, *Cathet Cardiovasc Diagn* (1994)**31**:95–101.

32 Foley JB, Brown RI, Penn IM, Thrombosis and restenosis after stenting in failed angioplasty: comparison with elective stenting, *Am Heart J* (1994)**128**:12–20.

33 Sutton JM, Ellis SG, Roubin GS et al, Major clinical events after coronary stenting. The multicenter registry of acute and elective Gianturco-Roubin stent placement, *Circulation* (1994)**89**:1126–37.

34 Hollman J, Gruentzig AR, Douglas JS Jr, King SB III, Ischinger T, Meier B, Acute occlusion after percutaneous transluminal coronary angioplasty — a new approach, *Circulation* (1983)**68**:725–32.

35 Myler RK, Topol EJ, Shaw RE et al, Multiple vessel coronary angioplasty: classification, results and patterns of restenosis in 494 consecutive patients, *Cathet Cardiovasc Diagn* (1987)**13**:1–15.

36 Sinclair IN, McCabe CH, Sipperly ME, Baim DS, Predictors, therapeutic options and long-term outcome of abrupt reclosure, *Am J Cardiol* (1988)**61**:61G–66G.

37 Sugrue DD, Holmes DR Jr, Smith HC et al, Coronary artery thrombus as a risk factor for acute vessel occlusion during percutaneous transluminal coronary angioplasty: improving results, *Br Heart J* (1986)**56**:62–6.

38 Steffenino G, Meier B, Finci L et al, Acute complications of elective coronary angioplasty: a

review of 500 consecutive procedures, *Br Heart J* (1988)**59**:151–8.

39 Holms DR Jr, Holubkov R, Vlietstra RE et al, and the co-investigators of the National Heart, Lung, and Blood Institute percutaneous transluminal coronary angioplasty registry, Comparison of complications during percutaneous transluminal coronary angioplasty from 1977 to 1981 and from 1985 to 1986: the National Heart, Lung, and Blood Institute Percutaneous Transluminal Coronary Angioplasty Registry, *J Am Coll Cardiol* (1988)**12**:1149–55.

40 Tenaglia AN, Fortin DF, Frid DJ et al, Long-term outcome following successful reopening of abrupt closure after coronary angioplasty, *Am J Cardiol* (1993)**72**:21–5.

41 Jackman JD Jr, Zidar JP, Tcheng JE, Overman AB, Phillips HR, Stack RS, Outcome after prolonged balloon inflations of >20 minutes for initially unsuccessful percutaneous transluminal coronary angioplasty, *Am J Cardiol* (1992)**69**:1417–21.

42 Leitschuh ML, Mills RM Jr, Jacobs AK, Ruocco NA Jr, LaRosa D, Faxon DP, Outcome after major dissection during coronary angioplasty using the perfusion balloon catheter, *Am J Cardiol* (1991)**67**:1056–60.

43 Van der Linden LP, Bakx AM, Sedney MI, Buis B, Bruschke AUG, Prolonged dilatation with an autoperfusion balloon catheter for refractory acute occlusion related to percutaneous transluminal coronary angioplasty, *J Am Coll Cardiol* (1993)**22**:1016–23.

44 Sigwart U, Urban P, Golf S et al, Emergency stenting for acute occlusion after coronary balloon angioplasty, *Circulation* (1988)**78**:1121–7.

45 Haude M, Erbel R, Straub U, Dietz U, Schatz R, Meyer J, Results of intracoronary stents for management of coronary dissection after balloon angioplasty, *Am J Cardiol* (1991)**67**:691–6.

46 Roubin GS, Cannon AD, Agrawal SK et al, Intracoronary stenting for acute and threatened closure complicating percutaneous transluminal coronary angioplasty, *Circulation* (1992)**85**:16–27.

47 Kiemeneij F, Laarman GJ, van der Wieken R, Suwarganda J, Emergency coronary stenting with the Palmaz-Schatz stent for failed transluminal coronary angioplasty: results of a learning phase, *Am Heart J* (1993)**126**:23–31.

48 Ozaki Y, Keane D, Ruygrok P, de Feyter P, Stertzer S, Serruys PW, Acute clinical and angiographic results with the new AVE micro coronary stent in bailout management, *Am J Cardiol* (1995)**76**:112–16.

49 Vrolix M, Piessens J, for the European Wiktor Stent Study Group, Usefulness of the Wiktor stent for treatment of threatened or acute closure complicating coronary angioplasty, *Am J Cardiol* (1994)**73**:737–41.

50 Keane D, Roubin G, Marco J, Fearnot N, Serruys PW, GRACE—Gianturco-Roubin stent in Acute Closure Evaluation: substrate, challenges and design of a randomised trial of bailout therapy, *J Interven Cardiol* (1994)**7**:333–9.

51 Ray SG, Penn IM, Ricci DR et al, Mechanisms of benefit of stenting in failed angioplasty. Final results from the Trial of Angioplasty and Stents in Canada (TASC II), *J Am Coll Cardiol* (1995)**25**(suppl A):156A (abstr).

52 Holmes DR, Vlietstra RE, Smith HC et al, Restenosis after percutaneous transluminal coronary angioplasty (PTCA): a report from the PTCA registry of the National Heart, Lung, and Blood Institute, *Am J Cardiol* (1984)**53**:77C–81C.

53 Serruys PW, Luijten HE, Beatt KJ et al, Incidence of restenosis after successful coronary angioplasty: a time related phenomenon. A quantitative angiographic study in 342 consecutive patients at 1, 2, 3 and 4 months, *Circulation* (1988)**77**:361–72.

54 Nobuyoshi M, Kimura T, Nosaka H et al, Restenosis after successful percutaneous transluminal coronary angioplasty: serial angiographic follow-up of 229 patients, *J Am Coll Cardiol* (1988)**12**:616–23.

55 Le Feuvre C, Bonan R, Cote G et al, Five- to ten-year outcome after multivessel percutaneous transluminal coronary angioplasty, *Am J Cardiol* (1993)**71**:1153–8.

56 Mintz GS, Kovach JA, Javier SP, Ditrano CJ, Leon MB, Geometric remodeling is the predominant mechanism of late lumen loss after coronary angioplasty, *Circulation* (1993)**88**(suppl I):I–654 (abstr).

57 Popma JJ, Califf RM, Topol EJ, Clinical trials of restinosis after coronary angioplasty, *Circulation* (1991)**84**:1426–36.

58 Bittl JA, Sanborn TA, Tcheng JE, Siegel RM, Ellis SG, for the Percutaneous Excimer Laser Coronary Angioplasty Registry, Clinical success, complications and restenosis rate with excimer laser coronary angioplasty, *Am J Cardiol* (1992)**70**:1533–9.

59 Buchwald AB, Werner GS, Unterberg C, Voth E, Kreuzer H, Wiegand V, Restenosis after excimer laser angioplasty of coronary stenoses and chronic total occlusions, *Am Heart J* (1992)**123**:878–85.

60 Bertrand ME, LaBlanche JM, Leory F et al, Percutaneous transluminal coronary rotary ablation with rotablator (European experience), *Am J Cardiol* (1992)**69**:470–4.

61 Stertzer SH, Rosenblum J, Shaw RE et al, Coronary rotational ablation: initial experience in 302 patients, *J Am Coll Cardiol* (1993)**21**: 287–95.

62 Feld H, Schulhoff N, Lichstein E et al, Coronary atherectomy versus angioplasty: the CAVA study, *Am Heart J* (1993)**126**:31–8.

63 Virchow R, Der atheromatous Prozess der Arteries, *Wie Med Wochenschr* (1856)**6**:825–9.

64 Ross R, The pathogenesis of atherosclerosis — an update, *N Engl J Med* (1986)**314**: 488–500.

65 Macaya C, Serruys PW, Ruygrok P et al, for the Benestent Study Group, Continued benefit of coronary stenting versus balloon angioplasty: one-year clinical follow-up of Benestent trial, *J Am Coll Cardiol* (1996)**27**:255–61.

66 Faxon DP, Kelsey SF, Ryan TJ, McCabe CH, Detre K, Determinants of successful percutaneous transluminal coronary angioplasty: report from the National Heart, Lung, and Blood Institute Registry, *Am Heart J* (1984)**108**:1019–23.

67 Detre K, Holubkov R, Kelsey S et al, and the co-investigators of the National Heart, Lung, and Blood Institute's Percutaneous Transluminal Coronary Angioplasty Registry, Percutaneous transluminal coronary angioplasty in 1985–1986 and 1977–1981: the National Heart, Lung, and Blood Institute Registry, *N Engl J Med* (1988)**318**:265–70.

68 Ryan TJ, Faxon DP, Gunnar RM et al, Guidelines for percutaneous transluminal coronary angioplasty: a report of the American College of Cardiology/American Heart Association Task Force on Assessment of Diagnostic and Therapeutic Cardiovascular Procedures (Subcommittee on Percutaneous Transluminal Coronary Angioplasty), *J Am Coll Cardiol* (1988)**12**:529–45.

69 Kuntz RE, Baim DS, Defining coronary restenosis: newer clinical and angiographic paradigms, *Circulation* (1993)**88**:1310–23.

70 Kuntz RE, Gibson M, Nobuyoshi M, Baim DS, Generalized model of restenosis after conventional balloon angioplasty, stenting, and directional atherectomy, *J Am Coll Cardiol* (1993)**21**:15–25.

71 Serruys PW, Azar AJ, Sigwart U et al, on behalf of the Benestent group, Long-term follow-up of 'stent-like' (≤ 30% diameter stenosis post) angioplasty: a case for provisional stenting, *J Am Coll Cardill* (1996)**27**(**suppl A**):15A (abstr).

72 Colombo A, Almagor Y, Maiello L, Khlat B, Gianrossi R, Finci L, Coronary stenting: results with different indications, *Circulation* (1993)**88** (**suppl I**):I–122 (abstr).

73 Remetz MS, Gallup DS, Rosen RE, Cabin HS, Cleman MW, Results of unplanned Palmaz-Schatz coronary stent placement after suboptimal balloon angioplasty: a report from the New Approaches to Coronary Intervention (NACI) Registry, *Circulation* (1993)**88**(**suppl I**):I–122 (abstr).

74 Kimura T, Nosaka H, Yokoi H, Iwabuchi M, Nobuyoshi M, Serial angiographic follow-up after Palmaz-Schatz stent implantation: comparison with conventional balloon angioplasty, *J Am Coll Cardiol* (1993)**21**:1557–63.

75 Rodriguez AE, Santaera O, Larribau M et al, Coronary stenting decreases restenosis in lesions with early loss in luminal diameter 24 hours after successful PTCA, *Circulation* (1995)**91**:1397–1402.

76 Israel DH, Adam PC, Stein B, Chesebro JH, Fuster V, Antithrombotic therapy in the coronary vein graft patient, *Clin Cardiol* (1991)**14**: 283–95.

77 Laird-Meeter K, van Domburg R, van den Brand M, Lubsen J, Bos E, Hugenholtz PG, Incidence, risk, and outcome of reintervention

after aortocoronary bypass surgery, *Br Heart J* (1987)**57**:427–35.

78 Lytle BW, Loop FD, Cosgrove DM et al, Fifteen hundred coronary reoperations, *J Thorac Cardiovas Surg* (1987)**93**:847–59.

79 Aueron F, Gruentzig A, Distal embolisation of a coronary artery bypass graft atheroma during percutaneous transluminal coronary angioplasty, *Am J Cardiol* (1984)**53**:953–4.

80 Cote G, Myler RK, Stertzer SH et al, Percutaneous transluminal angioplasty of stenotic coronary artery bypass grafts: 5 years' experience, *J Am Coll Cardiol* (1987)**9**:8–17.

81 Douglas JS JR, Gruentzig AR, King SB III et al, Percutaneous transluminal coronary angioplasty in patients with prior coronary bypass surgery, *J Am Coll Cardiol* (1983)**2**:745–54.

82 Liu MW, Douglas JS, Lembo NJ, King SB III, Angiographic predictors of a rise in serum creatine kinase (distal embolization) after balloon angioplasty of saphenous vein coronary artery bypass grafts, *Am J Cardiol* (1993)**72**:514–17.

83 Reeder GS, Bresnahan JF, Holmes DR Jr et al, Angioplasty for aortocoronary bypass graft stenosis, *Mayo Clin Proc* (1986)**61**:14–19.

84 Platko WP, Hollman J, Whitlow PL, Franco I, Percutaneous transluminal angioplasty of saphenous vein graft stenosis: long term follow up, *J Am Coll Cardiol* (1989)**14**:1645–50.

85 Popma JJ, Leon MB, Mintz GS et al, Results of coronary angioplasty using the transluminal extraction catheter, *Am J Cardiol* (1992)**70**:1526–32.

86 Meany TB, Leon MB, Kramer BL et al, Transluminal extraction catheter for the treatment of diseased saphenous vein grafts: a multicenter experience, *Cathet Cardiovasc Diagn* (1995)**34**:112–20.

87 Untereker WJ, Litvack F, Margolis JR et al, and ELCA Investigators, Excimer laser coronary angioplasty of saphenous vein grafts, *Circulation* (1991)**84**(suppl II):II–249 (abstr).

88 Strauss BH, Natarajan MK, Batchelor WB et al, Early and late quantitative angiographic results of vein graft lesions treated by excimer laser with adjunctive balloon angioplasty, *Circulation* (1995)**92**:348–56.

89 Selmon MR, Hinohara T, Vetter JW et al, Experience with directional coronary atherect-

omy; 848 procedures over 4 years, *Circulation* (1991)**84**(suppl II):II–80 (abstr).

90 Kaufmann UP, Garratt KN, Vlietstra RE, Holmes DR, Transluminal atherectomy of saphenous vein aortocoronary bypass grafts, *Am J Cardiol* (1990)**65**:1430–3.

91 Holmes DR Jr, Topol EJ, Califf RM et al, for the CAVEAT-II Investigators, A multicenter randomized trial of coronary angioplasty versus directional atherectomy for patients with saphenous vein bypass graft lesions, *Circulation* (1995)**91**:1966–74.

92 Lefkovits J, Holmes DR, Califf RM et al, for the CAVEAT-II Investigators, Predictors and sequelae of distal embolization during saphenous vein graft intervention from the CAVEAT-II trial, *Circulation* (1995)**92**:734–40.

93 Keane D, de Jaegere P, Serruys PW, Structural design, clinical experience and current indications of the coronary Wallstent, *Cardiol Clin* (1994)**12**:689–97.

94 Keane D, Buis B, Reifart N et al, Clinical and angiographic outcome following implantation of the new Less Shortening Wallstent in aortocoronary vein grafts: introduction of a second generation stent in the clinical arena, *J Intervent Cardiol* (1994)**7**:557–64.

95 Wong SC, Baim DS, Schatz RA et al, for the Palmaz-Scahtz Stent Study Group, Immediate results and late outcomes after stent implantation in saphenous vein graft lesions: the multicenter US Palmaz-Schatz stent experience, *J Am Coll Cardiol* (1995)**26**:704–12.

96 Wong SC, Popma JJ, Pichard AD et al, Comparison of clinical and angiographic outcomes after saphenous vein graft angioplasty using coronary versus 'biliary' tubular slotted stents, *Circulation* (1995)**91**:339–50.

97 Strauss BH, Serruys PW, Bertrand ME et al, Quantitative angiographic follow-up of the coronary Wallstent in native vessels and bypass grafts (European experience—March 1986 to March 1990), *Am J Cardiol* (1992)**69**:475–81.

98 Urban P, Sigwart U, Golf S, Kaufmann U, Sadeghi H, Kappenberger L, Intravascular stenting for stenosis of aortocoronary venous bypass grafts, *J Am Coll Cardiol* (1989)**13**: 1085–91.

99 Douglas JS Jr, Savage MP, Bailey SR et al, SAVED Trial Investigators, Randomized trial

of coronary stent and balloon angioplasty in the treatment of saphenous vein graft stenosis, *J Am Coll Cardiol* (1996)**27**(**suppl A**):178A (abstr).

100 Bell MR, Berger PB, Bresnahan JF, Reeder GS, Bailey KR, Holmes DR Jr, Initial and long-term outcome of 354 patients after coronary balloon angioplasty of total coronary artery occlusions, *Circulation* (1992)**85**:1003–11.

101 Hamm CW, Kupper W, Kuck K-H, Hoffman D, Bleifeld W, Recanalization of chronic, totally occluded coronary arteries by new angioplasty systems, *Am J Cardiol* (1990)**66**:1459–63.

102 Melchior JP, Meier B, Urban P et al, Percutaneous transluminal coronary angioplasty for chronic total coronary artery occlusion, *Am J Cardiol* (1987)**59**:535–8.

103 Ellis SG, Shaw RE, Gershony G et al, Risk factors, time course and treatment effect for restenosis after successful percutaneous transluminal coronary angioplasty of chronic total occlusion, *Am J Cardiol* (1989)**63**:897–901.

104 Warren RJ, Black AJ, Valentine PA, Manolas EG, Hunt D, Coronary angioplasty for chronic total occlusion reduces the need for subsequent coronary bypass surgery, *Am Heart J* (1990)**120**:270–4.

105 Goldberg SL, Colombo A, Maiello L, Borrione M, Finci L, Almagor Y, Intracoronary stent insertion after balloon angioplasty of chronic total occlusion, *J Am Coll Cardiol* (1995)**26**: 713–19.

106 Sirnes PA, Golf S. Myreng Y et al, for the SICCO Study Group, Stenting in chronic coronary occlusion (SICCO): a multicenter, randomized, controlled study, *J Am Coll Cardiol* (1996)**27**(**suppl A**):139A (abstr).

107 Black AJ, Anderson HV, Roubin GS, Powelson SW, Douglas JS, King SB III, Repeat coronary angioplasty: correlates of a second restenosis, *J Am Coll Cardiol* (1988)**11**:714–18.

108 Dimas AP, Grigera F, Arora RR et al, Repeat coronary angioplasty as treatment for restenosis, *J Am Coll Cardiol* (1992)**6**:1310–14.

109 Joly P, Bonan R, Palisaitis D et al, Treatment of recurrent restenosis with repeat percutaneous transluminal coronary angioplasty, *Am J Cardiol* (1988)**61**:906–8.

110 Quigley PJ, Hlatky MA, Hinohara T et al, Repeat percutaneous transluminal coronary angioplasty and predictors of recurrent restenosis, *Am J Cardiol* (1989)**63**:409–13.

111 Sigwart U, Puel J, Mirkovitch V, Joffre F, Kappenberger L, Intravascular stents to prevent occlusion and restenosis after transluminal angioplasty, *N Engl J Med* (1987)**316**:701–6.

112 Sigwart U, Kaufman U, Goy JJ et al, Prevention of coronary restenosis by stenting, *Eur Heart J* (1988)**9**(**suppl C**):31–7.

113 Urban P, Sigwart U, Kaufman U, Kappenberger L, Restenosis within coronary stents: possible effect of previous angioplasty, *J Am Coll Cardiol* (1989)**13**(**suppl A**):107A (abstr).

114 Erbel R, Haude M, Hopp HW et al, on behalf of the REST Study Group, REstenosis STent (REST)-Study: randomized trial comparing stenting and balloon angioplasty for treatment of restenosis after balloon angioplasty, *J Am Coll Cardill* (1996)**27**(**suppl A**):139A (abstr).

115 Hartzler GO, Rutherford BD, McConahay DR et al, Percutaneous transluminal coronary angioplasty with and without thrombolytic therapy for treatment of acute myocardial infarction, *Am Heart J* (1983)**106**:965–73.

116 Grines CL, Browne KF, Marco J et al, for the Primary Angioplasty in Myocardial Infarction Study Group, A comparison of immediate angioplasty with thrombolytic therapy for acute myocardial infarction, *N Engl J Med* (1993)**328**:673–9.

117 Gibbons RJ, Holmes DR, Reeder GS, Bailey KR, Hopfenspirger MR, Gersh BJ, for the MAYO Coronary Care Unit and Catheterization Laboratory Groups, Immediate angioplasty compared with the administration of a thrombolytic agent followed by conservative treatment for myocardial infarction, *N Engl J Med* (1993)**328**:685–91.

118 Zijlstra F, de Boer MJ, Hoorntje JCA, Reiffers S, Reiber JHC, Suryapranata H, A comparison of immediate coronary angioplasty with intravenous streptokinase in acute myocardial infarction, *N Engl J Med* (1993)**328**:680–4.

119 Ellis SG, O'Neill WW, Bates ER, Walton JA, Nabel EG, Topol EJ, Coronary angioplasty as primary therapy for acute myocardial infarction 6 to 48 hours after symptom onset: report of an initial experience, *J Am Coll Cardiol* (1989)**13**:1122–30.

120 O'Keefe JH Jr, Rutherford BD, McConahay DR et al, Early and late results of coronary angioplasty without antecedent thrombolytic therapy for acute myocardial infarction, *Am J Cardiol* (1989)**64**:1221–30.

121 Bedotto JB, Kahn JK, Rutherford BD et al, Failed direct coronary angioplasty for acute myocardial infarction: in-hospital outcome and predictors of death, *J Am Coll Cardiol* (1993)**22**:690–4.

122 Stone GW, Rutherford BD, McConahay DR, Hartzler GO, Direct coronary angioplasty in acute myocardial infarction: outcome in patients with single vessel disease, *J Am Coll Cardiol* (1990)**15**:534–43.

123 Roubin GS, Agrawal SK, Dean LS, What are the predictors of acute complications following coronary artery stenting? Single institutional experience, *J Am Coll Cardiol* (1991)**17** (suppl A):281A (abstr).

124 Heuser RR, Breaking the barrier: stenting in acute myocardial infarction, *Cathet Cardiovasc Diagn* (1994)**33**:46.

125 Neumann FJ, Walter H, Richardt G, Schmitt C, Schömig A, Coronary Palmaz-Schatz stent implantation in acute myocardial infarction, *Heart* (1996)**75**:121–6.

126 Le May MR, Labinaz M, Beanlands RSB et al, Intracoronary stenting in the setting of myocardial infarction, *J Am Coll Cardiol* (1996)**27** (suppl A):69A (abstr).

127 Monassier JP, Elias J, Meyer P, Morice MC, Royer T, Cribier A, STENTIM I: the French Registry of Stenting at Acute Myocardial Infarction, *J Am Coll Cardiol* (1996)**27**(suppl A):68A (abstr).

128 Lefèvre T, Morice MC, Karrillon G, Aubry P, Zemour G, Valeix B, Coronary stenting during acute myocardial infarction. Results from the Stent Without Coumadin French Registry, *J Am Coll Cardiol* (1996)**27**(suppl A):69A (abstr).

129 Romero M, Medina A, de Lezo JS et al, Elective stent implantation in acute coronary syndromes induced by thrombus containing lesions, *J Am Coll Cardiol* (1996)**27**(suppl A):69A (abstr).

130 Colombo A, Hall P, Nakamura S et al, Intracoronary stenting without anticoagulation accomplished with intravascular ultrasound guidance, *Circulation* (1995)**91**:1676–88.

131 Morice MC, Commeau P, Monassier JP et al, Coronary stenting without coumadin. Phase II, III, IV, and V. Predictors of major complications, *Eur Heart J* (1995)**16**(suppl):290 (abstr).

132 Elias J, Monassier JP, Carrie D et al, Final results of phases II, III, IV and V of Medtronic Wiktor stent implantation without coumadin, *J Am Coll Cardiol* (1996)**27**(suppl A):15A (abstr).

133 de Jaegere P, Mudra H, Almagor Y et al, for the MUSIC Study Investigators, In-hospital and 1-month clinical results of an international study testing the concept of IVUS guided optimised stent expansion alleviating the need of systemic anticoagulation, *J Am Coll Cardiol* (1996)**27** (suppl A):137A (abstr).

134 Hausmann D, Erbel R, Alibelli-Chemarin MJ et al, The safety of intra-coronary ultrasound. A multicenter survey of 2207 examinations, *Circulation* (1995)**91**:623–30.

135 Morice MC, Valeix B, Marco J et al, Preliminary results of the MUST trial. Major clinical events during the first month, *J Am Coll Cardiol* (1996)**27**(suppl A):137A (abstr).

136 Lablanche JM, Bonnet JL, Grollier G et al, Combined antiplatelet therapy without anticoagulation after stent implantation; the Ticlopidine Aspirin Stent Evaluation (TASTE) Study, *J Am Coll Cardiol* (1996)**27**(suppl A):137A (abstr).

137 Serruys PW, Emanuelsson H, Macaya C et al, Benestent-II pilot study: in-hospital results of phase 1, 2, 3, 4, *Eur Heart J* (1995)**16** (suppl):290 (abstr).

138 The EPIC Investigators, Use of a monoclonal antibody directed against the platelet glycoprotein IIb/IIIa receptor in high-risk coronary angioplasty, *N Engl J Med* (1994)**330**:956–61 (abstr).

139 Topol EJ, Bonan R, Jewitt D et al, Use of a direct antithrombin, Hirulog, in place of heparin during coronary angioplasty, *Circulation* (1993)**87**:1622–9.

140 Cohen DJ, Krumholz HM, Sukin CA et al, for the Stent Restenosis Study Investigators, In-hospital and one-year economic outcomes after coronary stenting or balloon angioplasty. Results from a randomised clinical trial, *Circulation* (1995)**92**:2480–7.

7

The significance and evaluation of myocardial viability in coronary artery disease

Samer R Dibs and Andrew J Buda

'We are always getting ready to live, but never living.'

Ralph Waldo Emerson, Journals, 1834.

Ischemic cardiomyopathy, hibernation, stunning: historical background and definitions

In 1970, Burch and colleagues[1] at Tulane University introduced the term 'ischemic cardiomyopathy' to describe 'degenerative changes of the myocardium due to inadequate blood supply' with resultant cardiac dilatation and congestive heart failure. They noted that its onset is usually *but not always* associated with angina pectoris that increases in severity and that there is gradual cardiac enlargement, with *or without* the development of one or more myocardial infarctions with scar formation. Since 1970, we have come to realize that much of the left ventricular dysfunction associated with coronary artery disease does not reflect myocardial necrosis and may be reversible. Myocardial *hibernation*, a term coined by Rahimtoola,[2] describes reduced myocardial contractility and metabolism to match the reduced blood supply of a prolonged stage of ischemia, thus preventing myocardial necrosis and allowing return of myocardium to a normal or near-normal state on restoration of an ade-

quate blood supply. On the other hand, myocardial *stunning*, a term coined by Braunwald and Kloner,[3] describes myocardial dysfunction and biochemical and ultrastructural changes occurring for a prolonged period following an acute ischemic insult of insufficient severity or duration to produce myocardial necrosis.

In this chapter, we will discuss the clinical significance of myocardial viability in chronic coronary artery disease and the role of single-photon cardiac imaging in its assessment.

Viable dysfunctional myocardium: hibernation, stunning, or both?

Myocardial hibernation and stunning may coexist or overlap in the clinical setting. Myocardial dysfunction following an acute episode of ischemia, such as acute infarction or simply stress-induced ischemia, may be superimposed on chronic myocardial dysfunction secondary to severe coronary artery disease. Moreover, it has been suggested that the myocardial dysfunction seen in chronic coronary artery disease may represent repeated stunning following repeated episodes of ischemia.

In an attempt to elucidate the mechanisms of myocardial dysfunction in chronic coronary artery disease, Vanoverschelde et al.[4] studied 26 patients with angina and chronic occlusion of a major coronary artery but without known previous infarction using positron emission tomography (PET), with N13-ammonia, C11-acetate, and F18-fluorodeoxyglucose to measure regional myocardial blood flow, oxidative metabolism, and exogenous glucose uptake, respectively. In patients with normal wall motion in the collateral-dependent segments, regional blood flow, oxidative metabolism, and glucose uptake were similar among collateral-dependent and remote segments. In contrast, in patients with abnormal wall motion in the collateral-dependent segments, regional blood flow and oxidative metabolism were lower and glucose uptake was higher in collateral-dependent segments compared with remote segments. However, absolute regional blood flow, oxidative metabolism, and glucose uptake were similar among collateral-dependent segments of patients without and those with segmental dysfunction. This was interpreted as a lack of chronic reduction in resting blood flow to chronically dysfunctional but viable myocardial segments, contrary to the definition of myocardial 'hibernation'. Furthermore, collateral-dependent myocardial blood flow increased after dipyridamole infusion to a larger extent in patients without than in those with segmental dysfunction, reflecting reduced collateral flow reserve in the latter group. Thus, the authors concluded that repeated episodes of ischemia during daily life and postischemic stunning may be the mechanism of chronic myocardial dysfunction in this group of patients.

It is, nevertheless, important to note that the group with collateral-dependent segmental dysfunction had larger mean left ventricular end-diastolic and end-systolic volume indices and mean rate-pressure product than the group without segmental dysfunction. Thus, myocardial demand may have been elevated in the viable, collateral-dependent segments as well as in the remote segments of the former

group. In fact, myocardial blood flow was increased in the normal remote segments of the group with segmental dysfunction compared with the group without segmental dysfunction. This raises the distinct possibility that, although resting blood flow to the dysfunctional segments was 'in the normal range', it may not have been appropriate for the workload.

A universal definition of ischemia is not available,[5] but the concept of supply–demand imbalance is widely accepted. Therefore, chronic ischemia (decrease in blood supply relative to demand), rather than chronic hypoperfusion (absolute decrease in blood supply), remains an important factor in chronic left ventricular dysfunction associated with coronary artery disease. Moreover, regardless of whether chronic myocardial dysfunction (without necrosis) in coronary artery disease is due to chronic ischemia (hibernation) or follows repeated acute ischemia (repeated/persistent stunning), correction of ischemia is likely to have a beneficial effect. Consequently, assessment of myocardial viability is essential to comprehensive and effective management in chronic coronary artery disease with left ventricular dysfunction.

Myocardial viability: is postrevascularization functional improvement the 'gold standard'?

In clinical practice, myocardial viability is determined not in individual myocytes but rather in regions or segments of the left ventricle. While improvement of function after coronary revascularization can be considered proof of viability in a region, lack of that improvement does not exclude viability. An 'infarcted' region of the left ventricle may contain both viable and necrotic myocytes. Depending on the proportion and distribution of viable myocytes in such a region, myocardial contraction may or may not be possible after correction of ischemia.

The complexities of transmural myocardial function are illustrated in a study by Myers et al.,[6] who investigated the contribution of different layers of the myocardium to total left ventricular wall thickening using epicardial echocardiography in an open-chest canine model. At rest, the fractional contributions to total wall thickening of the inner, middle, and outer thirds of the myocardium were estimated from the experimental data to be 58%, 25%, and 17%, respectively (Figure 7.1). After isoproterenol administration, total wall thickening increased but the fractional contributions of the different layers were not significantly changed. Given the relatively large contribution of subendocardial thickening to ventricular wall thickening, it is possible that a region with subendocardial scar and overlying hibernating myocardium, for example, may not show appreciable improvement in function at rest after coronary revascularization. However, with inotropic stimulation or during exercise, functional improvement in that region may be seen because of increased thickening of the viable outer layers of the ventricular wall.

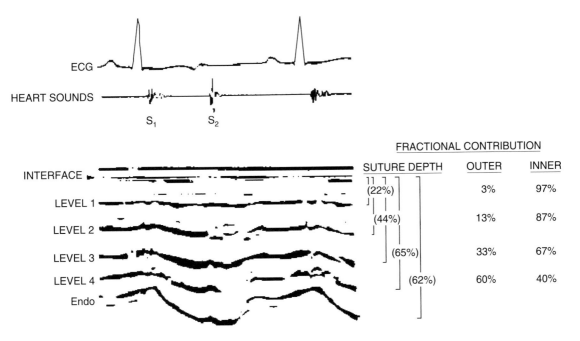

Figure 7.1
Example of echocardiographic tracings from one experiment in which four sutures were placed in the myocardial wall to serve as echocardiographic targets. The fractional contributions (to total thickening) of the inner and outer walls, defined at different depths by the four sutures, are illustrated on the right side of the figure. A gradient of wall thickening is evident, increasing from the epicardium to the endocardium, in close agreement with the combined results from all the experiments. The term INTERFACE refers to the epicardium and ENDO refers to the endocardial surface. (Reprinted with permission from Myers JH et al, Direct measurement of inner and outer wall thickening dynamics with epicardial echocardiography, Circulation (1986) **74***: 164–72.)[6]*

Accordingly, the assessment of myocardial functional reserve may complement rest studies in the determination of viability.

In patients with chronic coronary artery disease, identification of viable myocardium that will improve in function postrevascularization remains the primary goal for the clinician. Improvement of regional wall motion and hence overall left ventricular function may be expected to result in decreased morbidity from congestive heart failure, arrhythmia, thromboembolism and enhanced survival. Nevertheless, lack of improvement in function of viable myocardium following revascularization does not preclude other beneficial effects of revascularization, including possible improvement in angina, ventricular arrhythmia, and ventricular remodeling.

Potential revascularization benefits unrelated to regional wall motion improvement

Coronary revascularization may have a significant antiarrhythmic role given the prominent proarrhythmic effects of myocardial ischemia when superimposed on the susceptible substrate of admixed viable and necrotic tissue in the infarct region. In this regard, Margonato et al.[7] studied 60 patients with chronic stable angina and previous myocardial infarction using stress/rest technetium-99m sestamibi single-photon emission computed tomography (SPECT) for perfusion and, in the last 26 patients, F18-fluorodeoxyglucose (FDG) SPECT for metabolism. Half of the patients consistently developed ventricular arrhythmias (≥ 10 ectopic beats/minute, couplets, nonsustained tachycardia) with exercise, while the other half did not, although coronary artery disease severity was similar in the two groups. Partial sestamibi defect reversibility and FDG uptake in the infarct area were more common in patients with than in those without exercise-induced arrhythmias ($p < 0.001$). The authors concluded that in patients with myocardial infarction, ventricular arrhythmias appear to be triggered by transient ischemia occurring within an area with partial necrosis and a large amount of viable myocardium.

Coronary revascularization may also have a role in preventing infarct expansion and subsequent left ventricular dilatation, given the potential role of viable myocardium in limiting ventricular remodeling after acute myocardial infarction. We prospectively followed left-ventricular end-diastolic volume index by echocardiography in 45 patients with myocardial infarction.[8] Left ventricular volume increased from 1 week to 6 weeks in patients with acute Q-wave infarction but not in those with acute non-Q-wave infarction or in control patients with remote infarction (Figure 7.2). There was a strong correlation between the change in the left ventricular end-diastolic volume index and the peak creatine phosphokinase level. However, after correcting for infarct size, as measured by peak creatine phosphokinase level, there was still a significant impact of the type of infarct on the degree of remodeling. Our data indicated that ventricular remodeling does not occur, at least for the first 6 weeks, in non-Q-wave infarction, unlike Q-wave infarction, probably secondary to more limited and often nontransmural myocardial necrosis.

In further support of this concept, Vannan et al.[9] followed 44 patients with uncomplicated thrombolysed first Q-wave anterior myocardial infarction. Based on the defect severity on rest Tc-99m sestamibi SPECT performed at hospital discharge, patients were separated into those with more preserved and less preserved infarct zone viability. Over the subsequent 12 months, there was progressive increase in left ventricular end-diastolic volume index and decline in left

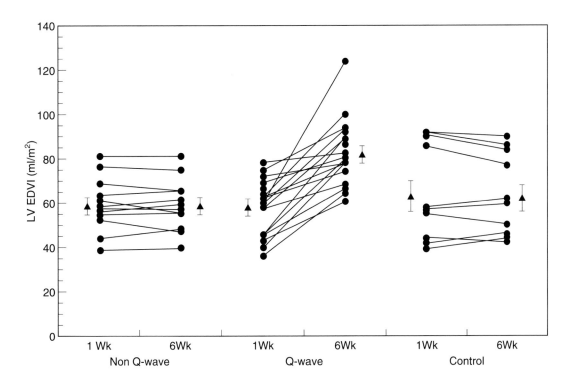

Figure 7.2
Change in left ventricular end-diastolic volume index from week 1 to week 6 in the three study groups.
▲ mean; I SEM; LVEDVI left ventricular end-diastolic volume index. (Reprinted with permission from
Irimpen AM et al, Lack of ventricular remodeling in non-Q-wave myocardial infarction, Am Heart J (1996)
***131**: 466–71.)[8]*

ventricular ejection fraction in both groups. However, despite similar infarct zone extent, those patients with more preserved infarct zone viability had significantly less deterioration in global left ventricular size and function over time.

It should be noted that in the studies by Irimpen[8] and Vannan,[9] initial patient assessment was early after acute myocardial infarction, a time when myocardial stunning may be superimposed on myocardial hibernation. Whether ischemic viable myocardium in chronic coronary artery disease with left ventricular dysfunction plays a role in preventing left ventricular dilatation is less clear.

Whereas dysfunctional viable myocardial segments may not regain resting function after coronary revascularization because of ventricular wall mechanics, it is possible, as discussed previously, that they will be functional when stimulated, for example during exercise. In a recent preliminary report, Trani et al.[10] presented data on 21 patients with prior myocardial infarction who had rest-redistribution thallium-201 SPECT and dobutamine echocardiography before and after coronary revascularization. Infarct zones were judged to be viable based on scintigraphic defect Tl-201 uptake and wall motion abnormality improvement with dobutamine. When only the revascularized infarct zones were considered, 8 out of 14 viable and 1 out of 16 nonviable infarct zones showed improvement in resting wall motion. Of the 6 viable infarct zones that were persistently asynergic after revascularization, all showed improved Tl-201 uptake and 5 out of 6 retained contractile reserve on dobutamine echocardiography. The investigators suggested that such infarct zones with myocardial viability but no contractile recovery could reflect an admixture of fibrosis and focal areas of viable cells. However, to our knowledge, no data are available on exercise echocardiography postrevascularization to evaluate myocardial segments judged to be viable preoperatively. It would be useful to determine whether viable but persistently asynergic segments exhibit improved wall motion with exercise.

Myocardial viability: a better outcome with revascularization

There is abundant evidence, although largely retrospective, of revascularization-related improvement in perfusion and, more importantly, in function of dysfunctional regions identified as viable before revascularization. We will present that evidence when discussing the various single-photon imaging techniques for assessment of myocardial viability.

There is also increasing evidence of additional benefits of revascularization when a significant amount of ischemic viable myocardium is identified preoperatively. Eitzman et al.[11] retrospectively evaluated the clinical outcome in 82 patients with coronary artery disease and left ventricular dysfunction who had positron emission tomography (at rest) for assessment of myocardial viability in consideration for coronary revascularization. The patients were classified according to whether they had evidence of

viability by PET (decreased blood flow with preserved metabolism) and whether they had subsequent coronary revascularization. The four patient groups did not differ significantly with respect to left ventricular ejection fraction and number of stenosed vessels. However, the patient group with evidence of viability but no subsequent revascularization had a higher combined event rate (death, myocardial infarction, cardiac arrest, late revascularization because of new symptoms) than each of the other patient groups. Although unknown factors such as stress-induced ischemia could have influenced patient prognosis, this study seemed to suggest that patients with coronary artery disease and left ventricular dysfunction who have evidence of ischemic, viable myocardium at rest are at increased risk of having an adverse cardiac event if not revascularized. Those findings have been supported by other studies using PET[12,13] and rest-redistribution Tl-201 SPECT.[14] Although a prospective, randomized trial of revascularization after viability assessment would provide solid scientific proof, this may not be feasible because of ethical considerations.[15]

Thallium-201 imaging for assessment of myocardial viability

Multiple thallium injection and imaging protocols for assessment of myocardial viability have been studied (Figure 7.3). These protocols are discussed below.

Stress–4-h redistribution (conventional protocol)

In 1977, Pohost et al.[16] established in 10 patients with stable angina undergoing exercise stress testing the clinical utility of serial imaging after a single dose of thallium-201 administered

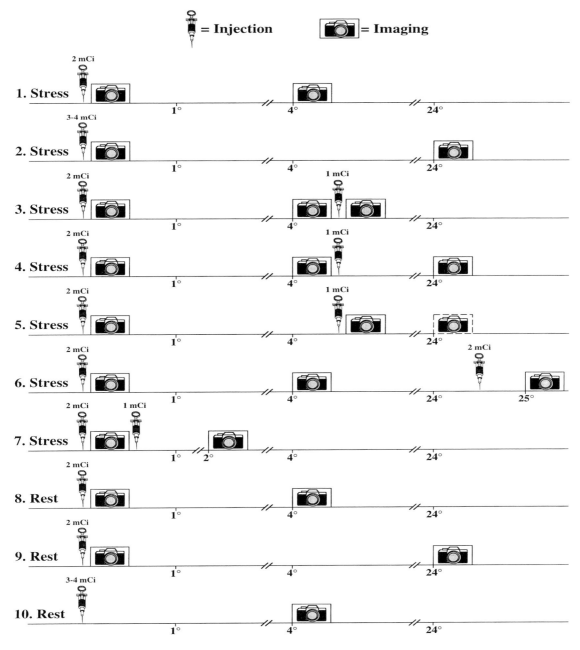

Figure 7.3
Representative thallium-201 stress (1–7) and rest (8–10) protocols. (1) Stress–4-h redistribution (conventional protocol). (2) Stress–24-h redistribution. (3) Stress–4-h redistribution–reinjection. (4) Stress–4-h redistribution–reinjection–24-h redistribution. (5) Stress–4-h reinjection. (6) Stress–4-h redistribution–24-h reinjection. (7) Stress–immediate reinjection. (8) Rest–4-h redistribution. (9) Rest–24-h redistribution. (10) 4-h redistribution (rest). Protocols 3 and 8 (with quantitative analysis) are recommended for identification of myocardial viability. (Technical assistance by Khoa Vo, BS.)

at peak exercise. Defects at 10 minutes after exercise which disappeared partially or completely (redistribution) within 1–6 hours after exercise corresponded to areas supplied by significantly stenosed coronary arteries. On the other hand, persistent defects were noted in areas corresponding to Q-wave leads on the electrocardiogram and akinetic segments on the ventriculogram, considered to represent old myocardial infarction. Upon reviewing individual patient data, it is evident that persistent defects were also seen in areas supplied by a significantly stenosed coronary artery in a patient with wall motion abnormalities on the ventriculogram but no abnormal Q-waves on the electrocardiogram, possibly reflecting the presence of hibernating myocardium, an unknown concept at the time of the study. Moreover, the authors recognized that in 'scar' regions with no (qualitative) increase in Tl-201 activity over time, some Tl-201 may have been taken up initially by residual viable cells.

Subsequent studies[17,18] comparing post-exercise 3–4-h redistribution scans with separate-injection rest scans in the same patients demonstrated a higher frequency of defects[17] and, often, a larger size of defects[18] on redistribution scans. These findings suggested that 4-h redistribution imaging postexercise overestimates myocardial necrosis, limiting its role in the assessment of myocardial viability.

An early study by Rozanski et al.[19] of 25 consecutive patients undergoing CABG suggested that exercise (3–6-h)-redistribution thallium imaging may play a role in differentiating viable from nonviable asynergic myocardial segments, thus predicting the functional response of these segments to coronary revascularization. However, in later studies 45–75% of myocardial segments with a fixed thallium defect before coronary revascularization showed a normal perfusion pattern, suggesting

viability, when exercise-redistribution thallium study was repeated after coronary bypass surgery[20] or coronary angioplasty.[21] Furthermore, PET studies of perfusion (N13-ammonia) and glucose utilization (F18-fluorodeoxyglucose) in glucose-loaded[22] and fasting[23] patients demonstrated residual tissue metabolic activity, indicating viability, in 38–58% of segments with a fixed thallium defect.

The severity of fixed defects on conventional exercise-redistribution thallium imaging has been evaluated in an attempt to enhance the identification of myocardial viability. Less severe fixed defects are more likely to show a normal thallium perfusion pattern postrevascularization.[20] Also, the majority of mild or moderate fixed defects (thallium activity 50–84% relative to a normal reference region) show evidence of myocardial viability by metabolic PET and gated MRI.[24–26] However, up to half of severe fixed defects (relative activity <50%) also show evidence of myocardial viability.[24–26] Therefore, myocardial segments with severe fixed thallium defects would require further work-up (such as metabolic PET or thallium reinjection) to determine viability.

Reverse redistribution has also received attention in the context of myocardial viability assessment in chronic coronary artery disease. Marin-Neto et al.[27] studied 39 patients with coronary artery disease who demonstrated reverse redistribution on postexercise 3–4-h redistribution thallium SPECT imaging. Reverse redistribution was defined as ≥10% decrease in relative Tl-201 activity between stress and redistribution images and included appearance of a new defect on redistribution images or worsening of a defect apparent on stress images. In 82% of regions with reverse redistribution, thallium reinjection immediately after redistribution imaging resulted in ≥10% increase in relative Tl-201 activity between redistribution and reinjection images, suggesting viability. Regions with reverse redistribution which showed improved thallium activity after reinjection were less likely to be associated with abnormal Q-waves and akinetic or dyskinetic wall motion and more likely to be associated with critically stenosed or totally occluded coronary arteries and collateral circulation. In the 16 patients (of 39) who underwent PET imaging with F18-fluorodeoxyglucose (glucose utilization) and O15-water (blood flow), the same regions with reverse redistribution and improved thallium uptake after reinjection manifested normal or mismatch patterns of FDG uptake and blood flow. The investigators concluded that reverse redistribution in chronic coronary artery disease usually reflects viable myocardium.

Similar conclusions were reached by Soufer et al.[28] who studied 32 patients with chronic coronary artery disease and reverse redistribution on exercise-redistribution thallium planar imaging using F18-FDG/N13-ammonia PET imaging.

The mechanisms for the phenomenon of reverse redistribution in chronic coronary disease have not been defined yet, although accelerated wash-out of thallium from the infarct zone, where there is an admixture of viable and necrotic tissue, has been hypothesized.[28]

Stress–late redistribution

Gutman et al.[29] performed serial thallium-201 postexercise imaging in 59 consecutive patients with coronary artery disease. Early (<1 h), average (3–5 h), and late (18–24 h) redistribution were seen in 14%, 32%, and 21%, respectively, of defects present on stress images. There was a significant correlation between the time to completed redistribution and the severity of stenosis in the coronary artery supplying the segment with the defect (Figure 7.4). Segments with defects showing late redistribution were less likely to be akinetic or dyskinetic and less likely

to be associated with abnormal Q-waves on ECG compared with segments with fixed defects (over 24 h). Further or complete thallium redistribution at 8–24 h in patients with incomplete redistribution at 4 h was similarly demonstrated by Cloninger et al.[30] Late redistribution occurred more commonly in patients without history or ECG evidence of prior myocardial infarction, none of whom had regional akinesis or dyskinesis on contrast left ventriculogram.

Among 118 consecutive patients with fixed defects (involving ≥ 2 of total 20 segments) at 4 h postexercise, 18–72-h redistribution (in ≥ 2 segments) occurred in 35% of patients and 19% of segments.[31] Performing stress and late redistribution imaging only (eliminating 4-h redistribution imaging) allowed the identification of the vast majority of reversible stress defects.[31]

In a study of 21 patients undergoing coronary artery bypass grafting or percutaneous transluminal coronary angioplasty,[32] 95% of segments with stress defects exhibiting late redistribution (18–72 h) on pre-revascularization thallium SPECT showed improved stress perfusion on thallium SPECT postrevascularization. However, 37% of segments with stress defects exhibiting no late redistribution prerevascularization also showed improved thallium activity on stress images postrevascularization. The latter findings, suggesting overestimation of myocardial nonviability by poststress late redistribution imaging, were attributed by the authors to revascularization 'referral bias' — that is, preferential referral for revascularization of those patients without evidence of prior myocardial infarction and with clinical or electrocardiographic evidence of myocardial ischemia.

In concert with the above findings, among patients with coronary artery disease and impaired left ventricular function, PET detected tissue metabolic activity, and hence viability, in

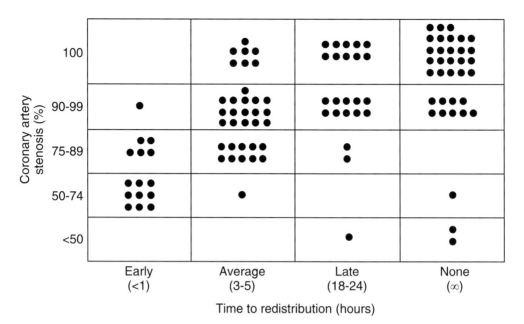

Figure 7.4
*Correlation between degree of coronary artery stenosis and time to redistribution of Tl-201 stress-induced defects (r = 0.56, p = 0.001). (Reprinted with permission from Gutman J et al, Time to completed redistribution of thallium-201 in exercise myocardial scintigraphy: relationship to the degree of coronary artery stenosis, Am Heart J (1983) **106**: 989–95.)[29]*

51% of segments with fixed defects on 24-h redistribution thallium SPECT.[33] Nevertheless, when thallium activity was visually scored on 24-h images, very severe (near-complete) defects were unlikely to exhibit metabolic activity on PET whereas mild defects were very likely to show metabolic activity.[33]

It should be noted that due to lower image count density, late images are usually inferior in quality to 3–4-h images. That may be a significant disadvantage in obese patients and in women with large breasts because of increased soft tissue photon attenuation. While increasing image acquisition time could increase image count density, motion artefacts may ensue.

Stress–4-h redistribution–reinjection

As mentioned previously,[17,18] performing two separate injections of thallium at stress and at rest on 2 different days has an advantage over single injection at stress (stress–4-h redistribution) in detection of myocardial viability. Hence, a modified double-injection technique was proposed in patients with coronary artery disease,[34] using reinjection (second injection) of thallium immediately after 3–4-h post-stress redistribution imaging, and performing reinjection imaging 10–15 min thereafter. Tamaki et al.[35] found that segments with fixed defects that improved postreinjection were less likely than those with fixed defects that did not improve postreinjection but were more likely than those with reversible defects to have severe wall motion abnormalities and to be associated with abnormal Q-waves on ECG.

In a leading study by Dilsizian et al.[36] of 100 patients with known coronary artery disease, 49% by qualitative analysis (and 40% by quantitative analysis) of irreversible (fixed) defects on redistribution images demonstrated improved (or normal) thallium activity on reinjection images (Figures 7.5 and 7.6). In a subset of 20 patients who underwent coronary angioplasty, the response to revascularization of regions with persistent (irreversible or partially reversible) defects on pre-revascularization redistribution images was analyzed. Of those regions showing enhanced thallium activity on reinjection images before angioplasty, 87% had normal thallium activity on both stress and redistribution images and improved wall

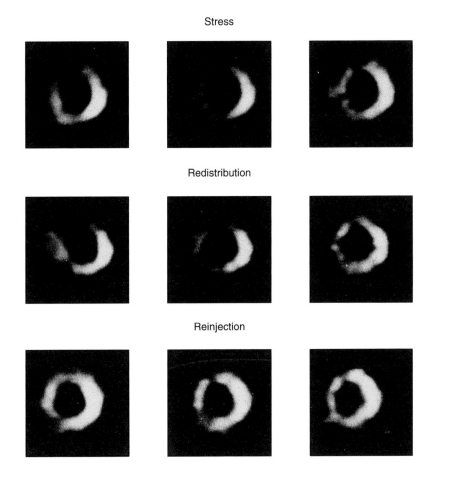

Figure 7.5
*Short-axis thallium tomograms during stress, redistribution, and reinjection imaging in a patient with coronary artery disease. The tomographic sections are 4 pixels thick from apex (left) to base (right). There were extensive abnormalities in anterior and septal perfusion during stress imaging that persisted on redistribution imaging but improved markedly on reinjection imaging. (Reprinted with permission from Dilsizian V et al, Enhanced detection of ischemic but viable myocardium by the reinjection of thallium after stress–redistribution imaging, N Engl J Med (1990) **323**: 141–6.)[36]*

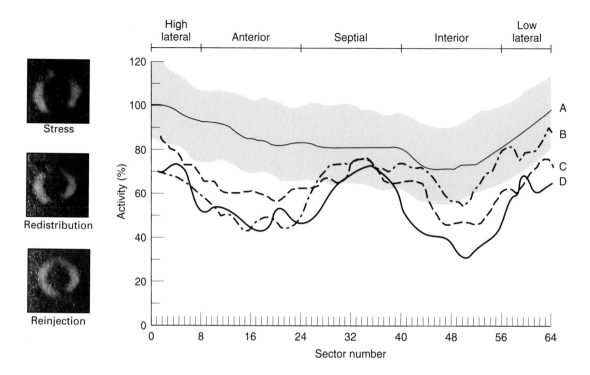

Figure 7.6

Quantitative analysis of regional thallium activity. The redistribution (line C) and reinjection (line B) curves are shown as a percentage of the activity in the sector with peak activity during stress imaging (line D). In this patient, the myocardial sectors in the anterior and high lateral regions with abnormal perfusion (that is, below the normal range) during exercise testing continued to have abnormal perfusion on the redistribution study but improved on reinjection imaging. The abnormal perfusion evident in the myocardial sectors in the inferior and low lateral regions during exercise testing was partially reversed on the redistribution study, and it returned to normal on reinjection imaging. The normal range (mean ± 2 SD for normal subjects) is denoted by the shaded area with the centered line (A). (Reprinted with permission from Dilsizian V et al, Enhanced detection of ischemic but viable myocardium by the reinjection of thallium after stress–redistribution imaging, N Engl J Med (1990)323: 141–6.)[36]

motion at rest after angioplasty. In contrast, all regions showing persistent defects on reinjection images before angioplasty again demonstrated persistent perfusion defects and resting wall motion abnormalities after angioplasty.

Similarly, in 24 patients referred for coronary bypass surgery, Ohtani et al.[37] showed thallium activity enhancement (defect 'fill-in') after reinjection in 47% of fixed defects on 3-h post-exercise redistribution images. The sensitivities

of preoperative exercise-redistribution-reinjection imaging for predicting postoperative improvement in perfusion on redistribution images and wall motion at rest were 94% and 89%, respectively, which were significantly higher than the sensitivities of preoperative exercise-redistribution (only) imaging (69% and 62%, respectively). However, the specificities of preoperative exercise-redistribution-reinjection imaging in predicting postoperative improvement in perfusion and wall motion were only 54% and 50%, respectively, and not significantly different from the specificities of exercise-redistribution imaging (65% and 67%, respectively). Those results suggest no improvement in regional perfusion and wall motion post-CABG in some regions considered viable by thallium reinjection imaging preoperatively, but do not necessarily imply that thallium reinjection imaging was false in determining viability. As discussed earlier, lack of improvement in resting regional function may be due to necrosis involving the inner (subendocardial) layers of the ventricular wall with residual viability in the outer layers. Also, regional perfusion may not be expected to become normal in regions with nontransmural necrosis.

Further work by the same group[38] supports the accuracy of thallium reinjection imaging in determining presence of viability. Of all segments showing fixed defects on the 3-h redistribution scans in 18 patients with coronary artery disease, the reinjection scan exhibited thallium activity enhancement in 42% and no such enhancement in 58%. All segments with enhanced thallium activity after reinjection demonstrated FDG uptake on PET, consistent with residual viability, and 65% of them showed improved wall motion after coronary bypass surgery. Moreover, 25% of segments with no enhancement postreinjection were also PET viable, and improved in wall motion after coronary bypass surgery. The possibility of overestimation of nonviability by thallium reinjection imaging was raised.[38]

There are possible limitations to using only the change in relative thallium activity from redistribution images to reinjection images for myocardial viability assessment.[24,25,38] Regional relative thallium activity is determined as per convention. The myocardial region with the maximum (peak) thallium activity (mean counts per pixel) on the stress images is used as the normal reference region in each patient and the same corresponding regions in the redistribution and reinjection images are used as the reference regions for those studies. The thallium activity in all other myocardial regions is then expressed as a percent of the activity measured in the reference region on each of the stress, redistribution, and reinjection images.

Bonow et al.[24] studied 16 patients with chronic stable coronary artery disease who underwent both exercise-redistribution-reinjection thallium SPECT and resting F18-fluorodeoxyglucose and O15-water PET. They found that among the regions with irreversible thallium defects on exercise-redistribution imaging, 12% of regions with increase in relative thallium activity after reinjection had no FDG uptake and, more importantly, 59% of regions with no increase in relative thallium activity after reinjection had FDG uptake. When irreversible defects on redistribution images were graded in severity according to their level of relative thallium activity — mild (60–84% of peak activity), moderate (50–59% of peak activity), and severe (<50% of peak activity) — the discordance between postreinjection increase in relative thallium activity and resting FDG uptake was found to be greatest in those regions with only mild or moderate irreversible thallium defects on redistribution images, in which the vast majority (84–91%) showed FDG uptake while less than half (42–47%) showed an increase in relative thallium activity postreinjection. On the other hand, among regions with severe irreversible defects on redistribution images, 51% were classified as viable by PET and 51% were classified as viable by thallium reinjection, with concordance in 88% of regions: 45% viable and 43% nonviable (scar). The authors concluded that combined assessment in exercise-redistribution fixed defects of level of thallium activity on redistribution images (mild or moderate defects = viable) and change of level of thallium activity from redistribution to reinjection images (severe defects with enhanced activity postreinjection = viable) provides comparable viability data (with few exceptions) to FDG uptake by PET.

The same group proposed that assessing the increase in regional absolute thallium activity (rather than the change in regional relative thallium activity) from redistribution images to reinjection images may improve myocardial viability determination.[25] In each patient, of the myocardial regions determined to be normal on the stress images, the region with the maximum increase in thallium activity from redistribution to reinjection was used as the normal reference region for that patient. The increase in thallium activity from redistribution to reinjection in all other myocardial regions was expressed as a percent of the increase in the normal reference region and termed regional 'differential uptake'. In 150 patients with chronic stable coronary artery disease who underwent exercise-redistribution-reinjection thallium SPECT,[25] irreversible thallium defects on redistribution images were graded in severity, as in the previous study.[24] All regions with mild or moderate irreversible defects demonstrated ≥50% differential uptake after reinjection, regardless of whether or not relative thallium activity increased postreinjection (Figures 7.7 and 7.8). On the other hand, among regions with severe irreversible defects, the vast majority of those with increase in relative thallium activity postreinjection had differential uptake ≥50%, whereas the vast majority of those with no increase in relative thallium activity postreinjection had differential uptake <50% (Figures 7.7 and 7.8). In 15 patients who also underwent F18-fluorodeoxyglucose and O15-water PET at rest, the results of differential uptake and FDG for viability assessment

in regions with irreversible defects on redistribution images were concordant in 81% of mild-to-moderate defects and 67% of severe defects. Those findings further supported the role of grading the severity of thallium defects on redistribution and measuring the change in thallium activity with reinjection in the assessment of myocardial viability.

Clinicopathologic correlation has come from a study of 37 patients with left anterior descending coronary artery disease who had exercise-redistribution-reinjection planar Tl-201 scintigraphy before coronary artery bypass grafting and transmural left ventricular anterior wall biopsy intraoperatively.[39] Among the 15 patients with irreversible thallium defects in the left anterior descending coronary artery perfusion territory on their exercise-redistribution images, there was a significant inverse relation between the amount of myocardial interstitial fibrosis and the level of relative Tl-201 activity in the defect region on redistribution images and, to a stronger degree, on reinjection images.

Several modifications in the original stress-redistribution-reinjection protocol have been studied, some of which are discussed below.

Stress–4-h redistribution–reinjection–24-h redistribution

Dilsizian et al.[40] compared this protocol, where imaging is performed late following reinjection (which is done at 4 hours poststress), with the original protocol, where imaging is performed immediately following reinjection. Among regions with irreversible thallium defects on stress-redistribution imaging, only 3% to 11% (by qualitative and quantitative analysis, respectively) of regions with no increase in relative thallium activity immediately postreinjection showed improvement at 24 hours. Hence, the authors concluded, 24-h delayed (compared with immediate) imaging after reinjection offers

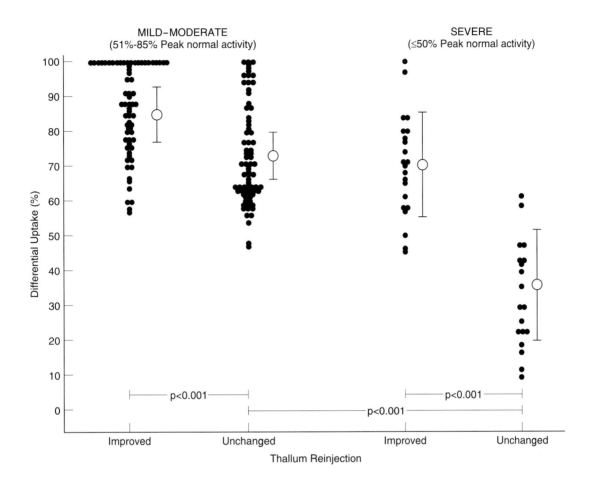

Figure 7.7
Plots show differential regional uptake of thallium after reinjection based on analysis of changes in magnitude of regional thallium activity in regions with irreversible thallium defects on redistribution imaging. Left panel: regions with mild-to-moderate reduction in thallium activity on redistribution images (ranging from 51% to 85% of peak normal activity). Right panel: regions with severe reduction in thallium activity (≤50% of peak activity). Within each panel, regions are further subdivided on the basis of improved or unchanged relative thallium activity after reinjection. Mild-to-moderate defects in which relative thallium activity was unchanged after reinjection had significantly greater increase in absolute thallium activity than severe defects in which relative thallium activity was unchanged after reinjection. (Reprinted with permission from Dilsizian V et al, Regional thallium uptake in irreversible defects. Magnitude of change in thallium activity after reinjection distinguishes viable from nonviable myocardium, Circulation *(1992)* **85**: 627–34.)[25]

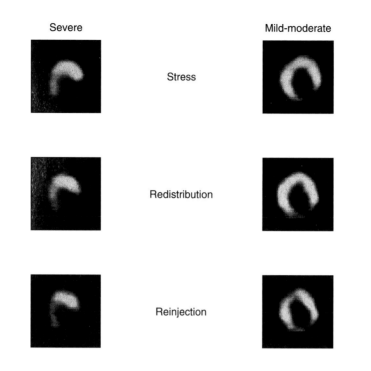

Figure 7.8

Single short-axis tomographic planes of stress, redistribution, and reinjection are presented from two different patients with coronary artery disease. Both patients have inferolateral thallium defects that appear irreversible on redistribution and reinjection images. Left panel: severe irreversible thallium defect after reinjection (27% of peak normal activity) in which the increase in absolute thallium activity was only 29% of normal. Right panel: mild-to-moderate thallium defect, although irreversible after reinjection by relative analysis (62% of peak normal activity), had an increase in absolute thallium activity that was 88% of normal. (Reprinted with permission from Dilsizian V et al, Regional thallium uptake in irreversible defects. Magnitude of change in thallium activity after reinjection distinguishes viable from nonviable myocardium, Circulation *(1992)* **85***: 627–34.)[25]*

little additional information regarding myocardial viability in regions with an irreversible thallium defect on 3–4-h redistribution images.

Stress–4-h reinjection

Because of logistical difficulties for a busy nuclear cardiology laboratory from the standard reinjection protocol, some laboratories eliminated 3–4-h redistribution imaging and started performing stress and 3–4-h reinjection

imaging only. However, Dilsizian and Bonow[41] demonstrated that 8% of regions with reduced relative thallium activity (by quantitative analysis using a normal reference group) on exercise images show complete or partial reversibility (redistribution) at 3–4 hours but exhibit apparent thallium wash-out (due to low differential uptake: defined above) after reinjection (Figures 7.9 and 7.10). Therefore, if 3–4-h redistribution imaging was eliminated, those regions would appear to have irreversible thallium defects,

Stress

Redistribution

Reinjection

24 Hour

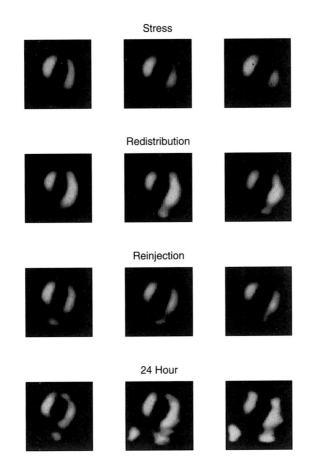

Figure 7.9
Thallium tomograms showing an example of apparent wash-out after reinjection due to low differential uptake. Three consecutive 3-pixel-thick short-axis tomograms from apex to base are displayed for stress (top), redistribution, reinjection, and 24 hours (bottom). There are extensive thallium perfusion abnormalities in anterior, septal, and inferior regions on stress images. Anterior and inferior thallium abnormalities persist on redistribution, reinjection, and 24-h studies. However, in septum, there is evidence of thallium redistribution at 3–4 hours; thallium appears to wash out in septum on reinjection images but again redistributes at 24 hours. Early (3–4-h) and late (24-h) images are comparable. (Reprinted with permission from Dilsizian V, Bonow RO, Differential uptake and apparent ^{201}Tl washout after thallium reinjection. Options regarding early redistribution imaging before reinjection or late redistribution imaging after reinjection, Circulation *(1992)* **85***: 1032–8.)[41]*

falsely implying nonviability. Such regions represent one-quarter of all regions with exercise-redistribution reversible defects. The same regions again appear reversible postreinjection if 24-h redistribution images are obtained. Thus, Dilsizian and Bonow recommended using either stress-redistribution-reinjection imaging (original protocol) or stress-reinjection-24-h imaging for assessment of myocardial viability.[41]

Nevertheless, some investigators have argued that the relatively small number of regions

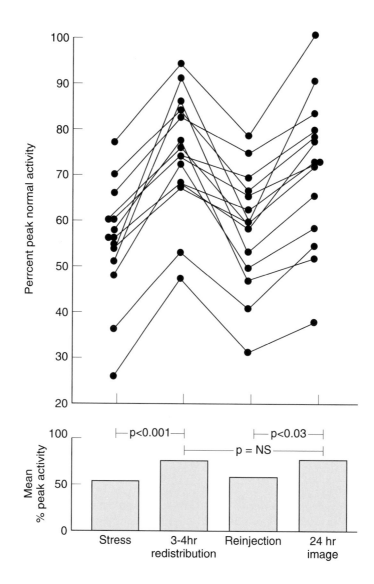

Figure 7.10

*Relative regional thallium activity (presented as a percentage of normal activity) in 14 regions demonstrating phenomenon of apparent thallium wash-out due to low differential uptake. Top panel: plot of individual data points displayed for stress, 3–4-h redistribution, reinjection, and 24-h images. Bottom panel: bar graphs of mean thallium activity in relation to each of four corresponding images. If 3–4-h redistribution images were eliminated and reinjection images were acquired alone, these regions would be incorrectly designated irreversible. On 24-h images, redistribution is again apparent, indicating reversibility of defect, and relative thallium activity is similar to that observed on 3–4-h redistribution studies. (Reprinted with permission from Dilsizian V, Bonow RO, Differential uptake and apparent ^{201}Tl washout after thallium reinjection. Options regarding early redistribution imaging before reinjection or late redistribution imaging after reinjection, Circulation (1992) **85**: 1032–8.)[41]*

where the interpretation of a defect may change from reversible to irreversible if redistribution imaging is eliminated does not justify the additional logistical costs.[42] In fact, using an exercise–4-h reinjection imaging protocol, He et al.[42] found that administering isosorbide dinitrate immediately after exercise imaging enhanced detection of ischemic but viable myocardium: 26% of apparently fixed defects on exercise–4-h reinjection images were reversible when nitrate was administered. The apparent improvement is presumably due to increase in coronary blood flow to ischemic myocardial regions.

Furthermore, in the above-mentioned study by Dilsizian and Bonow,[41] the majority of regions with falsely irreversible defects by stress-reinjection imaging had thallium activity $\geq 50\%$ peak normal (Figure 7.10). Thus, with the stress–4-h reinjection protocol, classifying mild or moderate irreversible defects as viable might further minimize any potential underestimation of viability.

Stress–4-h redistribution–24-h reinjection

Kayden et al.[43] showed that imaging 30–45 minutes after thallium reinjection at 24 hours yields 52% reversibility of stress defects, compared with 25% stress defect reversibility with 2–4-h redistribution imaging and 35% stress defect reversibility with 24-h redistribution imaging. Among patients with reversible defects on 2–4-h redistribution imaging, 10–14% showed fixed rather than reversible defects on 24-h redistribution imaging and 24-h reinjection imaging. In a subsequent study, there was no significant difference in results between imaging 30 minutes or 4 hours after thallium reinjection at 48–72 hours poststress.[44]

The separate-day thallium reinjection protocol deserves further investigation regarding its prediction of functional recovery post-revascularization as well as comparison with established methods for assessment of myocardial viability.

Stress–immediate reinjection

This protocol entails immediate thallium-201 reinjection following stress imaging and repeat imaging 1 hour later.[45] The advocates of such modification of the original reinjection protocol argued that it would reduce total imaging time and improve convenience for the patient. Using planar thallium imaging and questionable definitions for viability (normal or hypokinetic systolic wall motion) and nonviability (akinetic or dyskinetic systolic wall motion), the above protocol yielded 89% sensitivity and 46% specificity for detection of 'viability'.[46] Correlation with PET, established thallium protocols for viability assessment, or functional response to coronary revascularization is lacking.

The usefulness of an earlier proposed protocol[47] in which thallium-201 is reinjected immediately after stress imaging and imaging is repeated after 4 hours has been controversial.[47,48]

Rest–4-h redistribution

In 1979, Gewirtz et al.[49] performed serial imaging over 2–4 hours after thallium-201 injection at rest in 20 patients with severe coronary artery disease ($\geq 75\%$ luminal diameter narrowing) and no evidence of acute myocardial ischemia. Of the defects present on the initial scans (5–10 minutes postinjection), 57% filled in completely or partially, three-quarters doing so within the first 30–45 minutes. Transient defects were more likely than normal segments but less likely than persistent defects to be associated with electrocardiographic evidence of previous myocardial infarction. Transient defects and normal segments were both less likely than persistent defects to be associated with akinesis or dyskinesis on left ventriculography. Transient defects were more likely than normal segments to be associated with ≥75% diameter stenosis and less likely than persistent defects to be associated with complete occlusion on coronary arteriography. Thus, serial imaging after thallium injection at rest was found to be better than single immediate imaging, which would overestimate myocardial scar.

In 22 patients with stable or unstable angina but no acute ischemia who underwent resting thallium injection and serial imaging over 2–4 hours before and (7–10 days) after coronary bypass surgery, 77% of segments showing a transient defect on preoperative imaging normalized postoperatively, no longer showing a defect on the initial (10-minute) images.[50] Unexpectedly, 67% of segments showing a persistent defect on preoperative imaging also demonstrated no defect on the initial images postoperatively. The segments with a persistent defect preoperatively that improved with coronary revascularization were unlikely to be associated with abnormal Q-waves on the electrocardiogram. Therefore, persistent thallium defects on serial imaging at rest, particularly when not associated with Q-waves, may also not represent myocardial scar.

Immediate and 4-hour redistribution imaging after thallium injection at rest was performed before coronary artery bypass grafting in 26 patients with coronary artery disease and left ventricular dysfunction studied by Iskandrian and coworkers.[51] Patients with no or reversible resting thallium defects preoperatively were more likely than those with fixed defects (75% versus 20%) to show ≥5% improvement in left ventricular ejection fraction with coronary revascularization. The authors noted that abnormal Q-waves on the resting ECG and improvement in left ventricular ejection fraction after sublingual nitroglycerin on radionuclide ventriculography were less useful in predicting response of left ventricular function to coronary revascularization.

Mori et al.[52] performed rest–4-h redistribution thallium-201 planar imaging with quantitative analysis prior to coronary revascularization (PTCA or CABG) in 17 patients with previous anterior myocardial infarction (associated with severe hypokinesis, akinesis, or dyskinesis) and ≥90% left anterior descending coronary artery stenosis. Among myocardial regions exhibiting resting thallium redistribution, 79% had improvement in wall motion with revascularization. Moreover, 38% of myocardial regions not showing resting thallium redistribution also had improvement in wall motion with revascularization. Nevertheless, these regions without resting thallium redistribution but with wall motion improvement had higher regional thallium activity on the redistribution images than the regions without resting thallium redistribution that did not have improvement in wall motion. Those results suggested that presence of thallium redistribution or high thallium activity in absence of redistribution may predict functional improvement with revascularization, and hence viability, of severely asynergic myocardium.

Similarly, Ragosta et al.[53] studied 21 patients with coronary artery disease and left ventricular ejection fraction <35% who were referred for CABG and who underwent preoperative and postoperative planar thallium-201 rest–3-h redistribution imaging. Based on quantitative analysis of preoperative rest-redistribution images, one of three patterns of viability was identified in each myocardial segment: normal (no defect or defect with complete redistribution), mildly reduced (defect with partial redistribution or mild — 50–75% peak thallium activity — persistent defect), and severely reduced (severe — <50% peak thallium activity — persistent defect). Among severely asynergic (severely hypokinetic, akinetic, or dyskinetic) segments, 62% of those with normal viability and 54% of those with mildly reduced viability improved in function after surgery, compared with only 23% of those with severely reduced viability. When only severely asynergic segments with preoperative thallium defect and postoperative improvement in thallium activity (suggesting adequate and sustained revascularization and no perioperative infarct) were considered, the predictive value of a positive (normal or mildly reduced) preoperative viability test for functional improvement was 73% and the predictive value of a negative (severely reduced) preoperative viability test for lack of functional improvement was 77%. Moreover, with respect to global left ventricular function, patients with more than seven (of a total of 15) segments that were viable but asynergic had a significant improvement in left ventricular ejection fraction (from 27% to 41%), whereas patients with ≤ 7 viable, asynergic segments had no significant change in left ventricular ejection fraction. The investigators concluded that rest-redistribution thallium imaging may be helpful in the selection of patients with low ejection fraction who would benefit most from coronary artery bypass grafting. It should be noted that three-quarters of the patients in this study were included after presenting with acute myocardial infarction or unstable angina. Therefore, the above findings may not be readily extrapolated to patients with chronic coronary artery disease.

Pace et al. studied the phenomenon of reverse redistribution in relation to viability assessment on rest–4-h redistribution thallium scintigraphy.[54] As with stress–4-h redistribution thallium scintigraphy, two patterns of reverse redistribution were identified: pattern A with normal thallium activity on the initial images and reduced thallium activity on the redistribution images; and pattern B with reduced thallium activity on the initial images and further reduced thallium activity on the redistribution images. In 19 patients with coronary artery disease who had rest–4-h redistribution imaging before coronary revascularization (9 CABG, 10 PTCA),[54] segments with pattern B reverse redistribution were more commonly associated with abnormal Q-waves and akinesis/dyskinesis (before revascularization) than segments with pattern A reverse redistribution. Among segments with abnormal wall motion that demonstrated reverse redistribution, all those with pattern A but only 40% of those with pattern B had improved wall motion after revascularization. Although these results came from a small patient group with a small number of segments showing reverse redistribution, they suggested that dyssynergic segments with pattern A reverse redistribution at rest may be considered viable.

A few modifications to the original rest–redistribution protocol have been used. They are described below.

Rest–late redistribution

In 14 patients with coronary artery disease and regional wall motion abnormalities at rest due to previous myocardial infarction, thallium imaging was performed prior to successful coronary revascularization (CABG or PTCA) 10 minutes and 16 hours after thallium injection at rest.[55] However, scientigraphic criteria for viability were not clearly defined and data on defect reversibility were not provided. Therefore, it is unknown whether performing redistribution imaging late after resting injection has an advantage over standard 4-h redistribution imaging.

4-h redistribution (rest)

In 20 patients with coronary artery disease who underwent FDG metabolic imaging at rest and single-time thallium imaging 3 hours after thallium injection at rest, 'fixed' thallium defects were defined as segments with <50% peak thallium activity.[56] Significant FDG uptake suggesting metabolic viability was seen in 23% of fixed thallium defects; however, no data on thallium viable/FDG nonviable segments were provided and no data on functional response to revascularization were available.

Comparative studies of thallium-201 protocols for assessment of myocardial viability

The two most promising thallium-201 protocols for viability assessment, namely stress–4-h redistribution–reinjection and rest–4-h redistribution, have been compared.[57,58]

Both protocols using thallium SPECT imaging with quantitative analysis were performed 1–2 weeks apart in 41 patients with chronic stable coronary artery disease who had an irreversible thallium defect on postexercise 3–4-h redistribution images.[57] Among irreversible thallium defects, 79% showed concordance in the results of the two protocols regarding viability or nonviability. The concordance between stress–redistribution–reinjection and rest–redistribution improved further when the severity of reduction in thallium activity within irreversible defects was considered. In 20 patients who underwent PET at rest with F18-fluorodeoxyglucose and O15-water, the concordance between PET and stress–redistribution–reinjection was higher than that between PET and rest–redistribution among severe irreversible defects showing discordance between the two

thallium protocols, with the latter protocol generally underestimating viability. However, given the small number of such defects (20% of all severe irreversible defects but only 3% of all myocardial regions), an underestimation of viability by rest–redistribution is likely to have negligible clinical relevance.

As expected, the stress component of stress–redistribution–reinjection allowed better detection of coronary artery disease. There was a significant association between the severity of thallium activity reduction during stress, but not at rest, and percent coronary artery stenosis. Therefore, for assessment of viability as well as inducible ischemia specifically, stress–redistribution–reinjection imaging has an obvious advantage over rest–redistribution imaging.

Similar results on the high concordance of stress–redistribution–reinjection and rest–redistribution quantitative thallium SPECT imaging for myocardial viability assessment were reported in patients with coronary artery disease and regional left ventricular dysfunction at rest due to previous myocardial infarction.[58]

On the other hand, a multicenter study[44] in patients undergoing exercise testing who had at least one stress thallium defect compared planar imaging ≥30 minutes after thallium reinjection (immediately following conventional redistribution imaging) at 3–4 hours poststress with imaging ≥30 minutes after reinjection at 48–72 hours poststress. Among fixed defects on conventional stress–redistribution images, there was a higher prevalence of improvement in thallium activity with reinjection at 48–72 hours (36%), compared with reinjection at 3–4 hours (27%). However, since the imaging protocols were tested in two different groups of consecutive patients undergoing exercise stress testing (rather than in the same patients), definitive conclusions cannot be made regarding the superiority of one protocol over the other.

Technetium-99m sestamibi imaging for assessment of myocardial viability

Because technetium-99m sestamibi was originally believed not to undergo clinically significant redistribution (unlike thallium-201), most studies of its use in viability assessment have involved single-time imaging after resting administration.

In patients with prior myocardial infarction, Rocco et al.[59] showed that 26% of vascular territories with markedly reduced (qualitative) technetium-99m sestamibi activity on resting planar images have normal wall motion. Moreover, sestamibi activity improved after coronary bypass surgery (suggesting viability) in 92% of vascular territories with reduced sestamibi activity preoperatively, including all vascular territories with markedly reduced sestamibi activity. It was concluded that even markedly reduced technetium-99m sestamibi activity on visual analysis should not necessarily be considered evidence of myocardial scar.

Altehoefer et al.[60] studied 46 patients with coronary artery disease and severe wall motion abnormalities who underwent Tc-99m sestamibi SPECT imaging 1–2 hours after injection at rest and F18-deoxyglucose PET imaging on the same day at rest. Among segments with a resting Tc-99m sestamibi defect, 23% showed FDG uptake in the area of the defect and another 24% showed FDG uptake in the periphery of the defect only. Those results indicated that Tc-99m sestamibi overestimates the extent of myocardial scar. When resting defects were grouped according to the degree of Tc-99m sestamibi activity reduction (in percentage of peak activity), 80% of severe ($\leq$30% of peak activity) defects, 48% of moderate (31–50% of peak activity) defects, and 31% of mild (>50% of peak activity) defects were considered non-

viable on the basis of reduced FDG uptake. Thus, in this study even quantitative analysis with severity grading of resting sestamibi defects could not reliably differentiate viable from nonviable myocardium. Subsequent studies have confirmed the overestimation of myocardial necrosis by Tc-99m sestamibi compared with PET.[61–63]

Marzullo et al.[64] followed 14 patients with regional wall motion abnormalities at rest due to previous myocardial infarction who had resting Tc-99m sestamibi planar imaging before undergoing coronary revascularization (CABG or PTCA). Segments with <55% peak activity (that is, >2.5 standard deviations below normal activity) were considered nonviable by sestamibi. Among dyssynergic segments, the sensitivity and specificity of sestamibi in the prediction of postrevascularization functional improvement were 83% and 68%, respectively. Again, sestamibi appeared to provide suboptimal information regarding viability.

Prolonged infusion of Tc-99m sestamibi at rest was suggested (instead of the usual bolus injection) to allow for greater uptake by viable but hypoperfused myocardial cells; however, data on this are limited.[65]

Administration of nitrate (orally or by infusion) before resting Tc-99m sestamibi bolus injection appears to enhance the detection of ischemic viable myocardium, presumably due to improvement in coronary and collateral blood flow and possibly due to (transient) improvement in regional dysfunction (with resultan attenuation of sestamibi defect).[66–68] In patients with previous myocardial infarction and left ventricular dysfunction, there is excellent agreement between (pre-revascularization) nitrate-induced improvement in the extent of resting global sestamibi defect and revascularization-related improvement in resting left ventricular ejection fraction.[66,68] Among segments with severely reduced sestamibi activity at rest in patients with coronary artery disease and left ventricular dysfunction, 87% of those with significant increase in sestamibi activity after nitrate showed wall motion improvement after coronary revascularization, whereas 89% of those without significant increase in sestamibi activity after nitrate did not show wall motion improvement after coronary revascularization.[67]

Electrocardiographic gated acquisition of Tc-99m sestamibi SPECT, which offers the potential for assessment of both myocardial perfusion and function (wall motion and wall thickening) from a single study, has been evaluated for the assessment of myocardial viability.[69] In 58 patients referred for myocardial perfusion imaging, sestamibi was injected at peak stress (treadmill exercise or adenosine infusion) and sestamibi ECG-gated SPECT images were acquired 30 minutes to 1 hour later, thus showing stress perfusion/rest function. 'Reversibility' of a stress perfusion defect, defined as the presence of normal or mildly reduced resting wall motion or normal or mildly reduced resting wall thickening, was taken to indicate viability by gated sestamibi. Compared with stress sestamibi–rest thallium-late redistribution thallium imaging for the assessment of defect reversibility (indicating viability), gated sestamibi imaging showed excellent agreement in patients without previous myocardial infarction but not in patients with previous myocardial infarction. Gated sestamibi nonviability/thallium viability is probably due to the reduced wall motion and thickening seen with chronic ischemia (myocardial hibernation) or following acute stress-induced ischemia (myocardial stunning). On the other hand, gated sestamibi viability/thallium nonviability is possibly due to mixture of viable myocardium and scar with no reversible ischemia and may be minimized if all mild-to-moderate irreversible thallium defects are considered as viable. Therefore, in patients with previous myocardial infarction,

gated sestamibi is suboptimal for the assessment of myocardial viability.

Although there is minimal technetium-99m sestamibi redistribution over time, there is now some evidence that it may be detectable and clinically relevant for the assessment of myocardial viability.[62,70] Acquisition of (pre-stress) 4-h redistribution images (in addition to 45–60-min images) after resting sestamibi injection reduced the overestimation of stress defect irreversibility by Tc-99m sestamibi and improved the concordance regarding reversibility/irreversibility of stress defects between thallium stress–redistribution–reinjection imaging and sestamibi imaging from 71% to 82%.[62] In eight patients with coronary artery disease and left ventricular dysfunction who underwent coronary revascularization (CABG or PTCA), the results of pre-revascularization rest–redistribution Tc-99m sestamibi imaging were analyzed.[70] Among myocardial segments with wall motion abnormalities that showed severe (<50% of peak activity) Tc-99m sestamibi defects on the initial images (1 hour after resting injection), 83% of those with defect reversibility on the 5-h delayed images had wall motion improvement after revascularization, whereas 96% of those with defect irreversibility on the 5-h delayed images had no wall motion improvement after revascularization. Among myocardial segments with wall motion abnormalities and moderate (≥50% of peak activity) Tc-99m sestamibi defects on the initial images, 85% of those with reversible defects on the delayed images showed wall motion improvement after revascularization; however, data on the functional response to revascularization of segments with wall motion abnormalities and moderate irreversible defects were not provided. Thus, delayed Tc-99m sestamibi imaging following rest injection may lessen the disadvantage of sestamibi in assessing myocardial viability.

Comparative studies of technetium-99m sestamibi and thallium-201 for assessment of myocardial viability

Technetium-99m sestamibi rest imaging has been compared with thallium-201 protocols used in myocardial viability assessment (Figure 7.11). In 20 patients with coronary artery dis-ease and impaired left ventricular function with previous myocardial infarction and at least one irreversible defect on exercise–redistribution thallium-201 imaging, Cuocolo et al.[72] showed increased thallium activity after thallium rein-jection in 47% of segments with irreversible thallium defects on redistribution. In compari-son, among segments with irreversible thallium defects on redistribution, only 18% appeared as reversible defects on technetium-99m sestamibi stress–rest imaging. Thus, in this study using qualitative analysis, planar technetium imaging

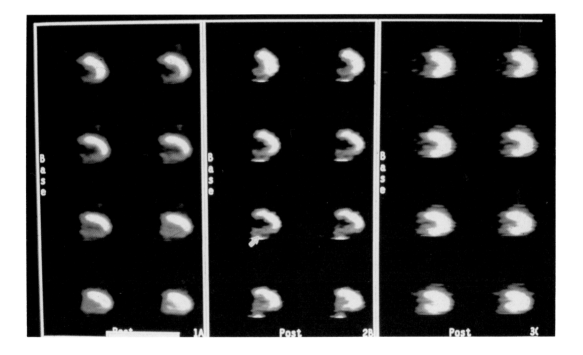

Figure 7.11

Technetium-99m sestamibi compared with thallium-201 for assessment of myocardial viability: overestimation of myocardial scar. Vertical long-axis tomographic images in a patient with exertional chest pain: stress sestamibi (left panel), rest sestamibi the following day (middle panel), and 24-h redistribution rest thallium a few days later (right panel). Note thallium uptake in the inferior wall region with fixed sestamibi defect. Cardiac catheterization showed the right coronary artery totally occluded in its proximal portion and filling distally by collaterals, and normal inferior wall motion. (Courtesy of Dr Alan M Taylor II.)[71]

was inferior to planar thallium imaging in the assessment of myocardial viability.

Taking >50% (of peak) activity as an indicator of 'clinically significant' viability, Anagnostopoulos et al.[73] found a significantly greater number of viable segments by thallium-201 4-h redistribution imaging after resting thallium reinjection 24 hours post-stress than by technetium-99m sestamibi imaging 1 hour after resting sestamibi injection (73% versus 59%) in patients with prior myocardial infarction and impaired left ventricular function, but no difference in patients with normal left ventricular function and no prior myocardial infarction.

On the other hand, a few studies suggest that with quantitative analysis, Tc-99m sestamibi imaging may provide viability information similar to Tl-201 imaging. Dilsizian et al.[62] showed that when irreversible sestamibi defects (on rest–stress imaging) were graded in severity (similarly to irreversible thallium defects on stress–redistribution–reinjection imaging) and mild-to-moderate defects (51–85% of peak activity) were considered viable, there was less overestimation of necrosis by Tc-99m sestamibi and the overall concordance in viability/nonviability between sestamibi SPECT imaging and thallium SPECT imaging was 93%. Taking >60% (of peak) activity as an indicator of viability, Udelson et al.[74] showed no significant difference in positive and negative predictive values for postrevascularization improvement of severe regional dysfunction between 3–4-h rest redistribution thallium SPECT imaging (75% and 92%, respectively) and 1-h rest sestamibi SPECT imaging (80% and 96%, respectively).

In summary, the role of technetium-99m sestamibi imaging with quantitative analysis and defect severity grading (compared with thallium-201) in the assessment of myocardial viability remains controversial. Nevertheless, its potential usefulness in certain patient populations warrants further investigation.

Acquisition of 4-h rest–redistribution sestamibi images,[62] administration of sestamibi as a 1-h infusion,[65] and administration of nitrate before sestamibi injection[67] have been reported to provide viability information comparable to thallium imaging; however, confirmation of those findings is needed.

Thallium-201/technetium-99m sestamibi imaging for assessment of myocardial viability

A separate-acquisition dual-isotope protocol was proposed by Berman and coworkers.[75] Thallium-201 is injected at rest (before exercise test) and resting thallium images are acquired after 10 minutes and again after 3–4 hours or 24–48 hours to allow thallium redistribution, whereas technetium-99m sestamibi is injected at peak exercise and stress sestamibi images are acquired after 15–30 minutes. Therefore, this protocol includes rest-redistribution thallium imaging for assessment of myocardial viability and rest thallium/stress sestamibi imaging for assessment of stress-induced ischemia. With regards to the latter, concerns about image comparability (with different isotopes) and cumulative cost have been raised.

Other technetium-99m imaging agents

Bisi et al.[76] compared exercise–rest technetium-99m teboroxime planar imaging with exercise–redistribution–reinjection thallium-201 planar imaging for the assessment of myocardial viability (stress defect reversibility) in 10 patients with previous myocardial infarction but normal overall left ventricular function. In that limited study, administration of sublingual isosorbide dinitrate prior to Tc-99m teboroxime rest injection and imaging seemed to improve detection of viable myocardium with teboroxime so that it became similar in accuracy to thallium-201.

Matsunari et al.[77] compared 2-day exercise–rest technetium-99m tetrofosmin SPECT imaging with exercise–redistribution–reinjection thallium-201 SPECT imaging for the assessment of myocardial viability in 25 patients with coronary artery disease and impaired regional or global left ventricular function. By visual analysis, overall concordance regarding viability (reversible defect) and nonviability (irreversible defect) between tetrofosmin and thallium was only 60%, with the former underestimating myocardial viability compared with the latter. However, with quantitative analysis, overall concordance for viability (reversible defect or mild-to-moderate (>50% peak activity) irreversible defect) and nonviability (severe ($\leq$50% peak activity) irreversible defect) improved to 90%.

In spite of those encouraging results, data are lacking on the usefulness of Tc-99m teboroxime or Tc-99m tetrofosmin for predicting wall motion response to coronary revascularization.

Radiolabeled fatty acids

Several radioiodinated fatty acids have been introduced for the assessment of myocardial fatty acid metabolism, and hence metabolic viability in chronic coronary artery disease.[78] Of those, iodine-123 15-iodophenyl pentadecanoic acid (IPPA) has been under clinical investigation for the longest time. Prior to coronary bypass surgery in 15 patients with coronary artery disease and resting left ventricular ejection fraction <35%, Murray et al.[79] performed continuous planar gamma-camera imaging over 25 minutes

following rest injection of IPPA. IPPA early wash-out (reflecting beta oxidation) or IPPA accumulation (reflecting esterification to triglycerides and phospholipids) were taken as evidence of myocardial viability. Using results of transmural left ventricular biopsies obtained during subsequent coronary bypass surgery as the gold standard for myocardial viability, IPPA scan sensitivity and specificity for viability were 92% and 86%, respectively. After coronary revascularization, resting and/or exercise systolic regional wall motion improved in 80% of IPPA-viable infarct segments but also in 33% of IPPA-nonviable infarct segments. In 23 patients with coronary artery disease and segmental or global left ventricular dysfunction referred for coronary revascularization, Hansen et al.[80] performed SPECT imaging in the 36 minutes following rest injection of IPPA. Regional IPPA metabolism in an intermediate range, slower than normal regions but faster than infarct regions, was taken as evidence of myocardial ischemia, although the imaging technique in this study may have resulted in artificially larger fractions of the left ventricle being in the intermediate metabolic range.[80] In fact, among patients receiving complete revascularization, >87% of the left ventricle was in the intermediate metabolic range in all patients with $\geq$5% increase in left ventricular ejection fraction postrevascularization but also in 30% of patients with <5% increase in left ventricular ejection fraction postrevascularization. Although the above studies suggest a possible role for IPPA in myocardial viability assessment, additional investigation is needed.

Compared with IPPA, iodine-123 15-iodophenyl 3-methyl pentadecanoic acid (BMIPP) shows considerably longer myocardial retention, and hence may be more suitable for SPECT imaging. Nevertheless, little is known of the role of BMIPP in myocardial viability assessment in chronic coronary artery disease.[81,82] SPECT metabolic imaging with iodine-123 16-iodo 3-methyl hexadecanoic acid (MIHA) has also been studied, but clinical data thus far are limited.[83]

FDG single-photon imaging

Höflin and coworkers[84] were the first to show that imaging of the positron-emitting F18-fluorodeoxyglucose is feasible with a gamma camera. That finding opened the door for research on technical modifications of the generally available gamma camera (such as the use of a special high-energy collimator) to allow the assessment of myocardial glucose metabolism, and hence viability.[56,85–89]

Burt et al.[56] compared FDG-SPECT and FDG-PET in 20 patients with coronary artery disease who had myocardial segments exhibiting thallium uptake <50% (of maximum uptake) on thallium-SPECT 3 hours after resting thallium injection. Considering FDG uptake by SPECT or PET of more than 50% (of maximum uptake) in the above myocardial segments as probable evidence of viability, the investigators found 92% overall concordance for viability and nonviability between FDG-SPECT and FDG-PET. Although FDG-PET images show myocardial wall margins more distinctly and depict wall thickness more accurately than FDG-SPECT images, there appeared to be little clinically relevant difference in detection of segments with FDG uptake between the two techniques. Therefore, FDG single-photon imaging is an exciting area in the field of myocardial viability assessment. Studies comparing FDG single-photon imaging with thallium myocardial viability protocols and correlating this technique with improvement of left ventricular function following coronary revascularization will help define its future role in viability determination.

The bigger challenge: true prediction of nonviability

We have discussed in detail the different single-photon imaging techniques for the assessment of myocardial viability, with their strengths and weaknesses. In particular, the inadequacies of conventional thallium-201 stress–redistribution imaging have been exposed. The results of viability assessment with newer thallium protocols have been presented. Of these protocols, stress–redistribution–reinjection and rest–redistribution, in combination with quantitative analysis, are currently the most useful for identification of myocardial viability, with the former providing the additional benefit of identification of stress-induced myocardial ischemia and possibly a slight advantage in identification of myocardial viability. Optimal timing of thallium reinjection requires further investigation. Experience with the use of pharmacologic stress instead of exercise stress is relatively limited. The usefulness of technetium-99m sestamibi for viability determination has been controversial; however, newer developments in sestamibi imaging as described and other technetium-99m imaging agents are encouraging. Radiolabeled fatty acids and FDG SPECT imaging offer promise for the detection of metabolic viability.

It may be evident by now that the limitations of single-photon imaging techniques are mostly in accurate identification of nonviable myocardium. In other words, the matter in doubt is usually not whether what is determined to be viable by single-photon imaging is truly viable. More commonly, the question is whether what is believed to be nonviable by single-photon imaging is truly nonviable. Therefore, the primary goal in clinical studies of viability assessment has been to minimize the overestimation ('overcalling') of nonviable myocardium or scar.

This again raises the issue of what should be considered the gold standard for myocardial viability determination. As we have stated, improvement in ventricular function following coronary revascularization is the most clinically relevant 'gold standard'. However, we have discussed the potential limitation of evaluating only resting function pre- and postrevascularization, as has been done in almost all studies of myocardial viability. For the theoretical and practical reasons presented earlier in this chapter and given the difference in physiologic conditions during rest and activity, we propose that future viability studies assess ventricular function during exercise, particularly postrevascularization, for optimal assessment of viability. It is conceivable that some of the myocardial regions that remain dysfunctional at rest in spite of coronary revascularization (commonly thought to be 'nonviable') may improve in function with exercise, thus indicating residual viability.

Along with enhanced assessment of functional response to revascularization, more data are needed on the time course of improvement or deterioration in wall motion following successful and sustained revascularization. Hence, the optimal time for evaluation of ventricular function postrevascularization may be determined. The contribution of postischemic stunning to ventricular dysfunction in chronic coronary artery disease deserves further investigation as well.

When in doubt...

Here is a scenario that the clinical cardiologist may face. LJ is a 55-year-old man who presented with worsening angina at exertion and rest. He had suffered a myocardial infarction in 1990. The patient was hypertensive and a heavy smoker with chronic obstructive pulmonary disease. Medications included atenolol, diltiazem, clonidine and albuterol. The physical exam was noncontributory. ECG showed sinus rhythm, incomplete right bundle branch block, and old inferoposterior infarction. Serial ECGs and cardiac enzymes ruled out acute myocardial infarction. Cardiac catheterization was performed. Coronary arteriography showed 40% stenosis of the left main coronary artery, 70% stenosis of the left anterior descending coronary artery, 60% stenosis of the left circumflex coronary artery, and total occlusion of the right coronary artery. Left ventriculography showed inferobasal and inferoapical hypokinesis, and resting left ventricular ejection fraction was 38%. A rest–redistribution thallium study was performed to assess myocardial viability in the right coronary artery territory with images obtained using a dual-headed gamma camera early and 4 hours after resting injection of 3 mCi of Tl-201. An irreversible defect in the inferolateral wall was seen (Figure 7.12). Because of clinical suspicion of residual viability, a metabolic study was performed the following day after glucose loading and resting injection of 10 mCi of F18-deoxyglucose, using the same dual-headed gamma camera equipped with high-energy collimators. Tracer activity was seen in the inferolateral wall similar to the anterior and septal walls (Figure 7.12), indicating viable myocardium. Coronary artery bypass grafting was performed with three grafts: SVG to PDA, SVG to OM1, and LIMA to LAD. Following coronary revascularization, the patient's resting left ventricular ejection fraction improved to 45%.

This case illustrates two basic concepts in medicine applicable to myocardial viability assessment:

(1) there is no perfect diagnostic test, and
(2) diagnostic tests complement but do not replace clinical judgment.

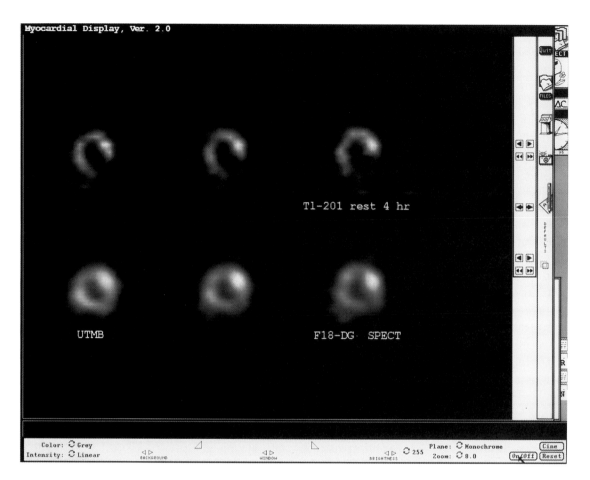

Figure 7.12

Midventricular short-axis images with 4-h rest redistribution thallium-201 SPECT and resting fluorine-18-deoxyglucose SPECT in a patient with crescendo angina. Note FDG uptake (by SPECT) in the inferolateral wall region with rest redistribution thallium defect. (Courtesy of Dr Javier Villanueva-Meyer, University of Texas Medical Branch, Galveston, TX.)

References

1 Burch GE, Giles TD, Colcolough HL, Ischemic cardiomyopathy, *Am Heart J* (1970)**79**:291–2.

2 Rahimtoola SH, A perspective on the three large multicenter randomized clinical trials of coronary bypass surgery for chronic stable angina, *Circulation* (1985)**72**(suppl V):123–35.

3 Braunwald E, Kloner RA, The stunned myocardium: prolonged, postischemic ventricular dysfunction, *Circulation* (1982)**66**:1146–9.

4 Vanoverschelde JLJ, Wijns W, Depré C et al, Mechanisms of chronic regional postischemic dysfunction in humans: new insights from the study of noninfarcted collateral-dependent myocardium, *Circulation* (1993)**87**:1513–23.

5 Hearse DJ, Myocardial ischemia: can we agree on a definition for the 21st century? *Cardiovasc Res* (1994)**28**:1737–44.

6 Myers JH, Stirling MC, Choy M, Buda AJ, Gallagher KP, Direct measurement of inner and outer wall thickening dynamics with epicardial echocardiography, *Circulation* (1986)**74**:164–72.

7 Margonato A, Mailhac A, Bonetti F et al, Exercise-induced ischemic arrhythmias in patients with previous myocardial infarction: role of perfusion and tissue viability, *J Am Coll Cardiol* (1996)**27**:593–8.

8 Irimpen AM, Tenaglia AN, Shin DJ, Buda AJ, Lack of ventricular remodeling in non-Q-wave myocardial infarction, *Am Heart J* (1996)**131**:466–71.

9 Vannan M, Kettle A, Coakely A, Griffith J, Udelson JE, Influence of infarct zone viability on left ventricular remodeling in the year following first anterior myocardial infarction, *Circulation* (1995)**92**(suppl):I–286 (abstr).

10 Trani C, Lombardo A, Giordano A et al, Residual contractile reserve in viable myocardium with persistent asynergy after revascularization, *J Am Coll Cardiol* (1996)**26**(suppl):98A (abstr).

11 Eitzman D, Al-Aouar Z, Kanter HL et al, Clinical outcome of patients with advanced coronary artery disease after viability studies with positron emission tomography, *J Am Coll Cardiol* (1992)**20**:559–65.

12 Di Carli MF, Davidson M, Little R et al, Value of metabolic imaging with positron emission tomography for evaluating prognosis in patients with coronary artery disease and left ventricular dysfunction, *Am J Cardiol* (1994)**73**:527–33.

13 Lee KS, Marwick TH, Cook SA et al, Prognosis of patients with left ventricular dysfunction, with and without viable myocardium after myocardial infarction. Relative efficacy of medical therapy and revascularization, *Circulation* (1994)**90**:2687–94.

14 Gioia G, Powers J, Heo J, Iskandrian AS, Prognostic value of rest-redistribution tomographic thallium-201 imaging in ischemic cardiomyopathy, *Am J Cardiol* (1995)**75**:759-62.

15 Gould KL, Does positron emission tomography improve patient selection for coronary revascularization? *J Am Coll Cardiol* (1992)**20**:566–8.

16 Pohost GM, Zir LM, Moore RH, McKusick KA, Guiney TE, Beller GA, Differentiation of transiently ischemic from infarcted myocardium by serial imaging after a single dose of thallium-201, *Circulation* (1977)**55**:294–302.

17 Blood DK, McCarthy DM, Sciacca RR, Cannon PJ, Comparison of single-dose and double-dose thallium-201 myocardial perfusion scintigraphy for the detection of coronary artery disease and prior myocardial infarction, *Circulation* (1978)**58**:777–88.

18 Ritchie JL, Albro PC, Caldwell JH, Trobaugh GB, Hamilton GW, Thallium-201 myocardial imaging: a comparison of the redistribution and rest images, *J Nucl Med* (1979)**20**:477–83.

19 Rozanski A, Berman DS, Gray R et al, Use of thallium-201 redistribution scintigraphy in the preoperative differentiation of reversible and nonreversible myocardial asynergy, *Circulation* (1981)**64**:936–44.

20 Gibson RS, Watson DD, Taylor GJ et al, Prospective assessment of regional myocardial perfusion before and after coronary revascular-

ization surgery by quantitative thallium-201 scintigraphy, *J Am Coll Cardiol* (1983)**1**:804–15.

21 Liu P, Kiess MC, Okada RD et al, The persistent defect on exercise thallium imaging and its fate after myocardial revascularization: does it represent scar or ischemia? *Am Heart J* (1985)**110**:996–1001.

22 Brunken R, Schwaiger M, Grover-McKay M, Phelps ME, Tillisch J, Schelbert HR, Positron emission tomography detects tissue metabolic activity in myocardial segments with persistent thallium perfusion defects, *J Am Coll Cardiol* (1987)**10**:557–67.

23 Tamaki N, Yonekura Y, Yamashita K et al, Relation of left ventricular perfusion and wall motion with metabolic activity in persistent defects on thallium-201 tomography in healed myocardial infarction, *Am J Cardiol* (1988)**62**:202–8.

24 Bonow RO, Dilsizian V, Cuocolo A, Bacharach SL, Identification of viable myocardium in patients with chronic coronary artery disease and left ventricular dysfunction. Comparison of thallium scintigraphy with reinjection and PET imaging with ^{18}F-fluorodeoxyglucose, *Circulation* (1991)**83**:26–37.

25 Dilsizian V, Freedman NMT, Bacharach SL, Perrone-Filardi P, Bonow RO, Regional thallium uptake in irreversible defects. Magnitude of change in thallium activity after reinjection distinguishes viable from nonviable myocardium, *Circulation* (1992)**85**:627–34.

26 Perrone-Filardi P, Bacharach SL, Dilsizian V, Maurea S, Frank JA, Bonow RO, Regional left ventricular wall thickening. Relation to regional uptake of ^{18}fluorodeoxyglucose and ^{201}Tl in patients with chronic coronary artery disease and left ventricular dysfunction, *Circulation* (1992)**86**:1125–37.

27 Marin-Neto JA, Dilsizian V, Arrighi JA et al, Thallium reinjection demonstrates viable myocardium in regions with reverse redistribution, *Circulation* (1993)**88**:1736–45.

28 Soufer R, Dey HM, Lawson AJ, Wackers FJTh, Zaret BL, Relationship between reverse redistribution on planar thallium scintigraphy and regional myocardial viability: a correlative PET study, *J Nucl Med* (1995)**36**:180–7.

29 Gutman J, Berman DS, Freeman M et al, Time to completed redistribution of thallium-201 in exercise myocardial scintigraphy: relationship to the degree of coronary artery stenosis, *Am Heart J* (1983)**106**:989–95.

30 Cloninger KG, De Puey EG, Garcia EV et al, Incomplete redistribution in delayed thallium-201 single photon emission computed tomographic (SPECT) images: an overestimation of myocardial scarring, *J Am Coll Cardiol* (1988)**12**:955–63.

31 Yang LD, Berman DS, Kiat H et al, The frequency of late reversibility in SPECT thallium-201 stress-redistribution studies, *J Am Coll Cardiol* (1990)**15**:334–40.

32 Kiat H, Berman DS, Maddahi J et al, Late reversibility of tomographic myocardial thallium-201 defects: an accurate marker of myocardial viability, *J Am Coll Cardiol* (1988)**12**:1456–63.

33 Brunken RC, Mody FV, Hawkins RA, Nienaber C, Phelps ME, Schelbert HR, Positron emission tomography detects metabolic viability in myocardium with persistent 24-hr single-photon emission computed tomography ^{201}Tl defects, *Circulation* (1992)**86**:1357–69.

34 Rocco TP, Dilsizian V, McKusick KA, Fischman AJ, Boucher CA, Strauss HW, Comparison of thallium redistribution with rest 'reinjection' imaging for the detection of viable myocardium, *Am J Cardiol* (1990)**66**:158–63.

35 Tamaki N, Ohtani H, Yonekura Y et al, Significance of fill-in after thallium-201 reinjection following delayed imaging: comparison with regional wall motion and angiographic findings, *J Nucl Med* (1990)**31**:1617–23.

36 Dilsizian V, Rocco TP, Freedman NMT, Leon MB, Bonow RO, Enhanced detection of ischemic but viable myocardium by the reinjection of thallium after stress-redistribution imaging, *N Engl J Med* (1990)**323**:141–6.

37 Ohtani H, Tamaki N, Yonekura Y et al, Value of thallium-201 reinjection after delayed SPECT imaging for predicting reversible ischemia after coronary artery bypass grafting, *Am J Cardiol* (1990)**66**:394–9.

38 Tamaki N, Ohtani H, Yamashita K et al, Metabolic activity in the areas of new fill-in

after thallium-201 reinjection: comparison with positron emission tomography using fluorine-18-deoxyglucose, *J Nucl Med* (1991)**32**: 673–8.

39 Zimmermann R, Mall G, Rauch B et al, Residual ^{201}Tl activity in irreversible defects as a marker of myocardial viability. Clinicopathological study, *Circulation* (1995)**91**:1016–21.

40 Dilsizian V, Smeltzer WR, Freedman NMT, Dextras R, Bonow RO, Thallium reinjection after stress-redistribution imaging. Does 24-hr delayed imaging after reinjection enhance detection of viable myocardium? *Circulation* (1991)**83**:1247–55.

41 Dilsizian V, Bonow RO, Differential uptake and apparent ^{201}Tl washout after thallium reinjection. Options regarding early redistribution imaging before reinjection or late redistribution imaging after reinjection, *Circulation* (1992)**85**: 1032–8.

42 He Z-X, Darcourt J, Guignier A et al, Nitrates improve detection of ischemic but viable myocardium by Tl-201 reinjection SPECT, *J Nucl Med* (1993)**34**:1472–7.

43 Kayden DS, Sigal S, Soufer R, Mattera J, Zaret BL, Wackers FJ, Thallium-201 for assessment of myocardial viability: quantitative comparison of 24-hr redistribution imaging with imaging after reinjection at rest, *J Am Coll Cardiol* (1991)**18**:1480–6.

44 Inglese E, Brambilla M, Dondi M et al, Assessment of myocardial viability after thallium-201 reinjection or rest-redistribution imaging: a multicenter study, *J Nucl Med* (1995)**36**:555–63.

45 Van Eck-Smit BLF, Van Der Wall EE, Kuijper AFM, Zwinderman AH, Pauwels EKJ, Immediate thallium-201 reinjection following stress imaging: a time-saving approach for detection of myocardial viability, *J Nucl Med* (1993)**34**:737–43.

46 Van Eck-Smit BLF, Van Der Wall EE, Zwinderman AH, Pauwels EKJ, Clinical value of immediate thallium-201 reinjection imaging for the detection of ischaemic heart disease, *Eur Heart J* (1995)**16**:410–20.

47 Kiat H, Friedman JD, Wang FP et al, Frequency of late reversibility in stress-redistribution thallium-201 SPECT using an early reinjection protocol, *Am Heart J* (1991)**122**:613–19.

48 Galli M, Marcassa C, Thallium-201 redistribution after early reinjection in patients with severe stress perfusion defects and ventricular dysfunction, *Am Heart J* (1994)**128**:41–52.

49 Gewirtz H, Beller GA, Strauss HW et al, Transient defects of resting thallium scans in patients with coronary artery disease, *Circulation* (1979)**59**:707–13.

50 Berger BC, Watson DD, Burwell LR et al, Redistribution of thallium at rest in patients with stable and unstable angina and the effect of coronary artery bypass surgery, *Circulation* (1979)**60**:1114–25.

51 Iskandrian AS, Hakki AH, Kane SA et al, Rest and redistribution thallium-201 myocardial scintigraphy to predict improvement in left ventricular function after coronary artery bypass grafting, *Am J Cardiol* (1983)**51**:1312–16.

52 Mori T, Minamiji K, Kurogane H, Ogawa K, Yoshida Y, Rest-injected thallium-201 imaging for assessing viability of severe asynergic regions, *J Nucl Med* (1991)**32**:1718–24.

53 Ragosta M, Beller GA, Watson DD, Kaul S, Gimple LW, Quantitative planar rest-redistribution ^{201}Tl imaging in detection of myocardial viability and prediction of improvement in left ventricular function after coronary bypass surgery in patients with severely depressed left ventricular function, *Circulation* (1993)**87**:1630–41.

54 Pace L, Cuocolo A, Marzullo P et al, Reverse redistribution in resting thallium-201 myocardial scintigraphy in chronic coronary artery disease: an index of myocardial viability, *J Nucl Med* (1995)**36**:1968–73.

55 Marzullo P, Parodi O, Reisenhofer B et al, Value of rest thallium-201/technetium-99m sestamibi scans and dobutamine echocardiography for detecting myocardial viability, *Am J Cardiol* (1993)**71**:166–72.

56 Burt RW, Perkins OW, Oppenheim BE et al, Direct comparison of fluorine-18-FDG SPECT, fluorine-18-FDG PET and rest thallium-201 SPECT for detection of myocardial viability, *J Nucl Med* (1995)**36**:176–9.

57 Dilsizian V, Perrone-Filardi P, Arrighi JA et al, Concordance and discordance between stress-redistribution-reinjection and rest-redistribution thallium imaging for assessing viable myocardium. Comparison with metabolic activity by

positron emission tomography, *Circulation* (1993)**88**:941–52.

58 Galassi AR, Centamore G, Fiscella A et al, Comparison of rest-redistribution thallium-201 imaging and reinjection after stress-redistribution for the assessment of myocardial viability in patients with left ventricular dysfunction secondary to coronary artery disease, *Am J Cardiol* (1995)**75**:436–42.

59 Rocco TP, Dilsizian V, Strauss HW, Boucher CA, Technetium-99m isonitrile myocardial uptake at rest. II. Relation to clinical markers of potential viability, *J Am Coll Cardiol* (1989)**14**:1678–84.

60 Altehoefer C, Kaiser H-J, Dörr R et al, Fluorine-18 deoxyglucose PET for assessment of viable myocardium in perfusion defects in ^{99m}Tc-MIBI SPET: a comparative study in patients with coronary artery disease, *Eur J Nucl Med* (1992)**19**:334–42.

61 Sawada SG, Allman KC, Muzik O et al, Positron emission tomography detects evidence of viability in rest technetium-99m sestamibi defects, *J Am Coll Cardiol* (1994)**23**:92–8.

62 Dilsizian V, Arrighi JA, Diodati JG et al, Myocardial viability in patients with chronic coronary artery disease. Comparison of ^{99m}Tc-sestamibi with thallium reinjection and ^{18}F fluorodeoxyglucose, *Circulation* (1994)**89**: 578–87.

63 Soufer R, Dey HM, Ng CK, Zaret BL, Comparison of sestamibi single-photon emission tomography with positron emission tomography for estimating left ventricular myocardial viability, *Am J Cardiol* (1995)**75**: 1214–19.

64 Marzullo P, Sambuceti G, Parodi O, The role of sestamibi scintigraphy in the radioisotopic assessment of myocardial viability, *J Nucl Med* (1992)**33**:1925–30.

65 Miron SD, Finkelhor R, Bahler R, Sodee DB, Bellon EM, Use of Tc-99m sestamibi infusion for detection of hibernating myocardium. A preliminary report, *Clin Nucl Med* (1995)**20**: 440–5.

66 Bisi G, Sciagrà R, Santoro GM, Fazzini PF, Rest technetium-99m sestamibi tomography in combination with short-term administration of nitrates: feasibility and reliability for prediction of postrevascularization outcome of asynergic

territories, *J Am Coll Cardiol* (1994)**24**:1282–9.

67 Maurea S, Cuocolo A, Soricelli A et al, Enhanced detection of viable myocardium by technetium-99m-MIBI imaging after nitrate administration in chronic coronary artery disease, *J Nucl Med* (1995)**36**:1945–52.

68 Bisi G, Sciagrà R, Santoro GM, Rossi V, Fazzini PF, Technetium-99m-sestamibi imaging with nitrate infusion to detect viable hibernating myocardium and predict postrevascularization recovery, *J Nucl Med* (1995)**36**:1994–2000.

69 Chua T, Kiat H, Germano G et al, Gated technetium-99m sestamibi for simultaneous assessment of stress myocardial perfusion, postexercise regional ventricular function and myocardial viability. Correlation with echocardiography and rest thallium-201 scintigraphy, *J Am Coll Cardiol* (1994)**23**:1107–14.

70 Maurea S, Cuocolo A, Soricelli A et al, Myocardial viability index in chronic coronary artery disease: technetium-99m-methoxy isobutyl isonitrile redistribution, *J Nucl Med* (1995)**36**:1953–60.

71 Taylor AM II, Merhige ME, Optimal identification of myocardial viability with SPECT: 24 hour redistribution thallium scintigraphy is superior to rest sestamibi imaging, *J Nucl Med* (1993)**34(suppl)**:23P (abstr).

72 Cuocolo A, Pace L, Ricciardelli B, Chiariello M, Trimarco B, Salvatore M, Identification of viable myocardium in patients with chronic coronary artery disease: comparison of thallium-201 scintigraphy with reinjection and technetium-99m-methoxyisobutyl isonitrile, *J Nucl Med* (1992)**33**:505–11.

73 Anagnostopoulos C, Laney R, Pennell D, Proukakis H, Underwood R, A comparison of resting images from two myocardial perfusion tracers, *Eur J Nucl Med* (1995)**22**:1029–34.

74 Udelson JE, Coleman PS, Metherall J et al, Predicting recovery of severe regional ventricular dysfunction. Comparison of resting scintigraphy with ^{201}Tl and ^{99m}Tc-sestamibi, *Circulation* (1994)**89**:2552–61.

75 Berman DS, Kiat H, Friedman JD et al, Separate acquisition rest thallium-201/stress technetium-99m sestamibi dual-isotope myocardial perfusion single-photon emission computed

tomography: a clinical validation study, *J Am Coll Cardiol* (1993)**22**:1455–64.

76 Bisi G, Sciagrà R, Santoro GM, Zerauschek F, Fazzini PF, Sublingual isosorbide dinitrate to improve technetium-99m-teboroxime perfusion defect reversibility, *J Nucl Med* (1994)**35**:1274–8.

77 Matsunari I, Fujino S, Taki J et al, Myocardial viability assessment with technetium-99m-tetrofosmin and thallium-201 reinjection in coronary artery disease, *J Nucl Med* (1995)**36**:1961–7.

78 Knapp FF Jr, Kropp J, Iodine-123-labelled fatty acids for myocardial single-photon emission tomography: current status and future perspectives, *Eur J Nucl Med* (1995)**22**:361–81.

79 Murray G, Schad N, Ladd W et al, Metabolic cardiac imaging in severe coronary disease: assessment of viability with iodine-123-iodophenylpentadecanoic acid and multicrystal gamma camera, and correlation with biopsy, *J Nucl Med* (1992)**33**:1269–77.

80 Hansen CL, Heo J, Oliner C, Van Decker W, Iskandrian AS, Prediction of improvement in left ventricular function with iodine-123-IPPA after coronary revascularization, *J Nucl Med* (1995)**36**:1987–93.

81 Tamaki N, Tadamura E, Kawamoto M et al, Decreased uptake of iodinated branched fatty acid analog indicates metabolic alterations in ischemic myocardium, *J Nucl Med* (1995)**36**:1974–80.

82 Matsunari I, Fujino S, Taki J et al, Impaired fatty acid uptake in ischemic but viable myocardium identified by thallium-201 reinjection, *Am Heart J* (1996)**131**:458–65.

83 Marie PY, Karcher G, Danchin N et al, Thallium-201 rest-reinjection and iodine-123-MIHA imaging of myocardial infarction: analysis of defect reversibility, *J Nucl Med* (1995)**36**:1561–8.

84 Höflin F, Ledermann H, Noelpp U, Weinreich R, Rösler H, Routine ^{18}F-2-deoxy-2-fluoro-D-glucose (^{18}F-FDG) myocardial tomography using a normal large field of view gamma-camera, *Angiology* (1989)**40**:1058–64.

85 Williams KA, Taillon LA, Stark VJ, Quantitative planar imaging of glucose metabolic activity in myocardial segments with exercise thallium-201 perfusion defects in patients with myocardial infarction: comparison with late (24-hr) redistribution thallium imaging for detection of reversible ischemia, *Am Heart J* (1992)**124**:294–304.

86 Bax JJ, Visser FC, van Lingen A, Huitink JM et al, Feasibility of assessing regional myocardial uptake of ^{18}F-fluorodeoxyglucose using single-photon emission computed tomography, *Eur Heart J* (1993)**14**:1675–82.

87 Drane WE, Abbott FD, Nicole MW, Mastin ST, Kuperus JH, Technology for FDG SPECT with a relatively inexpensive gamma camera. Work in progress, *Radiology* (1994)**191**:461–5.

88 Kalff V, Van Every B, Lambrecht RM et al, Planar cardiac F-18 fluorodeoxyglucose imaging with a conventional gamma camera, *Med J Aust* (1994)**161**:413–17.

89 Martin WH, Delbeke D, Patton JA et al, FDG-SPECT: correlation with FDG-PET, *J Nucl Med* (1995)**36**:988–95.

8

Hibernating myocardium

Stephen Campbell

Introduction

In the normal heart myocardial metabolism is predominantly aerobic and myocardial oxygen consumption is overwhelmingly created by myocardial contraction.[1] This demands an efficient blood supply and it is likely that, in normal circumstances, myocardial demand probably never outstrips supply.[2] However, in the presence of supply limitations, owing to fixed and/or dynamic obstruction, blood flow may not be able to meet the requirements of the myocardium, resulting in ischaemia.[3]

In experimental isolated cardiac muscle preparations, developed tension declines after 1 minute of ischaemia and the decline is complete within 5 to 10 minutes.[4] Furthermore, it has long been known that interruption of the blood supply to an area of myocardium in the intact animal leads to a rapid cessation of regional contraction and indeed passive bulging, as the rest of the heart continues to contract.[5] If ischaemia is sufficiently prolonged, it leads to infarction with irreversible cellular change and permanent loss of contractile function.[6,7] If ischaemia is relieved before infarction develops, functional recovery will usually occur. Until fairly recently, infarction was considered to be the main mechanism causing sustained left ventricular dysfunction in ischaemic heart disease.[8] However, since the 1980s, it has been recognized increasingly that the myocardium may exhibit more subtle responses to ischaemia. It is now known that the functional recovery of the myocardium after a period of intense ischaemia, which is then relieved by restoration of blood flow in time to avoid significant infarction, may sometimes proceed very slowly, resulting in a prolonged period of dysfunction. During this period the myocardium is said to be 'stunned'.[9] However, if myocardial perfusion is chronically impaired, but remains sufficient to maintain tissue viability, a related, but apparently distinct state of impaired myocardial function may exist; this is known as 'hibernation'.[10–12]

The term hibernating myocardium was first coined by Rahimtoola.[13] It was a concept that he had been developing for some time, as a result of observations of the functional response to coronary revascularization surgery, but at first it was not fully accepted.[11] The essence of myocardial hibernation is that there is a state of persistently impaired contractile function at rest attributed to reduced coronary blood flow that can be partially or completely normalized if the relationship between myocardial oxygen supply and demand is altered either by improving blood flow and/or reducing demand. Rahimtoola argued that hibernation may represent a metabolic and functional adaptation of the myocardium to reduced myocardial blood flow to avert necrosis.[11] A key feature of this chronic ischaemic state is that it is largely painless and is manifested clinically mainly by left ventricular dysfunction.

Pathophysiology of hibernation

Although there is considerable evidence to support the concept of myocardial hibernation,[10–12] the underlying pathophysiology remains something of an enigma. This is largely because of the lack of a good experimental model. Experiments of acute coronary artery occlusion in dogs have shown that regional myocardial function, as assessed by systolic wall thickening, is directly related to local blood flow, particularly to the subendocardium.[14] This has led to the formulation of the concept of myocardial perfusion-contraction matching. Furthermore, the concept has been shown to hold at rest, during exercise, at different heart rates and, importantly in relation to hibernation, during moderately prolonged (5-hour) periods of induced low-flow perfusion.[14] Restoration of flow levels leads to complete, albeit delayed, recovery of function after such periods. Unfortunately, however, no good experimental model exists for more prolonged periods (days, weeks, months or even years) of low flow to mimic the postulated situation in clinical hibernation.[11] Indeed, the existence of a true chronic, resting low-flow state must remain in some doubt. In an important study of patients with coronary arterial occlusion, but no evidence of prior infarction, Vanoverschelde et al.[15] investigated resting myocardial blood flow, using N13 ammonia and positron emission tomography (PET). They found no differences in flow between normally functioning and dysfunctional, collateral-dependent, left ventricular segments. However, they did show that the dysfunctional segments remained metabolically active and had reduced collateral-dependent flow reserve in relation to collateral-dependent but normally contracting segments, as well as normally supplied and con-

tracting segments. In those patients restudied after revascularization, regional left ventricular function improved significantly, fulfilling the functional definition of hibernation. In 30 patients with coronary heart disease and previous myocardial infarction, Marinho et al.[16] also recently demonstrated that mean myocardial blood flow, as assessed by PET using O-15 water (derived from inhaled O-15 carbon dioxide), was within the normal range in 59 dysfunctional left ventricular segments that subsequently improved after coronary artery bypass grafting (CABG). These recent results have called into question the existence of a chronic state of reduced flow *in vivo* and suggest instead that hibernation may not be as distinct from stunning as was once thought. It may, at least in part, be due to the cumulative effects of repeated episodes of ischaemia, a phenomenon termed repetitive stunning.[17,18] Another important feature of the Vanoverschelde study[15] was that the left ventricular segments that showed chronic dysfunction also exhibited ultrastructural changes in biopsy specimens (taken at the time of CABG), characterized by a reduction in contractile elements (myofibrils) and an increase in glycogen. In a further study from the same group,[19] immunohistochemical analysis of the left ventricular biopsy samples revealed that the cellular structural changes probably represented a form of de-differentiation. Similar findings (loss of myofibrils and accumulation of glycogen) have been found in myocardial biopsy specimens in patients with the rare ALCAPA (Anomalous origin of the Left Coronary Artery from the Pulmonary Artery) syndrome,[20] which has also been proposed as a model for chronic hibernation.[12,20]

The metabolic processes underlying chronic hibernation remain unclear. Observations in intact instrumented pigs for 3 hours after creation of an 80% stenosis in the left anterior descending coronary artery (LAD) showed the expected reduction in regional myocardial blood flow, particularly to the endocardial area, and reduction in regional myocardial oxygen consumption.[21] Known metabolic indicators of ischaemia — reduced coronary venous pH, increased coronary venous PCO_2 and increased regional lactate production — were present initially. But within 1 hour, the coronary venous pH and PCO_2 had returned to pre-stenosis levels and over the 3-h period lactate production declined, and indeed reverted to consumption, despite maintenance of the vessel constriction. Regional myocardial function was examined in a small subgroup in this study: it declined then stabilized at a lower level than that of the controls. This implies that contractile dysfunction may be an adaptive response of the myocardium to a reduced blood supply, to offset the potentially damaging consequences of ischaemia. Similar experiments in pigs[22] have shown that after 1 hour of coronary flow reduction there is an initial fall in high-energy phosphates, adenosine triphosphate (ATP) and creatine phosphate (CrP). But within 30 minutes the level of CrP had recovered, despite maintenance of ischaemia, and remained stable for the 1-h duration of the experiment. The ATP level remained depressed but stable. These changes were noted during both mild (20–25% flow reduction) and moderate (40–45% flow reduction) ischaemia. The initial depression of high-energy phosphates was more marked in the latter state and there was a transmural gradient of severity, with the subendocardial region exhibiting the greatest reductions. Further studies by the same group[23] incorporated an additional ischaemic stress, atrial pacing at around 50 bpm higher than the intrinsic heart rate, on the low-flow ischaemia model in the intact pig. This added stress produced no significant change in ATP levels but caused a fall in the 'recovered' CrP levels. There was also a switch back to net production of lactate.

These results imply that the sustainedly ischaemic myocardium may somehow downregulate its energy requirements but is still able, to a limited extent, to meet an additional demand. This hypothesis is further supported by the demonstration, again in a pig model, that moderately ischaemic myocardium is capable of an inotropic response to short-term intracoronary infusions of dobutamine, even after 90 minutes of sustained reduction in coronary flow.[24] These workers confirmed the adaptive changes in CrP and lactate metabolism noted previously by Pantely et al.[22] and the observations of Arai et al.[23] that these are reversed by altering the myocardial supply–demand situation. The increased demand appeared to be met largely by anaerobic metabolism. However, this process has its limitations. If intracoronary dobutamine is infused in the pig model for prolonged periods, levels of ATP and glycogen decline, contractile function deteriorates (after initial improvement), and myocardial necrosis begins.[25] In addition, at least in the experimental model, a threshold value of subendocardial blood flow of $0.15\,\mathrm{ml.min^{-1}/g^{-1}}$ can be determined. Above this, the aforementioned adaptive metabolic features of hibernation can develop, but below this flow level the adaptive mechanisms are overwhelmed. Serious depletion of myocardial high-energy phosphates occurs, ultimately leading to irreversible cellular changes and infarction.[25] Thus, many of the metabolic features of so-called acute hibernation have been characterized in relatively short-term experimental models, but it remains uncertain whether the same processes operate in the chronic clinical state. Furthermore, the precise mediators of the process remain obscure. One possible candidate is locally generated adenosine. Certainly, it seems to have a role in the related process of ischaemic preconditioning,[26] although studies of its role in short-term hibernation appear contradictory. In an isolated piglet heart preparation, Offstad et al.[27] showed no effect of adenosine receptor blockade with 8-p-sulphonyl theophylline on the metabolic and functional response to a 2-h period of low coronary flow, followed by reperfusion. They also showed no response to stimulation or blockade of potassium ATP channels. However, recent studies in an isolated guinea-pig heart model of hibernation[28] showed that blockade of adenosine receptors, again with 8-p-sulphonyl theophylline, attenuated the recovery of cytosolic energy levels during 60 minutes of ischaemia. Impairment of the processes of hibernation was not complete, however. Major differences in methodology may account for these differing results. Thus, the role of adenosine in hibernation remains uncertain. While it may be involved, it is certainly not the sole mediator of the metabolic downregulation that appears to be the hallmark of hibernation. Another possible factor in hibernation is alteration of responsiveness to calcium. However, recent studies in intact pigs have shown that hibernating myocardium remains responsive to an intracoronary infusion of calcium, albeit at a somewhat lower level than nonischaemic myocardium.[29] Therefore, at present, the detailed control mechanisms involved in hibernation remain unknown.

Methods of detection of hibernating myocardium

Until fairly recently our ability to distinguish viable, but dysfunctional and possibly hibernating, mycocardium from dysfunctional and non-viable (infarcted) myocardium prospectively was very limited. And even now it remains less than perfect. Of course, a retrospective assessment can be made following revascularization by CABG or percutaneous transluminal coronary angioplasty (PTCA). Thus a region of the left ventricle that appeared dysfunctional before revascularization and appears to improve, or even normalize after revascularization is assumed to be viable, so long as loading conditions, adrenergic state, global cardiac movement, and so on have not led to artefactual changes. Indeed, such functional improvement is still considered to be the hallmark of hibernation and one against which other methods of detection must be matched. It has been claimed that around one-third of patients with preoperative left ventricular dysfunction show significant improvement after CABG.[30] The important task is to be able to identify, pre-revascularization, those areas that are viable and that will potentially benefit from this procedure. Relatively simple methods include electrocardiography, particularly noting the presence or absence of Q-waves, and contrast angiography.[30] The latter allows assessment of coronary artery patency and global and regional ventricular function, most usefully before and after GTN, in association with post-extra-systolic potentiation or after catecholamine administration. However, these methods lack precision and angiography in particular is not suitable for serial studies. Therefore, attention has been focused on other functional and metabolic imaging modalities that are considered to give more precise information about myocardial viability. Those most frequently used are myocardial perfusion scintigraphy, positron emission tomography (PET) and stress echocardiography. Magnetic resonance imaging (MRI) may also turn out to be important but at present it still has major limitations.

Myocardial perfusion scintigraphy, using thallium-201, has been in routine clinical use in the evaluation of patients with known or suspected coronary heart disease since the late 1970s, following reports of its ability to detect reversible myocardial ischaemia and areas of infarction.[31] The standard protocol in most centres, both with the original planar imaging and with the now frequently used single-photon emission computed tomographic (SPECT) imaging, involves administration of a single dose of thallium-201 by intravenous injection during stress, and imaging soon thereafter and again around 3–4 h later, after the process known as 'redistribution'. This is the 'stress–redistribution' protocol. Evidence of normal thallium-201 uptake during stress or redistribution into areas that had reduced or absent uptake during stress (defects) is considered to be a reliable indicator of viability.[30] Areas of myocardium that exhibit absent or reduced uptake during stress and still appear as defects on delayed imaging, 3–4 h later, have conventionally been considered to represent areas of infarction. However, they cannot all necessarily be considered nonviable, as some can be shown to take up thallium-201 normally after a further injection at rest.[32] Furthermore, many apparently persistent thallium-201 defects seen in standard stress–redistribution studies, as well as those that exhibit partial redistribution, may normalize or improve after successful revascularization with PTCA[33,34] or CABG,[35,36] indicating viability even when there was marked wall motion abnormality before revascularization.[35] Thus, although standard stress–redistribution thallium-201 scintigraphy is of value in establishing viability and, by inference, hibernation, it may underestimate left ventricular segmental dysfunction because of the phenomenon of delayed redistribution.[34,36] Further (late redistribution) imaging is one way of improving detection of viability. Accordingly, it has been shown that by imaging up to 72 h after the initial thallium-201 injection, around 50% or more of patients with partial or complete defects at 4 h may show improvement or normalization of these defects.[34,36,37] However, there are several problems with late imaging. One is a simple logistic one, as noted by Yang et al.[37] and emphasized in an accompanying editorial.[38]

Another is that image quality declines because of loss of activity,[34,38] although it has been claimed that more prolonged acquisition times may partly offset this problem.[36,37] However, even with late-redistribution imaging there may be an underestimate of viability. Kiat et al.[36] noted that 37% of persistent defects on late imaging demonstrated improvement after revascularization. One way of improving the detection of viable myocardium, using thallium-201, may be to administer a second dose after the 3–4-h redistribution study. A study of 100 patients with proven coronary heart disease Dilsizian et al[39] showed that 49% of 85 apparently fixed defects on the 3–4-h redistribution study, assessed qualitatively, exhibited uptake of thallium-201 after a second injection, given immediately thereafter, implying probable viability.[39] In addition, 56% of 87 partially redistributed defects also showed increased thallium uptake on reinjection. Interestingly, 10% of regions deemed normal on the redistribution scan showed evidence of wash-out and around half these, 5% of the total, were interpreted as being fixed defects after reinjection. In a small subgroup, who were examined before and after PTCA, uptake of thallium-201 on reinjection appeared to correlate well with other indicators of viability. These more recent findings essentially confirmed earlier data on thallium injection at rest.[32] However, these latter observations had not had much impact on practice, as most centres continued to use the standard stress–redistribution protocol, based on the studies of Pohost et al.[31] More recently, further reinjection studies have confirmed that it appears to improve prediction of viability, as shown by improvement in myocardial segmental perfusion and function after CABG.[40] In a comparison of reinjection after 2–4-h and 24-h thallium-201 imaging, image quality was found to be superior to that seen in the 24-h delayed redistribution scan.[41] Of 159 views with a fixed defect at 2–4 h, 79% were still fixed at 24 h and only 48% after subsequent reinjection. Thus a 24-h reinjection study appears to give a better evaluation of viability than a 24-h delayed redistribution study alone. However, it is unclear whether this is better than reinjection after the standard 3–4-h redistribution period and whichever is more logistically convenient may be the deciding factor. If the earlier reinjection protocol is used it remains important to include a redistribution scan either at 3–4 h or, possibly, 24 h[42] because of the changes that can occur after reinjection in areas showing early redistribution, as discussed previously. One final protocol that can be used with thallium-201 to detect viable myocardium involves elimination of the stress study and injection at rest followed by a redistribution study within 4 h of the injection.[43] This rest–redistribution protocol can identify areas of myocardium that will improve after revascularization but may significantly underestimate the extent of viable myocardium,[30] although quantitative analysis may improve its ability to detect viability.[44] Nevertheless, it provides no information about stress-induced reversible ischaemia. Therefore, to obtain maximal information using thallium-201, some form of stress, reinjection and redistribution study is probably the optimum protocol. Thallium-201 myocardial perfusion scintigraphy is being gradually superseded by myocardial perfusion scintigraphy using technetium-99m agents, particularly as SPECT becomes more widespread. Although their imaging properties are superior to those of thallium-201, these agents may not undergo significant redistribution, a property of thallium-201 which has proven useful for the detection of viability. Detection of reversible ischaemia usually requires two injections — one given during stress and one at rest. However, a single rest injection may be of some value in assessing viability. Early studies with technetium-99m

methoxybutyl isonitrile, given as a single injection at rest, demonstrated only a moderate relationship between myocardial uptake and wall motion, assessed by radionuclide ventriculography and used as a surrogate measure of viability.[45] In a very small comparative study (14 patients), Marzullo et al.[46] showed that rest technetium-99m sestamibi imaging was less accurate than rest–redistribution thallium-201 imaging and dobutamine echocardiography in detecting viability, as assessed by myocardial segmental response to revascularization. However, another comparative study of quantitative rest–redistribution thallium-201 and resting technetium-99m sestamibi imaging in 31 patients with coronary artery disease indicated considerable concordance of technetium-99m sestamibi and redistribution thallium-201 when standardized to peak activities.[44] Moreover, in 18 patients who were studied before and after revascularization, a cut-off of 60% of peak segmental activity for both agents accurately predicted reversibility of severe regional ventricular dysfunction after revascularization, thus identifying hibernating myocardium. Therefore, quantitative analysis of resting technetium-99m sestamibi imaging appears to give information on myocardial viability that is comparable to quantitative rest–redistribution thallium-201 imaging. Dilsizian et al.[47] compared two established radionuclide methods of assessing myocardial viability — thallium-201 stress–redistribution–reinjection imaging and PET (using O15-labelled water for flow and F-18-fluorodeoxyglucose (FDG) for metabolism) — with rest–stress–redistribution technetium-99m setamibi imaging in patients with chronic coronary heart disease. In the comparison with thallium-201 in 54 patients, technetium-99m sestamibi misidentified 23% of thallium defects as nonviable, when in fact they exhibited reversibility, and by inference viability, on thallium-201 imaging.

A subset of 25 patients underwent additional PET imaging which yielded results on viability that were largely concordant with the thallium-201 data, although the authors claimed that quantitative analysis of technetium-99m sestamibi uptake provided a greater measure of agreement with thallium-201 and PET data. Furthermore they claimed that, contrary to previous data, technetium-99m sestamibi demonstrated redistribution and analysis of 4-h redistribution images improved detection of viability. These results have recently been confirmed by others.[48] The ability of technetium-99m sestamibi to detect viable, hibernating myocardium may also be improved by administration at rest after an infusion of nitrate.[49,50] Thus it appears that technetium-99m sestamibi, despite its better imaging properties, probably underestimates the extent of viable, hibernating myocardium and may not be as effective as thallium-201, although this deficiency may be overcome by quantitative analysis of images and/or administration after nitrates. Another, recently introduced, technetium-99m perfusion agent is tetrofosmin. In a comparative study of thallium-201 stress–redistribution–reinjection and stress–rest technetium-99m tetrofosmin imaging in 25 patients with known coronary artery disease, the latter appeared to underestimate reversibility of perfusion defects in 35% and 37% of left ventricular segments, in a qualitative analysis; depending on whether imaging took place 1 or 3 h after the rest injection of tetrofosmin.[51] However, again by using a quantitative analysis and a threshold cut-off of 50% of peak segmental activity to denote a 'significant' defect, much better agreement was obtained between thallium-201 and technetium-99m tetrofosmin imaging, but the validity of this approach was not tested against another marker of viability such as PET or improvement of function after revascularization. So the role of this agent, like the other technetium-99m agents, remains uncertain in the assessment of myocardial viability.

Many authorities regard PET as the definitive investigation for hibernating myocardium but its relative lack of availability makes it of less practical use. Detection of viable, hibernating myocardium is achieved by demonstrating evidence of preserved metabolic activity, using F-18-fluorodeoxyglucose (FDG) as a marker of glucose utilization and associated reduced perfusion, using flow markers such as N-13-ammonia[30] or O-15-labelled water,[47] in the presence of regional left ventricular dysfunction. This is known as metabolism–perfusion 'mismatch'.[30] Tillisch et al.[52] found that 13 (81%) out of 16 left ventricular regions with such metabolism–perfusion mismatch at rest and decreased contractile function preoperatively showed improvement in contractile function post-CABG. PET imaging appears to be superior to routine stress–redistribution thallium-201 imaging for detection of viability[53] but yields similar results to thallium-201 reinjection studies.[47,54] PET also seems to be better than technetium-99m sestamibi in the detection of viability although, as discussed previously, quantitative analysis and assessment of apparent redistribution may improve the performance of technetium-99m sestamibi.[47] While metabolism–perfusion mismatch at rest on PET has been most consistently used to assess viability, PET can be used for rest–stress myocardial perfusion studies using N13-ammonia. In a recent study comparing this technique with FDG uptake, Tamaki et al.[55] showed the latter to be a better predictor of improvement in function, in response to revascularization, in 130 asynergic left ventricular segments in 43 patients. However, severe hypoperfusion at rest and hypoperfusion with no stress-induced reduction was a good predictor of irreversibly damaged myocardium. Although clinical comparative trials of PET assessment of FDG uptake have appeared to show its value as a predictor of viability, a recent *in vitro* study in isolated rat hearts has cast some doubt on its ability to act as a quantitative marker of glucose metabolism[56] and, by extension, its role as a true marker of viability in PET studies has been questioned.[57] To date, this issue is unresolved.

In experimental animals ischaemic myocardium has been shown to remain responsive to inotropic stimulation with dobutamine for some time.[24] This property has been utilized in stress echocardiography to detect hibernating myocardium, by assessing the responses of wall motion and myocardial thickening to a relatively low-dose intravenous infusion of dobutamine. The occurrence of normal or improved wall motion and systolic myocardial thickening in a dysfunctional left ventricular segment, in response to dobutamine, is taken to indicate viability.[12,30] Sometimes the response may be biphasic, with initial improvement with lower doses of dobutamine, followed by deterioration, caused by ischaemia, as the dose increases, but this would still imply viability. Initial studies of dobutamine echocardiography to detect myocardial viability were performed in patients soon after infarction, when the phenomenon of stunning, rather than hibernation, may be responsible for most reversible dysfunction. However, as discussed previously, the distinction between the two may be more apparent than real. Pierard et al.[58] demonstrated good agreement (around 80% concordance) between dobutamine echocardiography and PET for assessment of viability both in the acute phase and during follow-up in 17 post-MI patients. More recently, however, dobutamine echocardiography has been used to detect hibernating myocardium, as conventionally defined. Cigarro et al.[59] studied 49 patients with multivessel coronary artery disease and ventricular dysfunction using low-dose dobutamine (5–20 ug/kg/min increasing in 3-minute stages).

They concentrated on systolic wall thickening as an index of 'contractile reserve'. An improvement in thickening was seen in 49% of patients. Importantly, 73 (40%) of 184 akinetic left ventricular segments showed an improvement, whereas only 2 (5%) of 38 dyskinetic segments improved. Twenty-five patients underwent successful revascularization, mostly by CABG, and were studied before and 4 weeks after the procedure. Of 11 patients with evidence of contractile reserve, in response to preoperative dobutamine, 9 (82%) showed evidence of a postoperative improvement in regional contractility at rest. By comparison, 12 of 14 patients (86%) with a negative preoperative response showed no postoperative improvement in contractile function. It was concluded that low-dose dobutamine stress echocardiography reliably identifies hibernating myocardium. Conversely, it also seems to detect reliably irreversibly damaged myocardium. Detection of myocardial viability by assessing contractile response represents a different approach to those techniques that depend on blood flow and cellular metabolic activity. Therefore, it is of interest to note the results of three recent studies of dobutamine stress echocardiography and thallium-201 scintigraphy, using SPECT.[60-62] In the study of Panza et al.[60] echocardiography at rest and during low-dose dobutamine stress was performed via the transoesophageal approach and compared with standard thallium-201 stress–redistribution–reinjection scintigraphy in 30 patients with coronary heart disease and depressed left ventricular function (resting ejection fraction <45%). A total of 311 myocardial segments had resting wall motion abnormalities on echocardiography: 84% were assessed as viable by scintigraphy, versus 56% by stress echocardiography. Sixty-four per cent of the segments considered viable by thallium-201 showed contractile improvement with dobutamine compared with only 12% of those designated as nonviable with thallium-201. The overall rate of agreement between the two techniques for criteria of viability was 68%. Although thallium-201 identified a greater number of myocardial segments as being viable than dobutamine echocardiography, the response to the latter was significantly and directly related to the magnitude of thallium-201 uptake. No comparison was made with response to revascularization in this study. In the second comparative study,[61] 38 patients with coronary heart disease and left ventricular dysfunction (resting ejection fraction ⩽40%) underwent dobutamine/atropine stress transthoracic echocardiography and stress (using dobutamine/atropine)–redistribution–reinjection thallium-201 SPECT scintigraphy before CABG and then reassessment by rest and stress (in 32 patients) echocardiography 3 months after cardiac surgery. Fourteen of 126 akinetic left ventricular segments, noted preoperatively, showed evidence of viability on both low-dose dobutamine stress echocardiography and thallium-201 scintigraphy. Thirteen (93%) of these segments improved postoperatively. No segments were found to be viable on echocardiography alone, whereas 49 were considered viable on thallium alone but only 9 (18%) of these showed postoperative improvement. Of 44 severely hypokinetic segments, 19 appeared viable on preoperative stress echocardiography and 18 of these were also considered viable with thallium-201. Fifteen (79% of echocardiographically viable segments) of these showed postoperative improvement. Of the remaining 25 severely hypokinetic segments, none showed evidence of viability on stress echocardiography versus 22 with thallium-201. Only one (4% of echocardiographically nonviable segments) of these showed improvement postoperatively. The third recent study[62] involved a different approach. Resting SPECT thallium-201 scintigraphy and transthoracic echocardiography were used to identify 79 hypoperfused and hypokinetic or akinetic myocardial segments in 18 patients with coronary heart disease undergoing revascularization with PTCA or CABG. Forty-six of these dysfunctional segments demonstrated improved contractility on preoperative low-dose dobutamine stress echocardiography. Forty-two (91%) of these showed an improvement also after revascularization, whereas only 6 (18%) of the 33 dysfunctional segments that had shown no improvement with dobutamine preoperatively showed postoperative improvement. Further-more, mean resting thallium-201 uptake was significantly higher in segments showing improvement with dobutamine and/or revascularization than in those which did not demonstrate improvement. It seems probable that thallium-201 is more sensitive than low-dose dobutamine stress echocardiography in detecting 'absolute' myocardial viability. This may be because it detects viability by reason that its uptake merely requires sufficient local blood flow for delivery and cell membrane pump integrity. A contractile response to dobutamine depends on the integrity of the contractile apparatus. This evaluation of functional integrity may be a cruder measure of viability, but it is interesting to speculate that it may be of greater practical and clinical importance, as indicated by the response to revascularization in the study of Arnese et al.[61] Indeed, response to revascularization is an integral part of the original definition of hibernation proposed by Rahimtoola.[11,13] One limitation of standard transthoracic dobutamine echocardiography is that, in around 10% of patients, it is not possible to generate technically adequate images.[59] Transoesophageal echocardiography may reduce this problem and appears well tolerated[60] but is obviously more invasive. Examples of

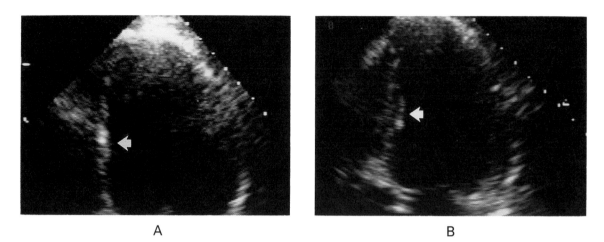

A   B

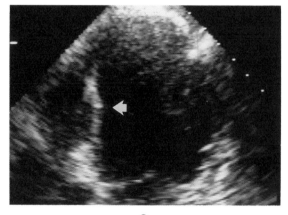

C

Figure 8.1

Two-dimensional echocardiographic end-systolic frames of the left ventricle in the apical 4-chamber view, in a 59-year-old man with a history of anterior myocardial infarction 6 years previously. He continued to have intermittent, but atypical, chest pain and equivocal exercise test results. Angiography demonstrated a proximally occluded left anterior descending coronary artery with only mild atheroma in the other vessels. Left ventricular function was reduced, with a global ejection fraction of 33%, with akinesis of the whole anterior wall. He underwent a dobutamine stress echocardiogram. The resting study (A) showed a dilated left ventricle with poor contractile function, including absence of septal thickening (arrowed). However, during a low-dose infusion of dobutamine, the septum showed very clear systolic thickening (arrowed) (B). As the dose of dobutamine was increased septal contractile function declined (arrowed) (C). This is an example of the biphasic response to an incremental dose infusion of dobutamine and indicates viability and hence hibernation. He has since undergone successful coronary artery bypass surgery. (Courtesy of Dr E Anagnostou.)

transthoracic stress echocardiographic studies are shown in Figures 8.1 and 8.2.

Although echocardiography is probably the current, and most practical, method of choice for evaluating myocardial viability on the basis of contractile function, in future other imaging modalities may emerge as equally or more important. One such modality is MRI. MRI

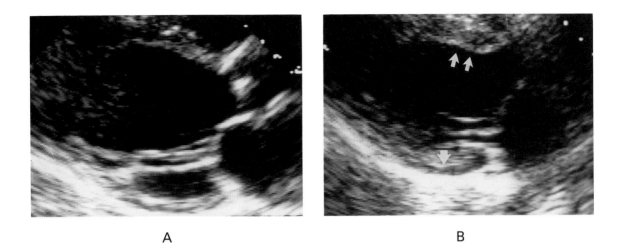

A   B

Figure 8.2
Two-dimensional echocardiographic end-systolic frames of the left ventricle in the left parasternal view in a 57-year-old man with a history of previous inferior myocardial infarction, angiographically documented triple-vessel coronary artery disease and poor left ventricular function (global ejection fraction 10%). He was originally referred for consideration for cardiac transplantation. (A) Echocardiography at rest confirmed the poor ventricular function. On infusion of low-dose dobutamine (B), a contractile response was evident in both the septum (small arrows) and the supposedly infarcted inferoposterior wall (large arrow). This demonstration of contractile reserve, probably because of hibernation, led to recommendation for revascularization, rather than cardiac transplantation. The patient underwent successful four-vessel coronary artery bypass grafting. (Echocardiograms courtesy of Dr E Anagnostou, patient details courtesy of Mr F Ciulli.)

was used in a recent study to assess myocardial end-diastolic thickness and systolic thickening, as indicators of viability, at rest and during a fixed low-dose dobutamine infusion. It was compared with FDG uptake by PET, at rest, in 35 patients with documented coronary heart disease.[63] Out of 2200 myocardial segments analysed, 482 were akinetic or dyskinetic at rest. Of these, 263 fulfilled the FDG-PET and MRI criteria (end-diastolic wall thickness $\geqslant 5.5$ mm or dobutamine-induced systolic wall thickening) for viability and 159 were not considered viable by either technique. The overall level of agreement was 88%. Discordance was noted in 60 segments, 24 were viable according to MRI but not by FDG-PET and the converse was found in the remaining 36 segments. Interestingly, 57 segments were found to be

viable by FDG-PET but showed no dobutamine contractile reserve. This discordance between metabolism and contractility is similar to that found with thallium-201 and stress echocardiography, as discussed previously. No data were available on response to revascularization. However, it would seem that MRI is a promising technique for assessment of viability, particularly as technology improves.

Clinical importance of hibernation

The clinical importance of myocardial hibernation lies in it being an indicator of the potential for recovery of function. It is well established that poor left ventricular function at rest is a major determinant of prognosis in patients with coronary heart disease and may be a contraindication to revascularization.[64] However, if there is evidence of ischaemia-related, and potentially reversible (hibernating) left ventricular dysfunction, patients may have most to gain from CABG.[64] In addition, identification of hibernation may help prevent some patients from being refused potentially beneficial revascularization, having been labelled previously as 'inoperable'. In such cases there is an acceptable level of risk of operative mortality and morbidity, even in the presence of severe resting left ventricular dysfunction.[65] Data on long-term survival in patients with impaired left ventricular function selected for revascularization on the basis of the presence of myocardial hibernation are not available. However, based on the surrogate improvement in regional and global left ventricular function,[66] the detection of hibernation may play a very important part in the selection of patients who would seem likely to benefit most from revascularization. The current diagnostic technique of choice is probably low-dose dobutamine stress echocardiography.[66]

If I had...

If I had coronary heart disease and significant left ventricular dysfunction I would very much like to know whether my myocardium was, in any way, potentially salvageable. I would regard the alternatives of continued medical treatment or cardiac transplantation as second best if hibernation could be proven. To detect any degree of myocardial hibernation that might respond to revascularization, I would expect to undergo a dobutamine stress echocardiogram or, if I were not a good echocardiographic subject, a stress–redistribution–reinjection thallium-201 scan. If hibernation was detected, and my coronary arteries were suitable for revascularization, I would hope to be offered either CABG or PTCA, depending on the coronary anatomy, and the skill of the operator(s)! The principles of the decision-making process in such a situation are illustrated in the simple algorithm shown in Figure 8.3.

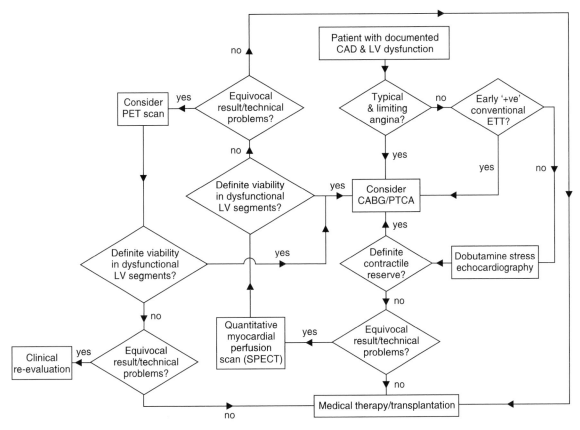

Figure 8.3
Assessment of patient with angiographically documented coronary artery disease (CAD) and associated left ventricular (LV) dysfunction. This algorithm emphasizes the importance of considering simple clinical features and the results of standard exercise testing in decision-making before those of more complex ancillary investigations. It also recognizes that echocardiographic and radionuclide investigations are subject to technical problems in some patients and can yield equivocal results.

References

1   Braunwald E, Sobel BE, Coronary blood flow and myocardial ischemia. In: Braunwald E, ed, *Heart disease: a textbook of cardiovascular medicine*, 4th edn (WB Saunders: Philadelphia, 1992)1161–91.

2   Factor SM, Bache RJ, Pathophysiology of myocardial ischemia. In: Schlant RC, Alexander RW, eds, *Hurst's The heart*, 8th edn (McGraw-Hill: New York, 1994)1033–53.

3   Hecht HH, Concepts of myocardial ischemia, *Arch Intern Med* (1949)**84**:711–29.

4   Shine KI, Douglas AM, Ricchiuti N, Ischemia in isolated interventricular septa: mechanical events, *Am J Physiol* (1976)**231**:1225–32.

5   Tennant R, Wiggers CJ, The effect of coronary occlusion on myocardial contractions, *Am J Physiol* (1935)**112**:351–6.

6   Armiger LC, Morphological changes in early myocardial ischaemic injury and infarction. In: Norris RM, ed, *Myocardial infarction: its presentation, pathogenesis and treatment* (Churchill Livingstone: London, 1982) 215–31.

7   Jennings RB, Sommers HM, Smyth GA, Flack HA, Linn H, Myocardial necrosis induced by temporary occlusion of a coronary artery in the dog, *Arch Pathol* (1960)**70**:68–78.

8   Heyndrickx GR, Wijns W, Melin JA, Regional wall motion abnormalities in stunned and hibernating myocardium, *Eur Heart J* (1993)**14 (suppl A)**:8–13.

9   Braunwald E, Kloner RH, The stunned myocardium: prolonged postischemic ventricular dysfunction, *Circulation* (1982)**66**:1146–9.

10 Braunwald E, Rutherford JD, Reversible ischemic left ventricular dysfunction: evidence for the 'hibernating myocardium' [editorial], *J Am Coll Cardiol* (1986)**8**:1467–70.

11 Rahimtoola SH, The hibernating myocardium [editorial], *Am Heart J* (1989)**117**:211–21.

12 Burn S, Caplin Jl, Myocardial hibernation, *Br J Hosp Med* (1995)**53**:395–402.

13 Rahimtoola SH, A perspective on the three large multicenter randomised clinical trials of coronary bypass surgery for chronic stable angina, *Circulation* (1985)**72(suppl V)**:123–35.

14 Ross Jr J, Myocardial perfusion-contraction matching: implications for coronary heart disease and hibernation, *Circulation* (1991)**83**: 1076–83.

15 Vanoverschelde J-LJ, Wijns W, Depre C et al, Mechanisms of chronic regional postischemic dysfunction in humans: new insights from the study of noninfarcted collateral-dependent myocardium, *Circulation* (1993)**87**:1513–23.

16 Marinho NVS, Keogh BE, Costa DC, Lammerstma AA, Ell PJ, Camici PG, Pathophysiology of chronic left ventricular dysfunction: new insights from the measurement of absolute myocardial blood flow and glucose utilization, *Circulation* (1996)**93**:737–44.

17 Bolli R, Myocardial 'stunning' in man, *Circulation* (1992)**86**:1671–91.

18 Buxton DB, Dysfunction in collateral-dependent myocardium: hibernation or repetitive stunning? [editorial] *Circulation* (1993)**87**: 1756–8.

19 Ausma J, Schaart G, Thone F et al, Chronic ischemic viable myocardium in man: aspects of dedifferentiation, *Cardiovasc Pathol* (1995)**4**:29–37.

20 Shivalkar B, Borgers M, Daenen W, Gewillig M, Flameng W, ALCAPA syndrome: an example of chronic myocardial hypoperfusion? *J Am Coll Cardiol* (1994)**23**:772–8.

21 Fedele FA, Gewirtz H, Capone RJ, Sharaf B, Most AS, Metabolic response to prolonged reduction of myocardial blood flow distal to a severe coronary stenosis, *Circulation* (1988)**78**: 729–35.

22 Pantely GA, Malone SA, Rhen WS et al, Regeneration of myocardial phosphocreatine in pigs despite continued moderate ischemia, *Circ Res* (1990)**67**:1481–93.

23 Arai AE, Pantely GA, Anselone CG, Bristow J, Bristow JD, Active downregulation of myocardial energy requirements during prolonged

moderate ischemia in swine, *Circ Res* (1991)**69**:1458–69.

24 Schulz R, Guth BD, Pieper K, Martin C, Heusch G, Recruitment of an inotropic reserve in moderately ischemic myocardium at the expense of metabolic recovery: a model of short-term hibernation, *Circ Res* (1992)**70**:1282–95.

25 Schulz R, Rose J, Martin C, Brodde O-E, Heusch G, Development of short-term myocardial hibernation: its limitation by the severity of ischemia and inotropic stimulation, *Circulation* (1993)**88**:684–95.

26 Marber M, Walker D, Yellon D, Ischaemic preconditioning: new insight into myocardial protection [editorial], *Br Med J* (1994)**308**:1–2.

27 Offstad J, Kirkeboen KA, Ilebekk A, Downing SE, ATP gated potassium channels in acute myocardial hibernation and reperfusion, *Cardiovasc Res* (1994)**28**:872–80.

28 Gao Z-P, Downey HF, Fan W-L, Mallet RT, Does interstitial adenosine mediate acute hibernation of guinea pig myocardium? *Cardiovasc Res* (1995)**29**:796–804.

29 Heusch G, Rose J, Skyschally A, Post H, Schulz R, Calcium responsiveness in regional myocardial short-term hibernation and stunning in the in situ porcine heart: inotropic responses to postextrasystolic potentiation and intracoronary calcium, *Circulation* (1996)**93**:1556–66.

30 Dilsizian V, Bonow RO, Current diagnostic techniques of assessing myocardial viability in patients with hibernating and stunned myocardium, *Circulation* (1993)**87**:1–20.

31 Pohost GM, Zir LM, Moore RH, McKusick KA, Guiney TE, Beller GA, Differentiation of transiently ischemic from infarcted myocardium by serial imaging after a single dose of thallium-201, *Circulation* (1977)**55**:294–302.

32 Blood DK, McCarthy DM, Sciacci RR, Cannon PJ, Comparison of single-dose and double-dose thallium-201 myocardial perfusion scintigraphy for the detection of coronary artery disease and prior myocardial infarction, *Circulation* (1978)**58**:777–88.

33 Liu P, Kiess MC, Okada RD et al, The persistent defect on exercise thallium imaging and its fate after myocardial revascularization: does it represent scar or ischemia? *Am Heart J* (1985)**110**:996–1001.

34 Cloninger KG, DePuey EG, Garcia EV et al, Incomplete redistribution in delayed thallium-201 single photon emission computed tomographic (SPECT) images: an overestimation of myocardial scarring, *J Am Coll Cardiol* (1988)**12**:955–63.

35 Rozanski A, Berman DS, Gray R et al, Use of thallium-201 redistribution scintigraphy in the preoperative differentiation of reversible and nonreversible myocardial asynergy, *Circulation* (1981)**64**:936–44.

36 Kiat H, Berman DS, Maddahi J et al, Late reversibility of tomographic myocardial thallium-201 defects: an accurate marker of myocardial viablity, *J Am Coll Cardiol* (1988)**12**:1456–63.

37 Yang LD, Berman DS, Kiat H et al, The frequency of late reversibility in SPECT thallium-201 stress-redistribution studies, *J Am Coll Cardiol* (1990)**15**:334–40.

38 Botvinick EA, Late reversibility: a viability issue [editorial], *J Am Coll Cardiol* (1990)**15**:341–4.

39 Dilsizian V, Rocco TP, Freedman NMT, Leon MB, Bonow RO, Enhanced detection of ischemic but viable myocardium by the reinjection of thallium after stress-redistribution imaging, *N Engl J Med* (1990)**323**:141–6.

40 Ohtani H, Tamaki N, Yonekura Y et al, Value of thallium-201 reinjection after delayed SPECT imaging for predicting reversible ischemia after coronary artery bypass grafting, *Am J Cardiol* (1990)**66**:394–9.

41 Kayden DS, Sigal S, Soufer R, Mattera J, Zaret BL, Wackers FJTh, Thallium-201 for assessment of myocardial viability: quantitative comparison of 24-hour redistribution imaging with imaging after reinjection at rest, *J Am Coll Cardiol* (1991)**18**:1480–6.

42 Dilsizian V, Bonow RO, Differential uptake and apparent ^{201}Tl washout after thallium reinjection: options regarding early redistribution imaging before reinjection or late redistribution imaging after reinjection, *Circulation* (1992)**85**:1032–8.

43 Gewirtz H, Beller GA, Strauss HW et al, Transient defects of resting thallium scans in patients with coronary artery disease, *Circulation* (1979)**59**:707–13.

44 Udelson JE, Coleman PS, Metherall J et al, Predicting recovery of severe regional ventricu-

lar dysfunction: comparison of resting scintigraphy with ^{201}Tl and ^{99m}Tc-sestamibi, *Circulation* (1994)**89**:2552–61.

45 Rocco TP, Dilsizian V, Strauss HW, Boucher CA, Technetium-99m isonitrile myocardial uptake at rest. II. Relation to clinical markers of potential viability, *J Am Coll Cardiol* (1989)**14**:1678–84.

46 Marzullo P, Parodi O, Reisenhofer B et al, Value of rest thallium-201/technetium-99m sestamibi scans and dobutamine echocardiography for detecting myocardial viability, *Am J Cardiol* (1993)**71**:166–72.

47 Dilsizian V, Arrighi Ja, Diodati JG et al, Myocardial viability in patients with chronic coronary artery disease: comparison of ^{99m}Tc-sestamibi with thallium reinjection and [18]Ffluorodeoxyglucose, *Circulation* (1994)**89**:578–87.

48 Maurea S, Cuocolo A, Soricelli A et al, Myocardial viability index in chronic coronary artery disease: technetium-99m-methoxy isobutyl isonitrile redistribution, *J Nucl Med* (1995)**36**:1953–60.

49 Bisi G, Sciagrà R, Santoro GM, Rossi V, Fazzini PF, Technetium-99m-sestamibi imaging with nitrate infusion to detect viable hibernating myocardium and predict postrevascularization recovery, *J Nucl Med* (1995)**36**:1994–2000.

50 Maurea S, Cuocolo A, Soricelli A et al, Enhanced detection of viable myocardium by technetium-99m-MIBI imaging after nitrate administration in chronic coronary artery disease, *J Nucl Med* (1995)**36**:1945–52.

51 Matsunari I, Fujino S, Taki J et al, Myocardial viability assessment with technetium-99m-tetrofosmin and thallium-201 reinjection in coronary artery disease, *J Nucl Med* (1995)**36**:1961–7.

52 Tillisch J, Brunken R, Marshall R et al, Reversibility of cardiac wall-motion abnormalities predicted by positron tomography, *N Engl J Med* (1986)**314**:884–8.

53 Brunken R, Schwaiger M, Grover-McKay M, Phelps ME, Tillisch J, Schelbert HR, Positron emission tomography detects tissue metabolic activity in myocardial segments with persistent thallium perfusion defects, *J Am Coll Cardiol* (1987)**10**:557–67.

54 Bonow RO, Dilsizian V, Cuocolo A, Bacharach SL, Identification of viable myocardium in patients with chronic coronary artery disease and left ventricular dysfunction: comparison of thallium scintigraphy with reinjection and PET imaging with ^{18}F-fluorodeoxyglucose, *Circulation* (1991)**83**:26–37.

55 Tamaki N, Kawamoto M, Tadamura E et al, Prediction of reversible ischemia after revascularisation: perfusion and metabolic studies with positron emission tomography, *Circulation* (1995)**91**:1697–705.

56 Hariharan R, Bray M, Ganim R, Doenst T, Goodwin G, Taegtmeyer H, Fundamental limitations of [18F]2-deoxy-2-fluoro-d-glucose for assessing myocardial glucose uptake, *Circulation* (1995)**91**:2435–44.

57 Clarke K, Veech RL, Metabolic complexities in cardiac imaging [editorial], *Circulation* (1995)**91**:2299–301.

58 Pierard LA, De Landsheere CM, Berthe C, Rigo P, Kulbertus HE, Identification of viable myocardium by echocardiography during dobutamine infusion in patients with myocardial infarction after thrombolytic therapy: comparison with positron emission tomography, *J Am Coll Cardiol* (1990)**15**:1021–31.

59 Cigarro CG, deFilippi CR, Brickner E, Alvarez LG, Wait MA, Grayburn PA, Dobutamine stress echocardiography identifies hibernating myocardium and predicts recovery of left ventricular function after coronary revascularization, *Circulation* (1993)**88**:430–6.

60 Panza KA, Dilsizian V, Laurienzo JM, Curiel RV, Katsiyiannis PT, Relation between thallium uptake and contractile response to dobutamine: implications regarding myocardial viability in patients with chronic coronary artery disease and left ventricular dysfunction, *Circulation* (1995)**91**:990–8.

61 Arnese M, Cornel JH, Salustri A et al, Prediction of improvement of regional left ventricular function after surgical revascularization: a comparison of low-dose dobutamine echocardiography with ^{201}Tl single-photon emission computed tomography, *Circulation* (1995)**91**:2748–52.

62 Perrone-Filardi P, Pace L, Prastaro M et al, Dobutamine echocardiography predicts improvement of hypoperfused dysfunctional

myocardium after revascularization in patients with coronary artery disease, *Circulation* (1995)**91**:2556–65.

63 Baer FM, Voth E, Schneider CA, Theissen P, Schicha H, Sechtem U, Comparison of low-dose dobutamine-gradient-echo magnetic resonance imaging and positron emission tomography with [^{18}F]fluorodeoxyglucose in patients with chronic coronary artery disease: a functional and morphological approach to the detection of residual myocardial viability, *Circulation* (1995)**91**:1006–15.

64 Loop FD, The surgical treatment of atherosclerotic coronary artery disease. In: Schlant RC, Alexander RW, eds, *Hurst's The heart*, 8th edn (McGraw-Hill: New York, 1994) 1367–80.

65 Mickleborough LL, Maruyama H, Takagi Y, Mohamed S, Sun Z, Ebisuzaki L, Results of revascularization in patients with severe left ventricular dysfunction, *Circulation* (1995)**92** (**suppl II**):II73–II79.

66 Vanoverschelde J-LJ, Gerber BL, D'Hondt A-M et al, Preoperative selection of patients with severely impaired left ventricular Function for coronary revascularization: role of low-dose dobutamine echocardiography and exercise-redistribution-reinjection thallium SPECT, *Circulation* (1995)**92**(**suppl II**):II37–II44.

9

Syndrome X

Richard Cooke

Introduction

No area of cardiology has attracted so much controversy as the association of chest pain resembling angina, electrocardiographic abnormalities suggestive of mycoardial ischaemia, and angiographically normal coronary arteries. The so-called paradox was first noted by Likoff et al. in 1967, and the term syndrome X was coined in an editorial by Kemp in 1973.[1,2]

A cardiac cause of pain is postulated but the evidence that this may occur is uncertain, after the exclusion of the small number of patients with epicardial spasm, and patients with pain due to increased wall tension or supply–demand mismatch such as occurs in dilated cardiomyopathy, left ventricular hypertrophy, valve disease, and various metabolic disorders. Significant stenoses have been detected in some cases by intravascular ultrasound. However, the underestimation of the extent of disease, or misinterpretations of the coronary angiogram are unlikely to be common sources of error where the angiogram shows no luminal irregularities.[3–5]

What is the evidence that chest pain may be cardiac despite the absence of angiographic evidence of disease and exclusion of well recognized cardiac pathology? One hypothesis is that this is a functional disorder due to impairment of the dilatory capacity of the coronary microvasculature. The hypothesis is reviewed in this chapter.

The population at risk

Patients with syndrome X are selected out for further cardiac investigations since their pain is considered to be 'typical' of angina.[6] The cardiac syndrome should be distinguished from the metabolic syndrome of the same name described by Reaven et al., despite recent reports suggesting similar pathogenesis between the two syndromes.[7–9]

It is clear that there is no general agreement about the population that should be studied, and the use of disparate groups has been a major impediment to research in this area. The incidence of syndrome X as defined is likely to be uncommon. Morise et al. reported an incidence in only four out of 109 (4%) female patients recruited over a 10-year period, although a higher proportion (25 out of 109, or 23%) had ST depression during treadmill testing in the absence of 'typical' symptoms.[10] Similarly, Rosano et al. reported an incidence of only 24 out of 189 (13%) consecutive patients, after excluding those with hypertension, valve disease, cardiomyopathy, and coronary artery spasm.[11]

Indeed the so-called paradox of syndrome X may be more illusory than previously thought, since in most patients it is likely that there are at least some atypical features in the history. In a report of 90 consecutive patients with syndrome X referred to a specialist clinic, atypical features were found in the majority.[12] Some authors doubt that pain which is 'typical' of angina ever occurs in the absence of significant angiographic stenoses, or obvious cardiac pathology.[13–15]

Similarly, ST segment depression during exercise testing is considered by many (but not all) to be an essential requirement (Figures 9.1).[16–18] However, it is well recognized that ST depression may be a nonspecific finding which does not invariably imply a diagnosis of myocardial ischaemia, and also that myocardial ischaemia may occur in the absence of ECG changes (Figure 9.2).[19] Although most authors exclude patients with epicardial spasm (Figure 9.3), ergonovine provocation is now used much less commonly in the United Kingdom because of previous reports of death due to refractory 'spasm'. However, the incidence of epicardial 'spasm' is likely to be low in patients whose angiograms show no luminal irregularities, and whose pain does not occur exclusively at rest.[20]

In pursuit of a microvascular cause of pain

Histological evidence of small vessel disease: a functional abnormality?

Suzuki et al. reported moderate or severe arteriosclerosis of the small intramyocardial vessels, due principally to medial thickening, in 18 of 19 (93%) syndrome X patients, but in only one of 10 (10%) controls with 'atypical' pain.[21] In addition, there was marked endothelial swelling of the capillaries, and perivascular fibrosis of the small arteries and arterioles. In view of the wide range of appearances obtained from normal hearts, the results should be interpreted with caution.[6] Moreover, the findings are in contrast to previous studies. Thus Shirey performed percutaneous punch biopsies of the

heart and found no evidence of microvascular disease in 14 patients with normal coronary angiograms and normal left ventricular function.[22] Similarly, Opherk et al. and Richardson et al. reported no histological evidence of small vessel disease on endomyocardial biopsies.[23,24] However, there are almost no pathological data about the resistance vessels between $100\,\mu m$ and $500\,\mu m$ in diameter, as these are beyond the reach of the endocardial biotope. These vessels are responsible for up to 50% of the microvascular resistance.[25]

Abnormalities of coronary blood flow: regional blood flow

Abnormalities of myocardial perfusion using single-photon emission scintigraphy are reported in between 13% and 98% of patients.[17,26,27] In at least one report the high incidence of abnormalities was due to selection bias, since in that particular practice an abnormal perfusion scan was a prerequisite for selection for coronary angiography.[17] A problem is that abnormalities may be due to a number of factors besides myocardial ischaemia, including previous infarction, cardiomyopathy, conduction disturbances, viral myocarditis, and thrombolytic therapy. In a well selected population, after exclusion of patients with hypertension, valve disease, and cardiomyopathy, Rosano et al. reported reversible thallium-201 perfusion defects in only four out of 24 (17%) patients.[28] Even in the small number of patients with abnormal perfusion scans, it is possible that the reported abnormalities may be due to an artefact such as soft tissue attenuation, nonuniformity of field, patient movement, and a variety of other technical factors.

In contrast to single-photon imaging which uses direct emitters of gamma radiation, positron emission tomography uses the principle of annihilation reaction and coincidence. It there-

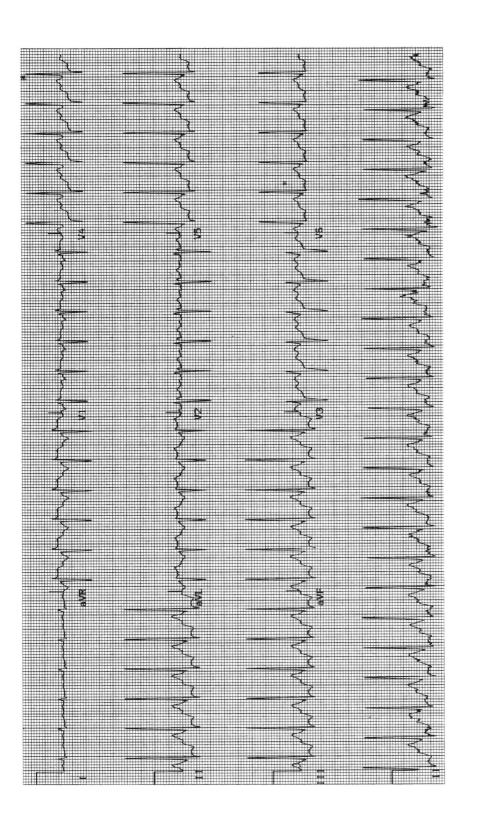
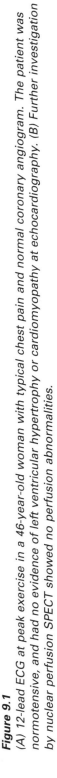

Figure 9.1

(A) 12-lead ECG at peak exercise in a 46-year-old woman with typical chest pain and normal coronary angiogram. The patient was normotensive, and had no evidence of left ventricular hypertrophy or cardiomyopathy at echocardiography. (B) Further investigation by nuclear perfusion SPECT showed no perfusion abnormalities.

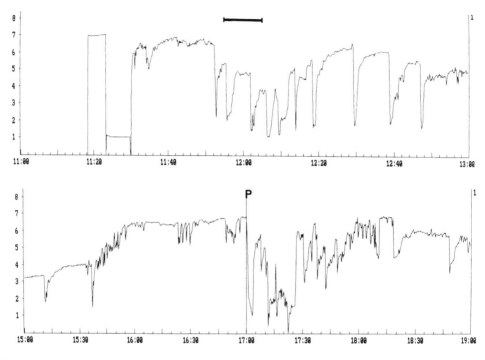

Figure 9.2

The diagnostic value of ambulatory pH monitoring in patients with unexplained chest pain. Gastro-oesophageal reflux occurs just before treadmill exercise testing (solid bar) and coincides with the reproduction of chest pain. A further episode of chest pain later in the day (marker P) was also associated with gastro-oesophageal reflux.

fore has a higher spatial resolution, and is not subject to attenuation artefact. Three studies using the technique in patients with syndrome X have shown no regional abnormalities of perfusion.[29–31] A great heterogeneity of flow was observed in one study using small ($<2.3\,cm^3$) tissue regions of interest and comparing their coefficients of variation, but there were no anatomical regional abnormalities of blood flow.[32]

Abnormalities of blood flow: the concept of myocardial flow reserve

The ability of the coronary vasculature to maintain flow over a wide range of perfusion pressures (50–120 mmHg) is known as autoregulation. If the coronary vasculature is maximally dilated, as occurs in response to exercise or pharmacological agents or pacing, autoregulation is lost and a steep, almost linear pressure–flow relationship results. The difference between autoregulated flow and flow at maximal vasodilatation is known as the myocardial flow reserve.[33]

Early studies using coronary sinus thermodilution catheters are limited by technical factors and a failure to test the technique on large numbers of asymptomatic volunteers because of its invasiveness. Inaccuracies may arise when the catheter displaces back into the coronary sinus.[34] In initial validation studies the catheter was sutured in place, but in later studies it was

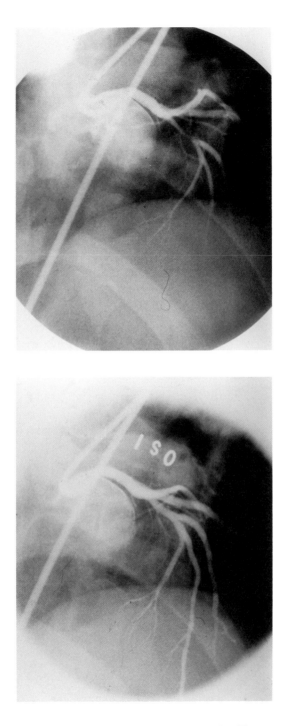

Figure 9.3
Spontaneous coronary artery spasm during coronary angiography. The operator was about to perform angioplasty when the administration of nitrates reversed the abnormality. Coronary artery spasm is an unusual cause of exertional chest pain particularly where the angiogram shows no evidence of plaques.

left untied, as in the clinical model, and there was only a weak correlation with actual flow.[35] The technique was validated against an electromagentic flow probe placed over vein bypass grafts intraoperatively, but in such a setting calibration is unreliable and flow was tested over only a narrow range.[36]

Various patient subgroups have been compared, defined by criteria such as their pain response after atrial pacing,[16] the presence or absence of 'typical' pain,[37] lactate production,[38] vasomotor response of the epicardial arteries,[39] or the results of radionuclide studies.[40] Often significant differences are found, but the results usually show wide overlap between the groups with large confidence intervals. Moroever, there are inconsistencies. Cannon et al. reported significantly lower flow reserves in patients who developed chest pain with atrial pacing than in patients who did not report pain, whereas Camici et al. found no significant differences using the same methods.[16,37] Similarly Opherk et al., using the argon inert gas clearance technique, reported significantly lower flow reserves in 21 patients with exertional chest pain, most of whom had ST depression on their exercise electrocardiogram, compared with controls with atypical chest pain.[23] In a similar study design, which used xenon and avoided sampling from the coronary sinus, Green et al. found no significant differences.[41]

Since positron emission tomography is a relatively noninvasive technique it may be used to quantify blood flow in apparently healthy volunteers. Recent studies using O^{15}-water positron emission tomography have shown no significant differences in blood flow between patients with syndrome X and asymptomatic volunteers.[29,31] Gallassi et al. reported a significantly lower flow reserve in the patient group than in controls (2.4 versus 3.9), but the differences were due to a higher basal flow in the patient group than in controls. There were no differences in absolute blood flow at peak stress.[32]

Geltman et al. used PET to separate patients into those with low and high flow reserves (<2.5 or >2.5). The incidence of chest pain during infusion of dipyridamole, or evidence of ischaemia by exercise electrocardiography or thallium-201 scintigraphy was similar in both groups.[29] Similarly, Rosen et al. reported no differences in blood flow comparing those with and without pain, or those with and without ST depression.[31]

The use of dipyridamole, which acts indirectly by causing the release of adenosine, as the stressor is a possible limitation. Chauhan et al. injected papaverine directly into the coronary arteries and reported significantly reduced flow reserves using intracoronary Doppler. However, the patient groups were not matched for age and gender, and the appropriateness of using transplant patients as the comparison group is questionable.[42] Holdright et al. and Egashira et al. found normal flow reserves in separate studies using papaverine.[43,44]

Vrints et al. measured the left epicardial coronary arterial diameters in response to acetylcholine, an endothelium-dependent vasodilator.[45] In 12 patients with typical pain, the luminal diameter decreased by up to one-third with graded infusions of 10^{-6}–10^{-4} M concentrations of drug. Nine had their usual chest pain induced, and five had significant ST depression. By comparision, in the remaining 12 patients with atypical pain, infusion of identical concentrations of drug induced either no change or mild dilatation. Only one patient in this group reported chest pain and none had ECG changes. Since the drug was used in higher concentrations than usual, it is possible that the effects observed were due to its direct vasoconstricting action on smooth muscle rather than as a result of endothelial dysfunction. Egashira et al. studied nine patients with syndrome X, and 10 controls with noncardiac chest pain, but excluded patients with hypercholesterolaemia and hypertension.[44] Although there was a normal initial vasodilatation of the epicardial arteries in response to acetylcholine in both groups (in contrast to Vrints et al.), the coronary flow reserves were significantly less in the patient group than in the controls (Table 9.1). One hesitates to conclude that endothelial dysfunction was the cause of chest pain, since the injection of papaverine caused the production of lactate and induced chest pain in every patient. At least one other study has shown no

Study			Population	Basal flow	Peak flow	MFR
Opherk (1981)[23]	argon	pacing	patients (21)	74 (13)	150 (37)*	2.0*
			controls (15)	78 (9)	300 (60)	3.8
Cannon (1983)[16]	thermo	pacing	group 1 (9)	58 (14)	85 (41)*	1.5*
			group 2 ((13)	63 (18)	117 (37)	1.9
Cannon (1987)[46]	thermo	pacing	patients (25)	63 (15)	134 (34)*	2.1*
			controls (15)	73 (13)	202 (45)	2.8
Greenberg (1987)[38]	thermo	pacing	patients (10)	81 (14)	124 (22)*	1.5*
			controls (17)	86 (30)	154 (42)	1.8
Bortone (1989)[39]	thermo	dipyridamole	group 1 (6)	128 (56)	153*	1.2*
			group 2 (7)	112 (24)	287 (143)	2.6
Camici (1991)[37]	thermo	pacing	patients (12)	56 (20)	90 (30)	1.6
			controls (10)	52 (16)	104 (30)	2.0
Camici (1992)[30]	PET ($^{13}NH_3$)	dipyridamole	group 1 (14)	88 (13)*	148 (29)*	1.7*
			group 2 (29)	112 (23)	302 (73)	2.7
Geltman (1990)[29]	PET (O_2)	dipyridamole	patients (17)	138 (46)	368 (201)	3.0
			controls (16)	125 (28)	462 (158)	3.8
Gallassi (1993)[32]	PET (O_2)	dipyridamole	patients (13)	124 (27)*	295 (75)	2.4*
			controls (7)	87 (7)	340 (82)	3.9
Holdright (1993)[43]	Doppler	papaverine	patients (25)	—	—	4.1
			controls (10)	—	—	>2.5
Egashira (1993)[44]	Doppler	acetylcholine	patients (9)	—	103 (77)*	2.3*
			controls (10)	—	345 (78)	4.5
		papaverine	patients (9)	—	366 (168)	4.7
			controls (10)	—	411 (92)	5.1
Chauhan (1994)[42]	Doppler	papaverine	patients (53)	63 (33)	—	2.7*
			controls (26)	54 (28)	—	5.2
Rosen (1994)[31]	PET (O_2)	dipyridamole	patients (29)	105 (25)	273 (81)	2.7
			controls (20)	100 (22)	300 (100)	3.1

Blood flows are expressed either as ml/min/100 g tissue or ml/min depending on the methodology.
*$p < 0.05$

Table 9.1
Myocardial flow reserve (MFR) in patients with normal coronary angiograms.

significant differences in flow reserves using acetylcholine in patients with syndrome X and controls with atypical chest pain.[47]

In pursuit of objective evidence of myocardial ischaemia

The search for confirmatory evidence of myocardial ischaemia has proved elusive. Myocardial ischaemia develops where there is an imbalance between the consumption of adenosine triphosphate and blood flow. This results in the almost immediate retention of hydrogen ions intracellularly and the net loss of potassium ions to the extracellular space,[19] followed by metabolic changes, the early loss of contractile function,[48] chest pain, and electrocardiographic changes in that order.[49]

Contractile dysfunction

A variety of techniques have been used to assess left ventricular contractile function in syndrome X. Echocardiography allows direct real-time imaging of myocardial wall thickening. This may be assessed at rest and more recently, with the help of computerized analysis and cine loop playback, after exercise or pharmacological stress. In an early report, Turiel et al. noted transient regional wall motion abnormalities using two-dimensional echocardiography in five out of 12 (42%) patients with syndrome X.[50] However, Picano et al. (in a study of 19 patients using dipyridamole), and Nihoyannopoulos et al. (in a study of 18 patients using exercise stress) reported no abnormalities of wall motion despite the occurrence of significant ST depression and chest pain in the majority of cases.[51,52]

However, the absence of a wall motion abnormality does not exclude myocardial ischaemia which is either patchy or confined to the subendocardium. Henein et al. reported abnormalities of left and right ventricular long axes shortening at rest in 70% of syndrome X patients and only 5% of controls.[53] The long axis function is mainly supported by subendocardial fibres which are particularly susceptible to ischaemia. The significance of these findings has yet to be determined. It should be noted that there was no correlation of abnormalities of long axis function with other evidence of ischaemia, including reversible perfusion abnormalities using single-photon scintigraphy.

The incidence of left ventricular dysfunction using radionuclide angiography varies from zero to 79% (Table 9.2). In most studies a failure of left ventricular ejection fraction to rise by a specified amount is taken to indicate an abnormality. The ejection fraction response depends on many factors besides contractile function, including the resting ejection fraction, the end-diastolic volume, workload, and gender.[54] Furthermore, a decrease in ejection fraction without real impairment in left ventricular contractility may occur where there is an inappropriate increase in afterload resulting in a preload–afterload mismatch.[61] Abnormalities of regional wall motion are a more reliable indicator of ischaemia and are less commonly reported. None the less the assessment of wall motion by radionuclide techniques is prone to technical error through the necessity to average several beats. It also relies on judgements made about endocardial motion rather than myocardial thickening. As with many of the techniques used to assess ischaemia in patients with normal angiograms, abnormalities are reported but there is rarely confirmatory evidence of ischaemia using complementary tests.

Levy et al. measured pulmonary artery diastolic pressure, a marker of left ventricular end-diastolic pressure, during treadmill exercise, and ambulatory monitoring using catheter mounted transducers.[62] There was a rise in

	Patients	Global	Regional	Total
Borer (1979)[55]	21	0	0	0
Berger (1981)[26]	31	12 (39%)	4 (13%)	
Gibbons (1981)[54]	60	27 (45%)	4 (7%)	
Osbakken (1983)[56]	21	8 (38%)	—	8 (38%)
Rozanski (1983)[57]	45	23 (51%)	29 (64%)	
Legrand (1985)[40]	18	5 (28%)	4 (22%)	
Cannon (1985)[58]	26	18 (69%)	12 (46%)	
Favaro (1987)[59]	32	22 (69%)	12 (37%)	
Camici (1991)[37]	12	0	0	0
Cannon (1991)[60] group 1	136	—	—	56 (41%)
group 2	56	—	—	7 (13%)
Taki (1994)[18]	14	11 (79%)	—	11 (79%)
Cannon (1994)[46]	49	—	—	11 (22%)

Table 9.2
Left ventricular dysfunction in patients with normal coronary angiograms: radionuclide studies.

pressure during exercise in only two of six patients, but in each case the rise was small and of similar magnitude to that observed in controls with atypical pain and normal ECGs. By comparison with patients with obstructive coronary disease in whom significant ST depression during ambulatory monitoring was invariably associated with a rise in pressure, episodes of ST depression in patients with normal angiograms were not associated with elevations in pressure.

Metabolic changes

The production of lactate is an important marker of ischaemia. This results from an increase in glycogenolysis under anaerobic conditions, and was first demonstrated by Clark et al. in the isolated frog heart, and later in humans by Cohen et al.[63,64] However, the clinical use of lactate measurements as evidence of myocardial ischaemia has a number of limitations. Firstly, the heart consumes as well as produces lactate and so uptake of lactate may be reduced by free

fatty acids, ketone bodies, insulin, heparin and other factors. Secondly, the concentrations of lactate in arterial blood may be small and differences between this and coronary sinus blood may be within the experimental error of the assay. Only the net production of lactate should be used to indicate ischaemia (Table 9.3).[65]

Greenberg et al. reported lactate production in 37% of 27 patients with normal coronary angiograms.[38] However, the group included a high proportion (70%) of patients with either poorly controlled hypertension or diabetes mellitus. In a study of 200 well selected patients from the National Institutes of Health, the incidence of lactate production was only 7%.[66] Other authors have reported no evidence of lactate production.[37,67]

Crake et al. measured coronary sinus oxygen saturation continuously during atrial pacing in 10 patients with syndrome X, and 11 controls with atypical pain.[68] Since the heart is a compulsory aerobe, any fall in saturation implies ischaemia due to an inadequacy of the coronary blood to deliver sufficient oxygen to meet the

	Patients	No. (%) lactate producers
Arbogast (1972)[69]	10	3 (30%)
Kemp (1973)[2]	100	22 (22%)
Boudoulas (1974)[70]	29	9 (31%)
Mammohansingh (1975)[71]	16	2 (13%)
Jackson (1978)[72]	25	0
Greenberg (1987)[38]	27	10 (37%)
Cannon (1991)[66] Group 1	141	14 (10%)
Group 2	59	0
Camici (1991)[37] Group 1	12	0
Group 2	10	0
Suzuki (1994)[21]	21	0

Table 9.3
Lactate production in patients with normal coronary angiograms.

metabolic requirements. In only two of the ten (20%) syndrome X patients, and in none of the controls was there a sustained fall in oxygen saturation similar to that observed with ischaemia in patients with confirmed obstructive coronary disease.

By contrast to controls, in whom there was an expected increase in carbohydrate oxidation during and after pacing, patients with syndrome X maintained a low level of carbohydrate oxidation but showed an increased uptake and oxidation of lipid substrates, and a reversed pattern of pyruvate and alanine exchange.[37] These changes were opposite to those expected with myocardial ischaemia and more consistent with abnormal sympathetic activation.

Unifying hypotheses

A number of hypotheses are advanced as possible mechanisms of pain. Adenosine is thought to be the link between myocardial ischaemia and chest pain,[73,74] although other mediators are postulated including acidosis and increased intracellular potassium.[75] It is suggested that inappropriate vasoconstriction of the small pre-arteriolar resistance vessels results in distal intramural arteriolar dilatation and compensatory release and 'spill over' of adenosine. Ischaemia results due to a steal effect and may be patchy or subendocardial. It is also postulated that pain may be due to the abnormal release of adenosine in the absence of ischaemia.[76] There is, however, no evidence to support these hypotheses since there are no methods currently available to measure transmural blood flow.[77]

One possible explanation of the wide overlap in blood flow responses between patients with syndrome X and uncomplaining and apparently healthy volunteers is that the former have lower pain thresholds. Adenosine was given by intravenous bolus injections to eight patients with normal coronary angiograms and reproduced their typical pain. Pain was also produced in nine patients with confirmed obstructive coronary disease, and 16 healthy controls, but the minimum dose at the onset of pain, and maximal tolerable doses of adenosine were significantly less in patients with normal coronary angiograms than in the other groups.[78]

Lowered stimulation thresholds have been shown using other agents besides adenosine, and may represent a more generalized abnormality of pain perception. Manipulation of a catheter or injection of normal saline in the right atrium,[79] pacing either the right atria or right ventricles at only five beats above resting heart rate, or injection of the coronary arteries with a single bolus of contrast commonly reproduces pain in patients but only rarely in controls.[80] Similarly Richter et al., and more recently Bradley et al. reported reduced stimulation thresholds compared with controls by inflating balloons in the body of the oesophagus,[81,82] and Turiel et al.,[50] but not Bradley et al.[82] reported reduced sensitivities to mechanical stimulation of the skin (Table 9.4).

Abnormalities of autonomic control are reported and these may affect coronary blood flow, and increase myocardial demand, and hence cause ischaemia and chest pain. Thus increased heart rates at rest, at maximal exercise, and during 24-hour ambulatory monitoring, have been reported,[84] although this is not a universal finding.[85] Similarly, plasma catecholamines were significantly higher immediately after exercise in patients with syndrome X than in healthy volunteers,[84,86] and there is also a suggestion that the QT interval, a marker of autonomic balance, is prolonged.[87] Rosano et al. assessed heart rate variability both in time and frequency during 24-hour Holter monitoring in a study of 26 syndrome X patients and 20 matched controls.[85] Significantly lower time domain parameters and spectral power suggested an autonomic imbalance in syndrome X compared with controls. A trend towards increased low-frequency to high-frequency spectral power ratios indicated a predominance of sympathetic activation. Such observations are consistent with the commonly reported, and well recognized clinically high levels of neuroticism in this patient group, and suggest possible mechanisms whereby disturbances of central function may produce physical symptoms. However, they stop far short of establishing a cause and effect.

A further hypothesis relates to the role of hormones, since a high proportion of patients with normal coronary angiograms are women. This has generated interest in the role of oestrogen in the pathogenesis of pain. Oestrogens have been shown to modulate the endothelial response to acetylcholine stimulation of endothelium relaxing factor (EDRF), and to

	Patients	Cardiac	Oesophageal	Cutaneous
Richter (1986)[81]	30		√	
Turiel (1987)[50]	12			√
Shapiro (1988)[79]	11	√		
Cannon (1990)[80]	36	√	√	
Bradley (1992)[82]	24		√	
Largerqvist (1992)[78]	8	√		
Chauhan (1994)[83]		√		

Table 9.4
Studies of pain perception in patients with chest pain despite normal coronary anatomy.

induce vascular smooth muscle relaxation in endothelial-free preparations.[88,89] They also have important effects on the release and uptake of catecholamines.[90] Sarrel et al. reported a high incidence of oestrogen deficiency in 30 female patients with syndrome X.[91] Twenty-five of the 30 had severe hot flushes (more than 20 episodes per day), and almost a half had migraine headaches. Eighteen (60%) had hysterectomies, half with preservation of ovaries, a rate that was considerably higher than the national average of 8–12%.

Rosano et al. reported biochemical evidence of ovarian insufficiency in 95 out of 107 (89%) consecutive female patients with syndrome X.[92] Forty-three (40%) of these had hysterectomies and in all but two the onset of symptoms was within a decade after hysterectomy. In those who did not have hysterectomies the onset of symptoms was either soon after the menopause or in the perimenopause. Of course, these observations do not account for the cause of pain in male patients with syndrome X, who account for about one-third of the total group. To add further confusion, Morise et al. reported that 15 out of 25 (58%) patients with abnormal exercise electrocardiograms were taking oral oestrogen replacement therapy, compared with only 25 out of 85 (29%) patients with normal or equivocal tests.[10]

Long-term outlook and therapeutic studies

The overall survival and freedom from cardiac events in the larger group of patients with normal coronary angiograms is excellent. Over a mean follow-up period of 6.3 years the 5-year survival in 1491 patients with normal coronary angiograms, or insignificant disease defined as less than 75% narrowing in any major vessel,

was 99%, and at 10 years was 98%. Patients with normal arteries differed significantly from those with insignificant disease only in their MI-free survival (99% versus 97% at 5 years, and 98% versus 90% at 10 years).[93] As in other studies, a fall in survival curves was noted after 5 years, which was most marked in patients with insignificant stenoses consistent with a higher incidence of disease progression in this group.[94,95]

There are little follow-up data for the subgroup of patients with 'typical' pain and significant ST depression during stress testing. In the CASS registry 843 exercise tests were available for analysis, of which 648 were normal, 125 showed >1 mm ST depression, and 70 showed ≥ 2 mm depression.[95] The electrocardiographic abnormalities had no predictive value for survival. Patients with left bundle branch block may comprise an important subgroup. In a study of 40 patients followed up over 4 years, 14 patients with LBBB were compared with patients whose ECGs showed ST depression alone. Left ventricular function was the same at baseline, but after 4 years there was a significant deterioration in patients with, but not in those without LBBB.[96] A similar deterioration in left ventricular performance in patients with LBBB was reported after a 6-year follow-up by Romeo et al.[97]

Morbidity remains high, despite the reassurance of an excellent long-term prognosis.[98] There are little controlled data about the use of conventional anti-anginal medications. However, it is likely that these are ineffective since many patients have tried them unsuccessfully before referral for angiography, and many continue to report symptoms on long-term follow-up.

Bugiardini et al., in a double-blind crossover placebo-controlled trial involving 12 syndrome X patients, reported a reduction of the number of ischaemic episodes (or perhaps more appropriately termed ST episodes) during ambulatory monitoring from 3.9 h (SD 1.8) to 0.7 h (SD 0.6) after propranolol, but not with verapamil.[99] Romeo et al. reported an increase in exercise tolerance during treadmill testing with acebutolol in 15 patients with syndrome X whose heart rate–blood pressure products increased by more than 1050 Hg.bt/min in the first stage, compared with other syndrome X patients.[100] However, verapamil increased the exercise tolerance in both groups, and after a mean follow-up of 5 years neither beta blockers nor verapamil had any important effect on symptoms.[97]

In a randomized, placebo-controlled cross-over trial involving 25 female patients with syndrome X, Rosano et al. reported a reduction of symptoms using 17β oestradiol over an 8-week period which just attained statistical significance.[101] In contrast to patients with confirmed obstructive coronary disease, there was no objective change in the maximum exercise tolerance during treadmill testing.[102]

Other investigators have studied the effects of alpha blockers. In a study of 10 syndrome X patients, Camici et al. reported a significant improvement in myocardial flow reserve, 2.2 (SD 0.6) to 3.5 (SD 1.2) using dipyridamole and $^{13}NH_3$ positron emission tomography after doxasosin.[103] However, in a previous study Galassi et al. found no important changes in exercise tolerance or in the number of ischaemic episodes during ambulatory monitoring with prazosin or clonidine.[104]

The most striking benefit has been with the antidepressant, imipramine. Sixty consecutive patients with normal coronary angiograms were entered by Cannon et al. into a double-blind placebo-controlled trial.[105] Twenty-three patients (38%) had abnormal exercise electrocardiograms, gated radionuclide blood pool scans, or both, and in 52 patients (87%) their usual pain was reproduced by right ventricular

pacing at 5 beats per minute above baseline or by the intracoronary infusion of adenosine. However, only 13 patients (22%) met the usual inclusion criteria for syndrome X. After only 3 weeks of active treatment there was a 50% reduction in the number, and the intensity ratings of symptom episodes. An improvement in mental state using standardized rating scales was observed in both patients receiving active treatment and patients who received placebo, suggesting that the beneficial effects may not have been related to changes in mental state. The observation that on repeat testing of right ventricular sensitivity there was a significant improvement while on imipramine but not on placebo suggests that the response may have been due to the effects of the drug on peripheral nerve receptors.

Conclusions

In the absence of a clear clinical definition, a unifying hypothesis relating to its pathogenesis, and an effective treatment, there is significant doubt about the utility of the term syndrome X. However, it is relevant to ask if the coronary angiogram is completely normal and what is the possibility that the chest pain may still be cardiac. After the exclusion of the small numbers of patients with epicardial spasm, and patients with noncoronary cardiac pathology, the case for a cardiac cause of pain relies principally on the demonstration of abnormalities of coronary blood flow. These are thought to be functional since there is no convincing histological evidence of small vessel disease. Studies using positron emission tomography show a wide spectrum of coronary flow reserves both in patients with normal coronary angiograms and in apparently healthy volunteers. The boundaries between normal and abnormal coronary flow reserve are therefore somewhat blurred. Some patients with normal coronary angiograms and low flow reserve may have low pain thresholds, which might account for their presentation with a condition which otherwise would have remained asymptomatic. This is rather speculative. That psychological factors are important is suggested by studies showing high levels of autonomic arousal, low pain thresholds, and favourable therapeutic responses to tricyclic antidepressants.

If I had . . .

I would be reassured of an excellent long-term event-free survival and only if my pain persisted, despite this reassurance, would I pursue further investigations. In the first instance, I would wish to know that there was no evidence of cardiomyopathy or significant valve pathology that had been missed, and would therefore request an echocardiogram. I would then wish to know if the coronary angiogram was completely normal or whether it showed evidence of plaque disease. If the angiogram showed plaques and if my pain was typical of angina and consistently related to exertion I would request a myocardial perfusion scan. However, only a large reversible defect would suggest an underestimation of the extent of disease and prompt further investigation by intravascular ultrasound. Alternatively if my pain was typical but occurred predominantly at rest, I might suspect coronary artery spasm. This would be unlikely if there was a poor response to nitrates but further investigations might include ambulatory ST analysis or stress echocardiography during voluntary overbreathing.

I would accept that my pain is likely to be noncardiac and would wish to see a gastroenterologist for investigations of the oesophagus, or a skilled physiotherapist who might identify sources of musculoskeletal pain. I should hope that I would recognize stress factors in my life that may be aggravating the situation but would accept that insight may often be lacking. I would try a course of imipramine as an empirical measure and if all else fails I would seek the help of a liaison psychiatrist who might help by providing cognitive and behavioural therapy.

Above all, in the absence of evidence of a definite cardiac abnormality, I would wish strong reassurance that my heart is normal. I would not wish to continue cardiac medication because my physician remained uncertain about the cause of my pain and did not wish to discount the unlikely diagnosis of a functional abnormality of the coronary microvasculature. Such uncertainty would be likely to make me more anxious and to reinforce my illness behaviour, which would be detrimental to my long-term prognosis.

References

1 Lifoff W, Segal BL, Kasparian H, Paradox of normal selective coronary arteriograms in patients considered to have unmistakable coronary heart disease, *N Eng J Med* (1967)**276**:1063–6.

2 Kemp HG, Vokoanas PS, Cohn PF, Gorlin R, The anginal syndrome associated with normal coronary arteriograms. Report of a six year experience, *Am J Med* (1973)**54**:735–42.

3 Isner MJ, Salem DN, Banas JS, Levine HJ, Long-term clinical course of patients with normal coronary arteriography: follow up study of 121 patients with normal or nearly normal coronary angiograms, *Am Heart J* (1981)**102**:645–53.

4 Davies SW, Winterton SJ, Rothman MT, Intravascular ultrasound to assess left main stem coronary artery lesion, *Br Heart J* (1992)**68**:524–6.

5 Ge J, Erbel R, Gerber T et al, Intravscular ultrasound imaging of angiographically normal coronary arteries: a prospective study in vivo, *Br Heart J* (1994)**71**:572–8.

6 Henderson A, Syndrome X, *Cardiovasc Focus* (1992)**30**:1–3.

7 Reaven G, Banting lecture 1988: role of insulin resistance in human diabetes, *Diabetes* (1988)**37**:1595–607.

8 Dean JD, Jones CJH, Hutchinson SJ, Peters JR, Henderson AH, Hyperinsulinaemia and microvascular angina, *Lancet* (1991)**337**:456–7.

9 Chauhan A, Foote, J, Petch MC, Schofield PM, Hyperinsulinaemia, coronary artery disease and syndrome X, *J Am Coll Cardiol* (1994)**23**:364–8.

10 Morise AP, Dalal JN, Duval RD, Frequency of oral oestrogen replacement therapy in women with normal and abnormal exercise electrocardiograms and normal coronary arteries by angiogram, *Am J Cardiol* (1993)**72**:1197–9.

11 Rosano G, Poole-Wilson PA, Collins P et al, Prevalence of syndrome X amongst 189 consecutive patients with angina and normal coronary arteries, *J Am Coll Cardiol* (1994) **(suppl)** **265A (abstr)**.

12 Kaski JC, Rosano GM, Collins P, Nihoyannopoulos P, Maseri A, Poole-Wilson PA, Cardiac syndrome X: clinical characteristics and left ventricular function. Long term follow up study, *J Am Coll Cardiol* (1995) **25**:807–14.

13 Proudfit WL, Shirey EK, Sones FM, Selective cine coronary arteriography: correlation with clinical findings in 1000 patients, *Circulation* (1966)**33**:901–10.

14 Waxler EB, Kimbiris D, Dreifus LS, The fate of women with normal coronary arteriograms and chest pain resembling angina pectoris, *Am J Cardiol* (1971)**28**:25–32.

15 Day LJ, Sowton E, Clinical features and follow up of patients with angina and normal coronary arteries, *Lancet* (1976)**14**:334–7.

16 Cannon RO, Watson RM, Rosing DR, Epstein SE, Angina caused by reduced vasodilator reserve of the small coronary arteries, *J Am Coll Cardiol* (1983)**1**:1359–73.

17 Tweddel AC, Hutton WM, Thallium scans in syndrome X, *Br Heart J* (1992)**68**:48–50.

18 Taki J, Nakajima K, Muramori A, Yoshi H, Shimizu M, Hisada K, Left ventricular dysfunction during exercise in patients with angina pectoris and angiographically normal coronary arteries (syndrome X), *Eur J Nucl Med* (1994)**21**:98–102.

19 Poole-Wilson PA, Angina-pathological mechanisms, clinical expression and treatment, *Postgrad Med J* (1983)**59(suppl 3)**:11–21.

20 Bertrand ME, LaBlanche JM, Tilmant PY et al, Frequency of provoked coronary arterial spasm in 1089 consecutive patients undergoing coronary angiography, *Circulation* (1982)**65**:1299–306.

21 Suzuki H, Takeyama Y, Koba S, Suwa Y, Katagiri T, Small vessel pathology and coronary hemodynamics in patients with microvascular angina, *Int J Cardiol* (1994)**43**:139–50.

22 Shirey EK, Correlative pathologic study of the coronary microcirculation with coronary arteriography, *Circulation* (1968)VI–179.

23 Opherk D, Zebe H, Weihe E et al, Reduced coronary dilatory capacity and ultrastructural changes of the myocardium in patients with angina pectoris but normal coronary arteriograms, *Circulation* (1981)63:817–25.

24 Richardson PJ, Rothman MT, Atkinson L, Baadrup U, Jackson G, The pathophysiology of angina pectoris with normal coronary arteriograms. Histopathological and metabolic correlations with coronary vasospasm, *Arch Mal Coeur* (1983)76:223–9.

25 Chilian WM, Eastham CL, Marcus ML, Microvascular distribution of coronary vascular resistance in beating left ventricle, *Am J Physiol* (1986)20:H779.

26 Berger HJ, Sands MJ, Davies RA et al, Exercise left ventricular performance in patients with chest pain, ischaemic appearing exercise electrocardiograms, and angiographically normal coronary arteries, *Ann Intern Med* (1981)94:186–91.

27 Kaul S, Newell JB, Chesler DA, Pohost GM, Okada RD, Boucher CA, Quantatative thallium imaging findings in patients with normal coronary angiographic findings and in clinically normal subjects, *Am J Cardiol* (1986)57:509–12.

28 Rosano GMC, Mavrogeni SI, Kaski JC et al, Reduced uptake and wash-out of thallium in patients with syndrome X, *Br Heart J* (1994)71 (suppl):64 (abstr).

29 Geltman EM, Henes CG, Senneff MJ, Sobel BE, Bergmann SR, Increased myocardial perfusion at rest and diminished perfusion reserve in patients with angina and angiographically normal coronary arteries, *J Am Coll Cardiol* (1990)16:586–95.

30 Camici PG, Gistri R, Lorenzoni R et al, Coronary reserve and exercise ECG in patients with chest pain and normal coronary angiograms, *Circulation* (1992)86:179–86.

31 Rosen SD, Uren NG, Kaski JC, Tousoulis D, Davies GJ, Camici PG, Coronary vasodilator reserve, pain perception, and sex in patients with syndrome X, *Circulation* (1994)90:50–60.

32 Galassi AR, Crea F, Araujo LI et al, Comparison of regional myocardial blood flow in syndrome X and one-vessel coronary artery disease, *Am J Cardiol* (1993)72:134–9.

33 Gould KL, Lipscomb K, Hamilton GW, Physiologic basis for assessing critical coronary stenosis. Instantaneous flow response and regional distribution during coronary hyperaemia as measures of coronary flow reserve, *Am J Cardiol* (1974)33:87–94.

34 Mathey DG, Chatterjee K, Tyberg JV, Lekven J, Brundage B, Parmley WW, A source of error in the measurement of thermodilution coronary sinus flow, *Circulation* (1978)57:779–86.

35 Weisse AB, Regan TJ, A comparison of thermodilution coronary sinus blood flows and krypton myocardial blood flows in the intact dog, *Cardiovasc Res* (1974)8:526–33.

36 Marcus ML, White CW, Coronary flow reserve in patients with normal coronary angiograms, *J Am Coll Cardiol* (1985)6:1254–6.

37 Camici PG, Marraccini P, Lorenzoni R et al, Coronary haemodynamics and myocardial metabolism in patients with syndrome X: response to pacing stress, *J Am Coll Cardiol* (1991)17:1461–70.

38 Greenberg MA, Grose RM, Neuburger N, Silverman R, Strain JE, Cohen MV, Impaired coronary vasodilator responsiveness as a cause of lactate production during pacing induced ischaemia in patients with angina pectoris and normal coronary arteries, *J Am Coll Cardiol* (1987)9:743–51.

39 Bortone AS, Hess OM, Eberli FR et al, Abnormal coronary vasomotion during exercise in patients with normal coronary arteries and reduced coronary flow reserve, *Circulation* (1989)79:516–27.

40 Legrand V, Hodgson J, Bates ER et al, Abnormal coronary flow reserve and abnormal radionuclide exercise test results in patients with normal coronary angiograms, *J Am Coll Cardiol* (1985)6:1245–53.

41 Green LH, Cohn PF, Holman BL, Adams DF, Markis JE, Regional myocardial blood flow in patients with chest pain syndromes and normal coronary arteriograms, *Br Heart J* (1978)40:242–9.

42 Chauhan A, Mullins PA, Petch MC, Schofield PM, Is coronary flow reserve in response to papaverine really normal in syndrome X? *Circulation* (1994)89:1998–2004.

43 Holdright D, Lindsay DC, Clarke D, Fox K, Poole-Wilson PA, Collins P, Coronary flow reserve in patients with chest pain and normal coronary arteries, *Br Heart J* (1993)**70**:513–19.

44 Egashira K, Inou T, Hirooka Y, Yamada A, Urabe Y, Takeshita A, Evidence of impaired endothelium dependent coronary vasodilation in patients with angina pectoris and normal coronary angiograms, *N Engl J Med* (1993)**328**:1659–64.

45 Vrints CJM, Bult H, Hitter E, Herman AG, Snoeck JP, Impaired endothelial dependent cholinergic coronary vasodilation in patients with angina and normal coronary angiograms, *J Am Coll Cardiol* (1992)**19**:21–31.

46 Cannon RO, Schenke WH, Leon MB, Rosing DR, Urqhart J, Epstein SE, Limited coronary flow reserve after dipyridamole in patients with ergonovine induced coronary vasoconstriction, *Circulation* (1987)**75**:163–74.

47 Holdright D, Clarke D, Lindsay D et al, Coronary flow reserve is not impaired in syndrome X, *J Am Coll Cardiol* (1992)**19**:211A (abstr).

48 Cobbe SM, Poole-Wilson PA, Continuous coronary sinus and arterial pH monitoring during ischaemia in coronary artery disease, *Br Heart J* (1982)**47**:369.

49 Hauser AM, Gangadharan V, Ramos RG, Gordon S, Timmis GC, Sequence of mechanical, electrocardiographic and clinical effects of repeated coronary artery occlusion in human beings: electrocardiographic observations during coronary angioplasty, *J Am Coll Cardiol* (1985)**5**:193–7.

50 Turiel M, Galassi AR, Glazier JJ, Kaski JC, Maseri A, Pain threshold and tolerance in women with syndrome X and women with stable angina pectoris, *Am J Cardiol* (1987)**60**:503–8.

51 Picano E, Lattanzi F, Masini M, Distante A, L'Abbate A, Usefulness of high-dose dipyridamole-echocardiography test for the diagnosis of syndrome X, *Am J Cardiol* (1987)**60**:508–12.

52 Nihoyannopoulos P, Kaski JC, Crake T, Maseri A, Absence of myocardial dysfunction during stress in patients with syndrome X, *J Am Coll Cardiol* (1991)**18**:1463–70.

53 Henein MY, Rosano GMC, Underwood R, Poole-Wilson PA, Gibson D, Relations between resting ventricular long axis function, the electrocardiogram, and myocardial perfusion imaging in syndrome X, *Br Heart J* (1994)**71**:541–7.

54 Gibbons RJ, Lee KL, Cobb F, Jones RH, Ejection fraction response to exercise in patients with chest pain and normal coronary arteriograms, *Circulation* (1981)**64**:952–7.

55 Borer JS, Kent KM, Bacharach SL et al, Sensitivity, specificity, and predictive accuracy of radionuclide cineangiography during exercise in patients with coronary artery disease, *Circulation* (1979)**60**:572–80.

56 Osbakken MD, Boucher CA, Okada RD, Bingham JB, Strauss W, Pohost GM, Spectrum of global left ventricular responses to supine exercise, *Am J Cardiol* (1983)**51**:28–35.

57 Rozanski A, Diamond GA, Berman D, Forrester JS, Morris D, Swan HJC, The declining specificity of exercise radionuclide ventriculography, *New Engl J Med* (1983)**309**:518–22.

58 Cannon RO, Bonow RO, Bacharach SL et al, Left ventricular dysfunction in patients with angina pectoris, normal epicardial coronary arteries, and abnormal vasodilator reserve, *Circulation* (1985)**71**:218–26.

59 Favaro L, Caplin JL, Fettiche JJ, Dymond D, Sex differences in exercise induced left ventricular dysfunction in patients with syndrome X, *Br Heart J* (1987)**57**:232–6.

60 Cannon RU, Schenke WH, Quyyumi A, Bonow RO, Efistein SE, Comparison of exersise testing with studies of coronary flow reserve in patients with microvascular angina, *Circulation* (1994) **89(Suppl III)** III77–81.

61 Ross JJ, Afterload mismatch and preload reserve: a conceptual framework for the analysis of ventricular function, *Prog Cardiovasc Dis* (1976)**182**:255–64.

62 Levy RD, Shapiro LM, Wright C, Mockus L, Fox KM, Syndrome X: the haemodynamic significance of ST segment depression, *Br Heart J* (1986)**56**:353–7.

63 Clarke AI, Gaddie R, Stewart CP, Anaerobic activity of the isolated frog's heart, *J Physiol* (1932)**75**:321.

64 Cohen LS, Elliott WC, Klein MD, Gorlin R, Coronary heart disease. Clinical, cinearterio-

graphic and metabolic correlations, *Am J Cardiol* (1966)**17**:153–68.

65 Camici PG, Ferrannini E, Opie LH, Myocardial metabolism in ischaemic heart disease: basic principles and application to imaging by positron emission tomography, *Prog Cardiovasc Dis* (1989)**32**:217–38.

66 Cannon RO, Schenke WH, Quyyumi A, Bonow RO, Epstein SE, Comparison of exercise testing with studies of coronary flow reserve in patients with microvascular angina, *Circulation* (1991)**83**(suppl III):III77–81.

67 Neill WA, Judkins MP, Dhindsa DS, Metcalfe J, Kassebaum DG, Kloster FE, Clinically suspect ischaemic heart disease not corroborated by demonstrable coronary artery disease, *Am J Cardiol* (1972)**29**:171–9.

68 Crake T, Canepa-Anson R, Shapiro L, Poole-Wilson PA, Continuous recording of coronary sinus oxygen saturation during atrial pacing in patients with coronary artery disease or with syndrome X, *Br Heart J* (1988)**59**:31–8.

69 Arbogast R, Bourassa MG, Myocardial function during atrial pacing in patients with angina pectoris and normal coronary angiograms, *Am J Cardiol* (1973)**32**:257–63.

70 Boudoulas H, Cobb TC, Leighton RF, Wilt S, Myocardial lactate production in patients with angina like chest pain and angiographically normal coronary arteries and left ventricle, *Am J Cardiol* (1974)**34**:501–5.

71 Mammohansingh P, Parker JO, Angina pectoris with normal coronary arteriograms: haemodynamic and metabolic response to atrial pacing, *Am Heart J* (1975)**90**:555–61.

72 Jackson G, Atkinson L, Clark M, Crook B, Armstrong P, Oram S, Diagnosis of coronary artery disease by estimation of coronary sinus lactate, *Br Heart J* (1978)**40**:979–83.

73 Sylven C, Beerman B, Jonzon B, Brandt R, Angina piectoris-like pain provoked by intravenous adenosine, *Br Med J* (1986)**293**:227–30.

74 Crea F, Pupita G, Galassi AR, Role of adenosine in pathogenesis of anginal chest pain, *Circulation* (1990)**81**:164–72.

75 Holdright DR, Rosano GMC, Sarrel PM, Poole-Wilson PA, The ST segment—the herald of ischaemia, the siren of misdiagnosis, or syndrome X? *Int J Cardiol* (1992)**35**:293–301.

76 Maseri A, Crea F, Kaski JC, Crake T, Mechanisms of angina pectoris in syndrome X, *J Am Coll Cardiol* (1991)**17**:499–506.

77 Ludman PF, Poole-Wilson PA, Myocardial perfusion in humans: what can we measure? *Br Heart J* (1993)**70**:307–14.

78 Lagerqvist B, Sylven C, Waldenstrom A, Lower threshold for adenosine-induced chest pain in patients with angina and normal coronary angiograms, *Br Heart J* (1992)**68**:282–5.

79 Shapiro LM, Crake T, Poole-Wilson PA, Is altered cardiac sensation responsible for chest pain in patients with normal coronary arteries? Clinical observation during cardiac catheterisation, *Br Med J* (1988)**296**:170–1.

80 Cannon RO, Cattau EL, Yakshe PN et al, Coronary flow reserve, oesophageal motility, and chest pain in patients with angiographically normal coronary arteries, *Am J Med* (1990)**88**:217–22.

81 Richter JE, Barish CF, Castell DO, Abnormal sensory perception in patients with oesophageal chest pain, *Gastroenterology* (1986)**91**:845–52.

82 Bradley LA, Richter JE, Scarinci IC, Haile JM, Schan CA, Psychosocial and psychophysical assessments of patients with unexplained chest pain, *Am J Med* (1992)**92**:5A-65S–73S.

83 Chauhan A, Mullin PA, Thuraisingham SI, Taylor G, Petch MC, Schofield PM, Abnormal cardiac pain perception in syndrome X, *J Am Coll Cardiol* (1994)**24**(2):329–35.

84 Galassi AR, Kaski JC, Pupita G, Vejar M, Crea F, Maseri A, Lack of evidence for alpha-adrenergic receptor-mediated mechanisms in the genesis of ischaemia in syndrome X, *Am J Cardiol* (1989)**64**:264–9.

85 Rosano GMC, Ponikowski P, Adamopoulos S et al, Abnormal autonomic control of the cardiovascular system in syndrome X, *Am J Cardiol* (1994)**73**:1174–9.

86 Marcomichelakis J, Taggart P, Gallivan S et al, Altered catecholamine response to exercise in syndrome X: a possible pathophysiological mechanism, *Br Heart J* (1993)**69**(suppl):P39 (abstr).

87 Rosen SD, Dritsas A, Bourdillon PJ, Camici PG, Analysis of the QT electrocardiographic interval in patients with syndrome X, *Am J Cardiol* (1994)**73**:971–2.

88 Nafziger AN, Herrington DM, Bush TC, Dehydroepiandrosterone and dehydroepiandrosterone sulphate: their relationship to cardiovascular disease, *Epidemiol Rev* (1991)**13**:267–93.

89 Mugge A, Riedel M, Barton M, Kuhn M, Lichtlen PR, Endothelium independent relaxation of human coronary arteries by 17 beta oestradiol in vivo, *Cardiovasc Res* (1995)**29**(11):1939–42.

90 Cheng DY, Gruelter CA, Chronic oestrogen alters responsiveness to angiotensin II and norephinephrine in female rat aorta, *Eur J Pharmacol* (1992)**215**:171–6.

91 Sarrel PM, Lindsay D, Rosano GM, Poole-Wilson PA, Angina and normal coronary arteries in women: gynaecologic findings, *Am J Obstet Gynaecol* (1992)**167**:467–71.

92 Rosano GMC, Kaski JC, Lindsay DC, Collins P, Sarrel PM, Poole-Wilson PA, Syndrome X in women is associated with oestrogen deficiency, *Eur Heart J* (1994)**16**(5):610–14.

93 Papanicolaou MN, Califf RM, Hlatky MA et al, Prognostic implications of angiographically normal and insignificantly narrowed coronary arteries, *Am J Cardiol* (1986)**58**:1181–7.

94 Proudfit WL, Bruschke AV, Jones FM, Clinical course of patients with normal or slightly or moderately abnormal coronary arteriograms: 10 year follow-up of 521 patients, *Circulation* (1980)**62**:712–17.

95 Kemp HG, Kronmal RA, Vliestra RE, Frye RL, Seven year survival of patients with normal or near normal coronary angiograms: a CASS registry study, *J Am Coll Cardiol* (1986)**7**:479–83.

96 Opherk D, Schuler G, Wetterauer K, Manthey J, Schwarz F, Kubler W, Four year follow up study in patients with angina pectoris and normal coronary arteriograms ('syndrome X'), *Circulation* (1989)**80**:1610–16.

97 Romeo F, Rosano GMC, Martuscelli E, Valente A, Long-term follow-up of patients initially diagnosed with syndrome X, *Am J Cardiol* (1993)**71**:669–73.

98 Potts SG, Bass CM, Psychological morbidity in patients with chest pain and normal or near normal coronary arteries: a long term follow up study, *Psychol Med* (1995)**25**(2):339–47.

99 Bugiardini R, Borghi A, Biagetti L, Puddu P, Comparison of verapamil versus propranolol therapy in syndrome X, *Am J Cardiol* (1989)**63**:287–90.

100 Romeo F, Gasspardone A, Ciavolella M, Gioffre P, Reale A, Verapamil versus acebutolol for syndrome X, *Am J Cardiol* (1988)**62**:312–23.

101 Rosano GMC, Sarrel PM, Poole-Wilson PA, Collins P, Symptomatic response to 17 beta oestradiol in women with Syndrome X, *J Am Col Cardiol* (1994)**6A**:702–4.

102 Rosano GMC, Lindsay D, Sarrel PM, Poole-Wilson PA, Collins P, Beneficial effects of oestradiol on exercise induced myocardial ischaemia in women with coronary artery disease, *Lancet* (1993)**342**:133–6.

103 Camici PG, Marraccini P, Gistri R, Salvadori PA, Sorace O, L'Abbate A, Adrenergically mediated coronary vasoconstriction with syndrome X, *Cardiovasc Drugs Ther* (1994)**8**(2):221–6.

104 Galassi AR, Kaski JC, Pupita G, Vejar M, Crea F, Maseri A, Lack of evidence for alpha-adrenergic receptor-mediated mechanisms in the genesis of ischaemia in syndrome X, *Am J Cardiol* (1989)**64**:264–9.

105 Cannon RO, Quyyumi AA, Mincemoyer R et al, Imipramine in patients with chest pain despite normal coronary angiograms, *N Engl J Med* (1994)**330**:1411–7.

10

Aspirin and heart failure: neither safe nor effective?

John GF Cleland

Introduction

The safety of aspirin in heart failure, the most common reason for which is coronary artery disease,[1] has recently been questioned. The SOLVD study,[2,3] of over 7000 patients with cardiac dysfunction with or without heart failure, suggested that the benefit of ACE inhibitors on mortality was lost with concomitant aspirin use.[2] Indeed, participants taking an ACE inhibitor and aspirin had a higher mortality than those taking aspirin and placebo.[2]

At least three possible explanations exist for the lack of apparent benefit from enalapril among those taking aspirin in the SOLVD trial. The lack of benefit from ACE inhibition among those taking aspirin could have occurred by chance. However the interaction was highly significant (p = 0.002). Alternatively, aspirin may genuinely negate the benefits of ACE inhibition, a potentially serious and costly interaction. Finally, it is possible that some of the mortality benefit from ACE inhibition can be achieved by aspirin alone and that ACE inhibitors confer no additional advantage. If this were the case, the less expensive option would be the more attractive one.

Should aspirin be administered to patients with heart failure and coronary disease?

The Aspirin Trialists recently suggested that the benefits of aspirin in patients with coronary artery disease were 'extraordinarily definitely established' based on a meta-analysis including a ISIS-2 study, that lasted only 35 days after acute myocardial infarction.[4,5] ISIS-2 is the only trial of aspirin to show a significant reduction in mortality in patients with ischaemic heart disease.

A meta-analysis of all the postinfarction, long-term antiplatelet agent trials published up to 1994 did suggest a reduction in mortality (about five lives saved per 1000 patients treated per year) with such treatment.[5] The level of statistical significance (p = 0.02) was not substantial considering the size of population studied.

The disparity between ISIS-2 and the other postinfarction trials suggests that the benefits of aspirin on mortality may be confined to the period immediately following myocardial infarction, a view that is supported by several long-term trials.[6–9] It should be stressed that it has not been established whether aspirin needs to be continued long term after myocardial infarction to maintain the initial benefit, or whether a short course gives rise to lasting benefits.

Six substantial trials[8–13] initiated treatment with aspirin more than 1 month after infarction. In these, a slightly higher percentage of patients died in the groups taking aspirin, and even the effect on vascular deaths was small (Table 10.1). Aspirin did appear to reduce nonfatal myocardial infarction, but the effect was not large.

The dispartiy between the effect on nonfatal myocardial infarction and death is worrying.

	PARIS-II[9] mortality (%)		AMIS[10] mortality (%)	
	placebo	aspirin	placebo	aspirin
Total mortality	114/1565 (7.3%)	111/1565 (7.1%)	219/2267 (9.7%)	246/2267 (10.9%)
HF absent	NA	NA	6.9	8.3
HF present	NA	NA	21.2	23.7
NYHA I	5.8	4.9	7.3	8.6
NYHA II	8.9	9.4	14.3	14.3
First infarct	6.2	5.9	8.1	9.2
>1 infarct	13.5	13.5	19.6	19.2
Digoxin: no	6.3	5.5	7.4	9.3
Digoxin: yes	13.7	15.6	21.0	20.8

Table 10.1
Effects of aspirin on total mortality in patients with and without evidence of heart failure after myocardial infarction. NB: NYHA I was attributed to all patients after mycardial infarction who did not exhibit features of heart failure.

The MONICA study indicated that a myocardial infarction under contemporary treatment was still associated with a 50% mortality at 30 days, mostly due to the high prehospital mortality rate.[14] Any agent that really reduces the incidence of myocardial infarction should be associated with at least a trend towards reduction in mortality. The fact that drugs can reduce nonfatal myocardial infarction artefactually is suggested by the CAST study,[15] in which nonfatal myocardial infarction was reduced by 43% in patients given flecainide or encainide (Table 10.2). There was a 238% increase in mortality with encainide and flecainide. The reduction in nonfatal myocardial infarction with these antiarrhythmic agents almost certainly reflected the fact that patients were dying of their infarcts before they reached hospital.

The long-term postinfarction trials also indicate a trend towards increased sudden death with aspirin (Table 10.3). It is possible that aspirin reduces nonfatal myocardial infarction by increasing prehospital deaths. About 25% of all myocardial infarctions are not associated with symptoms recognized as such.[18] Aspirin

	Death	Nonfatal MI
Placebo	3.5%	4.4%
Flecainide/ encainide	8.3%	2.5%
RExR	238% p < 0.0004	RRR 43% p = 0.05

Table 10.2
Rates of mortality and nonfatal MI in the CAST study.[15]

	Placebo	Aspirin
AMIS[10]	2.0%	2.7%
PARIS-I[8]	4.4%	5.6%
PARIS-II[9]	2.0%	2.4%
Swedish Angina[16]	3.0%	2.0%
US Physicians[17]	12 of 227 deaths	22 of 217 deaths

Table 10.3
Rates of sudden death aspirin in long-term postinfarction trials.

is an analgesic and may reduce the recognition of myocardial infarction. This would reduce the number of symptomatic, documented acute recurrent infarctions but increase the risk of sudden death due to failure to deliver adequate treatment, while leaving overall mortality unaffected.

The AMIS trial,[10] the largest aspirin study ever conducted in terms of years of patient exposure, showed a trend towards increased mortality with aspirin in most of the subgroups studied (*see* Table 10.1). Differences in baseline characteristics may have biased the AMIS study against aspirin, but the failure of aspirin to show significant benefit even among groups stratified for risk does not support this conjecture.[10] The PARIS-II[9] trial showed an overall trend towards benefit with aspirin but the trend was in the opposite direction among patients with heart failure or major ventricular dysfunction. The evidence supporting the long-term use of aspirin in patients with coronary disease and well preserved ventricular function was given further credence by data from the Swedish SAPAT study, in which patients with myocardial infraction were excluded.[16] Overall, the data suggest that long-term aspirin may indeed be helpful in patients with well preserved ventricular function but is possibly harmful in high-risk patients with major ventricular damage.

Aspirin is commonly used after coronary artery bypass grafting. It improves early graft patency but there is little evidence that it reduces the rate of infarction and no evidence that it reduces mortality (Table 10.4). Withdrawal studies suggest that continuation of aspirin beyond the first year is unnecessary (Tables 10.4 and 10.5).[22,24] Indeed the Veteran's trial suggested that all the benefit of aspirin on graft patency occurred within the first 9 days.[22] Graft occlusion or clinical events were no more frequent if aspirin was with-

drawn in the later studies.[24] Indeed, there was a trend towards more internal mammary artery graft failures in those randomized to continued aspirin therapy during years 2 and 3 (Table 10.5). This further supports the conjecture that aspirin may be helpful in the setting of acute vascular damage (in other words, myocardial infarction, unstable angina, early post-CAVG) but is of no benefit or possibly harmful at other times.

Although aspirin appears cheap, treating the side effects may not be. Patients taking aspirin are at a four-fold increased risk of gastrointestinal haemorrhage.[26] Aspirin may account for one-third of all major gastrointestinal haemorrhage in subjects over 60 years of age,[27] those most likely to have heart failure. Currently, of every 1000 patients taking aspirin, about two each year will have a major gastrointestinal bleed, leading to death in 10% of cases.[26,27] A considerably greater number of patients will have aspirin-induced dyspepsia. Prophylaxis and treatment of dyspepsia with H_2-antagonists or omeprazole and hospital management of haemorrhage is expensive.

Several of the long-term aspirin trials also noted that patients taking high-dose aspirin had a higher serum urea and uric acid.[9,10] As renal function is often precarious in patients with heart failure, this is of some concern. The effect of lower doses of aspirin on renal function in large long-term trials is unknown.

Evidence from large heart failure trials

A report from the SOLVD trialists suggested that aspirin may have a beneficial effect on mortality, although the administration of aspirin was not randomized (Table 10.6).[2] Careful scrutiny of the data suggests that the lowest mortality in both the treatment and prevention

Study	Number follow-up mean age	Comparisons	Nonfatal MI	Nonfatal stroke	Mortality
Brooks, 1985[19] & Gerschlick, 1988[20] Double-blind	320 78 months 54 years	aspirin 990 mg + dipyridamole **placebo**	n = 7 (angina = 49) n = 2 (angina = 45) ns	none	n = 9 n = 8 ns
Chesebro, 1984[21] Double-blind	407 12 months 56 years	aspirin 975 mg + dipyridamole **placebo**	none	not recorded	n = 5 n = 6 ns
VA Co-operative (Goldman), 1989[22] Double-blind	772 12 months 58 years	aspirin ± Dipyr/sulphinp or sulphinpyrozone **placebo**	6.5% 7.2% ns	n = 5 n = 3 ns	4.2% 3.3% ns
CABADAS, 1993 & 1994 (van der Meer [23])	948 12 months 58 years	aspirin aspirin + dipyridamole oral anticoagulants	8.1% 9.8% 7.8% ns	0.3% 2.0% 1.3% ns	2.6% 1.7% 1.0% ns
VA Co-operative (Goldman),1994[24] Withdrawal	334 24 months 60 years	aspirin continued after 1 year aspirin withdrawal	1.9% 1.7% ns	not recorded	1.9% 2.3%
Pfisterer, 1989[25] Partially blind	249 12 months 56 years	aspirin. 50 mg + dipyridamole phenprocoumon	n = 6 (4 perioperative) n = 8 (all perioperative) ns	n = 0 n = 1 ns	n = 3 n = 8 p > 0.05

Table 10.4
Aspirin and warfarin after CABG. Adapted from Cleland JGF, ed. Asymptomatic coronary artery disease and angina (Science Press: London, 1996).

Study	Interventions year 1		Outcome at 1 year			
Veteran's trial of CABG		death	MI	occlusions	IMA	
	aspirin	4.2%	2.8%	16%	6.0%	
	placebo	3.3%	1.4%	23%	5.4%	
		ns	ns	<0.03	ns	
	Interventions year 2–3		Outcome at year 2–3			
	aspirin continued[22]	death	MI	occlusions	IMA	
		1.9%	1.9%	4.8%	4.3%	
	aspirin withdrawn[24]	2.3%	1.7%	4.2%	2.5%	
		ns	ns	ns	ns	

Table 10.5
Veteran's trial and Veteran's withdrawal trial. IMA = Internal Mammary Artery.

arms of SOLVD was among patients taking placebo and aspirin (groups B1 and D1; Table 10.6). Assertion that aspirin is beneficial, based on these data, would logically lead one to withdraw the ACE inhibitor, at least if it were being given to reduce mortality rather than improve symptoms. This would be flying in the face of the data from properly constructed randomized controlled trials. If one accepts that enalapril is effective, based on a properly randomized comparison, then it is evident that the addition of aspirin is of little or no benefit (compare groups A1 and A2 and C1 and C2 in Table 10.6). However, the possible loss of benefit of ACE inhibition with the addition of aspirin (compare groups C1 with D1; $p = 0.002$) remains worrying. About 12% of patients in the SOLVD prevention and 16% in SOLVD treatment trials were taking warfarin. The higher percentage use in the treatment arm reflects the higher proportion of atrial fibrillation and the likely association between severity of heart failure and use of warfarin. Patients taking warfarin are less likely to receive aspirin. Thus the higher mortality in the aspirin nonusers may reflect the fact that they were a sicker population. Finally, it should be realized that the interaction described is with use of aspirin at baseline. No data are available on changing aspirin use during the study.

	Prevention		Treatment	
	enalapril	placebo	enalapril	placebo
APA+	A1: 12.7%	B1: 12.5%	C1: 34.8%	D1: 30.7%
APA−	A2: 17.4%	B2: 19.3%	C2: 35.2%	D2: 44.3%

Table 10.6
Interaction of enalapril and antiplatelet agents on mortality (%) in SOLVD. APA, antiplatelet agent.

Myocardial infarction and unstable angina were no less common among those taking aspirin in the SOLVD study placebo group,[3] although little significance can be put on this finding as patients at higher risk of infarction may have been more likely to receive aspirin. Aspirin had no effect in either direction on the benefits of ACE inhibitors on recurrent infarction and unstable angina. The V-HeFT studies suggested a reduction in thromboembolic events, not including myocardial infarction, with aspirin but not with warfarin. These were not randomized comparisons.[28]

The clinical trials suggest that stroke is not a very common event in heart failure patients, at least among the age groups incorporated into the landmark studies reported to date.[28–31]

All the postinfarction trials that have reported it show a trend towards less benefit from ACE inhibition among those taking aspirin, with the exception of the SAVE trial (Table 10.7).[32] However, even that showed a trend towards less benefit on a combined morbidity and mortality outcome among those taking captropril and aspirin.[32]

RRR with ACE inhibitors	Aspirin	No aspirin
SAVE (mortality/ morbidity)[32]	24% (20%)	14% (29%)
AIRE[33]	23%	37%
TRACE[34]	18%	22%
CONSENSUS-II[35]	Excess 23%	14% (p<0.05)
GISSI-3[36]	no data	no data
ISIS-4[37]	7.4%	9.5%

Table 10.7
Interaction between ACE inhibitors and aspirin on mortality post-MI.

Theoretical basis for the interaction between aspirin and ACE inhibitors in heart failure

The precise mechanism by which ACE inhibitors exert benefit in heart failure is unknown. Inhibition of angiotensin II formation and reduction in degradation of bradykinin or other peptides are candidates. Bradykinin stimulates increases in nitric oxide and prostaglandins, the latter of which may have vasodilating and platelet antiaggregatory properties. Vasodilating prostaglandins appear to be an important counter-regulatory pathway in patients with heart failure.[38]

The situation becomes even more complex when it is considered that reduction in angiotensin II might mediate the symptomatic and haemodynamic benefits of ACE inhibition but the mortality benefits might be mediated by the bradykinin pathway. Thus surrogate measures of the interaction on haemodynamics and such like may be a poor measure of clinical effect. The response of prostaglandin synthetic pathways to inhibitors may be very different in patients with heart failure compared with patients with coronary artery disease and good ventricular function.

Administration of indomethacin to patients with heart failure results in vasoconstriction, and a fall in cardiac output, renal blood flow and glomerular filtration rate.[38,39] Similar effects have been observed with aspirin.[40] Effects are more prominent among patients with hyponatraemia.[38]

Several studies had addressed the interaction of aspirin and other inhibitors of prostaglandin synthesis on cardiovascular function.[41] Although there is some controversy, many studies have now noted that the beneficial haemodynamic effects of ACE inhibitors are attenuated or abolished by cyclo-oxygenase inhibitors.

Conclusion

The data on the interaction of aspirin and ACE inhibitors are inconclusive. What should the clinician do when faced with the decision to use a combination of an ACE inhibitor and aspirin? It would be a great shame to throw away all the benefits of ACE inhibition because of concomitant therapy of unproved worth with potentially hazardous and costly side effects.

The best solution in the absence of adequate clinical data is to carry out a randomized clinical trial. The Warfarin Aspirin Study of Heart failure (WASH) trial has been set up to compare the effects of no antithrombotic treatment, aspirin and warfarin on mortality in patients with heart failure.[41] The trial should determine whether aspirin exerts significant harm or benefit in a population with heart failure predominantly caused by coronary heart disease.

If I had . . .

Would I take aspirin if I had heart failure due to coronary artery disease? The easy answer to this question is that I would allow someone else to decide. I certainly do not know of any data that indicate clearly whether aspirin is either safe or effective for the treatment of heart failure. If I were forced to decide for myself I think my position would be *primum non nocere*, therefore I would not take aspirin. I would be delighted, as I hope my cardiologist would be, if the decision was taken out of my hands and I were entered into a randomized controlled trial. Indeed, entry into such a trial appears to confer a survival advantage all by itself. Whether this is due to patient psyche or

compliance, improved levels of medical care or just trial selection is not clear, but it is a consistent finding.

The effects of aspirin on myocardial reinfarction, if real, are modest and there is no evidence of improvement in mortality rates during long-term therapy. Aspirin could take away the benefits of ACE inhibition and, on its own, may increase heart failure symptoms and impair renal function. The theoretical benefits of treatment are balanced by the potential for harm, leaving me with little enthusiasm for being on long-term aspirin.

Would I take warfarin instead of aspirin? No adverse interaction between warfarin and ACE inhibitors has been noted. Back in the 1940s warfarin was shown to reduce pulmonary embolism and possibly mortality in randomized controlled trials of in-hospital patients with severe heart failure.[42] Warfarin has been shown to reduce all-cause mortality after myocardial infarction, at least in some trials, although no subset data on heart failure exist.[43] Despite the fact that warfarin tends to be administered to sicker patients, its use was associated with a striking reduction in mortality in the CONSENSUS-1 study and in SOLVD.[42,44] The influence of age on warfarin prescribing, with younger patients having an intrinsically better prognosis, could account for the better outcome with this drug. Although the latter explanation is possible it seems, to me, improbable. Of course warfarin requires regular monitoring and also confers an additional bleeding risk, although the risk is low with appropriate precautions and a regimen that is not too aggressive. Therefore, on balance, if I could not enter a randomized trial and I had no contraindication to warfarin, I would take it.

What if I had a further myocardial infarction or episode of unstable angina while not taking aspirin or warfarin? The evidence in favour of aspirin for 6–12 weeks after infarction is compelling. I would take aspirin for 3 months and then revert to the above decision making process.

I would be prone to other complications of heart failure, in particular atrial fibrillation. Although observational experience in heart failure does not indicate that atrial fibrillation increases the risk of stroke, or that warfarin has any benefit on this outcome, the randomized trials of atrial fibrillation suggest the opposite. Patients with atrial fibrillation and heart failure, in the randomized trials, do not benefit from aspirin but have a dramatically reduced risk of stroke while taking warfarin. I would be disappointed not to receive warfarin if I had atrial fibrillation.

I recognize that my doctor has insufficient evidence to make any firm recommendations about aspirin, warfarin or neither. A randomized controlled trial is in progress. The old adage holds — 'when in doubt, randomize'.

References

1   Garg R, Yusuf S, Epidemiology of congestive heart failure. In: Barnett DB, Pouleur H, Francis GS. Congistive cardiac failure pathophysiology and treatment. (New York, Dekker, 1993).

2   Al-Khadra AS, Salem DN, Rand WM, Udelson JE, Smith JJ, Konstam MA, Effect on anti-platelet agents on survival in patients with left ventricular systolic dysfunction, *Circulation* (1995) **92**:I-665–6.

3   Yusuf S, Pepine CJ, Garces C et al, Effect of enalapril on myocardial infarction and unstable angina in patients with low ejection fractions, *Lancet* (1992)**340**:1173–8.

4   Antiplatelet Trialists' Collaboration, Secondary prevention of vascular disease by prolonged antiplatelet treatment, *Br Med J* (1988)**296**: 320–31.

5   Antiplatelet Trialists' Collaboration, Collaborative overview of randomised trials of antiplatelet therapy. I. Prevention of death, myocardial infarction, and stroke by prolonged antiplatelet therapy in various categories of patients, *Br Med J* (1994)**308**:81–106.

6   Elwood PC, Sweetnam PM, Aspirin and secondary mortality after myocardial infarction, *Lancet* (1979)**ii**:1313–15.

7   Elwood PC, Cochrane AL, Burr ML et al, A randomised controlled trial of acetylsalicylic acid in the secondary prevention of mortality from myocardial infarction, *Br Med J* (1974)**I**: 436–40.

8   The Persantine-Aspirin Reinfarction Study (PARIS) Research Group, Persantine and aspirin in coronary heart disease, *Circulation* (1980)**62**:449–62.

9   Klimt CR et al, Persantine-Aspirin Reinfarction Study. Part II. Secondary coronary prevention with persantine and aspirin, *J Am Coll Cardiol* (1986)**7**:251–69.

10   Aspirin Myocardial Infarction Study Research Group, A randomized, controlled trial of aspirin in persons recovered from myocardial infarction, *JAMA* (1980)**243**:661–8.

11   The Coronary Drug Project Research Group, Aspirin in coronary heart disease, *Circulation* (1980)**62**(**suppl V**):V59–62.

12   Breddin K et al, The German-Austrian Aspirin Trial: a comparison of acetylsalicylic acid, placebo and phenprocoumon in secondary prevention of myocardial infarction, *Circulation* (1980)**62**(**suppl V**):V63–71.

13   Vogel G, Fischer C, Huyke R, Prevention of reinfarction with acetylsalicylic acid. In: Nreddin K, Loew D, Ueberla K, Dorndorf W, Marx R, eds. *Prophylaxis of venous, peripheral, cardiac and cerebral vascular diseases with acetylsalicylic acid* (Stuttgart: Schattauer Verlag, 1981) 123–8.

14   Tunstall-Pedoe H, Kuulasmaa K, Amouyel P, Arveiler D, Rajakangas A-M, Pajak A, Myocardial infarction and coronary deaths in the World Health Organization MONICA project: registration procedures, event rates, and case-fatality rates in 38 populations from 21 countries in four continents, *Circulation* (1994)**90**:583–612.

15   Echt DS, Liebson PR, Mitchell LB et al, Mortality and morbidity in patients receiving encainide, flecainide, or placebo—the Cardiac Arrhythmia Suppression Trial, *New Engl J Med* (1991)**324**:781–8.

16   Jull-Moller S, Edvardsson N, Jahnmatz B, Rosen A, Sorensen S, Omblus R, Double-blind trial of aspirin in primary prevention of myocardial infarction in patients with stable chronic angina pectoris, *Lancet* (1992)**340**:1421–5.

17   Monson JE et al, Aspirin in the primary prevention of angina pectoris in a randomized trial of United States physicians, *Am J Med* (1990)**89**: 772–6.

18   Kannel WB, Abbott RD, Incidence and prognosis of unrecognised myocardial infarction: an update on the Framingham Study, *N Engl J Med* (1984)**311**:1144–7.

19   Brooks N et al, Randomised placebo controlled trial of aspirin and dipyridamole in

the prevention of coronary vein graft occlusion, *Br Heart J* (1985)**53**:201–7.

20   Gerschlick AH et al, Long term clinical outcome of coronary surgery and assessment of the benefit obtained with postoperative aspirin and dipyridamole, *Br Heart J* (1988)**60**:111–16.

21   Chesebro JH et al, Effect of dipyridamole and aspirin on late vein-graft patency after coronary bypass operations, *N Engl J Med* (1984)**310**:209–14.

22   Goldman S, Copeland J, Mortiz T et al, Improvement in early saphenous graft potency after coronary artery bypass surgery with antiplatelet therapy: results of a Veteran's Administration Cooperative Study, *Circulation* (1988)**77**:1324–32.

23   van der Meer J et al, Prevention of one-year vein-graft occlusion after aortocoronary-bypass surgery: a comparison of low-dose aspirin, low-dose aspirin plus dipyridamole, and oral anticoagulants, *Lancet* (1993)**342**:257–64.

24   Goldman S, Copeland J, Moritz T et al, Long-term graft patency (3 years) after coronary artery surgery: effects of aspirin. Results of a VA cooperative study, *Circulation* (1994)**89**:1138–43.

25   Pfisterer M et al, Trial of low-dose aspirin plus dipyridamole versus anticoagulants for prevention of aortocoronary vein graft occlusion, *Lancet* (1989)**ii**:1–7.

26   Sze PC, Reitman D, Pincus MM, Sacks HS, Chalmers TC, Antiplatelet agents in the secondary prevention of stroke: meta-analysis of the randomized control trials, *Stroke* (1988)**19**:436–42.

27   Faulkner G, Prichard P, Somerville K, Langman MJS, Aspirin and bleeding peptic ulcers in the elderly, *Br Med J* (1988)**297**:1311–13.

28   Dunkman WB, Johnson GR, Carson PE, Bhat G, Farrell L, Cohn JN, Incidence of thromboembolic events in congestive heart failure, *Circulation* (1993)**87**(suppl VI):VI94–101.

29   Cohn JN, Benedict CR, LeJemtel TH et al, Risk of thromboembolism in left ventricular dysfunction: SOLVD, *Circulation* (1992)**86**:(suppl I):I–252 (abstr).

30   Katz SD, Marantz PR, Biasucci L et al, Low incidence of stroke in ambulatory patients with heart failure: a prospective study, *Am Heart J* (1993)**126**:141–6.

31   Middlekauff HR, Stevenson WG, Stevenson LW, Prognostic significance of atrial fibrillation in advanced heart failure—a study of 390 patients, *Circulation* (1991)**84**:40–8.

32   Pfeffer MA, Braunwald E, Moye LA et al, Effect of captopril on mortality and morbidity in patients with left ventricular dysfunction after myocardial infarction, *N Engl J Med* (1992)**327**:669–77.

33   Ball SG, Hall AS, Mackintosh AF et al, Effect of ramipril and morbidity of survivors of acute myocardial infarction with clinical evidence of heart failure. *Lancet* (1993)**342**:821–8.

34   Kober L, Torp Pedersen C, Carlsen JE et al, A clinical trial of the angiotensin-converting-enzyme inhibitor trandolapril in patients with left ventricular dysfunction after myocardial infarction, *New Engl J Med* (1995)**333**:1670–6.

35   Nguyen KN, Aursnes I, Kjekshus J, Interaction between enalapril and aspirin on mortality after acute myocardial infarction: Subgroup analysis of the cooperative new scandinavian enalapril survival study II (CONSENSUS II). *Am J Cardiol* (1997)**79**:115–19.

36   De Vita C, Fazzini PF, Geraci E et al, GISSI-3: Effects of lisinopril and transdermal glyceryl binitrate singly and together on 6-week mortality and ventricular function after acute myocardial infarction. *Lancet* (1994)**343**:1115–22.

37   Collins R, Peto R, Flather M et al, A randomised factorial trial assessing early oral captopril, oral mononitrate, and intravenous magnesium sulphate in 58050 patients with suspected acute myocardial infarction, *Lancet* (1995)**345**:669–85.

38   Dzau VJ, Packer M, Lilly LS et al, Prostaglandins in severe congestive heart failure. Relation to activation of the renin-angiotensin system and hyponatremia, *N Engl J Med* (1984)**310**:347–52.

39   Gottlieb SS, Robinson S, Krichten CM, Fisher ML, Renal response to indomethacin in congestive heart failure secondary to ischemic or idiopathic dilated cardiomyopathy, *Am J Cardiol* (1992)**70**:890–3.

40   Riegger GAJ, Kahles HW, Elsner D, Kromer EP, Kochsiek K, Effects of acetylsalicylic acid

on renal function in patients with chronic heart failure, *Am J Med* (1991)**90**:571–5.

41   Cleland JGF, Bulpitt CJ, Falk RH et al, Is aspirin safe for patients with heart failure? *Br Heart J* (1995)**74**:215–19.

42   Cleland JGF, *Anti-coagulants and anti-platelet agents in heart failure* (Edinburgh: Churchill-Livingstone, 1996).

43   Cleland JGF, McMurray J, Ray S, *Prevention strategies after myocardial infarction* (London: Science Press, 1994) 1–92.

44   Al-Khadra AS, Salem DN, Rand WM, Udelson JE, Smith JJ, Konstam MA, Effect of warfarin anti-coagulation on survival in patients with left ventricular systolic dysfunction, *J Am Coll Cardiol* (1996)**27**(suppl A):140A.

11

Emotion, stress and the heart

Leisa J Freeman

Introduction

I am sure that we all follow the advice of Xenophanes — 'all of him sees, all of him listens'. Such ideals, however, often get lost when specialist attention is focused on a problem which is regarded as principally mechanical. It is easier to concentrate on defined areas of practice and while appreciating that a wider picture is often involved, cardiologists feel that other more variable and nebulous factors are not our concern. Nevertheless, the ways in which a patient perceives and responds to his or her surroundings are vitally important and no-one in cardiology will forget that classical description of angina pectoris, by John Hunter, exacerbated by a stressful board meeting at St George's Hospital.[1] The difficulty is that the effects of emotion and stress on the heart are viewed as vague and subjective and full of terminology that disenchants; furthermore, not everyone reacts in the same predictable fashion to a stressor.[2] Sir William Osler's famous statement comes to mind, that it is often more important to know what person has the disease than what disease the person has. These are difficult areas, but merit considerable attention for three reasons. First, the advent of new technology and methodology has produced increasing evidence to implicate psychosocial conflict, emotions and behavioural patterns in the pathogenesis and exacerbation of coronary artery disease, sudden death, cardiac arrhythmias and systemic hypertension. Second, multi-variate analysis has demonstrated that the standard risk factors are found in less than half of those who succumb to ischaemic heart disease.[3,4] Third, there are many patients whose symptoms are not associated with anatomical lesions and in whom failure to recognize the contribution of psychological factors to the aetiology of their complaints can lead to iatrogenic disease, chronic disability, the 'thick folder syndrome' and sometimes actual structural disease.

Definitions and methodologies

Stress is a word that produces considerable confusion, as it means stimulus or response to some, and interaction or complex combination of conditions to others. It is best to appreciate that the environment is a stressor requiring an adaptive response, the measured physiological response as strain, and stress as the psychophysiological degree of response observed during an interaction between the subject and the environment. The circulation is one of the response systems to stressors, which is mediated or modulated by the nervous system, partly on the basis of prior experience and is thus dependent on the context in which it occurs. Information concerning the effect of psychological stress is derived essentially from four broad areas: animal studies, laboratory mental stress testing, ongoing observational research (in health and disease states) and epidemiological studies. Since there are clearly substantial differences in host vulnerabilities to stressors, investigators have tried deliberately to impose a stressor so that they can scrutinize the physiological consequences during the anticipation of, administration of, and recovery from psychologically stressful stimuli.

Animal studies

Animal studies are highly valued because they lend themselves to tight experimental control of confounders such as diet and genetic background, as well as allowing direct inspection of the coronary arteries.[5,6]

Laboratory mental stress testing

Mental stress testing in the laboratory has been increasingly utilized as it allows precise control over stressors and assessment of any derangement of cardiovascular function in response to a stimulus and the particular qualities of the situation that provoke potentially dangerous reactions. Indeed, more complicated physiological measurements, such as positron emission tomography,[7] can also be made which are not possible with ambulatory monitoring. It has also been helpful in delineating cause and effect relationships that have been suggested from epidemiological research.[8,9] Steptoe and Vogele have distinguished five general categories of mental stress tests for use in the laboratory.[10] These are as follows:

- problem-solving tasks (for example mental arithmetic and quizzes);
- information-processing tasks (for example word identification, memory and vigilance);
- psychomotor tasks, with emphasis on accurate and complex behavioural responses (for example computer and video games);

- affective conditions, which include situations designed to elicit distress or some other emotional response from participants (for example stressful interviews, speech tasks). These situations often provoke larger cardiovascular reactions than problem-solving tasks but individuals vary in the type of material they find stressful and thus standardization can be a problem;
- aversive or painful conditions (for example cold pressor test).

Exaggerated cardiovascular reactions often occur in these tests that are out of all proportion to the energy requirement of the situation and must therefore be products of centrally generated autonomic or neuroendocrine stimulation. This is helpful in avoiding criticism of study design. Reliability, standardization, validity and consistency are now demanded of these stressors, providing better credibility for the responses they provoke.

Observational studies

Observational studies of people undergoing stressful experiences[11] with ambulatory monitoring of ST segment by Holter tape or blood pressure measurement have complemented studies of links between disease occurrence (for example myocardial infarction) and psychological state influenced by factors such as life events,[12] or job strain.[8] The MILIS (Multicenter Investigation of Limitation of Infarct Size) investigators found that emotion was more common than physical activity as a trigger for myocardial infarction.[13,14] Indeed the Northridge earthquake (Los Angeles, 1994) provoked a five-fold increase in sudden cardiac death, independent of physical exertion;[15] nonfatal myocardial infarction also increased after the earthquake, as did ventricular arrhythmias in patients with implantable defibrillators.

Epidemiological studies

Epidemiological studies that originally concentrated on the traditional risk factors (serum cholesterol, smoking and hypertension — especially in the presence of a strong family history) have been noteworthy by the fact that they account for less than 50% of the variance associated with coronary heart disease.[16–18] Indeed, puzzling studies were emerging that immigrants from the Indian subcontinent studied in the London boroughs of Brent and Harrow had a very high mortality and morbidity from coronary heart disease. This was despite the fact that, compared with whites, Asians consumed less saturated fat and cholesterol and more polyunsaturated fat and vegetable fibre. Their cholesterol and HDL levels were similar to those of a comparable white group and smoking rates were lower.[19] Findings such as these have stimulated the search to assess the contribution of psychological risk factors in cardiovascular disorders.

Psychosocial risk factors

Social isolation

Early studies showed that coronary heart disease rates were three-times higher among men who had experienced several lifetime job changes and geographic moves than among men with no such changes. The rates were four-times higher among men reared on farms who later moved to the city to take white-collar jobs compared with men who either stayed on the farm or took blue-collar jobs in the city.[20] In these studies, the findings were not attributable to differences in diet, smoking habits, physical activity, obesity, blood pressure, age or familial longevity. The difficulty then is to answer the question of whether the risk increases because of the mobility, because of the situation to which the person moves, or because of the characteristics predisposing certain persons to become mobile. Social isolation is found to be particularly important and is relevant when well established social support structures are lost after moving.[21] A prospective study has shown that social isolation, independent of other variables, was significantly associated with a high risk of subsequent myocardial infarction and/or cardiac death,[22] and provision of social support has improved the prognosis in coronary artery disease.[23] It is also seen as an important precursor of essential hypertension.[24]

Control and job strain

Work situations involving high demand but low control appear to have a significant influence on the development of coronary heart disease and hypertension,[25] which is in contrast to those for whom a high demand is associated with a high degree of control.[26] It has been difficult to disentangle the effects of control from those of particular types of work, or to determine whether selection factors such as individual preferences for different occupations (rather than the occupations themselves) are accountable. Thus, within many types of medical practice prejudged 'high-stress' areas of anaesthesiology and general practice have a higher coronary prevalence rate (11.9%) when compared with 'low-stress' areas of pathology and dermatology (3.2%). Nevertheless, laboratory experimental studies have compared the cardiovascular reactions associated with self- and externally paced work in randomized cohorts to assess the differences between controllable and uncontrollable conditions and support the importance of control.[9]

Animal studies have given further insight into the concept of high demand/low control. Instead of examining the effects of a single massive stressful event, monkeys were examined to judge the effect of chronic repeated social disruption — like working in a department with rapid changes of deans, departmental chairmen, hospital administrators, and so on. It was the first study to show that chronic social disruption impairs endothelium-dependent vascular responses of coronary arteries and even a low-cholesterol diet did not diminish the effect of this social disruption.[27] It was previously shown, by the same group, that chronic stress elevates the heart rate and exacerbates coronary artery atherosclerosis in monkeys.[28] In one group of young men who had survived myocardial infarction and returned to the same job situation, job strain was an independent predictor for subsequent coronary events,[29] although others have failed to confirm this.[30]

A worksite study of occupational stress has indicated that people in high-stress jobs have increased blood pressure throughout the day and night, which is a least consistent with a behaviourally mediated resetting of the tonic blood pressure level.[31] Job strain (lack of control) has been shown to be significantly related to hypertension with an estimated odds ratio of 3.1 (after controlling for all other variables).[32] This hypertension is sustained throughout day and night and is most marked in men who drink alcohol.[33] Alcohol does not have a significant effect on blood pressure at work in low-strain jobs.[34] Importantly, the left ventricular mass index (determined echocardiographically) is also found to be greater in those with job strain.[32]

Loss of 'wellbeing' (life-event stress)

There are difficulties with the concept that life-event stressors contribute to subsequent development of cardiovascular disorders, especially since much of this huge body of research is retrospective and those who report more stressful life events may subsequently experience a higher prevalence of these conditions as a function of more illness-reporting behaviour rather than a true difference in incidence rates. One prospective study questioned nearly 7000 middle-aged men (47–55 years) between 1970 and 1973 about their perceived stress levels (graded 1–6). After a mean follow-up of 11.8 years it found that 6% with a low level of stress (level 1–4) had sustained a nonfatal myocardial infarction or had died from coronary artery disease. The corresponding figure was 10% among those with high stress levels (level 5 and 6); the odds ratio was 1.5 after controlling for age and other risk factors.[35] The classic study of bereavement is very conclusive — 4486 widowers, aged 55 years and older were followed for 9 years after the death of their wives. In first 6 months of bereavement 213 widowers died, a rate 40% higher than would be expected for married men of the same age; in 67% of cases this was due to coronary artery disease.[36]

The consensus appears to suggest that life changes that deprive individuals of important sources of emotional security, self-esteem or a sense of identity (loss of wellbeing) are likely to be followed by a higher than normal risk of cardiovascular disease and cardiac death. A controlled trial of stress monitoring and subsequent intervention following myocardial infarction (in the survivors at 1 month) demonstrated a 47% decline in mortality over the first year in the psychologically treated group when compared with the control (no intervention) group.[37]

Psychological characteristics

Various psychological characteristics appear to increase cardiac vulnerability to stress.[38] A new British Heart Foundation project, which will include 1300 men and women aged 60–80 years in Edinburgh, has just commenced. This will investigate the psychological characteristics described below.

Angry and hostile behaviour

The type A behaviour pattern was originally described by Rosenman and Friedman in the 1950s and has been considered an independent risk factor in coronary artery disease of the same order of magnitude as blood pressure, serum cholesterol and smoking.[39] The Framingham study confirmed type A behaviour as an independent risk factor, but only for non-manual (white-collar) workers.[40] Rosenman has always maintained that its prevalence is increased by urbanization and by technological progress (and hence a move to nonmanual labour), which presents uniquely new challenges that were not experienced by previous generations and simpler societies.[41] The type A behaviour pattern has been a double-edged sword for the proponents of psychosocial risk factors in cardiovascular disease, as few forget the dynamic and competitive description of the person;[42] indeed, it has become common in daily usage, and is often voiced in an admiring tone. On the positive side, it has highlighted and popularized the concept that behaviour and personality are relevant in coronary artery disease, but the move away from the structured interview, specifically designed and validated to assess the behaviour complex, to short-hand questionnaires has meant that its role as an independent risk factor has lost ground. This is true especially in the UK after the British Regional Heart Study's failure to show a relationship between high scores on the Bortner Questionnaire and ischaemic heart disease.[43]

Yet the collective sigh of relief that perhaps it applied only to those on the other side of the Atlantic has been cut short, since the very use of questionnaires has allowed a better delineation of some of the relevant components of the type

A behaviour pattern — namely hostility and anger (often covert), which are enhanced when a situation threatens the individual with a perceived loss of control over his milieu — which brings us back to point made in the last section.[44] It does seem that special methods are needed to detect type A behaviour, since just affirming that one is more angry or hostile is not sensitive. In a recent study of asymptomatic air crew, self-reported hostility could not differentiate between cases with and without angiographically documented coronary artery disease, whereas hostility detected by a structured interview was discriminative.[45] Specific questionnaires that are widely used and validated are the Cook Medley Hostility scale[46] and the Anger Expression scale.[47] The methodologies and problems are well reviewed in *Anger, hostility and the heart*, published in 1994.[48]

Recalling a recent incident that provoked real anger has been used during cardiac catherization; vasoconstriction in narrowed coronary arteries was observed in association with high levels of anger, but there was no significant diameter change in non-narrowed coronary arteries.[49] Indeed, in some animal studies, the response to aggression is so intense that it impedes flow completely in the affected vessel.[50] Transient impairment of left ventricular function, as assessed noninvasively by radionuclide ventriculography, has also been seen following mental stress tests in a group of patients who had high anger and hostility characteristics as assessed by questionnaire and by the structured interview. Interestingly, LV dysfunction was also seen in the same group (and in three earlier nonresponders) following the interview![51] Indeed, the potency of anger and its recall is appreciated by the demonstration that more patients with documented coronary artery disease had a reduction in left ventricular ejection fraction (as assessed by MUGA scans) in response to anger than to exercise or mental arithmetic.[52]

The type B behaviour pattern is not merely the absence of type A response. Rather, it is a different set of coping behaviours and, of course, such individuals do also have coronary artery disease. Ambulatory ST Holter monitoring has shown that although type A and B patients may have similar daily ischaemic loads, type A subjects reported more episodes of ischaemia as painful as compared with type B individuals, in whom three-quarters of the episodes were asymptomatic.[53] Indeed, type B patients may be more likely to become depressed and this combination has been found to be associated with increased clinical events following myocardial infarction, even after controlling for other variables.[54]

Whilst there has been no consistent association between the type A personality and hypertension, suppressed anger and resentment are frequently detected. The hypertensive individual is noted to manifest a desire to please and a wish to be liked but while outwardly calm, the internal stance is that of unexpressed anger, tension, suspicion and hostility. It is postulated that the effect is mediated by the autonomic system, possibly in conjunction with high renin levels.[55]

Phobic anxiety

People with phobic anxiety feel anxious in specific situations and if these situations are avoided, they do not feel anxious. A prospective study of 1457 men at a North London hospital has shown that phobic anxiety (as detected by the Crown-Crisp questionnaire which asks about common phobias such as fear of enclosed spaces, going out alone, illness, heights and crowds) was strongly related to subsequent major ischaemic heart disease but was not associated with deaths from other causes. This was particularly clear in the case of fatal events and was independent of the contribution of other variables to the incidence of ischaemic heart disease. Furthermore, the study showed specifically that existing ischaemic heart disease did not in itself lead to heightened phobic anxiety. Their postulated mechanisms included hyperventilation and an exaggerated response of cortisol, adrenaline and noradrenaline to myocardial infarction in such individuals. Specifically, the increased risk could not be explained by an association with cholesterol concentration, measured haemostatic variables or blood pressure.[56] A score of 4 or more on the Crown-Crisp questionnaire (the same cut-off point as that used in the previous study) was also used in 33 999 American men to show that the age-adjusted relative risk of fatal coronary heart disease was 3.01 (95% confidence interval 1.3–6.9) and 6.08 (95% confidence interval 2.35–15.73) when confined to sudden death.[57] Animal studies have also shown that fear can produce substantial increases in coronary vascular resistance and markedly elevated levels of adrenaline and noradrenaline.[58,59]

Sudden cardiac death

The cohort studies described above[56,57] demonstrate the strong association between anxiety and fatal coronary heart disease, especially sudden cardiac death. Until now, anecdotal and retrospective assessments of exposure by proxy respondents have been utilized to infer an association between emotional stress and sudden cardiac death[60,61] and various mechanisms have been postulated.

Sudden death may occur in individuals without heart disease, but those with coronary heart disease are at greater risk. A variety of evidence suggests that activation of strong emotion often triggers sudden death, the pathophysiological mechanism of which is usually ventricular fibrillation.[62] The mechanism of tachyarrhythmias provoked by behavioural stress is still debated — it may be either a direct effect of catecholamines on the excitable properties of myocardium or an alteration in myocardial perfusion.[63] Animal studies have shown that while psychological stress produced a coronary vasoconstrictive effect in normal hearts, arrhythmias were not produced (even in the presence of coronary stenosis), but when there was a transient occlusion, there was a greater vulnerability to ventricular fibrillation. Moreover, this vulnerability is not related to the degree of ischaemia but rather to the presence of concomitant psychological stress.[64]

In a series of clinical and electrophysiological studies, Lown and colleagues identified precursors to fatal ventricular arrhythmia and sudden death, including intense psychologic stresses burdening daily life and recent important acute stressors that triggered arrhythmias.[65,66] Ventricular ectopy (>30 beats/min) in patients without previous infarction was found to be associated with high scores of anxiety, depression and social alienation,[67] but no relationship could be found in postinfarction patients.[68] On the other hand, diminished heart rate variability associated with behavioural factors was associated with increased sudden death. Diminished heart rate variability has been found in patients who are anxious and have panic disorders[69] and has been identified as a marker for sudden cardiac death in postinfarction patients,[70] as well as apparently normal individuals.[71,72] Heart rate variability is taken to provide a noninvasive estimate of autonomic tone to the heart[73] and markedly diminished variability is a significant predictor of mortality and implies reduced vagal tone as the mechanism for sudden cardiac death.

The occurrence of syncope or cardiac arrest precipitated by emotional stress (fear, anger, exercise fraught with emotions, awakening with a loud noise, etc.) in an otherwise healthy individual with a prolonged QT interval is a frequent and characteristic clinical presentation. It has been proposed as the classic example of sympathetic imbalance which lowers the arrhythmogenic threshold. In cats, life-threatening arrhythmias have been induced during a highly emotional situation, when the right stellate ganglion has been ablated, resulting in prolonged QT interval, and allowing increased left cardiac sympathetic activity, which is known to trigger malignant arrhythmias.[74] The role of reduced parasympathetic activity and increased sympathetic activity in coronary artery disease has been strongly supported[75–77] but some doubts have been expressed recently.[78]

Depression

Depression may increase cardiac vulnerability to stress and has been found to be an independent predictor of cardiac events 1 year after a diagnosis of coronary artery disease.[79,80] In the CAPS study, the combination of depression and diminished heart rate variability were associated with increased clinical events[54] and, as discussed above, may represent pathological alterations in cardiac autonomic control. Indeed, a five-fold higher mortality rate among depressed myocardial infarction survivors[81] should signal a turning point in the general perception of the role of psychosocial factors in the prognosis of coronary heart disease. Too often somatic complaints of fatigue, lethargy, insomnia and loss of appetite in patients postinfarction are ascribed only to their physical condition or medication and the possibility of depression is not considered.

Nixon should be credited with being one of the first to give a detailed description of exhaustion associated with cardiovascular conditions. Furthermore, he considered that there were two main emotional responses to exhaustion — one being rage and frustration, and the other insecurity with despair and hopelessness.[82,83] Nixon also pointed out that sleep disturbance, a well-known element of depression, was part of this pattern of exhaustion and other studies have found such sleep disturbances to be predictive of both future angina pectoris and myocardial infarction.[84,85] Cognitive therapies have shown good results as a clinical intervention for depression.[86] Pharmacological approaches also deserve serious consideration as potential interventions for psychosocial factors in coronary artery disease. The selective serotonin reuptake inhibitors are not only effective antidepressants but also have the potential to decrease sympathetic nervous system activation, aid in smoking cessation, decrease appetite, deplete platelet serotonin stores and decrease anger and aggression.[87]

Nonorganic disease

Thirty-two per cent of patients seen in a Manchester cardiology clinic recently were considered not to have organic heart disease and the physicians saw their principal task to be exclusion of organic disease rather than positive management for the problem.[88] While the knowledge that organic disease is not present may seem adequate to the physician, some patients are not reassured by negative investigations and it is they who have been found to have recognizable anxiety and depression — 33% of the Manchester patients were in this category, which is consistent with other studies.[89,90] Furthermore, follow-up of this group has shown that they continued to experience their somatic symptoms, as well as the symptoms of anxiety and depression, and the medical input was as great as for patients with organic disease.[91] Hospital outpatient clinics where, with the best will in the world, there is usually some time spent waiting, provide an ideal opportunity for screening patients by questionnaire for anxiety and depression. The recent joint report

of the Royal College of Physicians and Royal College of Psychiatrists[92] suggests that in those patients so identified, active treatment should be initiated by the hospital physician and continued by the GP, and be specifically directed at the anxiety, depression and fears of illness.[93] This, I suggest, should be irrespective of the presence of an underlying organic problem.

Gender differences

Depression and phobic anxiety are strongly associated with angina pectoris in women as well as in men, but in women passive dependency and suppressed hostility (not discussing anger) have been found to be related specifically to risk of cardiovascular disease and hypertension.[94] Death of a close and significant relative or divorce (but not other types of life-event changes) have been found to be associated with sudden cardiac death in women.[95]

Specific mental stress studies: myocardial ischaemia

Laboratory testing

The anecdotal evidence that mental stress and emotion produce angina has been well substantiated by laboratory testing and the prevalence of the ischaemic responses varies with the sensitivity of the assessment technique from about 20% using ST segment depression[96] to 70% with positron emission tomography of myocardial hypoperfusion.[7] Furthermore, mental stress-induced ischaemia resembles daily-life ischaemia,[97-99] in that both are often asymptomatic and occur at a lower heart rate and blood pressure than exercise-induced ischaemia. Indeed it has been shown recently that at a fixed level of myocardial oxygen demand, mental stress was associated with myocardial ischaemia, whereas the exercise response was nonischaemic.[100] This is exciting since the within-subject comparison study design means that the severity of fixed coronary disease and the myocardial oxygen demand is unchanged between the two situations and the only variable factor is a dynamic reduction in coronary blood flow in response to mental stress.

Such a dynamic component has been suggested for some time[101,102] and indeed Yeung et al.[103] reported direct angiographic visualization of coronary vasoconstriction during mental stress (anger), but only at sites of atherosclerotic plaques. In dogs increased vasomotor tone, mediated via alpha-adrenergic (noradrenaline transmitters) induces vasoconstriction in response to aggression.[104] This vasoconstriction persists well after heart rate and arterial blood pressure have recovered and the administration of an alpha blocker can avert this.[50,105] Beta blockers may help protect against mental stress-induced ischaemia,[100,106] perhaps by increasing the coronary reserve.[107]

Ambulatory monitoring, silent ischaemia, LV function

If laboratory stress-induced myocardial ischaemia, like the asymptomatic ST segment depression observed during Holter monitoring, is often not associated with pain, how relevant is it? A within-subject study (ST Holter monitoring) assessed during a stressful period compared with a nonstressful period found the episodes of asymptomatic ischaemia significantly higher during the stressor (and this was associated with higher noradrenaline and cortisol excretion) but the symptomatic ischaemic events were not significantly different (Figures 11.1 and 11.2).[11] Myocardial ischaemia in response to laboratory-induced mental stress also predicts episodes during daily life.[108,109] In an overview of recent studies of asymptomatic ischaemia in daily life, it is found to be an inde-

pendent predictor of an adverse outcome[110] — although if there is a reasonable exercise tolerance, *predominantly* asymptomatic ischaemia does not identify patients at subsequent risk of acute myocardial infarction or sudden death. Nevertheless, mental stress in postinfarction patients without heart failure produces impaired left ventricular function in the presence of asymptomatic ST depression;[111,112] this is independent of heart rate and blood pressure changes, cannot be predicted from exercise-induced changes, can last at least 10 minutes and is stable over long time periods.[113] Moreover, in patients with idiopathic dilated cardiomyopathy and heart failure, mental stress has been shown to increase left ventricular chamber stiffness and elevate left ventricular filling pressure.[114] In a retrospective study, emotionally deleterious events were found to precipitate or worsen heart failure in 49% of patients admitted to hospital.[115]

Prospect for risk stratification?
A small prospective study has assessed patients (with documented coronary artery disease) who developed transient left ventricular dysfunction in response to mental arithmetic (15 out of 30) and followed them up for 2 years. There were significantly more cardiac events in those who had electrographically silent left ventricular dysfunction in response to mental stress (9 out of 15) compared with those who did not (3 out of 15) — and this may be a good marker of abnormal cardiovascular reactivity to emotional and psychological stimuli with coronary artery disease and be useful for risk stratification.[116] It has been nicely shown that beta-endorphin levels are correlated with thermally measured pain thresholds in patients with coronary artery disease both at rest and after psychological stress (public speaking). Indeed stress very significantly raised the beta-endorphin level and this may be an explanation for the

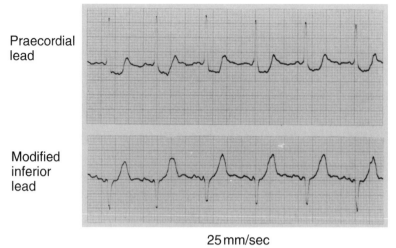

25 mm/sec

Diary entry: "9.00pm. Police called a few minutes ago to tell me
that my cousin's wife died in a fire. Feel very upset."

Figure 11.1
Diary entry of emotional upset and ST segment depression seen on Holter monitoring. No anginal symptoms were noted.

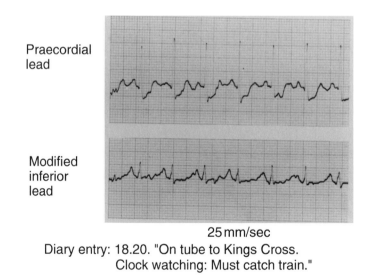

25 mm/sec

Diary entry: 18.20. "On tube to Kings Cross.
Clock watching: Must catch train."

Figure 11.2
The patient had attended the gym at 15.30, when his heart rate had risen to 130 bpm, but no ST segment depression was seen on Holter monitoring. This is in contrast to the elevation seen when the patient experienced emotional stress.

predominance of silent ischaemia during psychological stress in patients with coronary artery disease.[117]

Specific mental stress studies: hypertension

The role of stress in the development of essential hypertension has been hotly debated for many years but hurry, worry and anger have long been suggested to be important precursors for the development of hypertension. Acute exposure to such stressors, either in the laboratory or in normal daily life, can cause a transient elevation in blood pressure, but it has been difficult to demonstrate a sustained effect. Subjects with increased cardiovascular reactivity to acute stress may be at increased risk of developing hypertension and it is postulated that the repeated surges of blood pressure arising from the exposure to stress can cause structural changes in arterial walls and a sustained increase in vascular resistance.[118,119] While many support this hypothesis, it is not universally accepted and is probably not a useful clinical index of the course of future blood pressure.[120] The gold standard in hypertension is, increasingly, the use of continuous monitoring, which does not rely on intermittent blood pressure recordings with all the problems of interobserver variability and 'white coat' hypertension. Thus, two studies using intra-arterial monitoring have reported significant correlation between blood pressure variability during working hours and reactions to mental stress tests.[121,122] Behaviourally mediated resetting of the blood pressure level (elevated blood pressure both day and night — an accepted criterion for the diagnosis of hypertension) has already been discussed in response to occupational stress.[31]

Proposed mechanisms

Neuroendocrine mechanisms

There is a substantial body of research documenting the neuroendocrine responses to psychological stress.[123–126] The adrenocortical system responds to situations that lead to a high degree of uncertainty — associated with feelings of defeat, despair, loss and isolation. The sympatho-adrenal medullary system responds to situations that require attention and vigilance (fight–flight reaction). Clearly there is important interaction between the two axes. For example, cortisol appears to sensitize the heart to the toxicity of noradrenaline, either by increasing its extraneuronal uptake or by interfering with its subsequent degradation by catecho-O-methyl transferase; it is elicited by emotional stress and not by exercise.[127]

The combination of emotional stress, elevated neuroendocrine levels and coronary heart disease has now been documented with hypercoagulability (for example increased thromboxane B2),[128] elevated fibrinogen levels,[129] increased platelet aggregation,[130] accelerated atherosclerosis and high levels of free fatty acid,[131,132] and with myocardial ischaemia.[11]

Mental stress activates sympathetic nerves in the heart and other innervated organs, resulting in an increased cardiac and total body noradrenaline secretion, and increases myocardial oxygen requirements. The usual response of the coronary microcirculation to the increased myocardial oxygen demands of mental stress is vasodilatation, as manifested by a 26% reduction in coronary vascular resistance in patients with normal coronary arteries. In contrast, patients with early atherosclerosis of the left anterior descending coronary artery do not have vasodilatation in response to mental stress, despite increases in myocardial oxygen demand similar to those in patients with normal coronary arteries. The absence of vasodilatation is considered to be due to limitation of microvascular dilatation, since mental stress causes only minimal reductions in epicardial luminal diameter (average 12%).[133] Patients with atherosclerosis have impaired endothelium-dependent vasodilator function at the coronary microvascular level. Alpha and beta adrenoreceptor activation in the endothelium provokes release of endothelium-derived relaxing factors such as nitric oxide, which may normally oppose the vasoconstrictor effects of alpha-1 and alpha-2 adrenoreceptor activation in vascular smooth muscle. Thus, sympathetic nervous system activation by mental stress could result in a net microvascular constrictor effect in patients with coronary artery disease and dysfunctional microvascular endothelium.[134]

Sympathetic nervous system activity has also been found to be increased in borderline hypertension and is sustained over a 24-hour period. There are elevated plasma catecholamines and renin levels (which are also under sympathetic control),[114] and this correlates well with the finding that psychological stress induces sodium and fluid retention in men at high risk for hypertension.[135] Acute mental stress in patients with borderline hypertension also elicits significantly higher cortisol levels.[136] Since the sympathetic nervous system is the main pathway by which the brain influences blood pressure, any behavioural theory of hypertension must invoke the sympathetic nervous system as principal mediator.

Hyperventilation

Increased minute ventilation is part of the usual preparatory response in the flight–fight reaction; when there is no concomitant physical activity, hypocapnia develops. Emotion often triggers hyperventilation and an upper thoracic mode of breathing becomes a learned habit in such situations. It is a frequent concomitant of phobic anxiety (see above).

Role in angina pectoris

Nixon has long noted the presence of hyperventilation in patients with cardiovascular disease and exhaustion[83] and its presence has been documented in over half of a series of patients with angina pectoris and angiographically documented coronary artery disease,[137,138] and also in patients postinfarction.[139] It clearly exacerbates the underlying arterial disease; in a recent study, hyperventilation produced shorter times to ischaemic threshold and reduced exercise tolerance, despite the same atherosclerotic involvement of the coronary tree.[140]

Role in syndrome X, coronary vasospasm and normal coronary arteries

The role of hyperventilation in nonorganic chest pain has been recognized since 1871, when it was termed Da Costa's syndrome, and subsequently it has had many other eponymous names. It continues to be found in many patients with chest pain and normal coronary arteries,[141] in so-called syndrome X,[142] and in patients with variant angina due to coronary artery spasm.[143] Indeed, in variant angina it has been long used as one of the best provocative tests[144] and is acknowledged as a potential trigger mechanism for alteration in coronary tone in daily life, in response to emotional stress.[145] One can speculate about the aetiological role of hyperventilation when it is seen in such a wide spectrum of cardiovascular disorders,[146,147] but failure to recognize and treat certainly exacerbates existing coronary artery disease, possibly provoking earlier intervention than would otherwise be merited on the basis of the coronary artery lesions. It is probably an important cause of the 'thick-folder syndrome', since chest pain continues and it also provokes a wide range of other somatic complaints. Indeed, reassurance that the pain is not organic does little to alleviate the continuing morbidity experienced by the patient, who finds it difficult to differentiate the pain in the chest from impending coronary artery disease,[148,149] and unless he or she is taught to avoid hyperventilation, a vicious circle ensues. In a recent review, three-quarters of a group of patients with non-cardiac chest pain or benign palpitations continued to complain of a limitation of their activities and persistent disability at 3-year follow-up[150] and others have confirmed continued high rates of visits to their physician.[151] There is also a suggestion that, certainly in some patients with chest pain and normal coronary arteries, there is an abnormal cardiac pain perception.[152]

Physiological effects of hyperventilation

Hyperventilation affects myocardial oxygen supply in humans by a combination of an increase in the oxygen affinity of the blood due to the Bohr effect, and coronary vasoconstriction that decreases blood flow (Figure 11.3).[153] This has been documented in patients with coronary artery disease[154] and elegantly confirmed using intracoronary Doppler catheters for the measurement of coronary flow velocity.[142] This group found that both hyperventilation and mental stress produced a reduction in coronary flow velocity in syndrome X patients, in the absence of any significant changes in the diameter of the left anterior descending coronary artery. Furthermore, they documented that both stressors significantly elevated noradrenaline levels. Early hyperventilation-induced ST segment depression is due to increased oxygen demand, as indicated by an increase in rate pressure product, and delayed hyperventilation-induced ST segment depression is probably related to a primary reduction in coronary blood flow.[154] This reduction is probably due to constriction of the small resistance vessels, which have been shown to cause myocardial ischaemia.[155] In addition, Henderson states that EDRF activity is likely to be impaired in such a situation[156] and there may be an abnormality in adenosine metabolism in the myocardium.[157] As mentioned earlier, animal studies have shown that chronic social disruption impairs endothelium-dependent vascular responses.[27]

Treatment

Coronary artery disease

Efforts to reduce the hostile, competitive and impatient behaviour in type A individuals[158] have led to improved prognosis in coronary artery disease. Learning new ways to deal with anger could add an extra dimension to preventive healthcare. People who behave in a hostile manner tend to have higher levels of cholesterol and LDL, which may be lowered by appropriate therapy (for example, stress management) and standard risk factor management (for example smoking, cholesterol, hypertension) is, of course, synergistic with this and not antagonistic.[159,160] Debate continues about its effectiveness,[161] but stress management programmes, as part of cardiac rehabilitation (postinfarction, angioplasty or bypass surgery), have been found to produce significant reductions in anxiety, depression and improvements in general psychological wellbeing.[162] Some of the early benefits may not be seen so clearly 1 year later.[163] The spouse/partner is clearly recognized as having a very important role in rehabilitation and should be fully included, since they may be the single most important factor in recovery.[164,165]

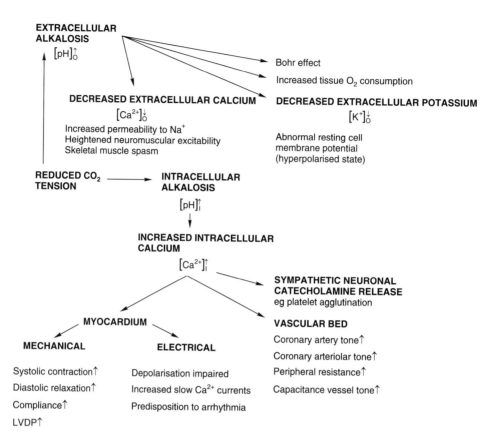

Figure 11.3

The mechanism by which hyperventilation, causing a fluctuating reduction of the blood CO_2 tension, induces vasomotor instability and disturbances of function [ ]$_o$ extracellular concentration, eg $[K^+]_o\downarrow$ decreased concentration of extracellular ionized potassium. [ ]$_i$ intracellular concentration, eg $[Ca^{2+}]_i\uparrow$ increased intracellular concentration of ionized calcium. LVDP left ventricular end-diastolic pressure. (Courtesy of Abbasi, personal communication.) (Reproduced with permission from Postgrad Med J(1985) **61***: 957–61.)*

Heart failure

In heart failure it is understandable that the extent and speed of physical activity, restricted social, leisure and family life can be correlated to quality of life and the emotional distress perceived by the patient.[166] As discussed above, emotional stress may impair left ventricular filling in such patients.[114] In a group of patients with heart failure (NYHA II and III), stress management and cognitive therapy have been shown to improve significantly exercise tolerance, functional capacity and quality of life compared with placebo or digoxin.[167]

Hypertension

Various studies have looked specifically at antihypertensive drugs in patients who have augmented cardiovascular and sympathetic nervous response to mental stress and have found that an ACE inhibitor alone,[168] or combined with verapamil,[169] successfully suppressed the augmented responses, whereas nifedipine worsened the situation. Patel has found success with stress management in mild hypertension[170] and concomitant falls in noradrenaline, renin and dopamine beta-hydroxylase have also been documented.[171] This effect importantly persists throughout the day, suggesting a resetting of the tonic blood pressure level,[172] but other studies have not be able to replicate this.[173]

Gender difference

Mental stress has been found to induce greater rises of blood pressure in postmenopausal women than in premenopausal women or in men and the mean ambulatory blood pressure at work is elevated compared with premenopausal women.[174] Since the use of HRT does not increase blood pressure and there may even be a slight fall in hypertensive patients,[175] treatment with HRT should clearly be considered. In postmenopausal women with coronary artery disease, the acute administration of sublingual oestradiol diminishes ischaemia (as measured by exercise time and time to ST segment depression on treadmill exercise testing) in similar proportions to that seen with sublingual GTN.[176] In women with syndrome X there appears to be a higher incidence of hysterectomy, and oestrogen replacement therapy often alleviates or reduces cardiac symptoms and enhances hyperaemic responses.[177] One can speculate that perhaps the microvasculature is less responsive to vasoconstrictive stimuli in the presence of oestrogen.

Guidelines on psychosocial care

Given the 1996 British Cardiac Society/College of Physicians guidelines on cardiac rehabilitation, which include psychosocial care,[178] it is worrying that a recent survey found that the number of psychologists to be found in rehabilitation schemes was negligible in the UK (putting us in the group with Poland, Turkey, Czechoslovakia, etc.) as compared to some of our other European partners.[179] It is should also be appreciated that there is a role for rehabilitation and counselling following bypass grafting, not only to detect and manage psychosocial risk factors, but also to identify those patients who have not improved following surgery because they are unwilling 'to relinquish the sick role' or have adopted 'resigned coping'.[180,181] Such emotional factors may account for 12–32% of those who fail to return to work within 1 year.[182] Clearly healthcare purchasers need to give this careful thought.

Conclusion

There is clear evidence to substantiate the role of stress and emotion as risk factors in coronary heart disease and, perhaps, to a lesser extent in hypertension. Obviously, such risk factors are not applicable in every case — but then, nor are the more traditional risk factors. It behoves us to seek those patients in whom there are psychosocial risk factors as assiduously as we do those who smoke, are obese or are hypercholesterlaemic, for the recognition and general discussion of psychosocial risk factors can be as valuable as the advice to lose weight or stop smoking. Perhaps taking the social history is no longer pursued as vigorously as we were taught as medical students, but time must be taken to ask about social isolation, control and job strain and loss of wellbeing. Anxiety, phobias, anger and hostility may be best screened by questionnaires, but if identified, then active treatment is indicated and we should not be slow in directing such patients towards colleagues who have the appropriate skills. Hopefully, psychologists or specifically trained nurses or occupational therapists will form part of an integrated approach so that they can be utilized in selected patients at any stage of their cardiovascular illness, rather than being limited to the postinfarction rehabilitation programme. Clearly this approach will run in tandem with the cardiological management and should not be viewed as less important or counterproductive to traditional management.

Differentiating 'ill-health' and depression is difficult and the use of a questionnaire as standard would be helpful in identifying individuals who would benefit from antidepressants, probably in the form of selective serotonin uptake inhibitors. Symptoms of hyperventilation must be sought specifically in the history and should be considered in all patients; perhaps a simple questionnaire, although not ideal and with problems of selectivity and specificity, might be helpful as a screen and such patients can be taught abdominal breathing — both at rest and with exercise.[139,183] Patients who do not have concomitant organic disease but in whom behaviour and emotion appear to be making a substantial contribution to cardiovascular symptoms should be directed early (by the assessing physician) towards appropriate therapy. The symptoms should not simply be dismissed since continuing morbidity will occupy further outpatient slots and acute beds and in the longer term early treatment will be more cost-effective.

If I had…

If I had angina I would like a standard cardiological work-up, which would of course include assessment of risk factors. I would expect my cardiologist to consider my social situation as well as screening me for depression and anxiety/phobias. Self-recognition of anger and hostility is unusual and so a questionnaire would enable an independent view to be taken. If my psychosocial risk factors were unusually high, and it was not thought that I could cope with them on my own, I would expect referral for appropriate counselling, in much the same way that I would expect a statin, for example, if diet did not control my hyperlipidaemia. As risk stratification, I would like a MUGA scan to look for any left ventricular dysfunction in response to mental arithmetic (which I know I would find extremely stressful). If I had depression, I would like to have a selective serotonin uptake inhibitor, which I would take in addition to aspirin and a beta blocker and, if I was postmenopausal, HRT. I would hope that any symptoms of hyperventilation would be assiduously sought and training given for abdominal breathing both at rest and with exercise.

References

1 Tuke D, *The mind upon the body, in health and disease* (J & A Churchill: London, 1872) 245.

2 Petch M, Triggering a heart attack, *Br Med J* (1996)**312**:459–60.

3 Mitchell R, What constitutes evidence on the dietary prevention of coronary heart disease? Cosy beliefs or harsh facts? *Int J Cardiol* (1984)**5**:287–98.

4 Oliver M, Prevention of coronary heart disease —propaganda, promises, problems, and prospects, *Circulation* (1986)**73**(1):1–9.

5 Manuck S, Kaplan J, Adams M, Clarkson T, Effects of stress and the sympathetic nervous system on coronary artery atherosclerosis in the cynomolgus macaque, *Am Heart J* (1988)**116**:328-33.

6 Dimsdale J, A new mechanism linking stress to coronary pathophysiology? [editorial] *Circulation* (1991) **84**(5):2201-2.

7 Deanfield J, Shea M, Kensett M et al, Silent myocardial ischaemia due to mental stress, *Lancet* (1984)**ii**:1001–4.

8 Karasek R, Theorell T, Schwartz J, Schnall P, Pieper C, Michela J, Job characteristics in relation to prevalence of myocardial infarction in the US HES and HANES, *Am J Public Health* (1988)**78**:910–18.

9 Bohlin G, Eliasson K, Hjemdahl P, Klein K, Fredrikson M, Frankenhauser M, Personal control over work pace: circulatory, neuroendocrine and subjective responses in borderline hypertension, *J Hypertens* (1986)**4**:295-305.

10 Steptoe A, Vogele C, Methodology of mental stress testing in cardiovascular research, *Circulation* (1991)**83**(suppl II):II-14–II-24.

11 Freeman L, Nixon P, Sallabank P, Reavely D, Psychological stress and silent ischaemia, *Am Heart J* (1987)**114**:477–82.

12 Johnson J, Hall F, Job strain, workplace social support, and cardiovascular disease: a cross sectional study of a random sample of the Swedish working population, *Am J Public Health* (1988)**78**:1336–41.

13 Toffler G, Stone P, Maclure M, Davis V, Robertson T, Analysis of possible triggers of acute myocardial infarction (the MILIS study), *Am J Cardiol* (1990)**66**:22–7.

14 Willich S, Lewis M, Lowel H, Arntz H, Schubert F, Shroder R, Physical exertion is a trigger of myocardial infarction, *N Engl J Med* (1993)**329**:1684–90.

15 Leor J, Poole K, Kloner R, Sudden cardiac death triggered by an earthquake, *N Engl J Med* (1996)**334**(7):413–19.

16 Weiss S, Krantz D, Mathews K, Coronary prone behaviour. In: Rowlands DJ, ed. *Recent advances in cardiology (9)*, (Churchill Livingstone: London, 1984) 241–58.

17 Jenkins C, Zyzanski S, Rosenman R, Risk of new myocardial infarction in middle-aged men with manifest coronary artery disease, *Circulation* (1976)**53**:342–47.

18 Kannel W, Eaker E, Psychosocial and other features of coronary heart disease: insight from the Framingham Study, *Am Heart J* (1986)**112**(5):1066–73.

19 McKeigue P, Adelstein A, Shipley M et al, Diet and risk factors for coronary heart disease in Asians in north-west London, *Lancet* (1985)**ii** 1086–90.

20 Syme S, Social and psychological risk factors in coronary heart disease, *Am Heart J* (1975)**44**(4):17–21.

21 Ruberman W, Weinblatt E, Goldberg J, Chaudhary B, Psychosocial influences on mortality after myocardial infarction, *N Engl J Med* (1984)**311**:552–9.

22 Orth-Gomer K, Rosengren A, Wilhelmsen L, Lack of social support and incidence of coronary disease in middle-aged Swedish men, *Psychosom Med* (1993)**55**(1):37-43.

23 Ornish D, Brown S, Scherwits L et al, Can lifestyle changes reverse coronary heart disease? The Lifestyle Heart Trial, *Lancet* (1990)**2**:129–33.

24 Prior I, Stanhope J, Evans J, Salmon C, The Tokelau Island Migrant study, *Int J Epidemiol* (1974)3:225–32.

25 Syme S, Control and health: a personal perspective. In: Steptoe A, Appels A, eds. *Stress, personal control and health* (Wiley: Chichester, 1989) 3–18.

26 Karasek R, Russel R, Theorell T, Physiology of stress and regeneration in job related cardiovascular illness, *J Human Stress* (1982)8:29–42.

27 Williams J, Vita J, Manuck S, Selwyn A, Kaplan J, Psychosocial factors impair vascular responses of coronary arteries, *Circulation* (1991)84(5):2146–53.

28 Kaplan J, Manuck S, Adams M, Weingand K, Clarkson S, Inhibition of coronary atherosclerosis by propranolol in behaviourally predisposed monkeys fed an atherogenic diet, *Circulation* (1987)76:1364–72.

29 Theorell T, Perski A, Orth-Gomer K, Hamsten A, de-Faire U, The effects of the strain of returning to work on the risk of cardiac death after a first myocardial infarction before the age of 45, *Int J Cardiol* (1991)30:61–7.

30 Hlatky M, Lam L, Lee K et al, Job strain and the prevalence and outcome of coronary artery disease, *Circulation* (1995)92:327–33.

31 Pickering T, Schnall P, Schwartz J, Pieper C, Can behavioural factors produce a sustained elevation of blood pressure? Some observations and a hypothesis, *J Hypertens* (1991)9(suppl 8):266–8.

32 Schnall P, Pieper C, Schwartz J et al, The relationship between 'job strain', workplace diastolic blood pressure and left ventricular mass index: results of a case-control study, *JAMA* (1990)263:1929–35.

33 Pickering T, Schwartz J, James G, Ambulatory blood pressure monitoring for evaluating the relationships between lifestyle, hypertension and cardiovascular risk, *Clin Exp Pharmacol Physiol* (1995)22:226–31.

34 Schnall P, Schwartz J, Landsbergis P, Warren K, Pickering T, Relation between job strain, alcohol, and ambulatory blood pressure, *Hypertension* (1992)19:488–494.

35 Rosengren A, Tibblin G, Wilhelmsen L, Self-perceived psychological stress and incidence of coronary artery disease in middle aged men, *Am J Cardiol* (1991)68:1171–5.

36 Parkes C, Benjamin B, Fitzgerald R, Broken heart: a statistical study of increased mortality among widowers, *Br Med J* (1969)i:740–3.

37 Frasure-Smith N, Prince R, The ischaemic heart disease life stress monitoring program: impact on mortality, *Psychosom Med* (1985)47:431–45.

38 Dimsdale J, A perspective on type A behaviour and coronary disease [editorial], *N Engl J Med* (1988)318:110–12.

39 Rosenman R, Brand R, Jenkins C, Friedman M, Straus R, Wurm M, Coronary heart disease in the Western Collaborative Group Study: final follow-up of $8\frac{1}{2}$ years, *JAMA* (1975)233:872–7.

40 Haynes S, Feinleib M, Kannel W, The relationship of psychosocial factors to coronary heart disease in the Framingham Study. III. 8 year incidence of CHD, *Am J Epidem* (1980) 3:37–58.

41 Rosenman R, Current status of risk factors and type A behaviour pattern in the pathogenesis of ischaemic heart disease. In: Dembroski T, Schmidt T, Blumchen G, eds. *Biobehavioural bases of coronary heart disease* (Karger: Basel, 1983) 5–12.

42 Freeman L, The mind and the heart. In: Julian D, Camm A, Fox K, Hall R, Poole-Wilson P, eds. *Diseases of the Heart* (Balliere Tindall, WB Saunders: London, 1989) 1500–9.

43 Johnson D, Cook D, Shaper A, Type A behaviour and ischaemic heart disease in middle aged British men, *Br Med J* (1987)295:86–9.

44 Eysenck H, *Smoking, personality and stress: psychosocial factors in the prevention of cancer and coronary heart disease* (Springer Verlag: New York, 1991).

45 Barefoot J, Patterson J, Haney T, Cayton T, Hickman J, Williams R, Hostility in asymptomatic men with angiographically confirmed coronary artery disease, *Am J Cardiol* (1994)74:439-42.

46 Cook W, Medley D, Proposed hostility and pharasaic-virtue scales for the MMPI, *J App Psychol* (1954)38:414–18.

47 Spielberger C, Johnson E, Russell S, Crane R, Jacobs G, Worden T, The experience and expression of anger: construction and validation of an anger expression scale. In: Chesney M, Rosenman R, eds. *Anger and hostility in*

cardiovascular and behavioural disorders (McGraw-Hill/Hemisphere: New York, 1985) 5–30.

48 Siegman A, Smith T, *Anger, hostility and the heart* (Lawrence Erlbaum: Hillsdale, 1994).

49 Boltwood M, Taylor C, Burke M, Grogin H, Giacomini J, Anger report predicts coronary artery vasomotor response to mental stress in atherosclerotic segments, *Am J Cardiol* (1993)**72**:1361–5.

50 Verrier R, Dickerson L, Autonomic nervous system and coronary blood flow changes related to emotional activation and sleep, *Circulation* (1991)**83**(suppl II):II-81–II-89.

51 Buss M, Jain D, Soufer R, Kerns R, Zaret B, Role of behavioural and psychological factors in mental stress induced left ventricular dysfunction in coronary artery disease, *J Am Col Cardiol* (1993)**22**:440–8.

52 Ironson G, Taylor C, Boltwood M et al, Effects of anger on left ventricular ejection fraction in coronary artery disease, *Am J Cardiol* (1992)**70**:281–5.

53 Freeman L, Nixon P, The effect of type A behaviour pattern on myocardial ischaemia during daily life, *Int J Cardiol* (1987)**17**:145–54.

54 Sloan R, Bigger T, Biobehavioural factors in cardiac arrhythmia pilot study (CAPS); review and examination, *Circulation* (1991)**83**(suppl II):II-52–II-57.

55 Cottingham E, Matthews K, Talbott E, Kuller L, Occupational stress, suppressed anger and hypertension, *Psychosom Med* (1968) **48**:249–60.

56 Haines A, Imeson J, Meade T, Phobic anxiety and ischaemic heart disease, *Br Med J* (1987)**295**:295–7.

57 Kawachi I, Colditz G, Ascherio A et al, Prospective study of phobic anxiety and risks of coronary heart disease in men, *Circulation* (1994)**89**:1992–7.

58 Arthur J, Gutterman D, Body M, Stress decreases coronary blood flow in the normal conscious cat, *Circulation* (1989)**80**(suppl II):II-310 (abstr.).

59 Gutterman D, Bonham A, Arthur J, Gebhart G, Marcus M, Body M, Central neural regulation of coronary blood flow. In: Buckley J, Ferrario C, eds. *Brain peptides and catecholamines in cardiovascular regulation* (Raven Press: New York, 1987)125–35.

60 Engel G, Sudden and rapid death during psychological stress: folklore or folk wisdom? *Ann Intern Med* (1971)**74**:771–82.

61 Lown B, Sudden cardiac death: biobehavioural perspective, *Circulation* (1987)**76**(suppl I): I-186–I-196.

62 Lown B, Verrier R, Rabinowitz S, Neural and psychologic mechanism and the problem of sudden cardiac death, *Am J Cardiol* (1977)**39**:890–902.

63 Da Silva R, Psychological stress and sudden cardiac death. In: Schmidt T, Dembroski T, Blumchen G, eds. *Biological and psychological factors in cardiovascular disease* (Springer-Verlag: Berlin/Heidelberg, 1986) 156–83.

64 Carpeggiani C, Skinner J, Coronary flow and mental stress, experimental findings, *Circulation* (1991)**83**(suppl II):II-90–II-93.

65 Lown B, Mental stress, arrhythmias and sudden death, *Am J Med* (1982)**72**:177–80.

66 Reich P, DeSilva R, Lown B, Murawski B, Acute psychological disturbances preceding life-threatening ventricular arrhythmias, *JAMA* (1981)**246**:233–5.

67 Katz C, Martin R, Landa B, Chadda K, Relationship of psychologic factors to frequent symptomatic ventricular arrhythmia, *Am J Med* (1985)**78**:589–94.

68 Follick M, Ahern D, Gorkin L et al, Relation of psychosocial and stress reactivity variables to ventricular arrhythmias in the cardiac arrhythmias pilot study (CAPS), *Am J Cardiol* (1990)**66**:63–7.

69 Yeragani V, Balon R, Pohl R et al, Decreased heart rate variability in panic disorder patients: a study of power-spectral analysis of heart rate, *Psychiatr Res* (1993)**46**:89–103.

70 Kleiger R, Miller J, Bigger J, Moss A, Decreased heart rate variability and its association with increased mortality after acute myocardial infarction, *Am J Cardiol* (1987)**59**:256–62.

71 Molgaard H, Sorensen K, Bjerregaard P, Attenuated 24-h heart rate variability in apparently healthy subjects, subsequently suffering sudden cardiac death, *Clin Auton Res* (1991)**1**:233–43.

72 Fei L, Anderson M, Katrisis D et al, Decreased heart rate variability in survivors of sudden

cardiac death not associated with coronary artery disease, *Br Heart J* (1994)**71**:16–21.

73 Pagani M, Lombardi F, Guzzette S et al, Power spectral analysis of heart rate and arterial pressure variabilities as a marker of sympathovagal interaction in man and conscious dog, *Circ Res* (1986)**59**:178–93.

74 Schwartz P, Zaza A, Locati E, Moss A, Stress and sudden death; the case of the long QT syndrome, *Circulation* (1991)**83**(**suppl II**):II-71–II-80.

75 Airaksinen K, Ikaheimo M, Linnaluoto M, Niemela M, Takkunen J, Impaired vagal heart rate control in coronary artery disease, *Br Heart J* (1987)**58**:592-7.

76 Hayano J, Sakakibara Y, Yamada M et al, Decreased magnitude of heart rate spectral components in coronary artery disease; its relation to angiographic severity, *Circulation* (1990)**81**:1217–24.

77 Hayano J, Yamada A, Kukai S et al, Severity of coronary atherosclerosis correlates with the respiratory component of heart rate variability, *Am Heart J* (1991)**121**:1070–9.

78 Nolan J, Flapan A, Reid J, Neilson J, Bloomfield P, Ewing D, Cardiac parasympathetic activity in severe uncomplicated coronary artery disease, *Br Heart J* (1994)**71**:515–20.

79 Carney R, Freedland K, Jaffe A, Insomnia and depression prior to myocardial infarction, *Psychosom Med* (1990)**52**:603–9.

80 Carney R, Saunders R, Freedland K, Stein P, Rich M, Jaffe A, Association of depression with reduced heart rate variability in coronary artery disease, *Am J Cardiol* (1995)**76**:562–4.

81 Frasure-Smith N, Lesperance F, Talajic M, Depression following myocardial infarction: impact on 6-month survival, *JAMA* (1993)**270**:1819–25.

82 Nixon P, The human function curve, *Practitioner* (1976)**217**:765–70, 935–44.

83 Nixon P, The responsibility of the cardiological mapmaker, *Am Heart J* (1980)**100**:139–43.

84 Appels A, The year before myocardial infarction. In: Dembroski T, Schmidt T, Blumchen G. eds. *Biobehavioural bases of coronary heart disease* (Karger: Basel, 1983) 18–35.

85 Jenkins C, Recent evidence supporting psychologic and social risk factors for coronary disease, *N Engl J Med* (1976)**294**:987–94,1033–8.

86 Hollon S, Sheltpon R, Davis D, Cognitive therapy for depression: conceptual issues and clinical efficacy, *J Consult Clin Psychol* (1993)**61**:270–5.

87 Williams R, Chesney M, Psychosocial factors and prognosis in established coronary artery disease: the need for research on interventions, *JAMA* (1993)**270**(15):1860–1.

88 Hamilton J, Campos R, Creed F, Anxiety, depression and management of medically unexplained symptoms in medical clinics, *J R Coll Physicians* (1996)**30**:18–20.

89 Fitzpatrick R, Hopkins A, Referrals to neurologist for headaches not due to structural disease, *J Neurol Neurosurg Psychiatry* (1981)**44**:1061–7.

90 van Hemert A, Hengeveld M, Bolk J, Rooigans H, Vandenbrouke J, Psychiatric disorders in relation to medical illness among patients of a general medical out-patient clinic, *Psychol Med* (1993)**23**:167–73.

91 Speckens A, van Hemert A, Bolk J, Hengeveld M, Unexplained physical symptoms: medical and psychiatric outcome at one year follow up. Poster presentation, *Dutch C-L psychiatry conference*: Amsterdam, 1993.

92 Royal College of Physicians/Royal College of Psychiatrists, *The psychological care of mental patients. Joint report* (Royal College of Physicians/Royal College of Psychiatrists: London, 1995).

93 Klimes I, Mayou R, Pearce M, Coles L, Fagg J, Psychological treatment for atypical non-cardiac chest pain: a controlled evaluation, *Psychol Med* (1990)**100**:450–547.

94 Hallstrom T, Lapidus L, Bengtsson C, Edstrom K, Psychosocial factors and risk of ischaemic heart disease and death in women: a twelve year follow up of participants in the population study of women in Gothenburg Sweden, *J Psychosom Res* (1986)**30**:451–9.

95 Talbott E, Kuller L, Perper J, Murphy P, Sudden unexpected death in women. Biologic and psychosocial origins, *Am J Epidemiol* (1981)**114**:671–82.

96 Schifer F, Hartley L, Schulman C et al, The quiz electrocardiogram: a new diagnostic and

research technique for evaluating the relation between emotional stress and ischaemic heart disease, *Am J Cardiol* (1976)**37**:41–7.

97 Deanfield J, Selwyn A, Chierchia S et al, Myocardial ischaemia during daily life in patients with stable angina: its relation to symptoms and heart rate changes, *Lancet* (1983)**ii**:753–8.

98 Deanfield J, Shea M, Selwyn A, Clinical evaluation of transient myocardial ischaemia during daily life, *Am J Med* (1985)**79**:18–24.

99 Freeman L, Nixon P, Time to rethink the syndrome of angina pectoris—implications from ambulatory Holter monitoring, *Quart J Med* (1987)**62**:25–32.

100 Legault S, Freeman M, Langer A, Armstrong P, Pathophysiology and time course of silent myocardial ischaemia during mental stress: clinical, anatomical, and physiological correlates, *Br Heart J* (1995)**73**:242–9.

101 Freeman L, Nixon P, Dynamic factors in angina pectoris, *Am Heart J* (1985)**110**:1087–91.

102 Schiffer F, Hartley H, Schulman C, Abelmann W, Evidence for emotionally induced coronary arterial spasm in patients with angina pectoris, *Br Heart J* (1980)**44**:62–6.

103 Yeung A, Vekshtein V, Krantz D et al, The effect of atherosclerosis on the vasomotor response of coronary arteries to mental stress, *N Engl J Med* (1991)**325**:1551–6.

104 Billman G, Randell D, Mechanisms mediating the coronary vascular response to behavioural stress in dogs, *Circulation* (1981)**48**:214-23.

105 Camici P, Marraccini P, Gistri R, Salvadori P, Sorace O, L'Ababate A, Adrenergically mediated coronary vasoconstriction in patients with syndrome X, *Cardiovasc Drug Ther* (1994)**8**:221–6.

106 Bairey C, Krantz D, DeQuattro V, Berman D, Rozanski A, Effect of beta blockade on low heart rate related ischemia during mental stress, *J Am Coll Cardiol* (1991)**17**:1388–95.

107 Bortone A, Hess O, Gaglione A et al, Effect of intravenous propranolol on coronary vasomotion at rest and during dynamic exercise in patients with coronary artery disease, *Circulation* (1990)**81**:1255–35.

108 Krittayaphong R, Light K, Biles P, Ballenger M, Sheps D, Increased heart rate response to laboratory induced mental stress predicts frequency and duration of daily life ambulatory myocardial ischemia in patients with coronary artery disease, *Am J Cardiol* (1995)**76**:657–60.

109 Legault S, Langer A, Armstrong P, Freeman M, Usefulness of ischemic response to mental stress in predicting silent myocardial ischemia during ambulatory monitoring, *Am J Cardiol* (1995)**75**:1007–11.

110 Mulcahy D, Purcell H, Patel D, Fox K, Asymptomatic ischaemia during daily life in stable coronary disease: relevant or redundant? *Br Heart J* (1994)**72**:5–8.

111 LaVeau P, Rozanksi A, Krantz D et al, Transient left ventricular dysfunction during provocative mental stress in patients with coronary artery disease, *Am Heart J* (1989)**118**:1–8.

112 Rozanski A, Bairey N, Krantz D et al, Mental stress and the induction of silent myocardial ischemia in patients with coronary artery disease, *N Engl J Med* (1988)**318**:1005–12.

113 Mazzuero G, Temporelli P, Tavazzi L, Influence of mental stress on ventricular pump function in post infarction patients; an invasive hemodynamic investigation, *Circulation* (1991)**83**(suppl II):II-145–II-54.

114 Giannuzzi P, Shabetai R, Imparato A et al, Effects of mental exercise in patients with dilated cardiomyopathy and congestive heart failure: an echocardiographic Doppler study, *Circulation* (1991)**83**(suppl II)II-155–II-165.

115 Tapp W, Levin B, Natelson B, Stress induced heart failure, *Psychosom Med* (1983)**45**:171–6.

116 Jain D, Burg M, Soufer R, Zaret B, Prognostic implications of mental stress-induced silent left ventricular dysfunction in patients with stable angina pectoris, *Am J Cardiol* (1995)**76**:31–5.

117 Sheps D, Ballenger M, DeGent G et al, Psychological responses to a speech stressor: correlation of plasma beta-endorphin levels at rest and after psychological stress with thermally measured pain threshold in patients with coronary artery disease, *J Am Coll Cardiol* (1995)**25**:1499–503.

118 Folkow B, Cardiovascular structural adaptation: its role in the limitation and maintenance of primary hypertension. In: Mathews K, Weiss S, Detre T, eds. *Handbook of stress, reactivity*

and cardiovascular disease (Wiley: New York, 1986) 11–34.

119 Jerns S, Bergbrant A, Hedner T, Hansson L, Enhanced pressor responses to experimental and daily life stress in borderline hypertension, *J Hypertens* (1995)**13**:69–79.

120 Carroll D, Smith G, Sheffield D, Shipley M, Marmot M, Pressor reactions to psychological stress and prediction of future blood pressure: data from the Whitehall II study, *Br Med J* (1995)**310**:771–6.

121 Parati G, Pomidossi G, Casadei R et al, Comparison of the cardiovascular effects of different laboratory stressors and their relationship with blood pressure variability, *J Hypertens* (1988)**6**:481–8.

122 Floras J, Assan M, Joes J, Sleight P, Pressor responses to laboratory stresses and day time blood pressure variability, *J Hypertens* (1987)**5**:715–19.

123 Mason J, A review of psychoendocrine research on the pituitary adrenal cortical system and on the sympathetic-adrenal medullary system, *Psychosom Med* (1968)**30**:576–607, 631–53.

124 Henry J, Stephens P, *Stress, health and the social environment. A sociobiologic approach to medicine* (Springer Verlag: New York, 1977).

125 Frakenhauser M, Psychoneuroendocrine approaches to the study of stressful person-environment transactions. In: Seyle, ed. *Seyle's guide to stress research vol 1* (Van Nostrand Reinhold: New York, 1980).

126 Dimsdale J, Ziegler M, What do plasma and urinary measures of catecholamines tell us about human response to stressors? *Circulation* (1991)**83**(suppl II):II-36–II-42.

127 Steptoe A, Neural and endocrine factors in cardiovascular control. In: Steptoe A, ed. *Psychological factors in cardiovascular disorders* (Academic Press: London, 1981) 44–5.

128 Ushiyama K, Ogawa T, Ishii M, Ajisaka R, Sugishita Y, Ito I, Physiologic neuroendocrine arousal by mental arithmetic stress tests in healthy subjects, *Am J Cardiol* (1991)**67**:101–3.

129 Marmot M, Does stress cause heart attacks? *Postgrad Med J* (1986)**62**:683–6.

130 Grignani G, Soffiantino F, Zucchella M et al, Platelet activation by emotional stress in patients with coronary artery disease, *Circulation* (1991)**83**(suppl II):II-128–II-136.

131 Henry J, Mechanisms by which stress can lead to coronary heart disease, *Postgrad Med J* (1986)**62**:687–93.

132 Troxler R, Sprague E, Albanes R, Fuchs R, Thompson A, The association of elevated plasma cortisol and early atherosclerosis as demonstrated by coronary angiography, *Atherosclerosis* (1977)**26**:151–62.

133 Dakak N, Quyyumi A, Eisenhofer G, Goldstein D, Canon R, Sympathetically mediated effects of mental stress on the cardiac microcirculation of patients with coronary artery disease, *Am J Cardiol* (1995)**76**:125–30.

134 Tuck M, Stern N, Sowers J, Enhanced 24 hour norepinephrine and renin secretion in young patients with essential hypertension: relation with the circadian pattern of arterial blood pressure, *Am J Cardiol* (1985)**55**:112–15.

135 Light K, Koepke J, Obrist P, Willis P, Psychological stress induces sodium and fluid retention in men at high risk for hypertension, *Science* (1983)**220**:429–31.

136 al'Abisi M, Lovallo W, McKey B, Pincomb G, Borderline hypertensives produce exaggerated adrenocortical responses to mental stress, *Psychosom Med* (1994)**56**:245–50.

137 Freeman L, Nixon P, Timmons B, Legg C, Hyperventilation and angina pectoris, *J R Coll Physicians* (1987)**21**:46–50.

138 Freeman L, Hyperventilation and ischaemic heart disease. In: Grossman P, Janssen K, Vaitl D, eds. *Cardiorespiratory and cardiosomatic psychophysiology* (Plenum Press: London, 1986) 319–26.

139 Nixon P, Al-Abassi H, King J, Freeman L, Hyperventilation in cardiac rehabilitation, *Holistic Med* (1986)**1**:5–13.

140 Specchia G, Falcone C, Traversi E et al, Mental stress as a provocative test in patients with various clinical syndromes of coronary heart disease, *Circulation* (1991)**83**(suppl II):II-108–II-114.

141 Bass C, Wade N, Gardener W et al, Unexplained breathlessness and psychiatric morbidity in patients with normal and abnormal coronary arteries, *Lancet* (1983)**1**:605-8.

142 Chauhan A, Mullins P, Taylor G, Petch M, Schofield P, Effect of hyperventilation and men-

tal stress on coronary blood flow in syndrome X, *Br Heart J* (1993)**69**:516–24.

143 Girotti L, Crossato J, Messuti H et al, The hyperventilation test as a method for developing successful therapy in Prinzmetal angina, *Am J Cardiol* (1982)**49**:834–8.

144 Bugiardini R, Pozzati A, Ottani F, Morgagni G, Puddu P, Vasotonic angina: a spectrum of ischemic syndromes involving functional abnormalities of the epicardial and microvascular coronary circulation, *J Am Coll Cardiol* (1993)**22**:417–25.

145 Mortensen S, Nielsen H, Grossman P, Hyperventilation as diagnostic stress test for variant angina and cardiomyopathy: cardiovascular response, likely triggering mechanisms and psychophysiological implications. In: Grossman P, Janssen K, Vaitl D, eds. *Cardiorespiratory and cardiosomatic psychophysiology* (Plenum Press: London, 1986) 303–17.

146 Freeman L, Nixon P, Are progressive heart damage and coronary artery spasm linked with the hyperventilation syndrome? *Br Med J* (1985)**291**:851–2.

147 Freeman L, Nixon P, Does hyperventilation have any effect in patients with chest pain? *Br Heart J* (1988)**59**:102.

148 Freeman L, Nixon P, Chest pain and the hyperventilation syndrome—some aetiological considerations, *Postgrad Med J* (1985)**61**:957–61.

149 Bass C, Wade C, Hand D et al, Patients with angina with normal and near normal coronary arteries: clinical and psychosocial state 12 months after angiography, *Br Med J* (1983)**287**:1505–8.

150 Mayou R, Bryant B, Forfar C, Clark D, Non-cardiac chest pain and benign palpitations in the cardiac clinic, *Br Heart J* (1994)**72**:548–53.

151 Barksy A, Cleary P, Coeytaux R, Ruskin J, The clinical course of palpitations in medical outpatients, *Arch Intern Med* (1995)**155**:1782–8.

152 Chauhan A, Mullins P, Thuraisingham S, Taylor G, Petch M, Schofield P, Abnormal cardiac pain perception in syndrome X, *J Am Coll Cardiol* (1994)**24**:329–35.

153 Neil W, Hattenhauer M, Impairment of myocardial O_2 supply due to hyperventilation, *Circulation* (1975)**52**:854–8.

154 Ardissino D, De Servi S, Barberis P et al, Significance of hyperventilation-induced ST segment depression in patients with coronary artery disease, *J Am Coll Cardiol* (1989)**13**:804–10.

155 Pupita G, Maseri A, Kaski J et al, Myocardial ischaemia caused by distal coronary artery constriction in stable angina pectoris, *N Engl J Med* (1990)**323**:514–20.

156 Henderson A, Endothelium, for example, *J R Coll Physicians* (1996)**30**:42–51.

157 Holdright D, Lindsay D, Clarke D, Fox K, Poole-Wilson P, Collins P, Coronary flow reserve in patients with chest pain and normal coronary arteries, *Br Heart J* (1993)**70**:513–19.

158 Friedman M, Thoresen C, Gill J et al, Alteration of type A behaviour and its effect on cardiac recurrences in post myocardial infarction patients: summary results of the Recurrent Coronary Prevention Project, *Am Heart J* (1986)**112**:653–65.

159 Grossarth-Maticek R, Eysenck H, Creative novation behaviour therapy as a prophylactic treatment for cancer and coronary heart disease. Part I. Description of treatment, *Behav Res Ther* (1991)**29**:1–16.

160 Eysenck H, Grossarth-Maticek R, Creative novation behaviour therapy as a prophylactic treatment for cancer and coronary heart disease. Part II. Effects of treatment, *Behav Res Ther* (1991)**29**:17–31.

161 Pelosi A, Appleby L, Psychological influences on cancer and ischaemic heart disease, *Br Med J* (1992)**304**:1295–8.

162 Trzcieniecka-Green A, Steptoe A, Stress management in cardiac patients: a preliminary study of the predictors of improvement in quality of life, *J Psychosom Res* (1994)**38**:267–80.

163 van Elderen-van-Kemenade T, Maes S, vanden-Broek Y, Effects of a health education programme with telephone follow up during cardiac rehabilitation, *Br J Clin Psychol* (1994)**33**:367–78.

164 Beach E, Maloney B, Plocica A et al. The spouse: a factor in recovery after acute myocardial infarction, *Heart Lung* (1992)**21**:30–8.

165 Millar P, Wikkof R, MacMahon M et al, Personal adjustments and regime compliance

one year after myocardial infarction, *Heart Lung* (1989)**18**:339–46.

166 Mayou R, Blackwood R, Bryant B, Garnham J, Cardiac failure: symptoms and functional status, *J Psychosom Res* (1991)**35**:399–407.

167 Kostis J, Rosen R, Cosgrove N, Shindler D, Wilson A, Nonpharmacologic therapy improves functional and emotional status in congestive heart failure, *Chest* (1994)**106**:996–1001.

168 Saitoh M, Miyakoda H, Kitamura H, Kinugawa T, Kotake H, Mashiba H, Effects of an angiotensin converting enzyme inhibitor, alacepril, on cardiovascular and sympathetic nervous responses to mental stress in patients with essential hypertension, *Intern Med* (1993)**32**:691–4.

169 Nazzaro P, Merlo M, Manzari M, Cicco G, Pirrelli A, Stress response and antihypertensive treatment, *Drugs* (1993)**46(suppl 2)**:133–40.

170 Patel C, North W, Randomised controlled trial of hypertension, *Lancet* (1975)**ii**:93–9.

171 Stone R, Deleo J, Psychotherapeutic control of hypertension, *N Engl J Med* (1976)**294**:80–4.

172 Southam M, Agras W, Taylor C, Kraemer H, Relaxation training, blood pressure lowering during the working day, *Arch Gen Psychiatr* (1982)**39**:715–19.

173 Johnston D, Gold A, Kentish J et al, Effect of stress management on blood pressure in mild primary hypertension, *Br Med J* (1993)**306**:963–9.

174 Owens J, Stoney C, Mathews K, Menopausal status influences ambulatory blood pressure levels and blood pressure changes during mental stress, *Circulation* (1993)**88**:2794–802.

175 Lobo K, Estrogen replacement therapy and hypertension, *Postgrad Med* (1987)**14**:48–54.

176 Rosano G, Sarrel P, Poole -Wilson P, Collins P, Beneficial effect of oestrogen on exercise induced myocardial ischaemia in women with coronary artery disease, *Lancet* (1993) **342**:133–13.

177 Sarrel P, Lindsay D, Rosano G, Poole-Wilson P, Angina and normal coronary arteries in women: gynecologic findings, *Am J Obstet Gynecol* (1992)**167**:467–71.

178 Thompson D, Bowman G, Kitson A, de Bono D, Hopkins A, Cardiac rehabilitation in the United Kingdom: guidelines and audit standards, *Heart* (1996)**75**:89–93.

179 Maes S, Psychosocial aspects of cardiac rehabilitation in Europe, *Br J Clin Psychol* (1992)**31**:473–83.

180 Mayou R, The psychiatric and social consequences of coronary artery surgery, *J Psychosom Res* (1986)**39**:255–71.

181 Brown J, Rawlinson M, Relinquishing the sick role following open heart surgery, *J Health Soc Behav* (1975)**16**:12–27.

182 Cox T, Coronary heart disease and stress: psychosocial and behavioural factors in rehabilitation, *Physiotherapy* (1986)**72**:231–3.

183 Pinney S, Freeman L, Nixon P, Role of the nurse counsellor in managing patients with the hyperventilation syndrome, *J Roy Soc Med* (1987)**80**:216–18.

12

Atrial fibrillation

Johan EP Waktare and A John Camm

Introduction

Atrial fibrillation (AF) is so prevalent that it is sometimes perceived as an acceptable alternative to normal sinus rhythm (SR), but this impression is false. AF is the most common sustained arrhythmia and results in more hospital admissions than result from any or all forms of ventricular arrhythmias (Figure 12.1).[1] Hospitalization can result directly from symptoms of haemodynamic compromise, or complications such as stroke. The incidence of AF rises with increasing age, but dismissing it as an 'ageing phenomenon' belies the difficult management dilemmas posed by the elderly. The management of paroxysmal AF and of recurrent, persistent AF are two of the most challenging problems in clinical cardiology practice for which new interventional strategies are now available.

Although patients with AF may appear to be symptomatically well when treated with digoxin, or even on no drug treatment, all must be fully assessed. They require evaluation of the probability of successful long-term restoration of SR, and assessment of the best strategy for doing so. If conversion fails or is deemed not feasible, optimal rate control becomes the goal of treatment. This requires assessment of the best drug or other treatment strategy for that individual and subsequent monitoring. Finally, a thorough assessment of the risks versus benefits of thromboembolic prophylaxis is required, relating the patient's circumstances to the published evidence.

For many years the high prevalence of AF, its apparently subtle impact on patients when compared with other cardiac disorders, and the lack of effective therapies other than digoxin, resulted in little research into the condition. Critical appraisal of treatment has not been undertaken. Recently, however, interest has grown and our understanding of the mechanism, treatment and complications of AF has advanced considerably.

Classification of AF

The classification of AF is difficult. Some distinct subgroups can be identified, but in general the disorder represents a continuous spectrum. It is often unclear how to classify a patient until the clinical history has been observed for some time, and with time the behaviour of their AF may change considerably. Most importantly, any classification is only useful if it adds to the management of patients. With these caveats in mind, we propose the following as a helpful framework.

Patients are divided into those with acute (defined as present less than 48 hours) or chronic AF. The latter group are then subdivided into paroxysmal, persistent and permanent AF. The framework of the classification is illustrated in Figure 12.2, which describes briefly the accepted and emerging treatment options, and a detailed description of each group is provided in the discussion of management. A patient's subgroup is not fixed, as this

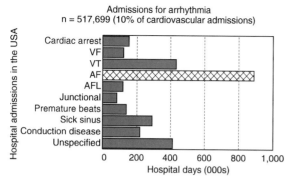

Figure 12.1
Number of hospital days due to different arrhythmias.

classification relates as much to an individual's current clinical priorities and the chosen approach to management, as it does to trying to describe distinct disorders.

The causes of AF?

Electrophysiology

According to the 'Multiple Wavelet Theory', AF is mediated by multiple meandering, interlacing re-entrant wavelets. This classic theory in electrophysiology was originally hypothesized by Moe more than 30 years ago.[2] Allesie and col-

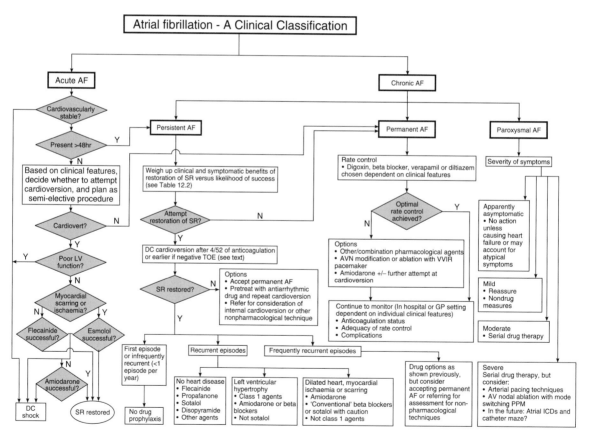

Figure 12.2
Atrial fibrillation – a clinical classification. (NB All patients also require assessment to thromboembolic prophylaxis (see text) and correction of any predisposing condition (see Table 12.1).)

leagues refined the model and demonstrated in living tissue that a leading circle of re-entry can exist in the absence of an anatomical obstacle,[3] which is required for the sustenance of AF. The model is based around the existence of a dynamic pattern of between six and 20 wave-fronts of depolarization traversing the atria at any one time. The path of each is constantly changing as it encounters fixed obstacles such as the atrioventricular ring and caval orifices (Figure 12.3), and temporary obstacles in the form of areas of refractoriness left by the passage of other wavelets. Wavelets encountering obstacles may divide, giving rise to two or more daughter wavelets, and the same occurs when a wavelet from an atrial free wall reaches the interatrial septum and continues simultaneously along the septum and the free wall of the other atrium. Wavelets entering a 'cul-de-sac' of

refractory and nonconducting tissue are extinguished, and if enough are extinguished simultaneously, the wavefront of depolarization originating from the automatic firing of the sinus node region is able to capture the entire atrial surface and restore SR. The likelihood of spontaneous reversion to SR is reduced if more wavelets are present simultaneously. From an electrophysiological perspective, therefore, the stability of AF is increased by a large atrial surface area, a short atrial effective refractory period (AERP) and slow atrial conduction. Spatial (across the atria) and temporal heterogeneity of the latter two properties will further promote the creation of multiple re-entrant pathways (Figures 12.4–12.6).

More recently, it has been hypothesized that a single atrial focus (which could be a macro-re-entrant circuit, a micro-re-entrant circuit or an

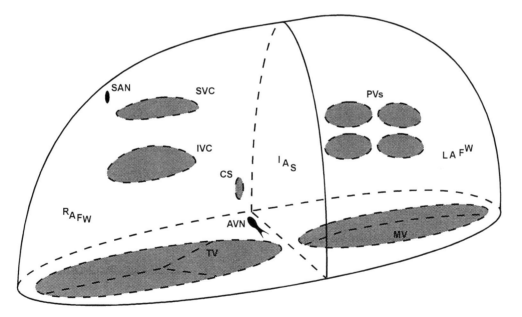

Figure 12.3
Schematic representation of the atria, demonstrating the anatomical obstacles which may facilitate re-entry. SVC superior vena cava, IVC inferior vena cava, CS coronary sinus, PVs pulmonary veins, TV tricuspid valve, MV mitral valve, IAS interatrial septum, LAFW left atrial free wall, RAFW right atrial free wall, SAN sinoatrial node, AVN atrioventricular node.

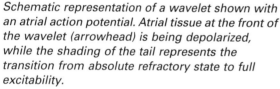

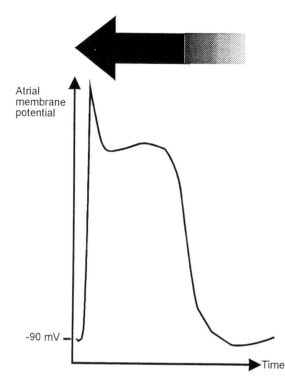

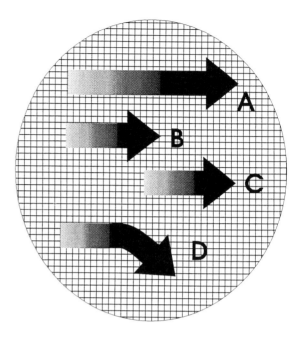

Figure 12.4
Schematic representation of a wavelet shown with an atrial action potential. Atrial tissue at the front of the wavelet (arrowhead) is being depolarized, while the shading of the tail represents the transition from absolute refractory state to full excitability.

Figure 12.5
Wavelets traversing atrial myocardium. (A) is normal. (B) is short because the atrial myocardium is slow-conducting (i.e. slow moving front). (C) is short because the atrial myocardium has a shorter refractory period (i.e. short tail). (D) is curved because the atrial myocardium has inhomogeneous conduction properties, with the tissue at its lower border being slow-conducting.

automatic focus) may create an ECG appearance identical to AF if there is inhomogeneous conduction through the rest of the atrium.[4] This is supported by experimental and human observations where regular, organized activity at relatively long cycle lengths (i.e. slow rates) can be documented in some regions of the atria, suggesting the existence of a 'mother' macro-re-entrant wavelet which continuously gives off daughter wavelets and sustains AF (Figure 12.7).[5,6] Recently the successful treatment of AF by limited radiofrequency ablation in three patients was reported.[7] In two of the patients there was a small focus responsible for

the AF, while the third required interruption of a macro-re-entrant circuit. Such limited lesions would not be expected to be effective according to the classic multiple wavelet theory, but at present it is uncertain if these novel findings represent isolated cases or if they are important in the genesis of AF in the wider population.

The onset and sustenance of AF are mediated by different electrophysiological abnormalities, illustrated by the existence of the distinct clinical subgroups. Those suffering from paroxysmal AF have atria prone to fibrillation but which sustain the arrhythmia poorly, whereas those with persistent AF may achieve long-term

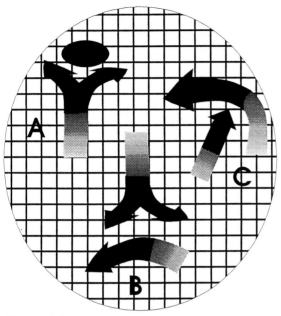

Figure 12.6
Behaviour of wavelets. (A) Wavelet dividing into two daughter wavelets on encountering a fixed obstacle (e.g. IVC oriface). (B) Wavelet dividing two daughter wavelets on encountering an area of refractory tissue left by another wavelet. (C) Wavelet extinguished by entering a 'cul-de-sac' of refractory tissue left by another wavelet.

restoration of SR with a single DC cardioversion and yet may never have reverted spontaneously.

Autonomic influences in AF

It has been proposed that paroxysmal AF is sometimes a disorder of autonomic tone.[8] There is a small subset of patients with paroxysmal AF that is vagally mediated.[9] The patients are typically male, in their 40s or 50s, do not have sinus node disease and are free from structural or coronary heart disease. Their episodes of paroxysmal AF last several hours and occur at times of high vagal tone, typically at night or after meals. In others, paroxysmal AF may be induced by high adrenergic tone, such as on waking, during exercise or periods of emotional stress. A predominance of adrenergic influences on the heart appears early in most forms of heart disease but, despite this, the adrenergically mediated variant is said to be less common than the former group.[9] However, these patients are more likely to have demonstrable cardiac disease.

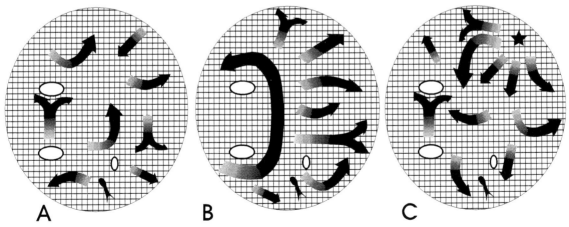

Figure 12.7
Possible mechanisms of AF. (A) Classic model of multiple wavelet re-entry. (B) AF sustained by a solitary mother wavelet, whose daughter wavelets exhibit chaotic conductance across the atria due to spatial and temporal inhomogeneity of conduction velocity and AERP. (C) AF sustained by a solitary focus in a similar way to (B). The focus may represent an automatic focus or a micro-re-entrant circuit.

The clinical role of the autonomic nervous system in the sustenance of AF has not been defined, but may be important as both increased sympathetic and parasympathetic tone shorten the refractory period of atrial pacemaker tissue,[10] and there is inhomogeneity of the distribution of vagal fibres over the atrial.[11]

Conditions predisposing to the onset of AF

A wide variety of acute illnesses predispose to the development of AF, and these are listed in Table 12.1. The mechanism varies and some conditions can induce the arrhythmia by several means. For example, in a patient with bronchopneumonia, the bacterial sepsis results in release of systemic toxins and increases myocardial work, but the bronchopneumonia can also cause hypoxia if it is severe, and a local pericarditis if it is adjacent to the heart.

Searching for and correcting these predisposing conditions form an important principle in the management of AF.

Conditions predisposing to the persistence of AF

The continuing presence of any of the conditions listed in Table 12.1 will make spontaneous reversion to SR, successful DC cardioversion, and the long-term maintenance of SR thereafter less likely. There are also clinical features that reduce the likelihood of long-term maintenance of SR, as listed in Table 12.2.

The duration of AF is now established as a powerful predictor of the likelihood of long-term maintenance of SR following cardioversion.[12–15] Changes in the electrophysiological properties of the atrial myocardium that may in part explain this phenomenon have recently been demonstrated in a goat model.[16] Episodes of induced AF lasting several days were associated with a reduction in the AERP and a maladaption of the AERP to changes in heart rate, both of which increase the stability of AF. Although interesting, these data leave many questions unanswered. The study only examined periods of AF lasting weeks and showed complete reversion to normal electrophysiological properties within days. Whether the severity of the abnormalities continued to evolve and

---

Myocardial disorders—myocardial infarction and ischaemia, myocarditis, cardiomyopathy, congestive heart failure, hypertrophy (due to hypertension, hypertrophic cardiomyopathy, etc.), cardiac surgery.
Conduction system disorders—sick sinus syndrome, intra-atrial conduction delay.
Irritation of the myocardium—intracardiac catheters, including central venous lines inadvertently advanced into the right atrium, pericarditis, adjacent pulmonary disorders (see below).
Valvular and congenital heart disease—particularly mitral stenosis.
Pulmonary disease—bronchopneumonia, pulmonary embolus, chronic airflow limitation, pulmonary fibrosis, carcinoma of the bronchus.
Endocrine disease—thyrotoxicosis, phaeochomocytoma.
Metabolic disturbance and toxins—electrolyte imbalance, alchohol.

Table 12.1
Illnesses and conditions predisposing to AF.

Persistence of any illness or condition responsible for onset of AF
Increasing duration of AF (especially >1 year)
Increasing age of patient
Left atrial enlargement (>42 mm), ventricular hypertrophy or ventricular dysfunction

Table 12.2
Clinical features predicting reduced likelihood of maintenance of SR after cardioversion.

whether it takes progressively longer for the atrial electrophysiology to revert to normal after more prolonged periods of AF is unknown, as is whether permanent changes in atrial electrophysiology occur. This information is required to explain why atria which have been in persistent AF for a month have a high likelihood of remaining in SR after DC cardioversion when compared with those in which AF has been present for 1 year. Indirect support for such changes comes from data showing that the time before return of mechanical atrial function, which varies from hours to months after cardioversion, is statistically related to the length of time that AF has been present,[17] but direct evidence is needed.

Atrial flutter

Unlike AF, atrial flutter (AFl) is mediated by a single macro-re-entrant circuit, which is stable and consistent (over time and between patients). In 'common AFl' (type I), the atrial rate is usually almost exactly 300 bpm unless the patient is on drugs which alter the atrial electrophysiology (e.g. Vaughan Williams class I anti-arrhythmic drugs). The impulse passes through a zone of slow conduction between the inferior vena cava and the atrioventricular node (AVN) and then around the right atrium. There is some debate as to whether the dominant route of depolarization is by encircling the caval orifices in a counterclockwise direction or by travelling clockwise around the triscuspid annulus. The rarer 'uncommon AFl' (type II) has a rate of 340–450 bpm and depolarization moves in a clockwise manner around the same circuit, or by a different circuit. Apart from the rate, the two may be distinguished by the precise morphology of the 'sawtooth' flutter waves in the inferior ECG leads. In common AFl they are characterized by a downsloping isoelectric portion, followed by a sharp downstroke and a less acute upstroke.

There is significant overlap with the population who suffer from AF, with some patients alternating between AF and AFl during episodes or between episodes of arrhythmia.

Sick sinus syndrome

The sick sinus syndrome (SSS) encompasses a number of clinical subgroups including sinus bradycardia, the 'tachy-brady' syndrome and sinus node chronotropic incompetence (i.e. failure of the heart rate to rise appropriately in response to stress). AF occurs commonly in this patient group, and the atrial electrophysiological abnormalities found in SSS are similar to those that may be found during SR in those who suffer from AF.

Pacing strategies in AF are discussed later, but it is important to emphasize the value of implanting an atrial or dual-chamber pacemaker in those with the SSS who require pacing. A number of studies have illustrated a reduction in subsequent permanent AF, stroke, heart failure and death in those whose atria are sensed and paced.[18-20] These studies suffered from treatment selection bias, but others using prospective randomization[21] or randomization by treatment centre[22] have confirmed reductions in all endpoints except mortality. When combined with an understanding of the electrophysiological advantages, there is ample evidence to support sensing and pacing the atrium routinely when pacing those with the SSS.

Why treat AF?

The goals of medical intervention in AF are reducing symptoms and improving prognosis, but this is made difficult by the sometimes subtle and nonspecific impact of the disease, and previously by a lack of knowledge regarding the long-term risks. It is important to review the treatment strategy from time to time to ensure that the regimen matches the evolving status of the atrial arrhythmia.

Symptoms

AF is usually perceived as fast, irregular palpitations but some patients do not notice the irregularity, and some are not aware at all of a change in their cardiac rhythm. In some, the predominant cause of palpitations is an intermittent large pulse volume following a long ventricular cycle. These long cycles may instead cause dizziness or syncope if they are very prolonged or if cardiac reserve is poor.

Patients may complain of a wide range of nonspecific symptoms, and exercise capacity is often significantly reduced. These symptoms result from a heart rate which is rapid, irregular and less responsive to physiological control, and because the loss of atrial systole reduces ventricular filling and cardiac output drops. In those with ischaemic heart disease, myocardial oxygen requirement is increased by the high

Variable	Relative risk (RR)
Age $\leq$ 60 years	1.0
Age 61–75 years	1.0
Age $\geq$ 76 years	1.3
History of hypertension	2.6
Duration of AF $\geq$1 year	0.7
Intermittent AF	0.9
Definite history of congestive cardiac failure	1.9
Recent congestive cardiac failure	3.2
Previous thromboembolism	2.7
Ischaemic heart disease	1.1

Table 12.3
Features associated with an increased risk for thromboembolism (using univariate analysis). When subjected to multivariate analysis, only a history of hypertension (RR 2.2), previous thromboembolism (RR 2.1) and recent congestive cardiac failure (RR 2.6) proved to be independent predictors of events. In those with none of these risk factors the event rate was 2.5% per year and these occurred exclusively in those older than 60 years. Modified from The Stroke Prevention in Atrial Fibrillation Investigators. Predictors of thromboembolism in atrial fibrillation: I. Clinical features of patients at risk. Ann Intern Med (1992) 116:1–5.[33]

heart rate, but coronary blood flow does not rise by the same amount. This imbalance is worsened by the increased heart rate reducing the net amount of time for diastolic coronary flow. Finally, there is evidence to suggest that AF itself induces left ventricular dysfunction.[23]

In some, AF may have apparently little or no symptomatic impact, particularly if it begins during an intercurrent illness. However, reversion to SR may still be associated with a marked improvement in general wellbeing and a retrospective awareness of previous limitations.

Sequelae

Thromboembolism

AF significantly increases the risk of systemic thromboembolism. This manifests principally as cerebral emboli, although limb and mesenteric emboli may also occur. The emboli arise from the fibrillating left atrium, and particularly the auricular appendage.[24–27] AF is associated with a six-fold rise in the incidence of stroke,[28] and the risk is increased even more if the patient also has mitral stenosis (relative risk 17-times controls),[29] heart failure or hypertension (both associated with a twelve-fold increase).[30] Readers are referred to a previous chapter from this series[31] for a more detailed discussion (*see also* Table 12.3). Recent large trials, recruiting a combined total of almost 4000 patients, have demonstrated a reduction of the risk of thromboembolism by two-thirds if patients are anticoagulated.[32]

For each patient a risk versus benefit calculation of anticoagulation is needed, and a decision whether or not to anticoagulate should be made in partnership with the patient following a full explanation of the pros and cons of treatment. It should be borne in mind that any underlying disease (valvular disorders, valve prostheses and dilated cardiomyopathy) may itself confer high thromboembolic risk and may justify long-term

anticoagulation irrespective of the outcome of the patient's AF. The decision must be regularly reviewed, especially in the light of any change in the patient's clinical circumstances. Having said all this, almost all with persistent or permanent AF and a significant proportion of those with paroxysmal AF should be anticoagulated.

Aspirin provides some protection, but is not as effective as formal anticoagulation with warfarin and does not provide adequate protection for those at significant risk.[34] Deciding the optimal intensity of anticoagulation has previously been complicated by the differing intensities of therapy having been used in different studies, and a lack of uniformity in the method of measuring prothrombin ratios between countries.[32] In a recently completed study the combination of anticoagulation at a target level of INR 1.2–1.5 with aspirin was associated with an incidence of stroke four-times higher than those treated with full anticoagulation.[35] Therefore, the balance of evidence now strongly suggests that for patients without other relevant disorders, an INR of 2.0–3.0 is optimal.[36] Careful control of anticoagulation therapy is important as it reduces haemorrhagic complications and increases the cost effectiveness of the treatment.[37]

Deterioration in ventricular function

Tachycardia-induced cardiomyopathy, reversible by successful reversion to SR or improved rate control, has been documented in those with AF,[38–41] as well as with SVT[42–46] and VT.[47–49] AF may therefore have a far more important effect on ventricular function than is currently appreciated. Patients presenting with heart failure and AF are usually assumed to have developed AF because of the heart failure and not the other way around. This is often despite there being no direct evidence for another cause of heart failure. In this situation, restoration of sinus rhythm is usually not considered feasible because of the heart failure and the duration of the AF, and sometimes monitoring of rate control is patchy. Even in those who have had careful rate control, ventricular function may improve following restoration of SR.[23] It may be that it is the irregularity of the heart rhythm which is responsible for this phenomenon, but at present the true magnitude of the problem and the mechanisms involved are unclear. Concern regarding the long-term impact on ventricular function does provide a powerful argument for the careful assessment, appropriate investigation and consideration of cardioversion for all patients discovered to have AF, including those who are apparently asymptomatic.

The onset of AF in those with pre-existing severe cardiac disease may be associated with a significant clinical deterioration. This is not unexpected as the adverse haemodynamic changes of AF will affect those with low reserves of cardiac function more severely. Although many of the features which adversely affect the chance of long-term success may be present, attempted restoration of SR should still be considered.

The management of different subgroups of AF

Acute AF

The management of patients with new-onset AF presents different priorities, risks and modes of treatment from those used for patients with chronic AF. The cut-off for new-onset AF is arbitrarily designated as 48-hours' duration, because AF is becoming less easy to convert and the risk of thromboembolism rises significantly around this time. Patients are often sufficiently symptomatic to need hospital admission. Severe haemodynamic compromise may ensue if the heart rate is rapid (for example, those

with Wolff-Parkinson-White syndrome or a short atrioventricular node refractory period), or the patient relies on atrial systole for ventricular filling (for example, those with mitral stenosis or hypertrophic cardiomyopathy). Whether or not this is the first episode of AF is immaterial to the immediate management, but consideration must be given separately to the longer-term management at a later stage if the AF does not terminate, recurs or has been present previously.

Whether and when to cardiovert

These decisions are dependent upon whether the underlying cause of the AF has been corrected (which will influence the risk of recurrence), the haemodynamic status of the patient, and the perceived likelihood of spontaneous reversion to SR. Unless haemodynamic collapse is present, observation for some hours with continuous ECG monitoring is advisable. This allows completion of relevant investigations, ensures that AF is sustained rather than occurring in paroxysms, and allows an opportunity for spontaneous reversion to SR. Detection of intermittent paroxysms of AF makes electrical cardioversion inappropriate.

During this period, rate control with intravenous or oral preparations of verapamil, diltiazem or beta blockers may be given. None of these is particularly effective in cardioverting AF on their own, although intravenous esmolol (an intravenous beta blocker with a very short half life) is effective in up to 50% of cases.[50] Digoxin has a significantly slower onset of action than other agents (median of 5.5 hours,[51] compared with less than 1 hour for agents such as intravenous diltiazem),[52] is ineffective in effecting cardioversion (efficacy no better than placebo),[51] and carries a small risk of proarrhythmia at DC cardioversion. However, as digoxin lacks negative inotropic actions, it may be safer in those with left ventricular impairment. Intravenous amiodarone via a central line is a valuable second-line agent for rate control in complex or resistant cases, and also has a high probability of effecting cardioversion. If the Wolff–Parkinson–White syndrome is suspected (rapid ventricular response rate, broad ventricular complexes), digoxin and verapamil should be avoided in view of the danger of the acceleration of ventricular rate[53,54] which causes haemodynamic deterioration and can lead to ventricular fibrillation. Flecainide and procainide, amongst others, provide a safe and effective alternative, or else electrical cardioversion can be used.

If any predisposing factors are not immediately correctable then limited attempts to restore SR may still be appropriate, but if AF recurs, rate control and thromboembolic prophylaxis should be pursued instead. Common examples of this scenario are following myocardial infarction or cardiac surgery, when the risks associated with many of the available antiarrhythmic drugs are particularly high. In these populations spontaneous reversion to SR often occurs as the myocardium heals over the following weeks, but otherwise patients can receive elective cardioversion at that stage.

What method for cardioversion?

If AF results in haemodynamic collapse then the best treatment is cardioversion by DC shock (under light general anaesthesia if still conscious). Usually, however, the patient feels unwell and is light-headed on exertion, but is not severely compromised at rest. In this setting, chemical cardioversion has several practical and theoretical advantages over DC shock. It avoids the inconvenience, discomfort and small risk associated with a general anaesthetic and DC shock. Antiarrhythmic drugs may, by their continued presence in the circulation, reduce the chance of early reversion to AF, but direct comparative data are absent. The delivery of electrical energy to the atria may theoretically cause endothelial disruption, and spontaneous echocardiographic contrast (sometimes called 'smoke', and a putative precursor of thrombus formation) has been documented following DC shock.[55,56] Transient impairment of left atrial appendage function[55] has been demonstrated—this site is thought to be the origin of most emboli—but only preliminary comparative studies with chemical cardioversion are available.[57,58] It is currently unclear whether DC cardioversion confers a higher risk of

Drug	Success rate in cardioversion/comments
Esmolol	Moderate (50%).[50] Short acting, safe in acute ischaemia. Good if high adrenergic tone
Verapamil	Poor (10%)[50]
Digoxin	Poor (no better than placebo)[51]
Propafanone	Moderate[59]
Flecainide	Good[59–61]
Amiodarone	Good,[62,63] but requires central line
Disopyramide	Moderate[64]

Table 12.4
Efficacy of drugs in cardioverting AF. Trials used different study populations and management protocols, making direct comparisons between drugs inappropriate.

thromboembolism than spontaneous or chemical cardioversion.

All patients should be considered for chemical cardioversion, but the choice of agent and route will depend on the clinician's preference, as well as familiarity with the different available agents (Table 12.4). Ibutalide is a new drug that will soon be licensed for use in the UK. It has novel electrophysiological effects and appears to be more efficacious than current agents, particularly for the cardioversion of AFl. Both chemical and electrical cardioversion carry a small risk of proarrhythmic events and bradycardia, particularly if electrolytes have not been corrected or shocks are not properly synchronized, and should therefore only be performed where appropriate resuscitation equipment is available.

Minimizing the risk of thromboembolism
A very low thromboembolic risk exists when AF has been present for only a few hours, but when it has persisted for several months anticoagulation is required for 1 month prior to cardioversion. Between these two extremes is a spectrum of increasing risk which must be assessed and managed carefully. An increased thromboembolic risk probably begins to appear as early as 12–24 hours, and certainly after 2 days a period of formal anticoagulation becomes mandatory. Not all subgroups are at equal risk, with higher rates of thromboembolism being apparent in those with structural heart disease. Transoesophageal echocardiography (TOE) can be a useful tool in risk-stratifying patients but emboli may still occur despite a negative study.[65] A common feature of those who experienced emboli in this series was the lack of thromboembolic prophylaxis, and the conclusion that can probably be drawn is that a negative TOE can allow earlier cardioversion but does not obviate the need for anticoagulation.

If heparin is begun within 24 hours of the onset of AF, cardioversion may be safely performed in uncomplicated cases. Heparin should be continued for 12 hours after cardioversion of any prolonged episode of AF, and a period of 3–4 weeks of oral anticoagulation should be considered if the patient has clinical features to suggest very high embolic risk. If there are features that indicate a high risk of recurrence of the AF, 3 months of anticoagulation is preferable, as more than 80% of recurrences occur within that time period.

Paroxysmal AF

Management of incidentally discovered and minimally symptomatic paroxysmal AF
Asymptomatic episodes of paroxysmal AF, sometimes prolonged, are seen relatively frequently on Holter recordings done for other purposes. Even in patients who suffer from symptomatic paroxysmal AF, only one-twelfth of episodes lasting more than 30 seconds are symptomatic.[66] There is little justification for antiarrhythmic, ventricular rate limiting or antithrombotic treatment in incidentally discovered paroxysmal AF. An important caveat to this statement is that paroxysmal AF must not account for atypical symptoms such as episodic weakness and lethargy, or be causing sequelae in the absence of symptoms by exacerbating heart failure or causing emboli. Silent cerebral infarction may be found in 15–48% of patients with AF,[67–70] underlining the need for awareness.

Even if a patient is symptomatic, lifestyle modifications including avoidance of stimulants such as caffeine, and of alcohol, should be used before instituting treatment. This is particularly true if episodes are infrequent, well tolerated or have a clear avoidable precipitant. Simple reassurance about the relatively benign nature of the disorder may be all that is required for some patients.

Approach to management of those requiring treatment

When planning the treatment of a patient, several strategies are available. The symptomatic impact of paroxysmal AF may be lessened by reducing the frequency of episodes or by minimizing the symptomatic impact of each episode. The latter objective may be achieved by preventing fast ventricular response rates during attacks, by regularizing the rhythm or by reducing the duration of attacks. The issues of preventing thromboembolism and deterioration of ventricular function also need to be considered, and may be a priority in some patients. These goals may now be accomplished by pharmacological and nonpharmacological means, as well as the lifestyle interventions mentioned above and the treatment of underlying predisposing conditions.

Drug treatment

If antiarrhythmic therapy is required, a wide range of effective agents are available, including Vaughan Williams class Ia agents (disopyramide[71] and quinidine[72]), class Ic agents (flecainide[73] and propafenone[74]), sotalol[75] (a beta blocker with class III activity) and amiodarone[76] (conventionally a class III agent but has multiple antiarrhythmic actions). The initial choice of agent is somewhat empirical, and dependent on which agents the clinician has practical experience with, but it must also take into account the features of the AF in specific patients. Those with paroxysmal AF occurring at times of high vagal tone will be excellent candidates for drugs with vagolytic effects, for example, disopyramide and quinidine. Conversely, those with structural heart disease or a clear pattern of adrenergic onset are more likely to benefit from beta blockers and propa-

fenone (which has some class II activity). In resistant cases, amiodarone can be a highly efficacious agent although its first-line use is usually precluded by photosensitivity and other side effects, and the long-term risk of thyroid dysfunction. Pulmonary fibrosis, the most feared complication of amiodarone, occurs occasionally as a hypersensitivity reaction after only a few tablets, but the risk of the usual form is dependent on the cumulative dose received and therefore can be minimized by using the lowest effective dose (200 mg daily, and sometimes as low as 50 mg/day).

Rate control during episodes usually takes a secondary place to the prevention of episodes since it requires the use of a second drug, but sotalol and amiodarone offer both properties. Acceleration of the ventricular response rate due to vagolytic effects or effects on AV nodal conduction may occur with disopyramide and quinidine. If the rhythm is converted to AFl by the antiarrhythmic agent, the flutter rate may also be slowed to a degree which allows 1:1 conduction of the atrial rhythm to the ventricle, causing a sudden increase of the ventricular rate and cardiovascular collapse.[77] In this situation, the use of an alternative drug is usually indicated, but if the agent is otherwise highly efficacious it may occasionally be appropriate to continue the current drug and add a rate limiting agent.

Nonpharmacological treatments
Pacing strategies
Atrial pacing may reduce the frequency of episodes of paroxysmal AF by several mechanisms. Increasing the atrial rate will reduce the frequency of atrial ectopic beats; it may also lessen their ability to initiate re-entry. Depolarization of the atria in a different direction may reduce the chance of initiating re-entrant circuits by avoiding anatomical obstacles and areas of electrophysiologically abnormal tissue near the

sinoatrial node. Finally, if paroxysmal AF is vagally mediated, atrial pacing provides improved symptomatic control.[9]

The optimal pacing mode in active patients for this indication is AAIR (rate responsive pacing of the atria, with no ventricular lead), unless the patient has coexistent AVN conduction disease. However, many clinicians prefer to implant a dual-chamber unit particularly if the patient may be a candidate for AV nodal ablation at a later stage. The baseline rate which does not cause symptoms yet reduces the likelihood of AF varies, but often lies between 70 and 90 beats per minute. The rate adapation algorithm should be programmed to ensure that the pacemaker rate exceeds the sinus rate at most times, although this is sometimes not tolerated. Drug therapy may be reduced or withdrawn, but the feasibility of this will be dependent on clinical circumstances. Implantation of a pacemaker also widens the range of agents available, if their use had previously been precluded by symptomatic bradycardia. At present pacing is used principally for those patients with paroxysmal AF in the context of SSS, but should be considered in other cases.

Pacing using two atrial leads has been proposed as a strategy to stabilize the atria in those with intra-atrial conduction delay, which manifests on the surface ECG as increased P-wave duration and abnormal morphology. The theoretical basis of this approach is to ensure that the entire atrial surface is rapidly depolarized, rendering the atria refractory to ectopic automatic firing and wavefronts emerging from areas of slow conduction. The initial results have been encouraging,[78] and larger studies are underway.

Surgery
The realization that macro-re-entry is the mechanism of AF has led to the development of surgical treatment for chronic AF. The 'maze operation' involves surgical division and reconstruction of the atria along predetermined lines (Figure 12.8). The aim is the creation of permanent barriers to conduction, forcing depolarization along narrow pathways leading away from the sinus node, none of which are otherwise interconnected and all of which are too narrow to allow re-entry. The follow-up[79] has shown this procedure to be highly successful, but complicated by substantial morbidity such as sinus node dysfunction (40% of postoperative patients require atrial pacing) and postoperative complications. Currently, it cannot be recommended unless all other treatment modalities fail and the patient remains highly symptomatic.

Techniques involving catheter ablation
AVN ablation with implantation of a mode-switching dual-chamber pacemaker has been used as a strategy for treating patients with drug-resistant paroxysmal AF, and has also been employed for other paroxysmal atrial arrhythmias such as ectopic atrial tachycardia. The creation of complete AVN block by nodal ablation makes the ventricle dependent on the pacemaker for transmission of atrial signals. The pacemaker is programmed with algorithms which attempt to determine whether the atrial electrical activity represents SR or a tachyarrhythmia. In the former situation it will pace in dual-chamber mode, but upon detecting an arrhythmia it will 'mode switch' to rate-responsive ventricular pacing (VVIR). When the sensed atrial signals suggest a return to SR, dual-chamber pacing is reinstituted. This approach appears to be highly successful in selected cases, but is not undertaken lightly as it renders the patient dependent upon a pacemaker for life.

Radiofrequency ablation is now used to treat atrial flutter and ectopic atrial tachycardias, and

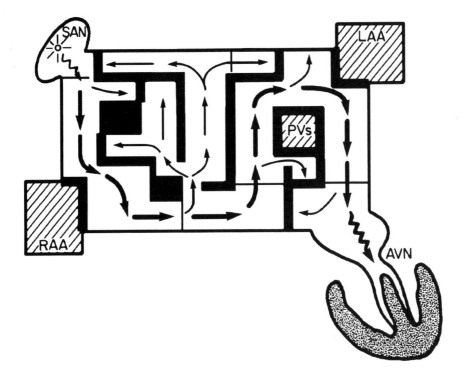

Figure 12.8
Surgical incisions made during the 'maze procedure'. SAN sinoatrial node, LAA left atrial appendage, PVs pulmonary veins, AVN atrioventricular node, RAA right atrial appendage. Reprinted with permission of the Futura Publishing Company.

may eventually become clinically feasible in AF. The procedure has been termed the 'catheter maze procedure', but the lines created do not attempt to recreate the surgical maze. Thus far Haissaguerre and colleagues have employed lines of punctate lesions predominantly in the right atrium,[80] while Swartz[81] has created linear burns mainly in the left atrium. Initial results are encouraging but at present the procedure is lengthy and difficult, and it is too early to judge what its role will be.

Atrial defibrillators

Over the last few years, implantable cardioverter defibrillators have become accepted treatment for malignant ventricular arrhythmias in appropriate cases. An atrial implantable defibrillator is currently undergoing clinical trials and other devices are under development. At present, devices are programmed not to work in automatic mode and shocks are somewhat painful, but initial experience suggest the device is safe and effective.

Persistent AF

Persistent AF refers to patients who remain in AF for more than 48 hours but are still capable of conversion to SR. Whether or not the patient has suffered from previous episodes of AF influences the management strategy and, in conjunction with the other clinical features and the patient's own preferences, determines how far to pursue attempts to restore SR.

Who should be cardioverted? Differentiating persistent and permanent AF

The most difficult decision in the management of patients presenting with persistent AF is to decide who has a high probability of long-term restoration of SR, and who has developed AF as an end-stage result of progressive structural and electrophysiological changes in the heart and is destined to remain in AF even if subjected to aggressive intervention.

The decision on how far to pursue restoration of SR must be made in consultation with the patient. It is determined by balancing the likelihood of success (*see* Table 12.2) and the benefits that will accrue from the restoration of SR, against the risks and inconvenience involved in trying (Table 12.5). Although attempting restoration of SR is inconvenient in the short term, it should be remembered that permanent AF requires lifelong treatment, and that the best opportunity to restore SR is soon after the onset of AF.

Protocol for anticoagulation and cardioversion

Published recommendations[36] suggest that patients should be anticoagulated (INR 2.0–3.0) for at least 3 weeks before and 1 month after cardioversion. The duration following cardioversion is based upon the average time until return of atrial mechanical systole, which is presumed to reflect an increased thromboembolic risk. However, this is not the sole issue when deciding management of a patient. AF has a significant risk of recurrence in the months following cardioversion, and the duration of anticoagulation should be calculated on a pragmatic basis, assessing when the inconvenience of continuing will not longer be justified by the reducing risk of recurrence. Since most recurrences occur within the first 3 months, this is a reasonable compromise for an 'average' patient, with a shorter period being appropriate if an underlying condition has been corrected or there is an increased risk of bleeding. Equally, a longer duration should be considered if there have been previous episodes of AF.

If AF has persisted for more than 1 week DC shock is generally used without attempting chemical cardioversion as drugs have a low cardioversion rate (with the possible exception of amiodarone).[82,83] Cardioversion is performed under general anaesthesia with full resuscitation equipment, including emergency pacing facilities, on hand (though these are needed very infrequently if safe practice is followed). Synchronized DC shocks are delivered at energies starting at 200 J and progressing immediately to 360 J if unsuccessful. More energy is delivered to the atria if an anteroposterior

Favouring attempting restoration of SR	Favouring accepting AF
Feel better, with improved exercise tolerance	No proarrhythmic risk from drugs
Eventual withdrawal of anticoagulation, antiarrhythmic and rate-limiting drugs	Avoid inconvenience and discomfort associated with hospitalization and general anaesthetic
No risk of AF-related myocardial dysfunction	May be eventual outcome anyway

Table 12.5
Factors that influence the decision of whether to attempt cardioversion of AF. Applicability of each of these varies between patients and with time.

(AP) field (with a paddle placed at the apex and the other to the right of the fourth thoracic vertebra) is utilized, and is therefore preferred if a backpaddle is available. If not, the patient should be rolled to allow an AP shock before abandoning the procedure if the sternum-apex shocks have failed. A minor degree of soreness over the paddle sites may occur despite good electrical contact, and usually no more than four shocks should be delivered. If the patient has been on digoxin it is conventionally discontinued 48 hours prior to cardioversion, but so long as the patient is not hypokalaemic or digitoxic, the risk of proarrhythmia is actually very small.

If DC cardioversion fails then patients should either be pretreated with antiarrhythmic drugs (usually amiodarone) before a further attempt, or referred for internal cardioversion. Internal cardioversion is performed using either a field between an electrode in the right atrium and one in the coronary sinus, when energies of 1–20 J are required,[84] or using a right atrial lead with an external paddle, where the required energy is comparable to standard external cardioversion.[85] Success rates are much higher than for external cardioversion, and the technique is particularly valuable in obese patients in whom it is difficult to deliver transthoracic electrical energy to the heart.[86] Obviously, the technique does not affect the chance of subsequent recurrence of AF.

Drug treatment—when, with what, and for whom?

Some 25% of patients remain free from recurrence of AF at 12 months without antiarrhythmic drug treatment,[72] and they are therefore unnecessary after a first episode of AF. Also, if AF recurs only at intervals of 1 year or more, many patients will wisely opt for occasional daycase cardioversion rather than take daily prophylactic drug treatment. However, antiar-

rhythmic drug treatment is usually indicated when AF becomes recurrent, and is also required when the initial cardioversion fails.

General guidelines for drug prophylaxis are given in Figure 12.2. As with other aspects of the management of AF, a wide range of antiarrhythmic agents have been shown to be effective. Using serial drug therapy and repeated cardioversion, 65% of patients may be maintained in SR for 2 years following cardioversions, at an expense of a mean of 1.8 DC cardioversions.[87] The patient population that develops persistent AF is older and more likely to have structural heart disease than those previously discussed. This heightens concern about potential proarrhythmic effects of treatment, which has been focused by data such as the meta-analysis of the efficacy of quinidine in preventing recurrence of AF following cardioversion.[72] Although quinidine reduced the rate of recurrence, it was also associated with a significant excess in total mortality.

Nonpharmacological strategies

Most of the techniques discussed under the 'nonpharmacologial strategies' subheading of the section on paroxysmal AF are equally applicable to recurrent persistent AF. Many of the relevant trials have recruited patients with both diagnoses, and this reflects the indistinct boundary between the two.

Permanent AF

If AF recurs repeatedly despite medical intervention, the physician and patient may agree that it is appropriate to abandon further attempts to restore SR. Similarly, if a patient is elderly, immobile and asymptomatic, or has an illness that limits life expectancy, the benefit of restoration of SR may not justify the inconvenience involved. Finally, AF that has been present for many years has a low likelihood of successful long-term reversion to SR, and cardioversion is only justified if there is a strong indication.

In all the above scenarios the goal of treatment has changed to minimizing the symptomatic impact of AF and reducing the risk of complications. Anticoagulation has already been discussed, leaving the issue of optimal rate control to improve symptoms and prevent tachycardia-induced cardiomyopathy.

Rate control
Drug treatments
Digoxin has been the agent traditionally used for this purpose, yet controls rate poorly during exercise (Figure 12.9). In view of this lack of efficacy, some have suggested that it should no longer be considered a first-line agent.[88] Numerous studies have shown improved rate control with diltiazem, verapamil and beta blockers. This has generally been paralleled by an improvement in exercise capacity and

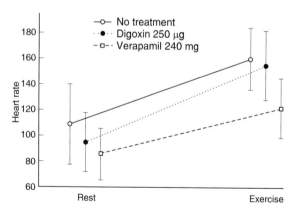

Figure 12.9
*Effect of digoxin and verapamil on heart rate at rest and during exercise. Note that although digoxin lowers heart rate at rest, during exercise it does not differ significantly from no treatment at all.
Modified from Lang RM et al, Superiority of oral verapamil therapy to digoxin in treatment of chronic atrial fibrillation,* Chest *(1983)* **83**:491–9.[89]

maximal oxygen uptake in the case of the two calcium channel antagonists, but not with beta blockers. To date, no studies have addressed the long-term effects of the different agents on outcomes such as left ventricular function.

In order to maximize compliance and minimize the impact of treatment on daily life, single-agent therapy and a once or twice daily dosing are preferred where possible. Alternatives include digoxin, sustained-release preparations of verapamil and diltiazem, and a range of agents with beta blocking activity. The choice of agent for particular patients must be tailored to their requirements. The principal issues are the quality of the rate control, the risk reduction for that patient and the side effect profile. Often, younger patients may tolerate one of the calcium channel antagonist best, whereas someone who has ischaemic heart disease would derive prognostic benefit from a beta blocker. Those who are inactive may achieve acceptable rate control with digoxin, and in those with significant left ventricular dysfunction the positive inotropic effect may be an advantage. In the latter group, the fact that digoxin has not been shown to provide a mortality benefit in a recent randomized trial including 7788 patients (Digitalis Investigators Group, personal communication), whereas the evidence in favour of beta blockers is accumulating,[90] should be remembered before making a decision. The use of combination therapy may be required to achieve adequate rate control, or if high-dose single-agent therapy is precluded by side effects. Amiodarone is also effective for rate control,[82] and because of its lack of negative inotropic action, may be helpful in those intolerant of other agents. An alternative in this situation and in other resistant cases are the nonpharmacological approaches discussed below.

Nonpharmacological treatment

Catheter radiofrequency ablation may be used in two separate ways for rate control in AF. The first technique is called AV nodal modification, and involves the creation of lesions in the region posteroinferior to the compact AV node in the right atrium. This is where the 'slow pathway' lies in those with dual AV nodal physiology (i.e. those who suffer from AV nodal re-entrant tachycardia), and the technique has been shown to provide rate control in those previously refractory to medical treatment.[91] There is some evidence to support the idea that a slow pathway is being ablated, but this is as yet unproven. (The adjective 'slow' appears paradoxical but actually refers to the conduction velocity of the pathway. Its refractory period is short and so it conducts more impulses per minute than the fast pathway.) The theoretical risk of inadvertent high-degree AV block is small since the burns are remote from the compact AV node, and this is borne out by initial experience. The other alternative is deliberately to ablate the AV node and implant a rate-responsive ventricular pacemaker. This has the advantage of creating a regular ventricular response rate and preventing symptomatic ventricular pauses, but at the expense of rendering the patient pacemaker dependent.

A surgical solution is the 'corridor operation', which allows preservation of sinus node control over ventricular rate. This operation involves surgically creating a corridor of atrial tissue running from the sinoatrial node to the AV node. In contrast to the maze procedure, the majority of the atrial mass is rendered electrically isolated and allowed to continue to fibrillate. If the original substrate for AF was SSS the operation is not worthwhile, but this may not always be apparent preoperatively.

Special considerations in the management of the elderly

The perception of many doctors of AF simply as an ageing phenomenon was alluded to in the introduction, but it should be remembered that the impact is by no means more benign.

Side effects of rate-limiting and antiarrhythmic drugs are more common in the elderly due to their reduced lean body mass, slower drug metabolism, and higher incidence of hepatic and renal impairment. Polypharmacy is more common, and increases the risk of drug interactions. The frequency of cardiac dysfunction rises with age, heightening concern regarding proarrhythmic events from prophylactic antiarrhythmic drugs. For these reasons, as well as the reduced likelihood that long-term side effects will become an issue, amiodarone deserves earlier consideration than it receives in younger patients.

The risk of haemorrhagic complications with anticoagulation increases significantly with age but so does the risk of stroke, and the decision of whether treatment is in the patient's interest can be particularly difficult for older patients. Relative contraindications include frequent falls, cognitive impairment which may hinder safe administration of the drug and logistic considerations, such as difficulty in travelling to the GP or anticoagulant clinic. For the fit and active elderly patient there is no doubt that anticoagulation is indicated, but for others a very careful risk versus benefit analysis is required.

If I had . . .

If I had atrial fibrillation, I would want to know that my physician had made a careful assessment of my overall cardiac and medical condition before deciding what management plan to pursue.

First, I would want to know the cause of my AF, and whether any adverse effects were present. A careful history would help, and might give some guide to possible later treatment. Next would come physical examination and appropriate investigations. The latter would start with a 12-lead ECG to confirm that I am in AF and not simply having frequent atrial or ventricular extrasystoles, and also to look for other features such as evidence of recent or remote myocardial infarction, myocardial ischaemia or left ventricular hypertrophy. Subsequent investigations would depend on my circumstances and past history, but a full blood count, serum electrolytes, thyroid function tests, a 24-hour ECG, a transthoracic echocardiogram, and a chest X-ray are mandatory.

With this information available I would like to discuss how to minimize the impact of AF on my current and long-term quality of life and health. I would hope that sinus rhythm might be restored and maintained, and would like to know what combination of lifestyle changes, drug and nonpharmacological strategies my physician thought appropriate.

I should be aware that despite the best treatment, there remains a significant risk that I may end up in permanent AF. In this eventuality, I would insist that my heart rate was monitored by Holter or exercise electrocardiography, and controlled using a simple regime of one or more drugs.

I would want to discuss the benefits and risks of anticoagulation, but would not be surprised if it were strongly recommended to me.

As my clinical course evolved, I might be exposed to tiered treatment strategies, possibly even culminating in a pacemaker implantation or a radiofrequency ablation procedure. The goals of my treatment may also change, and I hope that my physician would ask me what I wanted from treatment as we reached each new hurdle.

References

1   Bialy D, Lehmann MH, Schumacher DN, Steinman RT, Meissner MD, Hospitalization for arrhythmias in the United States: importance of atrial fibrillation, *J Am Coll Cardiol* (1992)**19**:41A (abstr).

2   Moe GK, On the multiple wavelet hypothesis of atrial fibrillation, *Arch Int Pharmcodyn Ther* (1962)**140**:183–8.

3   Allessie MA, Bonke FIM, Schopman FJG, Circus movement in rabbit atrial muscle as a mechanism of tachycardia. III. The 'leading circle' concept: a new model of circus movement in cardiac tissue without the involvement of an anatomical obstacle, *Circ Res* (1977)**41**:9–18.

4   Cox JL, Schuessler RB, Boineau JP, The surgical treatment of atrial fibrillation. I. Summary of the current concepts of the mechanisms of atrial flutter and atrial fibrillation, *J Thorac Cardiovasc Surg* (1991)**101**:402–5.

5   Cox JL, Canavan TE, Schuessler RB et al, The surgical treatment of atrial fibrillation. II. Intraoperative electrophysiologic mapping and description of the electrophysiologic basis of atrial flutter and atrial fibrillation, *J Thorac Cardiovasc Surg* (1991)**101**:406–26.

6   Ferguson TB Jr, Schuessler RB, Hand DE, Boineau JP, Cox JL, Lessons learned from computerized mapping of the atrium. Surgery for atrial fibrillation and atrial flutter, *J Electrocardiol* (1993)**26(suppl)**:210–19.

7   Haissaguerre M, Marcus FI, Fischer B, Clementy J, Radiofrequency catheter ablation in unusual mechanisms of atrial fibrillation: report of three cases, *J Cardiovasc Electrophysiol* (1994)**5**:743–51.

8   Coumel P, Paroxysmal atrial fibrillation: a disorder of autonomic tone? *Eur Heart J* (1994)**15**:9–16.

9   Coumel P, Neural aspects of paroxysmal atrial fibrillation. In: Falk RH, Podrid PJ, eds. *Atrial fibrillation: mechanisms and management* (Raven Press: New York, 1992)109–25.

10 Hutter OF, Trauwein W, Vagal and sympathetic effects on the pacemaker fibres in the sinus venosus of the heart. *J Gen Physiol* (1956)**39**:715–33.

11 Ninomiya I, Direct evidence of nonuniform distribution of vagal effects on dog atria, *Circ Res* (1966)**19**:576–83.

12 Bjerkelund C, Orning OM, An evaluation of DC shock treatment for atrial fibrillation, *Acta Med Scand* (1968)**184**:481–91.

13 Waris E, Kreus K, Salokannel J, Factors influencing the persistence of sinus rhythm after DC shock treatment of atrial fibrillation, *Acta Med Scand* (1971)**189**:161–6.

14 Van Gelder IC, Crijns HJ, van Gilst WH, Verwer R, Lie KI, Prediction of uneventful cardioversion and maintenance of sinus rhythm from direct-current electrical cardioversion of chronic atrial fibrillation and flutter, *Am J Cardiol* (1991)**68**:41–6.

15 Morris JJJ, Peter RH, McIntosh HD, Electrical cardioversion of atrial fibrillation: immediate and long term results and selection of patients, *Ann Intern Med* (1966)**65**:216–31.

16 Wijffels MCEF, Kirchhof CJHJ, Dorland R, Allessie MA, Atrial fibrillation begets atrial fibrillation: a study in awake chronically instrumented goats, *Circulation* (1995)**92**:1954–68.

17 Shapiro EP, Effron MB, Lima S, Ouyang P, Siu CO, Bush D, Transient atrial dysfunction after conversion of chronic atrial fibrillation to sinus rhythm, *Am J Cardiol* (1988)**62**:1202–7.

18 Markewitz A, Schad N, Hemmer W, Bernheim C, Ciavolella M, Weinhold C, What is the most appropriate stimulation mode in patients with sinus node dysfunction? *Pacing Clin Electrophysiol* (1986)**9**:1115–20.

19 Hesselson AB, Parsonette V, Perry G, Progression to atrial fibrillation from the DDD, DVI and VVI packing modes, *Pacing Clin Electrophysiol* (1990)**13**:564 (abstr).

20 Stangl K, Seitz K, Wirtzfeld A et al, Difference between atrial single chamber pacing (AAI) and ventricular single chamber pacing (VVI) with respect to prognosis and antiarrhythmic effect

in patients with sick sinus syndrome, *Pacing Clin Electrophysiol* (1990)**13**:2080–5.

21 Andersen HR, Thuesen L, Bagger JP, Vesterlund T, Thomsen PEB, Prospective randomized trial of atrial versus ventricular pacing in sick-sinus syndrome, *Lancet* (1994)**344**:1523-8.

22 Rosenqvist M, Brandt J, Schuller H, Long-term pacing in sinus node disease: effects of stimulation mode on cardiovascular morbidity and mortality, *Am Heart J* (1988)**116**:16–22.

23 van Gelder IC, Crijns HJ, Blanksma PK et al, Time course of hemodynamic changes and improvement of exercise tolerance after cardioversion of chronic atrial fibrillation unassociated with cardiac valve disease, *Am J Cardiol* (1993)**72**:560–6.

24 Jordan RA, Scheifley CH, Edwards JE, Mural thrombosis and arterial embolism in mitral stenosis: a clinicopathologic study of 51 cases, *Circulation* (1951)**3**:363–7.

25 Aschenberg W, Schluter M, Kremer P, Schroder E, Siglow V, Bleifeld W, Transesophageal two-dimensional echocardiography for the detection of left atrial appendage thrombus, *J Am Coll Cardiol* (1986)**7**:163–6.

26 Black IW, Chesterman CN, Hopkins AP, Lee LC, Chong BH, Walsh WF, Hematologic correlates of left atrial spontaneous echo contrast and thromboembolism in nonvalvular atrial fibrillation, *J Am Coll Cardiol* (1993)**21**:451–7.

27 Leung DY, Black IW, Cranney GB et al, Left atrial spontaneous echo contrast is a risk factor for future thromboembolic events in nonvalvular atrial fibrillation—results of a prospective study, *J Am Coll Cardiol* (1994)**23**:441A.

28 Wolf PA, Dawber TR, Thomas HE, Kannel WB, Epidemiologic assessment of chronic atrial fibrillation and risk of stroke: the Framingham study, *Neurology* (1978)**28**:973–7.

29 Solti F, Vecsey T, Kekesi V, Juhasz-Nagy A, The effect of atrial dilatation on the genesis of atrial arrhythmias, *Cardiovasc Res* (1989)**23**:882–6.

30 Wolf PA, Abbott RD, Kannel WB, Atrial fibrillation as an independent risk factor for stroke: the Framingham Study, *Stroke* (1991)**22**:983–8.

31 Chambers J, The cardiac investigation of transient ischaemic attacks and stroke. In: Jackson G, ed. *Difficult concepts in cardiology* (Martin Dunitz: London, 1994) 157–81.

32 Theiss W, Anticoagulants: when and how? *Pacing Clin Electrophysiol* (1994)**17**:1011–15.

33 The Stroke Prevention in Atrial Fibrillation Investigators, Predictors of thromboembolism in atrial fibrillation. I. Clinical features of patients at risk, *Ann Intern Med* (1992)**116**:1–5.

34 SPAF Investigators, Warfarin versus aspirin for prevention of thromboembolism in atrial fibrillation: Stroke Prevention in Atrial Fibrillation II Study, *Lancet* (1994)**343**:687–91.

35 SPAF Investigators, Adjusted-dose warfarin versus low-intensity warfarin plus aspirin for high risk patients with atrial fibrillation: Stroke Prevention in Atrial Fibrillation III randomised clinical trial. *Lancet* (1996)**348**:633–8.

36 Laupacis A, Albers G, Dunn M, Feinberg W, Antithrombotic therapy in atrial fibrillation, *Chest* (1992)**102**:426S–33S.

37 Gustafsson C, Asplund K, Britton M, Norrving B, Olsson B, Marke LA, Cost effectiveness of primary stroke prevention in atrial fibrillation: Swedish national perspective, *Br Med J* (1992)**305**:1457–60.

38 Grogan M, Smith HC, Gersh BJ, Wood DL, Left ventricular dysfunction due to atrial fibrillation in patients initially believed to have idiopathic cardiomyopathy, *Am J Cardiol* (1992)**69**:1570–3.

39 Haiat R, Halphen C, Stoltz JP, Leroy G, Soussana C, [Auricular fibrillation: a cause of reversible myocardiopathy]. [French], *Ann Cardiol Angeiol* (1987)**36**:417–19.

40 Peters KG, Kienzle MG, Severe cardiomyopathy due to chronic rapidly conducted atrial fibrillation: complete recovery after restoration of sinus rhythm, *Am J Med* (1988)**85**:242–4.

41 van Den Berg MP, van Veldhuisen DJ, Crijns HJ, Lie KI, Reversion of tachycardiomyopathy after beta-blocker, *Lancet* (1993)**341**:1667.

42 Corey WA, Markel ML, Hoit BD, Walsh RA, Regression of a dilated cardiomyopathy after radiofrequency ablation of incessant supraventricular tachycardia, *Am Heart J* (1993)**126**:1469–73.

43 Gillette PC, Smith RT, Garson A Jr et al, Chronic supraventricular tachycardia. A cur-

able cause of congestive cardiomyopathy, *JAMA* (1985)**253**:391–2.

44 Cruz FE, Cherix EC, Smeets JL et al, Reversibility of tachycardia-induced cardiomyopathy after cure of incessant supraventricular tachycardia, *J Am Coll Cardiol* (1990)**16**:739–44.

45 Leman RB, Gillette PC, Zinner AJ, Resolution of congestive cardiomyopathy caused by supraventricular tachycardia using amiodarone, *Am Heart J* (1986)**112**:622–4.

46 Damiano RJ Jr, Tripp HF Jr, Asano T, Small KW, Jones RH, Lowe JE, Left ventricular dysfunction and dilatation resulting from chronic supraventricular tachycardia, *J Thorac Cardiolvasc Surg* (1987)**94**:135–43.

47 Fyfe DA, Gillette PC, Crawford FA Jr, Kline CH, Resolution of dilated cardiomyopathy after surgical ablation of ventricular tachycardia in a child, *J Am Coll Cardiol* (1987)**9**:231–4.

48 Rakovec P, Lajovic J, Dolenc M, Reversible congestive cardiomyopathy due to chronic ventricular tachycardia, *Pacing Clin Electrophysiol* (1989)**12**:542–5.

49 Sternick EB, Bahia FC, Gontijo Filho B, Vrandecic MO, [Cardiomyopathy induced by incessant ventricular tachycardia ('tachycardiomyopathy'): cure after control of arrhythmia]. [Portuguese], *Arq Bras Cardiol* (1992)**58**:209–14.

50 Platia EV, Michelson EL, Porterfield JK, Das G, Esmolol versus verapamil in the acute treatment of atrial fibrillation or atrial flutter, *Am J Cardiol* (1989)**63**:925–9.

51 Falk RH, Knowlton AA, Bernard SA, Gotlieb NE, Battinelli NJ, Digoxin for converting recent-onset atrial fibrillation to sinus rhythm. A randomized, double-blinded trial, *Ann Intern Med* (1987)**106**:503–6.

52 Ellenbogen KA, Dias VC, Cardello FP et al, Safety and efficacy of intravenous diltiazem in atrial fibrillation of atrial flutter, *Am J Cardiol* (1995)**75**:45–9.

53 Gulamhusein S, Ko P, Carruthers SG, Klein GJ, Acceleration of the ventricular response during atrial fibrillation in the Wolff-Parkinson-White syndrome after verapamil, *Circulation* (1982)**65**:348–54.

54 Sellers TD Jr, Bashore TM, Gallagher JJ, Digitalis in the pre-excitation syndrome. Analysis during atrial fibrillation, *Circulation* (1977)**56**:260–7.

55 Grimm RA, Stewart WJ, Maloney JD et al, Impact of electrical cardioversion for atrial fibrillation on left atrial appendage function and spontaneous echo contrast: characterization by simultaneous transesophageal echocardiography, *J Am Coll Cardiol* (1993)**22**:1359–66.

56 Fatkin D, Kuchar DL, Thorburn CW, Feneley MP, Transesophageal echocardiography before and during direct current cardioversion of atrial fibrillation: evidence for 'atrial stunning' as a mechanism of thromboembolic complications, *J Am Coll Cardiol* (1994)**23**:307–16.

57 Abascal VM, Dubrey S, Ochoa MR, Davidoff R, Falk RH, Electrical vs pharmacologic cardioversion in atrial fibrillation: does the atrium really care? *Circulation* (1995)**92**(**suppl I**):591.

58 Manning WJ, Silverman DI, Katz SE et al, Temporal dependence of the return of atrial mechanical function on the mode of cardioversion of atrial fibrillation to sinus rhythm, *Am J Cardiol* (1995)**75**:624–6.

59 Suttorp MJ, Kingma JH, Jessurun ER, Lie AH, van Hemel NM, Lie KI, The value of class IC antiarrhythmic drugs for acute conversion of paroxysmal atrial fibrillation or flutter to sinus rhythm, *J Am Coll Cardiol* (1990)**16**:1722–7.

60 Donovan KD, Dobb GJ, Coombs LJ et al, Reversion of recent-onset atrial fibrillation to sinus rhythm by intravenous flecainide, *Am J Cardiol* (1991)**67**:137–41.

61 Nathan AW, Camm AJ, Bexton RS, Hellestrand KJ, Intravenous flecainide acetate for the clinical management of paroxysmal tachycardias, *Clin Cardiol* (1987)**10**:317–22.

62 Noc M, Stajer D, Horvat M, Intravenous amiodarone versus verapamil for acute conversion of paroxysmal atrial fibrillation to sinus rhythm, *Am J Cardiol* (1990)**65**:679–80.

63 Faniel R, Schoenfeld P, Efficacy of iv amiodarone in converting rapid atrial fibrillation and flutter to sinus rhythm in intensive care patients, *Eur Heart J* (1983)**4**:180–5.

64 Stewart DE, Ikram H, The use of intravenous disopyramide for the conversion of supraventri-

cular tachyarrhythmias, *N Z Med J* (1984)**97**:148–50.

65   Black IW, Fatkin D, Sagar KB et al, Exclusion of atrial thrombus by transesophageal echocardiography does not preclude embolism after cardioversion of atrial fibrillation: a multicenter study, *Circulation* (1994)**89**:2509–13.

66   Page RL, Wilkinson WE, Clair WK, McCarthy EA, Pritchett EL, Asymptomatic arrhythmias in patients with symptomatic paroxysmal atrial fibrillation and paroxysmal supraventricular tachycardia, *Circulation* (1994)**89**:224–7.

67   Petersen P, Madsen EB, Brun B, Pedersen F, Gyldensted C, Boysen G, Silent cerebral infarction in chronic atrial fibrillation, *Stroke* (1987)**18**:1098–100.

68   Ezekowitz MD, James KE, Nazarian SM et al, Silent cerebral infarction in patients with non-rheumatic atrial fibrillation. The Veterans Affairs Stroke Prevention in Nonrheumatic Atrial Fibrillation Investigators, *Circulation* (1995)**92**:2178–82.

69   Feinberg WM, Seeger JF, Carmody RF, Anderson DC, Hart RG, Pearce LA, Epidemiologic features of asymptomatic cerebral infarction in patients with nonvalvular atrial fibrillation, *Arch Intern Med* (1990)**150**:2340–4.

70   Guidotti M, Tadeo G, Zanasi S, Pellegrini G, Silent cerebral ischemia in patients with chronic atrial fibrillation—a case–control study, *Ir J Med Sci* (1990)**159**:96–7.

71   Hartel G, Louhija A, Konttinen A, Disopyramide in the prevention of recurrence of atrial fibrillation after electroconversion, *Clin Pharmacol Ther* (1974)**15**:551–5.

72   Coplen SE, Antman EM, Berlin JA, Hewitt P, Chalmers TC, Efficacy and safety of quinidine therapy for maintenance of sinus rhythm after cardioversion. A meta-analysis of randomized control trials, *Circulation* (1990)**82**:1106–16.

73   Pritchett EL, DaTorre SD, Platt ML, McCarville SE, Hougham AJ, Flecainide acetate treatment of paroxysmal supraventricular tachycardia and paroxysmal atrial fibrillation: dose-reponse studies. The Flecainide Supraventricular Tachycardia Study Group, *J Am Coll Cardiol* (1991)**17**:297–303.

74   Hamill SC, Wood DL, Gersh BJ, Osborn MJ, Holmes DR Jr, Propafenone for paroxysmal

atrial fibrillation, *Am J Cardiol* (1988)**61**:473–4.

75   Camm AJ, Paul V, Sotalol for paroxysmal supraventricular tachycardias [review], *Am J Cardiol* (1990)**65**:67A–73A.

76   Graboys TB, Podrid PJ, Lown B, Efficacy of amiodarone for refractory supraventricular tachyarrhythmias, *Am Heart J* (1983)**106**:870–6.

77   Feld GK, Chen P, Nicod PH, Fleck P, Meyer D, Possible atrial proarrhythmic effects of class 1c antiarrhythmic drugs, *Am J Cardiol* (1990)**66**:378–83.

78   Daubert C, Mabo P, Berder V, Gras D, Leclercq C, Atrial tachyarrhythmias associated with high degree interatrial conduction block: prevention by permanent atrial resynchronization, *Eur JCPE* (1994)**4**:35–44.

79   Cox JL, Boineau JP, Schuessler RB, Kater KM, Lappas DG, Five-year experience with the maze procedure for atrial fibrillation, *Ann Thorac Surg* (1993)**56**:814–23.

80   Haissaguerre M, Gencel L, Fischer B et al, Successful catheter ablation of atrial fibrillation, *J Cardiovasc Electrophysiol* (1994)**5**:1045–52.

81   Swartz JF, Pellersels G, Silvers J, Patten L, Cervantez D, A catheter-based curative approach to atrial fibrillation in humans, *Circulation* (1994)**90**:I335.

82   Blevins RD, Kerin NZ, Benaderet D et al, Amiodarone in the management of refractory atrial fibrillation, *Arch Intern Med* (1987)**147**:1401–4.

83   Gold RL, Haffajee CI, Charos G, Sloan K, Baker S, Alpert JS, Amiodarone for refractory atrial fibrillation, *Am J Cardiol* (1986)**57**:124–7.

84   Murgatroyd FD, Slade AKB, Sopher SM, Rowland E, Ward DE, Camm AJ, Efficacy and tolerability of transvenous low energy cardioversion of paroxsymal atrial fibrillation in humans, *J Am Coll Cardiol* (1995)**25**:1347–53.

85   Levy S, Lauribe P, Dolla E et al, A randomized comparison of external and internal cardioversion of chronic atrial fibrillation, *Circulation* (1992)**86**:1415–20.

86   Baker BM, Botteron GW, Smith JM, Low-energy internal cardioversion for atrial fibrilla-

tion resistant to external cardioversion, *J Cardiovasc Electrophysiol* (1995)**6**:44–7.

87 Crijns HJ, Van Gelder IC, van Gilst WH, Hillege H, Gosselink ATM, Lie KI, Serial anti-arrhythmic drug treatment to maintain sinus rhythm after electrical cardioversion for chronic atrial fibrillation or atrial flutter, *Am J Cardiol* (1991)**68**:335–41.

88 Falk RH, Leavitt JI, Digoxin for atrial fibrillation: a drug whose time has gone? *Ann Intern Med* (1991)**114**:573–5.

89 Lang RM, Klein HO, Weiss E et al, Superiority of oral verapamil therapy to digoxin in treat-ment of chronic atrial fibrillation, *Chest* (1983)**83**:491–9.

90 Packer M, Bristow MR, Cohn JN et al, The effect of carvedilol on morbidity and mortality in patients with chronic heart failure, *N Engl J Med* (1996)**334**:1349–55.

91 Feld GK, Fleck RP, Fujimura O, Prothro DL, Bahnson TD, Ibarra M, Control of rapid ven-tricular response by radiofrequency catheter modification of the atrioventricular node in patients with medically refractory atrial fibrilla-tion, *Circulation* (1994)**90**:2299–307.

13

To ablate or not to ablate?

Kim H Tan and Jaswinder S Gill

Introduction

The surgical ablation of an accessory pathway in a patient with Wolff–Parkinson–White syndrome in 1968 was the beginning of the age of ablation.[1] Developments in catheter techniques were ushered in by high-voltage direct-current ablation.[2] However, the uncontrolled and traumatic nature of this technique led to things being overtaken by newer energy sources, including radiofrequency ablation. The first report of a successful ablation using radiofrequency energy was in 1987,[3] and since that time the applications and success of this technique have increased exponentially. The technique can be applied to most forms of supraventricular tachycardia, including atrioventricular re-entrant tachycardia, atrioventricular nodal re-entrant tachycardia, atrial tachycardia and atrial flutter. Ventricular tachycardia particularly in patients with no evidence of structural heart disease, can also be successfully treated. The technique has advanced to the extent that it offers a curative treatment for many forms of arrhythmia which would normally require life-long treatment with toxic antiarrhythmic drugs. The question now is which forms of arrhythmia should be aggressively treated with catheter ablation and which should be managed by drugs? This chapter attempts to summarize the success and efficacy rates of catheter ablation, together with the problems, complications and costs of the technique. The focus of this chapter is on supraventricular tachycardia: it does not attempt to discuss ventricular arrhythmias.

General aspects of radiofrequency ablation

Apparatus and equipment

The technique requires a fully equipped catheter laboratory together with electrophysiology recording and stimulation set-up. The appropriate ablator and catheters are necessary. It is important that all staff are appropriately trained in the technique. This limits the number of centres where interventional electrophysiology can be practised. It is also necessary to have cardiothoracic surgical facilities close at hand, since complications such as cardiac perforation, although rare, have been described.

Size of the lesion

Application of radiofrequency energy results in damage to tissue of approximately 10 mm diameter. The necrosed myocardium gradually undergoes scar formation, which is sharply demarcated from the adjacent viable tissue. Newer catheters with irrigated tips or larger diameter (8 mm) tips and the use of high-output ablators can result in larger lesions.[4] Radiofrequency energy lesions do not appear to cause any significant dysfunction of the myocardium or cardiac enzyme release.

Potential complications of the technique are cardiac perforation, stroke, sudden death and long-term cardiac pacing. Fortunately these are rare for radiofrequency ablation. Currently, an ablation registry is maintained to monitor any side effects which would not be detected otherwise.[5]

Radiation exposure

Ablation procedures can take from less than 1 hour to several hours. In prolonged procedures, the radiation exposure to the operator and the patient can be considerable, although it may not be more than during coronary intervention. The use of more modern equipment and meticulous care in avoiding unnecessary screening will reduce doses.

Radiofrequency ablation of the atrioventricular junction

Initially, the technique of AV nodal ablation was used for all forms of supraventricular tachycardia, including those involving Wolff–Parkinson–White syndrome, AV nodal re-entry, atrial tachycardia and atrial flutter (Figure 13.1). With the advent of specific techniques for the ablation of these varities of arrhythmia, the uses of this treatment has become limited to the treatment of patients with atrial fibrillation refractory to other treatments, inappropriate sinus tachycardia, and atrial flutter/atrial tachycardia, where conventional treatments (including ablation) have failed.

The indications for this procedure are changing continually with improvements in catheter technology. There is now expectation that atrial fibrillation can be treated with preservation of sinus rhythm and normal atrioventricular conduction by the use of the catheter MAZE procedure. The technique is currently being researched in animal models, and will soon be possible in humans. Patients with atrial fibrillation and paroxysmal atrial fibrillation that is

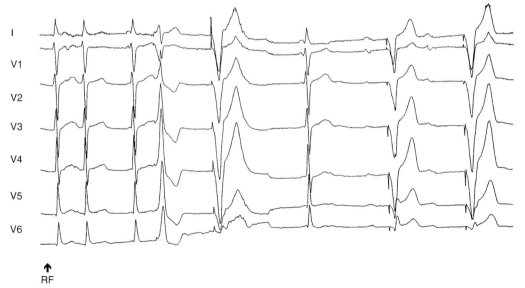

Figure 13.1

An example of ablation of the atrioventricular junction using radiofrequency energy. Following the initiation of radiofrequency energy, there is abolition of atrioventricular conduction and back-up ventricular pacing. A slow nodal escape rhythm was present after the end of energy delivery.

under reasonable control with drugs should await the arrival of these more complex procedures, when a definitive cure may be possible.

Atrioventricular re-entrant tachycardias

The first ablations of accessory pathways using radiofrequency energy were performed in 1986,[3] and since that time the use of this technique has expanded rapidly. Accessory pathways can be eliminated on the left side of the heart with success rates of over 90% at the first procedure and recurrence rates of less than 5%. On the right side of the heart, success rates are lower, but exceed 85% in experienced hands (Figure 13.2).[6] Many of these pathways which fail on the first occasion can be ablated at a second procedure. The techniques for mapping

of accessory pathways and determining the successful ablation site are now well established. Complication rates of the procedure are extremely low, and data from the Multicentre European Radiofrequency Survey[7] demonstrate arrhythmias in 0.81%, perforation/tamponade in 0.72%, AV block in 0.63%, pericardial effusion in 0.54%, pulmonary or cerebral embolism in 0.58% and vascular thrombosis in 0.36%. The procedure is therefore extremely safe and effective. This raises the question of whether all accessory pathways should undergo ablation or whether this technique should be reserved for particular patients. To address this question, we need to consider the risks and problems associated with accessory pathways. Accessory pathways can be overt — that is pre-excitation is present on the resting electrocardiogram (Wolff–Parkinson–White (WPW)) syndrome, and latent — where pre-excitation is intermit-

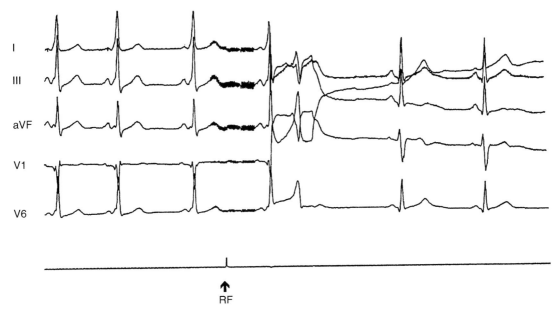

Figure 13.2
Ablation of Wolff–Parkinson–White syndrome. A left-sided accessory pathway. Within seconds of application of radiofrequency energy, there is disappearance of pre-excitation and narrowing of the QRS complex, inferring elimination of the pathway.

tently present and concealed, and is not found on the resting electrocardiogram, but tachycardia can occur as a consequence of retrograde conduction in the pathway resulting in circus movement tachycardia.

Risk of overt Wolff–Parkinson–White syndrome

The course of WPW syndrome can be extremely variable. Many patients remain free of symptoms for life and generally have a benign prognosis.[8] Some patients do not have retrograde conduction over the pathway and do not have tachycardias. However, 11% of patients with asymptomatic WPW will go on to experience reciprocating tachycardia, or atrial fibrillation over a median follow-up of 4 years.[9] Patients with full WPW syndrome experience tachycardias, some of which can be associated with light-headedness and syncope. Other patients can present with sudden death as the first manifestation of the syndrome. The estimated rate of sudden death is 1 per 1000 patient-years and is usually the result of atrial fibrillation being rapidly conducted to the venticle, causing ventricular fibrillation.[10] The incidence of atrial fibrillation is increased in patients with WPW syndrome and is thought to be due to the occurrence of a retrogradely conducted beat which falls in the vulnerable period of the atrium. Thus, risk stratification of patients with WPW syndrome presents a challenge. It is possible to subdivide patients with WPW into three main categories, which are described below.

Patients with severe symptoms
This group includes those who have suffered attacks of rapid atrial fibrillation, ventricular fibrillation or disabling attacks of tachycardia. These patients are at the highest risk of occurrence of sudden cardiac death. In such individuals it is important to perform a curative radiofrequency ablation, which will remove the risk of sudden cardiac death, as well as preventing attacks of tachycardia. If ablation is unsuccessful or is not available, the effect of class Ic and class III drugs in depressing accessory pathway conduction should be examined.

Patients with mild or moderate symptoms
This group includes those who have only infrequent and well tolerated attacks of tachycardia. The risk of sudden cardiac death is variable, and markers which will identify potential risk include:

- multiple pathways — two or more pattens of pre-excitation generally cause greater risk to the patient than single pathways;
- an RR interval of <250 ms in patients with spontaneous or induced atrial fibrillation, who are capable of rapid condution and therefore at risk of more malignant arrhythmia.

In these patients an invasive electrophysiological study is a useful means of studying the conduction properties and number of pathways. Multipolar catheters are placed in the high right atrium, the His bundle region and the right ventricle. Conduction is examined using anterograde and retrograde curves. An anterograde refractory period of the pathway <270 ms and a minimum RR interval of the pathway <250 ms during induced atrial fibrillation are associated with potentially dangerous pathways. Conduction within accessory pathways is subject to autonomic influence, therefore some authors have proposed that the maximal rate of conduction within the pathway should be studied following an isoprenaline infusion. However, this technique remains controversial.[11]

Patients with asymptomatic WPW

The degree to which these individuals need to be investigated is debatable. Clearly, the development of ventricular fibrillation in this group is a rare event, but can occur. Therefore, routine electrophyisological study is proposed by some centres. When this is done, approximately 20% of individuals will have a rapid ventricular response during atrial fibrillation with an RR interval <250 ms demonstrating the high sensitivity but low specificity of this parameter as a marker of risk.[9] Clearly, to subject patients who are asymptomatic and at low risk of any serious event to aggressive treatment would be unwarranted, but to miss investigation of such an individual who then suffers sudden cardiac death would be distressing. The investigation of these individuals requires some degree of judgement. Many electrophysiologists, knowing the relative simplicity of a curative ablation procedure, with its low complication rate, would decide to investigate the majority of these patients with a view to treatment if necessary.

Atrioventricular nodal re-entrant tachycardia

The basis of atrioventricular nodal re-entrant tachycardias is the presence of anatomically and functionally discreet pathways for conduction within the node. Selective ablation of one of these pathways and cure of AVNRT was achieved in the 1980s using open heart surgery.[12] The method was then modified and applied to catheter techniques, initially with DC energy and more recently with radiofrequency current. In the classical variety of AVNRT, the initial attempts at ablation were based on the fast pathway. This pathway is in the atrium above and anterior to the site of recording of the His bundle potential. Ablation in this territory is associated with an increase in the PR interval on the surface ECG and an increase in the AH interval on intracardiac recordings. Ablation of the pathway is also marked by a loss of the dual AV nodal physiology. Unfortunately, because of the close proximity of this pathway to the His bundle, the incidence of complete AV block is relatively high and has been reported in up to 21% of patients.[13] AV block is generally seen during the performance of the procedure, but delayed AV block has been described from 1–2 days to 6 months after the ablation. Other complications, such as pulmonary embolism, deep vein thrombosis and cardiac tamponade are rare. The recurrence rate of AVNRT after fast pathway ablation is approximately 10%.[14]

The high incidence of AV block with ablation of the fast pathway led to approaches based on the slow pathway. The slow pathway input to the atrioventricular node is inferior and posterior to the His bundle, and most of the pathways can be located around the os of the coronary sinus. The incidence of complete heart block with this technique is low, at around 1–2%.[15] Recurrence rates of tachycardia are around 5%, and most can be eliminated at a second procedure.[16]

AVNRT is generally not a life-threatening arrhythmia, therefore any consideration of ablation should be based on whether the degree of discomfort from the symptoms of arrhythmia exceed the risks and costs of ablation. Some patients do not find the risk of a pacemaker implantation acceptable and will refuse any offers of an ablation. However, the majority are willing to accept some degree of risk and will be willing to proceed with the ablation. The decision of whether or not to ablate will depend on the level of symptoms. If the patient has only one or two attacks every few years, then it would be unreasonable to proceed to an ablation, whereas with more frequent symtoms ablative therapy may be a better option.

Obviously, in patients with frequent symptoms and repeated admissions, ablation would be the best course of action. This is one of the few areas in which there is a study of cost efficacy of ablation compared with drug treatment in the management of drug refractory AVNRT.[17] This study clearly indicates that catheter ablation is more cost effective than life-long drug treatment, particularly if the arrhythmia involves recurrent hospital visits (Figure 13.3).

Atrial tachycardia and atrial flutter

Atrial tachycardias can be automatic or re-entrant. Automatic atrial tachycardias tend to be resistant to drug treatment and, if incessant, can cause a dilated cardiomyopathy. Therefore, ablation of the ectopic focus in these patients would appear to be an attractive alternative. Ablation of ectopic atrial foci has been reported in small numbers of patients by several groups. The mapping of the focus is undertaken by the method of activation mapping and the earliest activation site is sought. Ablation at such sites results in approximately 80–95% success rates if assessed by the noninducibility of tachycardia by isoprenaline infusion. However, recurrence occurs in approximately 20% of cases, although this may be due to development of another focus in some cases.[18,19]

Re-entrant forms of atrial tachycardia generally occur in the presence of atrial disease, in

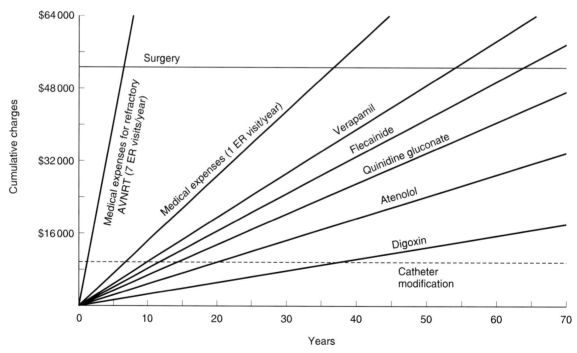

Figure 13.3
*A comparison of the cost of ablation for atrioventricular nodal re-entrant tachycardia with drug treatment. (Modified from Kabfleisch SJ et al, Comparison of the cost of radiofrequency catheter modification of the atrioventricular node and medical therapy for drug-refractory atrioventricular node reentrant tachycardia, J Am Coll Cardiol (1992)**19**:1583–7.[17])*

particularly previous atrial surgery. The opening of the right atrium for surgery, for example closure of an atrial septal defect, can lead to the formation of a scar around which the myocardium has differential conducting and electrophysiological properties. This can lead to circus movement tachycardia. The ablation target in these cases is the zone of slowed conduction which forms the basis of the tachycardia. Ablation at the exit point of this zone of slowed conduction can be successful in eliminating the tachycardia.[20] It is difficult to be sure of the acute and long-term results of ablation for these forms of tachycardia, but they are not as good as for automatic atrial rhythms. Thus for a patient with an atrial tachycardia, study of the mechanism is critical in determining the likely success of the ablation. This will also allow the operator to determine whether the arrhythmia is of left or right atrial origin and to plan the ablation appropriately. Considering the poor response of these forms of arrhythmia to drug therapy and the possibility of the development of cardiomyopathy in the incessant varieties, it would be reasonable to consider ablative treatment rather than drug therapy, when the complication rate is so low.

Atrial flutter comes in two varieties: common (type 1) or atypical (type 2). In common flutter, the re-entrant circuit occupies the right atrium and the hallmark is a zone of slowed conduction in the low right atrium. The atrium is activated down the free wall through this zone of slowed conduction, with upward activation of the atrial septum completing the circuit (Figure 13.4). Atrial flutter is generally poorly responsive to drug treatment and several groups have directed their attention to ablative treatment of this arrhythmia. It appears clear that lesions placed from the tricuspid valve annulus to the orifice of the inferior vena caval orifice can interrupt the circuit at the site of the zone of slowed conduction and remove the substrate

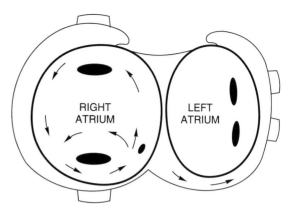

Figure 13.4
The circuit of common atrial flutter, with the anticlockwise rotation of activation in the right atrium. A zone of slowed conduction exists in the low right atrium.

for flutter to exist. Initial results for the ablation of flutter were poor, with only around 60% acute success rates and a high rate of recurrence following ablation.[21] However, the techniques for reliably and consistently performing atrial flutter ablation are currently being researched and impressive results are being reported by some groups.[22]

Atypical atrial flutter generally arises from circus movement around an anatomical obstacle, generally a scar. These arrhythmias frequently emerge following cardiac surgery and are frequently unresponsive to drug treatment. The approach to ablation of these rhythms is similar to re-entrant atrial tachycardias and only small number of patients have been reported. Success rates are likely to be lower than typical atrial flutter.

In patients with atrial flutter, although success rates of ablation are not currently high, the development of new catheters and techniques specifically for this arrhythmia appear to be improving treatment rapidly. It would therefore be reasonable to offer patients this therapy in the near future and avoid drug treatment, which in any case is not generally effective. Little is lost in attempting ablation, which should be performed in a centre with experience of the technique.

If I had . . .

If I had supraventricular tachycardia my initial concern would be to get an electrophysiological study so that the mechanism of the arrhythmia could be determined. If I had overt Wolff–Parkinson–White syndrome, it would be important to know the potential risks of the pathway, and I would prefer it to be ablated because of the small but significant risk of sudden cardiac death. If the pathway was not overt, my decision would be based on the degree of symptoms. If the episodes were infrequent (less than two prolonged attacks per year), prophylactic drug therapy might be tolerable. Attacks

more frequent than this would justify ablative treatment. Similar criteria apply to AVNRT, except that I would be a little more tentative because of the small risk of pacemaker implantation. Nevertheless, any frequency of attacks above two prolonged episodes per year would be strong motivation for curative therapy. With atrial tachycardia of an automatic nature, ablation would be my first choice. However, with atrial tachycardias of a re-entrant variety, although I would offer myself for an attempted ablation, my hopes of cure would not be high. In the case of atrial flutter, I would avoid ablation currently, until the techniques are perfected for achieving high success rates without the need for prolonged procedures. Similarly, I would have my atrial fibrillation treated medically until the methods for the performance of the intracardiac catheter MAZE procedure are perfected.

References

1 Cobb RF, Blumenschein SD, Sealy WC et al, Successful surgical interruption of the bundle of Kent in a patient with Wolff–Parkinson–White syndrome, *Circulation* (1968)**38**:1018–29.

2 Scheinman MM, Morady F, Hess DS et al, Catheter-induced ablation of the atrioventricular junction to control refractory supraventricular arrhythmias, *JAMA* (1982)**248**:851–5.

3 Huang SK, Bharati S, Graham A et al, Closed chest catheter desiccation of the atrioventricular junction using radiofrequency energy: a new method of catheter ablation, *J Am Coll Cardiol* (1987)**9**:349–58.

4 Langberg J, Gallagher M, Strickberger S, Temperature-guided radiofrequency catheter ablation using very large distal electrodes, *Circulation* (1993)**88**:245–9.

5 Evans G, Scheinman M, Zipes D et al, The Percutaneous Cardiac Mapping and Ablation Registry: final summary of results, *PACE* (1988)**11**:1621–6.

6 Calkins H, Kim Y, Schmaltz S et al, Electrogram criteria for identification of appropriate target sites for radiofrequency catheter ablation of accessory pathways, *Circulation* (1992)**85**:565–73.

7 Hindricks G, The Multicentre European Radiofrequency Survey (MERFS). Complications of radiofrequency catheter ablation of arrhythmias, *Eur Heart J* (1993)**14**:1644–53.

8 Klein GJ, Yee R, Sharma AD, Longitudinal electrophysiologic assessment of asymptomatic patients with the Wolff–Parkinson–White electrocardiographic pattern, *N Engl J Med*(1989)**320**:1229–32.

9 Leitch JW, Klein GJ, Yee R, Prognostic value of electrophysiology testing in asymptomatic patients with Wolff–Parkinson–White syndrome, *Circulation* (1990)**82**:1718–23.

10 Munger TM, Packer DL, Hammill SC et al, A population study of the natural history of Wolff–Parkinson–White syndrome in Olmsted County, Minnesota 1953–89, *Circulation* (1993)**87**:866–73.

11 Szabo TS, Klein GJ, Sharma AD et al, Usefulness of isoproterenol during atrial fibrillation in the evaluation of asymptomatic Wolff–Parkinson–White syndrome, *Am J Cardiol* (1989)**63**:187–92.

12 Ross DL, Johnson DC, Denniss AR et al, Curative surgery for atrioventricular junctional ('AV nodal') reentrant tachycardia, *J Am Coll Cardiol* (1985)**6**:1383–92.

13 Jazayeri MR, Hempe SL, Sra JS et al, Selective transcatheter ablation of the fast and slow pathways using radiofrequency energy in patients with atrioventricular re-entrant tachycardia, *Circulation* (1992)**85**:1318–28.

14 Lee MA, Morady F, Kadish A et al, Catheter modification of the atrioventricular junction in patients with atrioventricular nodal reentrant tachycardia, *N Engl J Med* (1989)**320**:426–33.

15 Lanberg JJ, Leon A, Borvanelli M et al, A randomised comparison of anterior and posterior approaches to radiofrequency catheter ablation of atrioventricular nodal reentry tachycardia, *Circulation* (1993)**87**:1551–6.

16 Kabfleisch SJ, Strickberger SA, Williamson B et al, Randomised comparison of anatomic and electrogram mapping approaches to ablation of the slow pathway of atrioventricular node reentrant tachycardia, *J Am Coll Cardiol* (1994)**23**:716–23.

17 Kabfleisch SJ, Calkins H, Langberg JJ et al, Comparison of the cost of radiofrequency catheter modification of the atrioventricular node and medical therapy for drug-refractory atrioventricular nodal reentrant tachycardia, *J Am Coll Cardiol* (1992)**19**:1583–7.

18 Kay GN, Chong F, Epstein L, Radiofrequency catheter ablation of primary atrial tachycardias, *J Am Coll Cardiol* (1993)**21**:910–19.

19 Walsh EP, Saul JP, Hulse JE et al, Transcatheter ablation of ectopic atrial tachycardia in young using radiofrequency current, *Circulation* (1992)**86**:1138–46.

20 Lesh M, Van Hare G, Epstein L, RF catheter ablation of atrial arrhythmias — results and mechanism, *Circulation* (1994)**89**:1074–9.

21 O'Nunain S, Linker NJ, Sneddon JF et al, Catheter ablation by low energy DC shocks for successful management of atrial flutter, *Br Heart J* (1992)**67**:67–71.

22 Cruz FES, Boghossian SH, Fagundes M et al, A randomised comparison of entrance and exit point from slow zone for radiofrequency ablation of common atrial flutter: efficacy and recurrences using a large tip electrode catheter, *J Am Coll Cardiol* (1996)**27**:189A (abstr).

14

Implantable cardioverter defibrillators

Neil Sulke

Introduction

The treatment of malignant ventricular arrhythmias that cause sudden cardiac death outside the hospital represents one of the most formidable challenges currently facing cardiology. Sudden cardiac death is one of the most common causes of mortality in the developed world and hopes that a pharmacological therapy can be found consistently to protect against this disorder have not materialized. At present, and for the foreseeable future, the use of electrical countershock is the mainstay of any attempt to terminate ventricular fibrillation as well as haemodynamically unstable ventricular tachyarrhythmias.

Atrial fibrillation is the most common cardiac arrhythmia and, contrary to widely held belief, this is a malignant arrhythmia resulting in considerable morbidity and mortality. New developments in the treatment of this problem using atrial implantable cardioverter defibrillators (ICDs) are a possible major advance in both the treatment and potential cure of these arrhythmias.

History of ICDs

Michel Mirowski is undoubtedly the 'father' of the implantable cardioverter defibrillator. His single-minded quest to develop this device started when his great mentor, Professor Horowitz, succumbed to a malignant arrhythmia as he was walking down the street. Mirowski demonstrated that internal defibrilla-

tion of the heart was possible using a ring electrode in the superior vena cava and an electrode in the left ventricle during cardiac surgery, when ventricular fibrillation was repeatedly terminated by this technique.

The first experimental implantable cardioverter defibrillator was implanted into a beagle dog and induced ventricular fibrillation successfully reverted. The first successful human implant was performed at the Johns Hopkins hospital in 1980.[1] The patient was a 57-year-old woman with refractory ventricular fibrillation. The first ICD was the AID defibrillator of Medrad, which was encased in titanium weighing 250 g with a volume of 145 ml. This device was designed to monitor cardiac electrical activity recognizing ventricular fibrillation and ventricular tachyarrhythmias with a sinusoidal waveform and it was then able to deliver corrective defibrillatory discharges. The lithium batteries gave it a capability of delivering 100 shocks. The first system used a sampled probability density function of the ventricular electrical activity and for all practical purposes ventricular fibrillation was identified by the absence of isoelectric potential segments. This system was deemed unreliable in later years. Interestingly however, this system is being resurrected in some modern devices.

Success of the initial implants, coupled with Mirowski's drive, led to approval of the first ICD by the US Food and Drug Administration in 1985 and there have now been nearly 70 000

ICD implants worldwide, with the annual implantation rate rising exponentially.

Technical aspects of ICDs

The device

The generator contains capacitors, batteries, integrated circuits and is encased in a titanium shell. Current commercially available devices weigh between 150 g and 200 g and have a volume of 59 ml to 100 ml. Good progress is being made by miniaturizing the batteries and capacitors and economically packing components, so that currently the smallest devices (Figure 14.1) are 52 ml and weigh just 140 g. Despite this size reduction, they are still capable of delivering 200 maximum output shocks and offer a full repertoire of therapy, with a life expectancy of 5 years.

The older, larger generators were initially implanted in an abdominal position with the device pocket created in the anterior or posterior rectus sheath. Various positions were tried,

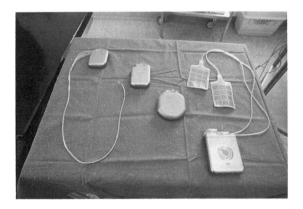

Figure 14.1
Miniaturization of ICDs. Foreground shows a device from 1988 to the smallest current device, the CPI 'Mini II'. Also shown are epicardial patch electrodes from the 1980s (left) and a current endocardial defibrillation electrode (right).

but many patients found it uncomfortable to lean over or sit forward. Reduction in the size of modern generators has allowed implantation in the pectoral position, usually beneath the pectoralis major muscle, but in large patients subcutaneous positioning is possible. Prior to 1990, adequate defibrillation thresholds were possible only with patches placed epicardially on the heart via thoracotomy, and this greatly increased the morbidity and mortality of the implantation procedure. Both epicardial and endocardial sensing and pacing electrodes were used, again complicating the procedure. However after 1990, electrode technology improved significantly, allowing endocardial placement of so called 'nonthoracotomy' electrodes. These electrodes incorporated a conventional tip, allowing pacing and sensing with a defibrillation coil more proximally and occasionally a further defibrillation coil in the mid-portion of the electrode. Some manufacturers utilized two electrodes and initially defibrillation thresholds were satisfactory only if the shock was 'triangulated' with a subcutaneous patch electrode placed over the cardiac apex (Figure 14.2). An electrode 'array' was developed to achieve improved thresholds and recently generators have been made available using 'hot can' technology, where the third coil (or second in some cases) is the device itself. Initial defibrillation thresholds using epicardial patches were achieved with as little energy as 5 J. With the latest devices, using endocardial electrode technology, these low thresholds are again being reached.

Arrhythmia detection

Tachycardia detection by all devices currently in use is based on rate criteria. Tachycardia is detected when a preset and programmable number of intervals exceed the detection rate limit and device therapy will be initiated.

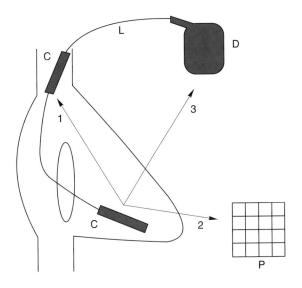

Figure 14.2
Different system configurations currently available for endocardial defibrillation. (C=coils; D=ICD generator; L=lead; P=subcutaneous patch or 'array'). Energy can thus be 'triangulated' between (1) coils, (2) coils and/or patch, or (3) coils and 'hot' or 'active' can, to lower the energy required for defibrillation.

Although there have been various developments to improve the sensitivity and specificity of detection algorithms, any tachycardia, whether it is supraventricular or ventricular, whether it is regular or irregular, will trigger device therapy. Thus the possibility of delivering a painful and potentially proarrhythmic shock exists in patients who have sinus tachycardia, supraventricular re-entrant tachycardias, atrial tachycardias, atrial flutter or fibrillation. Newer devices allow additional programming to avoid detection of sinus tachycardia by allowing tachycardia detection criteria to be fulfilled only if there is a sudden increase in heart rate in addition to a high rate. Rate stability criteria can now be programmed so that the device will examine the intervals between R waves and if the difference in successive intervals exceeds a preset value,

then therapy is inhibited by the device. This allows the device the potential to detect atrial fibrillation. However if there is intermittent sensing of ventricular fibrillation, the situation exists where the device will fail to deliver life-saving therapy. In addition, if the variability of the atrial fibrillation is less than the preset stability value, shock therapy will be delivered anyway.

Newer defibrillators are now incorporating dual-chamber pacemaker functions instead of the normal ventricular pacemaker functions of older devices and apart from allowing physiological pacing, accurate detection of atrial fibrillation is now assured in these devices. Thus, they should be selected in patients prone to atrial flutter or fibrillation or other atrial tachyarrhythmias. As mentioned earlier, the probability density function is also useful in detecting nonventricular arrhythmias and at least one new device has reincorporated this algorithm to improve tachycardia detection.

All modern ICDs incorporate an 'autosensing' facility which allows the minimum sensitivity setting to be used without oversensing the T wave and thus erroneously interpreting comparatively slow heart rates as tachycardias by 'double counting'. This feature is important as the amplitude of malignant ventricular fibrillation can be small and the autosensing feature rapidly increases the sensitivity of the device to half the level of the preceding R wave, until detection is continuous.

Delivery of therapy

Most modern ICDs allow different levels of therapy to be administered and this is a crucial method of increasing device longevity as well as avoiding the delivery of unpleasant and often unnecessary shocks. Thus therapy can be programmed into three or more 'tiers' and such devices are therefore called 'tiered therapy' devices. One therapy can be used for slow ventricular tachycardia, another for rapid ventricular tachycardia and finally another for ventricular fibrillation. The forms of therapy that are available are antitachycardia pacing, R-wave synchronized low-energy cardioversion and maximum energy defibrillation.

Antitachycardia pacing

In the late 1970s pacing extra stimuli were shown to be capable of terminating monomorphic ventricular tachycardia.[2] The problem with this mode of tachycardia termination is that there is a significant risk of acceleration of the tachyarrhythmia and also induction of ventricular fibrillation, in other words it can be a proarrhythmic therapy. However, with the possibility of defibrillator backup, successful termination of a ventricular tachyarrhythmia using antitachycardia pacing has both technical and clinical advantages. Antitachycardia pacing is a non-noxious stimulus, so that if recurrent well tolerated tachycardias occur termination is painless, and battery draining cardioversion or defibrillation is avoided, increasing the longevity of the implanted device.

There are several different techniques of antitachycardia pacing that can be programmed singularly or sequentially in most of the modern tiered-therapy ICDs. The first is programmed extra stimuli, in which pacing beats are introduced either singularly, doubly or in triplets to try to render part of the tachycardia circuit refractory, thus terminating the arrhythmia. The second is burst pacing, in which recurrent trains of extra stimuli (4–40 beats) are introduced at fixed coupling intervals. This is a rather 'scatter-gun' approach to tachycardia termination and is more likely to be proarrhythmic than the rather more subtle single, double or triple programmed extra sti-

muli. The third technique is what is known as ramp pacing, which delivers recurrent bursts of extra stimuli where the coupling intervals within the burst are progressively shortened. The first stimulus is timed as a programmable percentage of the tachycardia cycle length. This technique is known as adaptive stimulation. The more proarrhythmic ramp-burst pacing protocols can accelerate haemodynamically stable ventricular tachycardias into unstable malignant arrhythmias in up to 20% of cases, while antitachycardia pacing is effective in termination of the VT in up to 80% of cases. Increased success rates occur with slower monomorphic tachycardias and proarrhythmia is more likely in more rapid polymorphic tachycardias. Antitachycardia pacing has no effect on ventricular fibrillation.

Synchronized low-energy cardioversion

Most ventricular tachycardias can be safely reverted by timed low-energy shocks administered immediately after the peak of the R wave. This avoids the risk of proarrhythmia (induction of ventricular fibrillation) and also preserves battery life. Unfortunately, pain perception by most patients of timed cardioversion shocks of as low as 0.5 J is no different from that of a full-energy 34 J shock.

Defibrillation

As early as 1970 it was realized that for the heart to be reverted from ventricular fibrillation, a critical mass of myocardium has to be depolarized.[3] The earlier devices achieved the defibrillation threshold using a monophasic pulse and the energy was generated using a lithium carbide battery and a 120 µF capacitor with an initial voltage of about 700 V which was truncated after a fixed time (fixed duration ICDs) or after the voltage had dropped by a

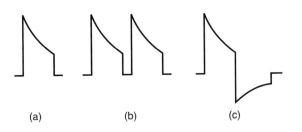

Figure 14.3
Different defibrillation waveforms. (A) Monophasic wave with 60% 'tilt'. (B) Sequential monophasic shocks with 60% tilt. (C) Biphasic shock with 60% tilt of each phase.

lation thresholds (DFT) using endocardial electrodes showed that the DFT could be decreased by almost 25% using a biphasic wave form (*see* Figure 14.3). This has allowed a shrinkage of newer devices as they need smaller capacitors and smaller batteries. This astute packaging means that device volumes are now such that implantation in the prepectoral area is routine and the procedure is little more demanding than implanting a pacemaker. Indeed some centres now use general anaesthetic only for a short period during VF induction to assess the defibrillation threshold of the implanted electrode and an increasing number use local anaesthesia and sedation only. The procedure is being undertaken more commonly in district general hospitals, although it is vital that appropriate patients are selected and the implanting clinicians have good awareness of how to program the device

fixed percentage (fixed tilt ICDs) (Figure 14.3). The maximum output of most modern ICDs is 34 J, although the latest 'ultra small' defibrillators have a maximum output of only 25 J. Intensive work on methods of lowering defibril-

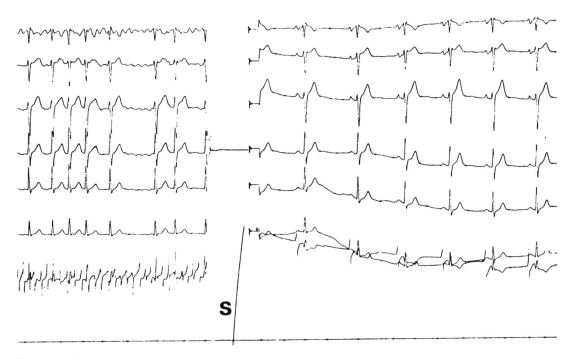

Figure 14.4
Example of endocardial atrial defibrillation from AF to sinus rhythm.

for optimal function, to minimize patient discomfort and to maximize device longevity. With new developments in the materials and dimensions of endocardial electrodes, use of active cans as a pole for shock delivery and biphasic waveforms, current defibrillation thresholds at implantation are now under 10 J and are likely to fall further in the near future, allowing further progress in miniaturization of ICDs. This will have marked clinical implications by reducing morbidity at implant as well as improving patient perception of the device by improving the cosmetic result.

Device diagnostic functions

Early devices provided little information about the onset of arrhythmias and therapy delivery but ICD Holters have become extremely sophisticated. Second-generation machines allowed telemetry of RR intervals during detection of tachycardia and immediately postdelivery of therapy, although it was soon obvious that this information was limited as only intervals sensed by the device were stored. More recently, the endocardial electrogram derived from the tip or proximal defibrillation electrode can be stored, allowing interpretation of the arrhythmia that induced the therapeutic response from the ICD. The latest devices will store several minutes of such electrograms and they can be divided into multiple tachycardia episodes providing useful information on the type of arrhythmia and the efficacy of both sensing and antitachycardia pacing algorithms. In addition, Holter functions allow trends in arrhythmias to be detected, possibly allowing adjustment in concurrent pharmacological therapy. Newer devices have greater storage capability and defibrillators incorporating dual-chamber pacemakers allow capture and storage of atrial electrograms,

increasing the sensitivity of diagnosis of ventricular arrhythmias.

Clinical aspects of ICDs

Patient selection

Cobb and colleagues[4] have suggested that patients who are successfully resuscitated following cardiac arrest have a 40% risk of recurrence of sudden cardiac death within 4 years. Patients with poor left ventricular function (ejection fraction <30%) and those with complex ventricular arrhythmias (polymorphic ventricular tachycardia, torsades des pointes or ventricular fibrillation) have a much higher risk of subsequent cardiac arrest. Thus, any patient with documented ventricular tachyarrhythmia should undergo invasive electrophysiological study to assess whether or not the arrhythmia is inducible. If ventricular tachycardia or fibrillation can be initiated using appropriate stimulation protocols, the patient is at increased risk of sudden cardiac death.[5] If the arrhythmia can be suppressed by antiarrhythmic drugs so that it is rendered noninducible at invasive electrophysiological study or on 24-hour ECG Holter monitoring, this suggests an improved outcome for the patient. If the tachycardia is slowed by antiarrhythmic drug therapy but is still inducible at EP study, this too suggests an improved prognosis.

What are the current indications for a defibrillator?

The current consensus for implantation of an ICD is as follows:

(1) Persistent inducibility of clinically relevant sustained ventricular tachycardia and/or ventricular fibrillation at electrophysiological study despite the use of drug, surgical or catheter ablation therapy.

(2) Recurrent spontaneous sustained VT and/ or VF in spite of antiarrhythmic drug therapy guided by invasive electrophysiological study or noninvasive methods, or when the use of drugs is not tolerated by the patient.

(3) One or more episodes of spontaneous sustained ventricular tachycardia or fibrillation in patients in whom electrophysiological testing or noninvasive techniques cannot be used to predict accurately the efficacy of nondevice therapy.

Ventricular ICDs should not be used in patients in whom ventricular tachycardia and/or fibrillation occurs in the setting of acute myocardial ischaemia or infarction, or in the presence of reversible toxic or metabolic aetiologies. In addition, patients with persistent recurrent malignant tachycardias should not have the device due to the psychological effects of rapidly recurrent defibrillator discharges. Other contraindications to ICD implantation include syncope of undetermined aetiology in a patient without inducible sustained ventricular tachyarrhythmias, or any surgical or psychiatric contraindications.

All patients should undergo routine haematological and biochemical tests (including thyroid function tests), echocardiography, chest X-ray and exercise electrocardiography as well as coronary angiography, to exclude potentially reversible causes for malignant ventricular arrhythmias. It should be noted that revascularization alone cures ventricular arrhythmias in only a few situations. An exception to this is critical left main stem disease. Most patients should undergo detailed electrophysiological study before contemplation of implantation of an ICD. This will often afford valuable information regarding device programming. The rates of the various tachyarrhythmias induced and their suscept-

ibility to paced termination, as well as possible information on numbers of extra stimuli and type of ramp or burst-pacing that is most efficacious, can be programmed into the device at implantation thus optimizing therapy as soon as possible.

Does the ICD decrease mortality from malignant ventricular arrhythmias?

Until recently there were no controlled randomized trials of ICD therapy versus pharmacological therapy in the treatment of malignant ventricular arrhythmias. All quoted evidence was registry data and this was compared with historical controls and universally confirmed the efficacy of ICDs in improving mortality.[6] With the improvement of Holter monitoring in second-generation ICDs, studies such as that of Bocker et al.[7] suggested that survival rate was 100% for sudden cardiac death, 97% for total arrhythmic death and 95% for all cardiac death in patients with ICDs implanted for life-threatening ventricular arrhythmias. However, this paper and many others assumed that any ventricular arrhythmia not treated with an ICD had a fatal outcome, which is manifestly untrue, and their conclusions have to be assessed with great caution. Unfortunately all implanters of ICDs have anecdotal cases of patients with recurrent ventricular arrhythmias and poor LV function, where the device discharged appropriately and reverted the arrhythmia for a few seconds, followed by persistent recurrence of the arrhythmia and the ultimate demise of the patient.

Several ongoing studies are comparing the efficacy of drug therapy with ICD therapy in patients with life-threatening ventricular arrhythmias. The Dutch study of Wever and colleagues[8] describes the outcome of patients randomized to antiarrhythmic drug therapy or ICD implantation. Mortality was 14% in the 29 ICD patients compared with 26% in 31 patients randomized to drug therapy, and this was highly statistically significant. The CASH study of Kuck and colleagues[9] compared ICD implantation with three different drug regimes—metoprolol, amiodarone, and propafenone. The safety and efficacy committee of the study has stopped the propafenone limb prematurely because of increased mortality. Preliminary results appear to favour the ICD strongly over both the remaining limbs, although these data have yet to be published.

The most striking results yet presented are those of the multicentre automatic defibrillator implantation trial (MADIT) of Moss and colleagues.[10] This large study, with a duration of 5 years, finally enrolled 196 patients. (Although this sounds a small number when compared with other major cardiology trials such as ISIS or GISSI, it should be remembered that the total number of ICD implants in the UK from 1990 to 1995 was less than 500.) Patients were enrolled if they had previous myocardial infarction (ejection fraction <35%), nonsustained ventricular tachycardia (3–30 beats) and were inducible into sustained ventricular tachycardia at EP study. Patients were excluded if they had significant comorbidity or severe heart failure or myocardial infarction within 3 weeks of the episode of ventricular tachycardia. Patients were randomized to 'conventional medical management' which could involve a series of drugs throughout the study period or to implantation of an ICD. It should be noted that the inducible ventricular tachycardia in almost all cases was monomorphic, which itself carries a better prognosis. Yet the findings were so significant that the trial was stopped prematurely in March 1996. It was found that there was a 54% reduction in mortality in the ICD group (15 deaths compared with 39 in the drug-trea-

ted group, p<0.009) and the reduction in deaths was shown to be in patients with sudden arryth mic cardiac death. Interestingly, 80% of patients with ICDs received shocks within 4 years and there was no perioperative mortality in the ICD-treated patients who all had endocardial systems implanted. These data appear unequivocally to favour device therapy for malignant arrhythmias over drug therapy with mortality reduction occurring in patients who were asymptomatic with nonsustained ventricular arrhythmias.

The two major amiodarone postinfarction trials, the European Myocardial Infarction Amiodarone Trial (EMIAT) and the Canadian Study (CAMIAT) with similar inclusion criteria to the MADIT study, showed that while amiodarone did reduce sudden cardiac death, there was no significant reduction in all-cause mortality suggesting that this drug may be proarrhythmic in some patients. In addition, nearly 50% of patients had to be taken off amiodarone due to adverse side effects within 2 years of commencement in both studies. It appears that there are now convincing data that suggest that prophylactic use of ICDs is indicated in some patients following myocardial infarction. This has major cost implications which will be discussed below.

Whether implantation of the ICD benefits a patient with severe left ventricular impairment is still open to question. Arrhythmic death in patients with congestive cardiac failure accounts for half the total mortality and many drugs have been shown to increase mortality if used in this subgroup of patients (for example flecainide and the CAST study). Many clinicians are concerned that an ICD may well avert sudden cardiac death secondary to a malignant arrhythmia, but that the patient may die soon afterwards from heart failure. However, some studies have shown that there is an improvement in survival, even in patients with severe left ventricular dysfunction.[11] The results of further trials in such patients are eagerly awaited.

Complications of ICD therapy

Perioperative mortality with epicardial ICDs was as high as 5%, often because patches were applied concurrently with coronary artery bypass grafting and/or valve surgery. Preoperative mortality with the latest transvenous epicardial systems is <0.5% and the transvenous approach is associated with a significantly shortened postoperative hospital stay.

Both techniques are at risk from the following complications:

(1) Device pocket infection, erosion or protrusion, always requiring explanation. It occurs in 1–5% of implants and is probably the most serious complication.
(2) Wound heamatoma.
(3) Lead fracture.
(4) Insulation break.
(5) Displacement causing malsensing.

All require reintervention. This is mandatory as inappropriate shocks can occur with defective sensing during normal sinus rhythm, including ventricular arrhythmias which could be fatal. Using transvenous endocardial electrodes can cause additional complications such as pneumothorax, haemothorax and rarely, pericardial tamponade. These electrodes too are susceptible to 'the subclavian crush syndrome' and this can induce device malfunction requiring explanation.

Psychological implications

Patients receiving ICDs are often told that they will receive an unpleasant stimulus and that the device will 'bring them back to life' after they have 'died' from their arrhythmia. Unsurprisingly, psychological complications are common. In a recent study undertaken at our institution, ICD patients who were compared with arrhythmia patients treated pharmacologically and patients implanted with dual-chamber pacemakers were shown to be significantly more depressed and anxious and to have a poorer quality of life. The most common complaint is fear of painful shocks and this can result in the patient refusing to get out of bed, in terror of inducing a noxious discharge. Anxiety and depression cloud their lives, resulting in an unacceptable quality of life. It is not uncommon for some patients to insist that the device is removed or switched off in spite of the risk of sudden cardiac death. A randomized study assessing the efficacy of interactive group counselling after ICD implantation has shown that anxiety and depression can be improved although only the latter was long-lasting, with little effect on general functional well-being.[12] This study also showed that the counselled patients appreciated the availability of experienced help and advice provided by a telephone help line.

It is important that preoperative counselling as well as postoperative counselling is available and that ICDs should not be implanted in patients who are potentially psychologically unstable.

Economic implications of ICD therapy

The cost of modern ICD generators and electrodes is between £15 000 and £20 000 at present. If these devices are implanted for the appropriate indications described above, the economic implications to the National Health Service in the UK and to healthcare throughout the world are vast. We must consider not only the cost of the initial implant, but also the fact that the longevity of these devices is 5 years at best, and recurrent changes of the generators (which cost between £10 000 and £14 000 in their own right) must also be taken into account. All manufacturers of these devices are currently recouping research and development costs and we must hope that in the very near future, with the prospect of an exponential rise in the rate of implantation of such devices, there will be a corresponding exponential fall in equipment costs so that all patients who are thought to require such intervention can receive it.

Atrial implantable cardioverter defibrillators

Potential use of atrial ICDs in patients with atrial fibrillation

The development of an implantable cardioverter defibrillator which is similar in size to a current dual-chamber pacemaker solely for reversion of atrial flutter and fibrillation is appealing. An atrial defibrillator would not have to respond instantly to the onset of tachycardia, allowing a longer charge time and requiring a smaller, lower voltage battery and smaller capacitors than those in ventricular ICDs. Good Holter functions would be required and it must be a dual-chamber device. These features could be incorporated into a generator of 30 ml or less in volume.

Incontrol Corporation has developed the first of such devices which has been implanted recently into human beings with atrial fibrillation. The maximum energy shock in this device is just 6 J and a proportion of patients with the device have failed to be cardioverted by this energy output. As stated previously, low-energy shocks are just as painful as high-energy ones and it is questionable whether patients with a comparatively nonlife-threaten-

ing arrhythmia will tolerate recurrent unpleasant shocks.

Studies of low-energy cardioversion using biphasic waveforms in human beings have shown that the defibrillation threshold can be as low as 1 J with dedicated electrodes placed in the coronary sinus, right atrial appendage and right ventricle.[13] Recurrent shock delivery for cardioversion of atrial arrhythmias in both humans and animals has been shown to be entirely safe if the energy delivery is synchronized on the R wave. However, postshock bradycardia occurs in 20% of patients and therefore postshock ventricular and atrial pacing is required in any atrial ICD.[14]

A recent study has shown that in selected patients with recurrent atrial fibrillation, repeated 'rapid' (within 24-hr) endocardial cardioversion does increase the ensuing period of sinus rhythm exponentially and thus atrial defibrillators may be a cure for atrial fibrillation in a subgroup of patients. This study has shown that a low defibrillation threshold, absence of sinus node dysfunction 24 hours after cardioversion, normal left atrial size, and specific atrial electrophysiology shown by either monophasic action potential recordings or atrial signal averaged ECG traces, all predispose to increasing periods of sinus rhythm as well as increasing efficacy of endocardial defibrillation of atrial fibrillation.[15]

In such patients high energy outputs would be unnecessary, although it must be remembered that during atrial fibrillation it is much less likely that patients will suffer altered levels of consciousness that allow them to tolerate unpleasant shocks, as in the case of ventricular defibrillators. Therefore it may be necessary that sedation is given prior to shock delivery. This could be indicated to the patient by a tone emitted from the device 5–15 minutes before delivery of the defibrillatory shock, allowing self-administration of sedatives, and ensuring the safe disposition of the patient (i.e., not driving or swimming) during shock delivery.

It must also be remembered that the energy requirements for cardioversion are greater in patients with chronic atrial fibrillation than in patients who have had acute atrial fibrillation induced at electrophysiological study (as in the vast majority of patients in whom endocardial defibrillation has been attempted). In my opinion, the problem of the high defibrillation thresholds required to revert atrial fibrillation must be resolved before atrial defibrillators can become an established treatment. However, our findings that rapid, recurrent cardioversion may be curative in up to 30% of patients with chronic atrial fibrillation require further investigation in patients with first-generation atrial ICDs.

If I had . . .

If I were unfortunate enough to suffer from survived sudden cardiac death or recurrent syncope due to malignant ventricular tachyarrhythmias, I would wish to undergo electrophysiological study to assess better the type of arrhythmia that I was suffering from and also whether and how it was pace-terminable. If I was appropriate for ICD implant I would wish to undergo counselling, informing me of every aspect of the implant procedure and my expected quality of life thereafter. I would want to be informed about the possibility of my driving a car with an implantable cardioverter defibrillator. (In the UK, if I have not suffered a device discharge for 3 months, I would be fit to drive with an ICD *in situ*.) I would enrol in an interactive counselling group long-term after implantation. I would hope that the device used was a tiered-therapy defibrillator allowing pace termination to try to decrease the number of noxious shocks that I might receive. I would also hope that concurrent medical therapy would keep the number of shocks to a minimum.

If I had suffered a myocardial infarction and was shown to suffer from nonsustained ventricular tachyarrhythmias, even if I was asymptomatic, I would hope for the above management.

If I was suffering from intractable chronic atrial fibrillation and was intolerant of all medication, I would request an appropriate work-up to be considered for an atrial implantable cardioverter defibrillator, assuming that the initial assessment defibrillation threshold was <20 J. If this was not the case, I may consider other forms of therapy such as the maze operation, but not ablation therapy at our current stage of knowledge and expertise. If I were shown to be an appropriate patient to benefit from an atrial defibrillator, I would ensure that I was on warfarin therapy until my episodes of atrial fibrillation became infrequent. I would hope to postpone such an implant until atrial defibrillator technology was sufficiently advanced, so that the energy required for defibrillation was <0.5 J and miniaturization of the devices to the size of a current pacemaker had been achieved.

References

1 Mirowski M, Reid PR, Mower MM et al, Termination of malignant ventricular arrhythmias with an implanted automatic defibrillator in human beings, *N Engl J Med* (1980)**303**:322.

2 Fisher J, Mehra R, Furman S, Termination of ventricular tachycardia with bursts of rapid ventricular pacing, *Am J Cardiol* (1978)**11**:94.

3 Schuder JC, Stoeckle H, Gold JC et al, Experimental ventricular defibrillation with an automatic and completely implanted system, *Trans Am Soc Artif Intern Organs* (1970)**16**:207.

4 Cobb LA, Weaver D, Fahrenbruch CE et al, Community-based interventions for sudden death. Impact limitation and changes, *Circulation* (1992)**85**:98.

5 Waller TJ, Kay HR, Spielman SR et al, A comparison of electrophysiologically guided antiarrhythmic drug therapy with beta-blocker therapy in patients with symptomatic sustained ventricular tachyarrhythmia, *J Am Coll Cardiol* (1987)**10**:83.

6 Mercando AD, Furman S, Johnston D et al, Survival of patients with the automatic implantable cardioventricular defibrillator, *Pacing Clin Electrophysiol* (1988)**11**:2059.

7 Bocker D, Bocker M, Isbruch F et al, Do patients with an implantable defibrillator live longer? *J Am Coll Cardiol* (1993)**21**:1638.

8 Wever EFD, Hauer RNW, Crijns HJGM et al, Dutch prospective randomised trial of implantable defibrillators as first-choice therapy in post-infarct sudden death survivors vs conventional therapy, *Eur J Cardiol* (1994)**15**:344.

9 Siebals J, Cappato R, Ruppel R and the CASH Investigators, ICD vs drugs in cardiac arrest survivors; preliminary results of the cardiac arrest study Hamburg, *Pacing Clin Electrophysiol* (1993)**16**:552.

10 Moss A, Hall J, Cannom D et al, Multicenter Automatic Defibrillator Implantation Trial (MADIT), *Pacing Clin Electrophysiol* (1993)**19**:364.

11 Fogoros NR, Elson JJ, Moosdorf R et al, Clinical efficacy of the automatic implantable cardioverter-defibrillator in prolonged survival in patients with severe underlying cardiac disease, *J Am Coll Cardiol* (1990)**16**:382.

12 Sulke N, Barakat K, Fiumicelli G et al, The efficacy of group counselling in patients with implantable cardioverter defibrillators, *Pacing Clin Electrophysiol* (1997) (*in press*).

13 Murgatroyd FD, Johnson EE, Cooper RS et al, Safety of low energy transvenous atrial defibrillation: world experience, *Circulation* (1994)**90**:1–14.

14 Keane D, Sulke N, Cooke R et al, Endocardial cardioversion of atrial flutter and fibrillation, *Pacing Clin Electrophysiol* (1993)**16**:928.

15 Sulke N, Kamalvand K, Tan K et al, A prospective evaluation of recurrent atrial endocardial defibrillation in patients with refractory chronic atrial flutter and fibrillation, *Pacing Clin Electrophysiol* (1996)**19**:624.

15

Resuscitation

Paul W Johnston and AA Jennifer Adgey

Introduction

Since the first report of successful resuscitation from out-of-hospital cardiac arrest,[1] there have been many attempts to improve survival. However, in recent years the survival rate for out-of-hospital ventricular fibrillation has remained static at 24–33%.[2] In an attempt to standardize treatment and improve outcome, several bodies have recommended guidelines for the management of cardiac arrest.[3,4] In doing so they have acknowledged that the inclusion or omission of certain treatments remains controversial.[3] This chapter will examine what is new in resuscitation and discuss the controversial issues, and will deal with basic life support and advanced life support techniques.

Cardiopulmonary resuscitation

History

The first report of closed chest cardiopulmonary resuscitation (CPR) was 36 years ago.[5] However, widespread training of the public only occurred after the Standards Conference on CPR in 1973.[6] Virtually complete acceptance of their concepts and recommendations resulted in the development of Basic Life Support teaching materials.

Physiology

It has been demonstrated experimentally that CPR results in a cardiac output of approximately 20% of prearrest cardiac output[7] and coronary and cerebral blood flows of less than 10% of normal levels.[8]

When closed chest compression was first described by Kouwenhoven et al. it was hypothesized that blood flow was caused by compression of the heart between the thoracic vertebrae and the sternum.[5] It was believed that this compression acted as an external pump allowing the sequential filling and emptying of cardiac chambers, and that the presence of valves favoured the forward flow of blood, in other words the 'cardiac compression' theory.

Other workers have challenged this explanation of blood flow during CPR. In an echocardiographic study in humans, Werner et al. found no significant change in LV diameter and no closure of the mitral valve during CPR.[9] It has also been shown in animals that there is no pressure gradient across the heart during chest compressions; equal RA and aortic pressures have been recorded.[10,11] However, Rudikoff et al. demonstrated a pressure difference between the intrathoracic and cervical venous systems and suggested that a pressure difference between the carotid arteries and the cervical veins provided the pressure gradient for cerebral blood flow.[11] Their explanation for this pressure difference was that it was caused by collapse of the jugular venous system.

Neimann et al. showed valve closure in the jugular veins using cineangiography during CPR.[10] These findings are consistent with the theory that the mechanism of blood flow during CPR is not due to cardiac compression but rather it is caused by a general increase in intrathoracic pressure, in other words the 'thoracic pump' model.[10]

More recently, evidence has accumulated which suggests that direct cardiac compression is an important mechanism for forward flow. In an extensively instrumented dog model, Maier et al. demonstrated left ventricular volume changes during high impulse CPR.[7] Using an active compression-decompression device, direct visualization of cardiac compression during CPR has been provided by transoesophageal echocardiography (TOE).[12] Therefore it is probable that both mechanisms described contribute to the beneficial effects of CPR.

Active compression-decompression

Based on the theory that active chest wall decompression would cause an increase in negative intrathoracic pressure and augment venous return, the active compression-decompression (ACD) device was developed. The idea for the device followed a report of a man being resuscitated from cardiac arrest by family members using a household plunger.[13]

This device consists of a handle, a force gauge and a suction cup. It is attached to the chest in the mid-sternal region. CPR is carried out in the standard way, except that active decompression is carried out at the end of the compression phase by lifting up the device.

Whereas coronary perfusion occurs only during passive decompression in ordinary CPR in most patients,[14] there is evidence that ACD leads to coronary flow in both active compression and active decompression.[13] There is evidence of increased coronary and cerebral blood flow in animals.[13,15] There is improved peak BP in animals[15] and man.[16,17] Improved cardiac output indicated by raised $ETCO_2$ has also been reported in man.[16-18] These haemodynamic improvements may be explained by beneficial effects of ACD on both the 'thoracic pump' model and the 'cardiac compression' model of CPR. Active decompression generates a greater negative intrathoracic pressure and increases venous return and intrathoracic fluid volume.[14,19] TOE studies have demonstrated increased end-decompression left ventricular volumes and transmitral flow.[12,20] This increased filling primes the heart for the active compression phase. There is also evidence that the ACD device delivers a high-energy impulse which causes direct compression of the right and left ventricles.[12]

In spite of the improved haemodynamics with ACD, it remains to be proven that the device will lead to improved survival. Several studies have compared ACD and standard CPR in humans.[16,21-24] Two studies on in-hospital arrests obtained a doubling of the return of spontaneous circulation (ROSC) and an improvement in neurological recovery in the ACD group.[21,22] In out-of-hospital cardiac arrest the results are mixed. Lurie et al. reported a strong trend to improved ROSC and hospital admission with ACD.[23] When the study was limited to a down-time of 10 minutes, the ACD resulted in an approximate doubling of admission and discharge rates. However, in a large study of 860 out-of-hospital cardiac arrests in two Californian cities, ACD was not found to be superior to standard CPR.[24] There was no improvement in ROSC, hospital admission rates, neurological state or discharge rates in either city. Also of note in this study was the short average time delay from activation of the emergency medical services to CPR — 6.4 minutes in Fresno and 4.0 minutes in San Francisco.

In conclusion, some human cardiac arrest studies have demonstrated that ACD improved short-term outcomes, that is ROSC,[21] ICU admission rates,[23] or 24-hour survival.[22] These positive results have tended to be for in-hospital arrests or in out-of-hospital arrests with a short down-time. No study has demonstrated an improvement in the important outcomes, that is neurologically intact survival and hospital discharge.

Defibrillation

Automated external defibrillators

One of the most important predictors of survival from out-of-hospital cardiac arrest is rapid defibrillation.[25] In Seattle, it was demonstrated that the time delay to defibrillation could be reduced by 5 minutes if performed by the 'first responder' to the cardiac arrest rather than by the usual paramedic service.[26]

Cummins et al. reviewed five controlled trials in which emergency medical technicians (EMTs) were taught to defibrillate and found odds ratios for improved survival ranging from 3.3 to 6.9.[27] In four of these five trials the EMTs were taught to recognize cardiac arrhythmias and to operate a manual defibrillator. In the remaining study, an automatic external defibrillator (AED) was employed which recognized the rhythm and delivered a DC shock when appropriate.

Three controlled trials have compared AEDs with manual defibrillators used by EMTs.[28–30] These studies found no significant difference between the hospital admission or discharge rates for cardiac arrest victims treated either by EMTs trained to recognize VF or by EMTs operating an AED. The delay to the first shock was significantly shorter in the AED group.

The successful use of AEDs by emergency medical technicians has raised the possibility of these devices being used by 'minimally trained individuals'. They have already been used successfully by family members of survivors of out-of-hospital cardiac arrest:[31] security staff at large public gatherings have also been successful in resuscitating out-of-hospital cardiac arrest victims.[32] Clearly, the use of such devices by laypersons could further reduce the time delay to defibrillation. The potential benefit of the AED has been recognized by the American Heart Association (AHA) Task Force on the Future of Cardiopulmonary Resuscitation.[33] The task force recommended that the AHA propose and support legislation and other measures to facilitate the availability and the use of AEDs in all public places where more than 10 000 people gather. It also recommended that legislation be enacted requiring all ambulances to be equipped with defibrillators and all 'first responders' to be trained in their use.

AEDs have a relatively high specificity for shockable rhythms but there have already been reports of the inappropriate delivery of DC shocks by these devices.[34,35] It is therefore essential that pulselessness is confirmed before an AED is attached to a patient. However, it is recognized that the 'pulse check' is one of the most frequently lost CPR skills.[36] There is therefore a potential role for a non-ECG sensor to confirm cardiac arrest independently before a shock is delivered. One of the earliest AEDs used a breath detector indirectly to confirm the absence of blood flow to the brain.[37] This sensor was subsequently abandoned because it led to a delay in the delivery of a DC shock, probably due to agonal respirations.[38] Another potential sensor to confirm pulselessness prior to defibrillation is the impedance cardiogram.[39]

Pad size and position

The use of adhesive ECG/defibrillator pads simplifies the process of defibrillation. The optimum size of these pads has been investigated. With larger pad sizes the transthoracic impedence is lower[40] and the delivered current is greater.[41] However, if the pad size is too large the current density is reduced and defibrillation effectiveness falls.[42] In an animal study, Ewy et al. investigated the effectiveness of defibrillation from 15 seconds of VF using a 50 J shock and three sizes of defibrillator pads.[41] The success rates for 8.0/8.0 cm, 12.8/12.8 cm and 13/20 cm pads were 59%, 83% and 33% respectively. In the clinical setting the optimum pad size has been investigated during defibrillation of patients from VF and VT.[43] Three pads sizes were compared — 8 cm/8 cm, 8 cm/12 cm, 12 cm/12 cm. It was found that transthoracic impedence was higher with the small pads than either the intermediate-size or large pads. Defibrillation by two 200 J shocks was successful in 55%, 75% and 100% of patients respectively.

Correct positioning of the adhesive ECG/defibrillator pads is essential. If the anterior–anterior approach is used then one electrode should be placed in the region of the cardiac apex and the other just beneath the right clavicle on the anterior chest wall to the right of the sternum. If the anterior–posterior approach is employed, the anterior electrode should be to the left of the sternum at the level of the fourth intercostal space and the posterior electrode should be between the shoulder blades. It is important also that the electrodes are applied firmly to the skin. In women the apex pad should be applied to the chest wall directly and not placed on top of or underneath the surface of the left breast.

Waveforms

Defibrillation is a lifesaving procedure but it has potential complications. The prognosis of patients who receive multiple shocks is reduced.[44] The effect of one, five or 10 synchronized (400 J) transthoracic shocks delivered at 30-second intervals was investigated in adult greyhounds.[45] More animals died of EMD or asystole as the number of shocks increased (0%, 44% and 71% respectively). In the animals receiving five or 10 shocks significant ST elevation was recorded 15 minutes and 1 hour after the shocks. Macroscopic cardiac damage at three days was minimal in the group given one shock and greater in those given 10 shocks than in those given five.

Trouton et al. examined the effects of defibrillation shocks on aerobic metabolism in an animal model.[46] They demonstrated transient failure of oxygen extraction in spite of hyperaemia, normal arterial O_2 content and increased cardiac work. They concluded that this finding could best be accounted for by a central effect of DC shocks on myocardial cellular respiration.

Use of internal defibrillation in humans has demonstrated that a biphasic waveform requires less energy than monophasic waveforms for successful defibrillation by automatic internal cardioverter-defibrillators (AICDs).[47] However, if more efficient waveforms were also to be associated with more injurious effects on myocardial function, they might not provide a true biological advantage. Osswald et al. addressed this problem in an animal model of internal defibrillation.[48] They demonstrated that the two biphasic waveforms tested were associated with less injurious effects on myocardial oxidative metabolism and haemodynamic performance than the monophasic waveform.

Two studies have examined the use of biphasic waveforms in transthoracic defibrillation.

Greene et al. compared the Edmark monophasic and the Gurvich biphasic waveforms in an EP laboratory.[49] They found that the biphasic waveform delivering a mean energy of 171 J was superior to the Edmark waveform delivering a mean 215 J in the successful conversion of VT and VF. Bardy et al. compared two truncated biphasic waveforms with a damped sine waveform for transthoracic defibrillation in patients undergoing AICD testing.[50] All waveforms were equally efficacious but the two biphasic waveforms delivered less energy (115 J and 130 J compared with 200 J).

Use of these waveforms could lead to lighter, smaller, more portable defibrillators with possibly less myocardial injury.

Oesophageal defibrillation

The oesophagus offers an alternative low impedance approach to defibrillation. It has been used for the DC cardioversion of atrial arrhythmias and requires significantly less energy and lower currents than the transchest approach.[51] It has also been used successfully to terminate VT and VF during electrophysiological studies.[52] It has been used as a 'rescue' defibrillation technique for refractory VF. Cohen et al. described the use of transoesophageal defibrillation in four patients in whom VF was successfully terminated after prolonged cardiac arrest.[53]

Pharmacotherapy

Adrenergic agonists

Coronary and cerebral blood flow during closed chest CPR fall to levels that are far below those necessary to meet the metabolic demands of the heart and brain.[54,55]

Adrenergic agonists have been used in the management of cardiac arrests since the beneficial effects of adrenaline on aortic diastolic pressure were first demonstrated in an animal model of CPR.[56] Coronary perfusion pressure (aortic diastolic pressure minus right atrial pressure) has been correlated highly with coronary blood flow[57] and is one of the best haemodynamic predictors of the return of spontaneous circulation both in animal models of cardiac arrest[57] and in man.[58] It has been demonstrated that adrenergic agonists can increase peripheral vascular resistance, raise aortic diastolic blood pressure, increase coronary perfusion pressure and improve cerebral and coronary blood flow during CPR.[56,57,59]

These positive haemodynamic effects are at the expense of decreased blood flow to other vital organs which can result in intrapulmonary shunting[60] causing arterial hypoxaemia, a reduced blood flow to the muscle and splanchnic bed resulting in a lactic acidosis,[59] and impaired renal perfusion.[61]

Adrenaline has been reported to increase the amplitude of the fibrillatory waveform in VF.[62] However, this effect does not decrease the energy requirements for defibrillation in animals with healthy hearts[63] or following coronary occlusion.[64] Indeed, beta-adrenergic stimulation may promote ventricular arrhythmias.[65,66]

Which agonist?

Adrenaline and noradrenaline have mixed adrenergic agonist effects, stimulating both of the subsets of the alpha and beta-adrenoreceptors. However, noradrenaline has less potent beta-adrenergic activity. By administering alpha and beta-blockers prior to adrenergic treatment in an animal model of CPR, it has been shown that most of the beneficial effects are the result of alpha-adrenergic stimulation.[67,68]

It is unclear if the beta-adrenergic effects are beneficial or harmful. Brown et al. reported that very large doses of adrenaline improved both coronary blood flow and the myocardial oxygen balance.[69] However, it is known that the fibrillating heart rapidly consumes oxygen[70] and beta-adrenergic stimulation may increase oxygen demand but not oxygen availability.[71,72] Two studies by Ditchey et al. also suggested the beta-adrenergic effects of adrenaline may be harmful.[73,74] They found that the combination of phenylephrine or adrenaline and the beta-blocker propranolol improved the haemodynamics and the balance between oxygen supply and demand in an animal model of VF, leading to higher levels of myocardial ATP and lower levels of lactate than in the control group. In contrast, high-dose adrenaline or phenylephrine alone worsened this balance.[73]

Several clinical trials have compared adrenaline with a more selective alpha-agonist and the results have been mixed.[75-78] Olson et al. reported that in patients with VF, adrenaline was superior to methoxamine in terms of rates of defibrillation, return of spontaneous circulation and hospital discharge.[75] However, Turner et al. reported no difference between 10 mg methoxamine and 1 mg adrenaline iv in the treatment of EMD.[76] In patients with VF, Lindner et al. found noradrenaline to be superior to adrenaline in causing ROSC and hospital discharge.[77] In contrast, Silfvast et al. found that up to 1.0 mg adrenaline and 2.0 mg phenylephrine were associated with similar rates of resuscitation in patients with cardiac arrest rhythms.[78]

What dose?

The current recommended dose of adrenaline is a 1 mg bolus repeated every 5 minutes as necessary. However, no prospective placebo-controlled trial of 'standard dose' adrenaline has been performed in cardiac arrest patients.[79] The effects of 'standard dose' adrenaline versus no adrenaline have been addressed in a large retrospective analysis of 1360 patients with witnessed out-of-hospital VF.[80] During the obser-vational period, some of the emergency medical staff were authorized to give standard doses of adrenaline and others were not. Adrenaline was given to 35% of patients and was associated with a significantly greater rate of ROSC and hospital admission. However, there was no significant difference in the hospital discharge rates between the two groups. Woodhouse et al. reported a trial of placebo versus high-dose and standard-dose adrenaline for cardiac arrest.[79] There was no significant difference in immediate survival or hospital discharge between patients receiving 1 mg adrenaline and those given placebo. The disappointing results with standard-dose adrenaline have led some workers to recommend the high dose.

The dose of 1 mg adrenaline is equivalent to 0.014 mg/kg in a 70 kg person. Recently, some animal studies have suggested beneficial effects with higher doses of adrenaline, up to 0.2 mg/kg (in other words, ten-times the standard dose).[54,69,81,82]

In uncontrolled trials in humans, high-dose adrenaline has been reported to improve aortic diastolic pressure,[83] coronary perfusion pressure[84] and return of spontaneous circulation.[85,86] Nevertheless no survival advantage was demonstrated in two small controlled trials, but they lacked the power to detect an important difference between groups.[87,88] Since then there have been four larger controlled trials.[89-92] One of the studies reported a significant increase in ROSC in the high-dose adrenaline group.[91] However, none of the studies found an increase in the hospital discharge rate with high-dose adrenaline. Brown et al. attempted to explain the difference between the promising experimental work and their disappointing controlled trial by the time delays to treatment.[89] In the experimental model the interval from arrest to administration of adrenaline was 13 minutes, compared with an average of 17 minutes in the clinical trial. In the subgroup of patients treated within 10 minutes there was a trend to greater hospital discharge rates. However, Steill et al. did not identify any subgroup that benefited from the higher dose.[90] A second possible explanation is that in contrast to the animal experiments, the majority of the patients would have significant coronary disease.[93] In the presence of fixed atherosclerotic plaques, high-dose adrenaline may worsen the balance between oxygen delivery and demand.

Adverse effects

In the nonarrested patient even 'standard-dose' adrenaline is associated with significant adverse effects. As little as 1.1 mg has been demonstrated to cause cardiac ischaemia in humans[94] and doses of 5 mg and 1 mg have been shown to cause severe pain and pulmonary oedema.[95] In a series of 15 patients suffering adverse effects of adrenaline a minimal lethal dose of 4 mg subcutaneously and maximum tolerated dose of 7–8 mg were reported.[96] Adrenaline has also been reported as causing sustained ventricular arrhythmias.[97]

In animal studies of cardiac arrest, high-dose adrenaline was associated with improved haemodynamics. However, immediately after the return of spontaneous circulation most animals demonstrated a hyperadrenergic state with severe tachycardia and hypertension.[98] Others have reported tachycardia associated with decreased inotropy following resuscitation with high-dose adrenaline.[99]

In spite of these adverse effects in animals and the reports of significant morbidity and mortality in the nonarrested patient, in the cardiac arrest setting Callaham et al. did not find any adverse effects postarrest of high-dose adrenaline on blood pressure, electrolytes, glucose level, acidosis, pulmonary oedema, ECG findings, CK or CKMB rise.[100] However, high-dose adrenaline has been associated with increased postarrest VT,[91] postresuscitation hypertension[89] and renal impairment.[61]

In view of the lack of evidence of benefit with high-dose adrenaline and the reports of significant morbidity, this therapy is not currently recommended. Furthermore, the administration of standard doses of adrenaline is not associated with improved longevity.

Antiarrhythmics

Lignocaine

Lignocaine has traditionally been recommended as an adjuvant for the treatment of VF resistant to DC shocks. More recently, its place in the management of VF has been relegated to a very late stage in one resuscitation protocol.[4]

Lignocaine has a membrane stabilizing effect and increases the ventricular fibrillation threshold.[101] In some animal studies it has also been reported to increase the defibrillation threshold, that is the energy required for successful defibrillation.[102,103] Dorian et al.[104] and Echt et al.[105] reported a concentration- dependent increase in the defibrillation energy requirement in normal dogs at therapeutic concentrations. However, Iyer et al. found no effect of lignocaine on the defibrillation threshold (DFT) in normal dogs.[106] Two studies have examined the effects of lignocaine on the DFT for internal defibrillation in humans.[107,108] Echt et al.[107] found that the defibrillation energy requirements were not elevated when the plasma concentration of lignocaine was less than 5 µg/ml (therapeutic range 1.2–5.5 µg/ml).[101] However, at higher plasma concentrations the defibrillation energy requirements were elevated. In the second study lignocaine did not alter the energy requirements for internal defibrillation.[108]

A possible explanation for the conflict between the experimental and clinical findings is that the anaesthetic regimen in animals may interact with lignocaine to raise the defibrillation threshold.[109,110] In the study by Kerber et al. lignocaine increased the defibrillation threshold more in the pentobarbitone-anaesthetized dogs (up to 60%) than in the chloralose-anaesthetized dogs (10–20%).[109] Natale et al. investigated the effects of three doses of lignocaine on the DFT in 36 halothane-anaesthetized pigs and the effects of the highest dose of lignocaine on a further eight pigs anaesthetized by barbiturates.[110] None of the doses of lignocaine affected the DFT in the halothane-anaesthetized pigs, whereas there was a significant increase in the barbiturate-anaesthetized pigs.

In humans, there is also evidence that the defibrillation threshold is not increased by lignocaine. Kerber et al. investigated factors which influence the success of defibrillation in 183 patients.[111] In the 26 patients with iv infusions of lignocaine running until the time of the arrest there was no increase in energy requirements for defibrillation. In addition, Lake et al. reported a beneficial effect of lignocaine on the defibrillation threshold in a randomized placebo-controlled trial of 20 patients undergoing myocardial reperfusion after CABG.[112]

There has been one randomized trial comparing lignocaine with adrenaline in out-of-hospital VF resistant to one 200 J DC shock. There was an increased incidence of asystole following lignocaine. However, there was no difference in the proportion of patients resuscitated or in the number of survivors.[113]

In conclusion, the decision to relegate lignocaine to a late stage (at least 7 minutes from the start of the resuscitative process) is not justified on present evidence.[114]

Buffers

It is well established that a respiratory or metabolic acidosis decreases myocardial contractility and impairs the cardiovascular response to catecholamines[115-117] and metabolic acidosis reduces VF threshold.[118,119] Consequently, buffer therapy in the form of sodium bicarbonate was recommended in the management of ventricular fibrillation.[6]

More recently, the use of sodium bicarbonate in a cardiac arrest setting has been challenged. The theoretical disadvantages are as follows:

- it worsens intracellular acidosis,[120]
- it produces hypernatraemia and hyperosmolarity,[120,121]
- and it shifts the oxygen dissociation curve to the left, increasing the affinity of haemoglobin for oxygen and reducing oxygen release in the tissues.[120]

It is intracellular acidosis that impairs cardiac contractility[116] and this may be exacerbated by sodium bicarbonate.[122] The explanation for this apparent paradoxical action is that carbonic acid (H_2CO_3) is a weak acid and it exists in equilibrium with dissolved CO_2. The effect of the addition of sodium bicarbonate is to drive the equilibrium equation to the right, increasing the concentration of extracellular dissolved CO_2. Bishop et al. have demonstrated that even small amounts of bicarbonate can significantly increase arterial P_{CO_2}.[123] This CO_2 can diffuse freely across the cell membrane, increasing the concentration of intracellular CO_2 and driving the equilibrium equation to the left causing intracellular acidosis:[120]

$$NaHCO_3 + H^+ \leftrightarrows Na^+ + H_2CO_3 \leftrightarrows Na^+ + H_2O + CO_2$$

Nevertheless, the combination of $NaHCO_3$ and hyperventilation to prevent the rise in Pa_{CO_2} can prevent intracellular acidosis.[124] Furthermore, Landow and Visner have demonstrated that the effect of $NaHCO_3$ on intramyocardial pH is biphasic.[125] There is an initial fall in intracellular pH followed by correction of the acidosis.

The production of CO_2 cannot be the only explanation for the initial increase in intracellular acidosis because CO_2-consuming buffers have also failed to improve intramyocardial pH.[126] It has been suggested that this is related to a fall in coronary perfusion pressure produced by the hyperosmolar solutions. Detrimental haemodynamic effects of hypertonic solutions have previously been reported[127,128] and may be mediated by both a vagal reflex and a direct action on the vessel wall.[127,129] Kette et al. examined the haemodynamic effects of Carbicarb, hypertonic sodium chloride and normal saline in an animal model of VF.[130] When compared with normal saline both the hypertonic solutions resulted in significantly reduced aortic pressures and coronary perfusion pressure during CPR and were associated with increased mortality.

Others have not found a detrimental effect of sodium bicarbonate. Bleske et al. found that administration of sodium bicarbonate had no effect on coronary perfusion pressure.[131] Their explanation for the difference between their study and those by Kette et al.[130] and Gazmuri et al.[126] was the dose used. Bleske et al.[131] administered the standard 1 mmol/kg whereas the other groups used much larger doses. Thus, when administered alone, sodium bicarbonate may decrease coronary perfusion in a dose-dependent manner.

There are no controlled trials of $NaHCO_3$ in the human cardiac arrest situation. In a retrospective study of 619 cardiac arrests there was no difference in survival between those receiving sodium bicarbonate and those who did not receive the buffer following standardization for the initial rhythm of VF and CPR time intervals.[132] However, in the survivors in whom electrolytes and arterial blood gases were performed there was no evidence of the major metabolic abnormalities described in the animal studies. Only 2% had hypernatraemia

$(Na^+ > 150)$ and 11% had a metabolic alkalosis compared with 10% in the no-buffer group with a metabolic alkalosis. A randomized controlled trial of the buffer Tribonat, which produces little CO_2, has been performed in 502 out-of-hospital cardiac arrests.[133] No difference in hospital admissions or discharge rates was found. The authors concluded that buffer therapy during out-of-hospital CPR did not improve outcome. However, Koster pointed out that in this study the dispatch-response time was short (mean 5.8 minutes) and the degree of acidosis was not very profound in either group.[134] Also, the confidence intervals were wide and the study was still consistent with an improvement of 40% in survival with the use of Tribonat.

In light of these results the AHA has revised their guidelines on the administration of sodium bicarbonate.[135] The European Resuscitation Council has also advised caution in the use of $NaHCO_3$.[136] They recommend that this buffer should only be administered with a pH < 7.0–7.1 and a base excess $\leqslant 10$. They further recommend that 'blind' administration of sodium bicarbonate should only take place after prolonged cardiac arrest (10–20 minutes).

Cerebral protection

A number of the new techniques described above can lead to an increased return of spontaneous circulation. However, the goal of resuscitation is neurologically intact survival to discharge.

In experimental total circulatory arrest brain oxygen stores are depleted in 15 seconds and energy stores within 5 minutes. However, individual neurones can survive up to 20 and possibly 60 minutes of normothermic circulatory arrest.[137] Safar postulated that cerebral recovery from circulatory arrest was hampered by cerebral perfusion failure, cerebral reoxygenation injury and cerebral intoxication resulting from derangement of extracerebral organs.[137] Attempts have been made to reduce the detrimental effects of the postresuscitation syndrome. However, results have been disappointing.

Standard brain-orientated support

This includes intensive-care monitoring, controlled ventilation, optimizing blood gases ($P_{O_2} > 100$ mmHg and $P_{CO_2} < 30$ mmHg), maintaining adequate arterial blood pressure, and avoiding hyperthermia. This standard brain-orientated support seems to improve prognosis in both animals and in humans when compared with 'usual' care.[137]

Other specific agents have been more disappointing.

Barbiturates

Among the first agents to be investigated were barbiturates. They had been demonstrated to reduce cerebral metabolism, oedema formation and intracranial pressure.[137] An initial study in monkeys with thiopental was promising,[138] but a controlled clinical trial has failed to confirm this finding.[139] In the Brain Resuscitation Clinical Trial I, 262 comatose survivors of cardiac arrest were randomized to receive standard brain-orientated intensive care or standard care with iv thiopental (30 mg/kg).[139] At 1 year there was no difference in mortality, survival with good cerebral recovery or survival with neurological damage.

Calcium antagonists

Calcium antagonists can reduce cerebral vasospasm and are suspected to reduce the intraneuronal liberation of calcium which accompanies cerebral reperfusion. Nimodipine has been shown to be beneficial in subarachnoid haemorrhage[140] but did not improve functional outcome in acute ischaemic strokes.[141] In a placebo-controlled trial of 150 consecutive patients resuscitated from out-of-hospital VF, nimodipine did not improve the 1-year survival rate.[142]

The second Brain Resuscitation Trial assessed another calcium antagonist, lidoflazine, in a randomized, placebo-controlled trial in the treatment of 520 comatose survivors of cardiac arrest.[143] At 6 months there was no difference between the two groups in mortality, survival with good cerebral recovery, or survival with neurological deficit. Thus, calcium antagonists cannot be routinely recommended postarrest.

Steroids

Glucocorticoids are effective in reducing cerebral oedema associated with focal neurological lesions. In view of this, steroids were used in the management of cerebral oedema accompanying trauma and hypoxia. The publication of prospective controlled studies showing no benefit from steroids in traumatic cerebral insult led the Brain Resuscitation Clinical Trial (Study I) group to analyse retrospectively their data for the effects of steroids on global brain ischaemia.[144] Of the 262 comatose cardiac arrest survivors, 192 received steroids (75% of the thiopental group and 72% of the control group). The steroid dosages were divided into low, medium and high. None of the three steroid groups had a significantly better neurological outcome than the group not receiving steroids.

If I had . . .

If I was to have out-of-hospital ventricular fibrillation, I would like to have it in a public place or in the presence of a bystander skilled in CPR (Figure 15.1). As a priority I would want someone to activate the emergency services. If there was to be any delay in the arrival of a defibrillator, I would want efficient CPR.

Defibrillation should be performed as early as possible either by an emergency medical technician, a paramedic or a physician. Particular attention should be paid to the ECG/defibrillator pad application and positions. To minimize myocardial damage, I would like a perfusing rhythm to be restored by one 200 J shock. However, if VF persisted after two 200 J and one 360 J shocks I would prefer to be managed by a physician. At this stage, I would want to be given 100 mg of lignocaine iv and then further 360 J DC shocks with CPR. If VF persisted after this treatment, I would want to be given a further antiarrhythmic iv such as mexiletine or amiodarone or bretylium tosylate in therapeutic doses, followed by further 360 J DC shocks and CPR. The arrest would now be prolonged and

50 mmol of 8.4% sodium bicarbonate should be considered for administration. If VF continued despite DC shocks, antiarrhythmics and sodium bicarbonate, I would wish to have endotracheal intubation and positive-pressure ventilation. The attempted resuscitation should be continued for at least 20 minutes with consideration of iv administration of magnesium/potassium blindly or adrenaline. If I was hypothermic, I would want the resuscitation attempt to be continued for at least 1 hour.

If immediate consciousness did not ensue after the correction of the VF, I would wish to have controlled ventilation for at least 24 hours with maintenance of normal oxygen saturation and mild hypocapnia. In addition, to reduce cerebral oedema, I would wish my physician

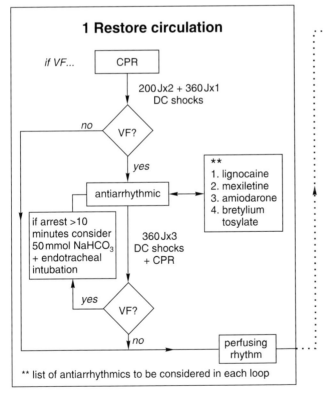

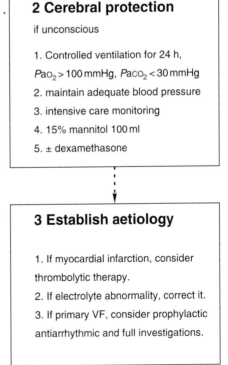

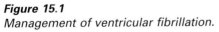

Figure 15.1
Management of ventricular fibrillation.

to consider mannitol followed by dexametha-sone. At 24 hours, I would wish to maintain spontaneous respiration.

The aetiology of the VF should be established. If it occurred in the setting of an acute myocardial infarction and the resuscitation was not traumatic, I would want to be given thrombolytic therapy. If the VF was due to an electrolyte abnormality (for example, hypokalaemia, hypomagnesaemia or hypocal-caemia), it should be corrected. If it occurred in the setting of chronic ischaemic heart disease, I would want to be given a prophylactic antiarrhythmic such as mexiletine until a full assessment could be performed; this would include coronary angiography, electrophysio-logical studies and assessment of late potentials. Long-term management, including consideration for an AICD, would depend on the aetiology.

References

1 Pantridge JF, Geddes JS, A mobile intensive-care unit in the management of myocardial infarction, *Lancet* (1967)**2**:271–3.

2 O'Nunain S, Ruskin J, Cardiac arrest, *Lancet* (1993)**341**:1641–7.

3 Emergency cardiac care committee and sub-committees, American Heart Association, Guidelines for cardiopulmonary resuscitation and emergency cardiac care, III Adult advance cardiac life support, *JAMA* (1992)**268**: 2171–295.

4 Guidelines for advanced life support. A statement by the Advanced Life Support Working Party of the European Resuscitation Council, *Resuscitation* (1992)**24**:111–21

5 Kouwenhoven WB, Jude JR, Knickerbocker GG, Closed chest cardiac massage, *JAMA* (1960)**173**:1064–7.

6 Standards for cardiopulmonary resuscitation (CPR) and emergency cardiac care (ECC), *JAMA* (1974)**227**:837–67.

7 Maier GW, Tyson GS Jr, Olsen CO et al, The physiology of external cardiac massage: high-impulse cardiopulmonary resuscitation, *Circulation* (1984)**70**:86–101.

8 Luce JM, Ross BK, O'Quin RJ et al, Regional blood flow during cardiopulmonary resuscitation in dogs using simultaneous and non-simultaneous compression and ventilation, *Circulation* (1983)**67**:258–65.

9 Werner JA, Greene HL, Janko CL, Cobb LA, Visualization of cardiac valve motion in man during external chest compression using two-dimensional echocardiography, *Circulation* (1981)**6**:1417–21.

10 Niemann JT, Rosborough JP, Hausknecht M, Garner D, Criley JM, Pressure-synchronized cineangiography during experimental cardio-pulmonary resuscitation, *Circulation* (1981)**64**:985–91.

11 Rudikoff MT, Maughan WL, Effron M, Freund P, Weisfeldt ML, Mechanisms of blood flow during cardiopulmonary resuscitation, *Circulation* (1980)**61**:345–52.

12 Pell AC, Pringle SD, Guly UM, Steedman DJ, Robertson CE, Assessment of the active compression-decompression device (ACD) in cardiopulmonary resuscitation using transoeso-phageal echocardiography, *Resuscitation* (1994)**27**:137–40.

13 Lindner KH, Pfenninger EG, Lurie KG, Schurmann W, Lindner IM, Ahnefeld FW, Effects of active compression-decompression resuscitation on myocardial and cerebral blood flow in pigs, *Circulation* (1993)**88**:1254–63.

14 Kern KB, Hilwig R, Ewy GA, Retrograde cor-onary blood flow during cardiopulmonary resuscitation in swine: intracoronary Doppler evaluation, *Am Heart J* (1994)**128**:490–9.

15 Chang MW, Coffeen P, Lurie KG, Shultz J, Bache RJ, White CW, Active compression-decompression CPR improves vital organ per-fusion in a dog model of ventricular fibrillation, *Chest* (1994)**106**:1250–9.

16 Cohen TJ, Tucker KJ, Lurie KG et al, Active compression-decompression. A new method of cardiopulmonary resuscitation. Cardiopulmon-ary Resuscitation Working Group, *JAMA* (1992)**267**:2916–23.

17 Guly UM, Robertson CE, Active decompres-sion improves the haemodynamic state during cardiopulmonary resuscitation, *Br Heart J* (1995)**73**:372–6.

18 Orliaguet GA, Carli PA, Rozenberg A, Janniere D, Sauval P, Delpech P, End-tidal carbon diox-ide during out of hospital cardiac arrest resus-citation: comparison of active compression-decompression and standard CPR, *Ann Emerg Med* (1995)**25**:48–51.

19 Shultz JJ, Coffeen P, Sweeney M et al, Evaluation of standard and active compres-sion-decompression CPR in an acute human model of ventricular fibrillation, *Circulation* (1994)**89**:684–93.

20 Tucker KJ, Redberg RF, Schiller NB, Cohen TJ, Active compression-decompression resuscita-tion: analysis of transmitral flow and left

ventricular volume by transesophageal echocardiography in humans. Cardiopulmonary Resuscitation Working Group, *J Am Coll Cardiol* (1993)**22**:1485–93.

21 Tucker KJ, Galli F, Savitt MA, Kahsai D, Bresnahan L, Redberg RF, Active compression-decompression resuscitation: effect on resuscitation success after in-hospital cardiac arrest, *J Am Coll Cardiol* (1994)**24**:201–9.

22 Cohen TJ, Goldner BG, Maccaro PC et al, A comparison of active compression-decompression cardiopulmonary resuscitation with standard cardiopulmonary resuscitation for cardiac arrests occurring in the hospital, *N Engl J Med* (1993)**329**:1918–21.

23 Lurie KG, Shultz JJ, Callaham ML et al, Evaluation of active compression-decompression CPR in victims of out-of-hospital cardiac arrest, *JAMA* (1994)**271**:1405–11.

24 Schwab TM, Callaham ML, Madsen CD, Utecht TA, A randomized clinical trial of active compression-decompression CPR vs standard CPR in out-of-hospital cardiac arrest in two cities, *JAMA* (1995)**273**:1261–8.

25 Weaver WD, Cobb LA, Hallstrom AP, Fahrenbruch C, Copass MK, Ray R, Factors influencing survival after out-of-hospital cardiac arrest, *J Am Coll Cardiol* (1986)**7**:752–7.

26 Weaver WD, Copass MK, Bufi D, Ray R, Hallstrom AP, Cobb LA, Improved neurological recovery and survival after early defibrillation, *Circulation* (1984)**69**:943–8.

27 Cummins RO, Ornato JP, Thies WH, Pepe PE, Improving survival from sudden cardiac arrest: the 'chain of survival' concept, *Circulation* (1991)**83**:1832–47.

28 Stults KR, Brown DD, Kerber RE, Efficacy of an automated external defibrillator in the management of out-of-hospital cardiac arrest: validation of the diagnostic algorithm and initial clinical experience in a rural environment, *Circulation* (1986)**73**:701–9.

29 Cummins RO, Eisenberg MS, Litwin PE, Graves JR, Hearne TR, Hallstrom AP, Automatic external defibrillators used by emergency medical technicians: a controlled clinical trial, *JAMA* (1987)**257**:1605–10.

30 Jakobsson J, Rehnqvist N, Nyqvist O, Clinical experience with three different defibrillators for resuscitation of out of hospital cardiac arrest, *Resuscitation* (1990)**19**:167–73.

31 Swenson RD, Hill DL, Martin JS, Wirkus M, Weaver WD, Automatic external defibrillators used by family members to treat cardiac arrest, *Circulation* (1987)**76(suppl IV)**:463 (abstr).

32 Weaver WD, Sutherland K, Wirkus MJ, Bachman R, Emergency medical care requirements for large public assemblies and a new strategy for managing cardiac arrest in this setting, *Ann Emerg Med* (1989)**18**:155–60.

33 Cobb LA, Eliastam M, Kerber RE et al, Report of the American Heart Association task force on the future of cardiopulmonary resuscitation, *Circulation* (1992)**85**:2346–55.

34 Ornato JP, Shipley J, Powell RG, Racht EM, Inappropriate electrical countershocks by an automated external defibrillator, *Ann Emerg Med* (1992)**21**:1278–81.

35 Sedgwick ML, Watson J, Dalziel K, Carrington DJ, Cobbe SM, Efficacy of out of hospital defibrillation by ambulance technicians using automated external defibrillators. The Heartstart Scotland Project, *Resuscitation* (1992)**24**:73–87.

36 Martin WJ, Loomis JH, Lloyd CW, CPR skills: achievement and retention under stringent and relaxed criteria, *Am J Public Health* (1983)**73**:1310–12.

37 Diack AW, Welborn WS, Rullman RG, Walter CW, Wayne MA, An automatic cardiac resuscitator for emergency treatment of cardiac arrest, *Med Instrum* (1979)**13**:78–81.

38 Cummins RO, Eisenberg MS, Stults KR, Automatic external defibrillators: clinical issues for cardiology, *Circulation* (1986)**73**:381–5.

39 Johnston PW, Anderson J, Adgey AAJ, A haemodynamic verification system for an automated external defibrillator, *Br Heart J* (1995)**73(suppl 3)**:10 (abstr).

40 Connell PN, Ewy GA, Dahl CF, Ewy MD, Transthoracic impedence to defibrillator discharge: effect of electrode size and electrode-chest wall interface, *J Electrocardiol* (1973)**6**:313–17.

41 Ewy GA, Horan WJ, Effectiveness of direct current defibrillation: role of paddle electrode size: II, *Am Heart J* (1977)**93**:674–5.

42 Ewy GA, Recent advances in cardiopulmonary resuscitation and defibrillation, *Curr Probl Cardiol* (1983)**8**:1–42.

43 Dalzell GWN, Cunningham SR, Wilson CM, Allen JD, Anderson J, Adgey AAJ, Ventricular defibrillation: the Belfast experience, *Br Heart J* (1987)**58**:441–6.

44 Dunn HM, McComb JM, MacKenzie G, Adgey AA, Survival to leave hospital from ventricular fibrillation, *Am Heart J* (1986)**112**:745–51.

45 Wilson CM, Allen JD, Bridges JB, Adgey AAJ, Death and damage caused by multiple direct current shocks: studies in an animal model, *Eur Heart J* (1988)**9**:1257–65.

46 Trouton TG, Allen JD, Young IS, Trimble ER, Adgey AA, Altered cardiac oxygen extraction, lactate production and coronary blood flow after large dose transthoracic DC countershocks, *PACE* (1993)**16**:1304–9.

47 Bardy GH, Ivey MD, Allen MD, Johnson G, Mehra R, Greene HL, A prospective randomised evaluation of biphasic versus monophasic waveform pulses on defibrillation efficacy in humans, *J Am Coll Cardiol* (1989)**14**:728–33.

48 Osswald S, Trouton TG, O'Nunain SS, Holden HB, Ruskin JN, Garan H, Relation between shock-related myocardial injury and defibrillation efficacy of monophasic and biphasic shocks in a canine model, *Circulation* (1994)**90**:2501–9.

49 Greene HL, DiMarco JP, Kudenchuk PJ et al, Comparison of monophasic and biphasic defibrillating pulse waveforms for transthoracic cardioversion, *Am J Cardiol* (1995)**75**: 1135–9.

50 Bardy GH, Gliner BE, Kudenchuk PJ et al, Truncated biphasic pulses for transthoracic defibrillation, *Circulation* (1995)**91**:1768–74.

51 Cochrane DJ, McEneaney DJ, Anderson JM, Adgey AA, Transoesophageal versus transchest DC cardioversion, *Q J Med* (1993)**86**:507–11.

52 Adgey AA, McKeown PP, Anderson J McC, Cardioversion and defibrillation: the esophageal approach. In: Vincent JL, ed. *Update in intensive care and emergency medicine 14*, 1st edn (Springer-Verlag: Berlin, 1991) 34–39.

53 Cohen TJ, Innovative emergency defibrillation methods for refractory ventricular fibrillation in a variety of hospital settings, *Am Heart J* (1993)**126**:962–8.

54 Brown CG, Werman HA, Davis EA, Hobson J, Hamlin RL, The effects of graded doses of epinephrine on regional myocardial blood flow during cardiopulmonary resuscitation in swine, *Circulation* (1987)**75**:491–7.

55 Taylor RB, Brown CG, Bridges T et al, A model for regional blood flow measurements during cardiopulmonary resuscitation in a swine model, *Resuscitation* (1988)**16**:107–18.

56 Redding JS, Pearson JW, Evaluation of drugs for cardiac resuscitation, *Anesthesiology* (1963)**24**:203–7.

57 Michael JR, Guerci AD, Koehler RC et al, Mechanisms by which epinephrine augments cerebral and myocardial perfusion during cardiopulmonary resuscitation in dogs, *Circulation* (1984)**69**:822–35.

58 Paradis NA, Martin GB, Rivers EP et al, Coronary perfusion pressure and the return of spontaneous circulation in human cardiopulmonary resuscitation, *JAMA* (1990)**263**:1106–13.

59 Ornato JP, Use of adrenergic agonists during CPR in adults, *Ann Emerg Med* (1993)**22**:411–16.

60 Tang W, Weil MH, Sun S et al, Epinephrine produces pulmonary A-V shunt during CPR, *Circulation* (1990)**82(suppl III)**:485 (abstr).

61 Mattana J, Singhal PC, High dose epinephrine in cardiopulmonary resuscitation, *N Engl J Med* (1993)**328**:735.

62 Livesay JJ, Follette DM, Fey KH et al, Optimizing myocardial supply/demand balance with alpha-adrenergic drugs during cardiopulmonary resuscitation, *J Thorac Cardiovasc Surg* (1978)**76**:244–51.

63 Yakaitis RW, Ewy GA, Otto CW, Taren DL, Moon TE, Influence of time and therapy on ventricular defibrillation in dogs, *Crit Care Med* (1980)**8**:157–63.

64 Otto CW, Yakaitis RW, Ewy GA, Effect of epinephrine on defibrillation in ischemic ventricular fibrillation, *Am J Emerg Med* (1985)**3**:285–91.

65 Harris AS, Otero H, Bocage AJ, The induction of arrhythmias by sympathetic activity before and after occlusion of a coronary artery in the canine heart, *J Electrocardiol* (1971) **4**:34–43.

66 Tisdale JE, Patel RV, Webb CR, Borzak S, Zarowitz BJ, Proarrhythmic effects of intravenous vasopressors, *Ann Pharmacother* (1995)**29**:269–81.

67 Yakaitis RW, Otto CW, Blitt CD, Relative importance of alpha and beta adrenergic receptors during resuscitation, *Crit Care Med* (1979)**7**:293–6.

68 Otto CW, Yakaitis RW, Blitt CD, Mechanism of action of epinephrine in resuscitation from asphyxial arrest, *Crit Care Med* (1981)**9**:321–4.

69 Brown CG, Taylor RB, Werman HA, Luu T, Ashton J, Hamlin RL, Myocardial oxygen delivery/consumption during cardiopulmonary resuscitation: a comparison of epinephrine and phenylephrine, *Ann Emerg Med* (1988)**17**:302–8.

70 Monroe RG, French G, Ventricular pressure-volume relationships and oxygen consumption in fibrillation and arrest, *Circ Res* (1960)**8**:260–6.

71 Ditchey RV, Lindenfeld J, Failure of epinephrine to improve the balance between myocardial oxygen supply and demand during closed-chest resuscitation in dogs, *Circulation* (1988)**78**:382–9.

72 Midei MG, Sugiura S, Maughan WL, Sagawa K, Weisfeldt ML, Guerci AD, Preservation of ventricular function by treatment of ventricular fibrillation with phenylephrine, *J Am Coll Cardiol* (1990)**16**:489–94.

73 Ditchey RV, Slinker BK, Phenylephrine plus propranolol improves the balance between myocardial oxygen supply and demand during experimental cardiopulmonary resuscitation, *Am Heart J* (1994)**127**:324–30.

74 Ditchey RV, Rubio-Perez A, Slinker BK, Beta-adrenergic blockade reduces myocardial injury during experimental cardiopulmonary resuscitation, *J Am Coll Cardiol* (1994)**24**:804–12.

75 Olson DW, Thakur R, Stueven HA et al, Randomized study of epinephrine versus methoxamine in prehospital ventricular fibrillation, *Ann Emerg Med* (1989)**18**:250–3.

76 Turner LM, Parsons M, Luetkemeyer RC, Ruthman JC, Anderson RJ, Aldag JC, A comparison of epinephrine and methoxamine for resuscitation from electromechanical dissociation in human beings, *Ann Emerg Med* (1988)**17**:443–9.

77 Lindner KH, Ahnefeld FW, Grunert A, Epinephrine versus norepinephrine in prehospital ventricular fibrillation, *Am J Cardiol* (1991)**67**:427–8.

78 Silfvast T, Saarnivaara L, Kinnunen A et al, Comparison of adrenaline and phenylephrine in out-of-hospital cardiopulmonary resuscitation. A double-blind study, *Acta Anaesthesiol Scand* (1985)**29**:610–13.

79 Woodhouse SP, Cox S, Boyd P, Case C, Weber M, High dose and standard dose adrenaline do not alter survival compared with placebo, in cardiac arrest, *Resuscitation* (1995)**30**:243–9.

80 Herlitz J, Ekstrom L, Wennerblom B, Axelsson A, Bang A, Holmberg S, Adrenaline in out-of-hospital ventricular fibrillation. Does it make a difference? *Resuscitation* (1995)**29**:195–201.

81 Kosnik JW, Jackson RE, Keats S, Tworek RM, Freeman SB, Dose-related response of centrally administered epinephrine on the change in aortic diastolic pressure during closed-chest massage in dogs, *Ann Emerg Med* (1985)**14**:204–8.

82 Chase PB, Kern KB, Sanders AB, Otto CW, Ewy GA, Effects of graded doses of epinephrine on both noninvasive and invasive measures of myocardial perfusion and blood flow during cardiopulmonary resuscitation, *Crit Care Med* (1993)**21**:413–19.

83 Gonzalez ER, Ornato JP, Garnett AR, Levine RL, Young DS, Racht EM, Dose-dependent vasopressor response to epinephrine during CPR in human beings, *Ann Emerg Med* (1989)**18**:920–6.

84 Paradis NA, Martin GB, Rosenberg J et al, The effect of standard- and high-dose epinephrine on coronary perfusion pressure during prolonged cardiopulmonary resuscitation, *JAMA* (1991)**265**:1139–44.

85 Barton C, Callaham M, High-dose epinephrine improves the return of spontaneous circulation rates in human victims of cardiac arrest, *Ann Emerg Med* (1991)**20**:722–5.

86 Goetting MG, Paradis NA, High-dose epinephrine improves outcome from pediatric cardiac arrest, *Ann Emerg Med* (1991)**20**:22–6.

87 Maha RJ, Yealy DM, Menegazzi JJ et al, High dose epinephrine in pre-hospital cardiac arrest: a preliminary report of 50 cases, *Ann Emerg Med* (1990)**19**:956 (abstr).

88 Sherman BW, Munger MA, Panacek EA, Foulke GE, High dose epinephrine in patients failing pre-hospital resuscitation, *Ann Emerg Med* (1991)**20**:949 (abstr).

89 Brown CG, Martin DR, Pepe PE et al, A comparison of standard-dose and high-dose epinephrine in cardiac arrest outside the hospital. The Multicenter High-Dose Epinephrine Study Group, *N Engl J Med* (1992)**327**:1051–5.

90 Stiell IG, Hebert PC, Weitzman BN et al, High dose epinephrine in adult cardiac arrest, *N Engl J Med* (1992)**327**:1045–50.

91 Callaham M, Madsen CD, Barton CW, Saunders CE, Pointer J, A randomized clinical trial of high-dose epinephrine and norepinephrine vs standard-dose epinephrine in prehospital cardiac arrest, *JAMA* (1992)**268**:2667–72.

92 Choux C, Gueugniaud PY, Barbieux A et al, Standard doses versus repeated high doses of epinephrine in cardiac arrest outside the hospital, *Resuscitation* (1995)**29**:3–9.

93 Kuller L, Cooper M, Perper J, Epidemiology of sudden death, *Arch Intern Med* (1972) **129**:714–19.

94 Hall A, Kulig K, Rumack B, Intravenous epinephrine abuse, *Am J Emerg Med* (1987)**5**:64–5.

95 Ersoz N, Finestone SC, Adrenaline-induced pulmonary oedema and its treatment. A report of two cases, *Br J Anaesth* (1971)**43**:709–12.

96 Freedman BJ, Accidental adrenaline overdosage and its treatment with piperoxan, *Lancet* (1955)**266**:575–8.

97 Morady F, Nelson SD, Kou WH et al, Electrophysiologic effects of epinephrine in humans, *J Am Coll Cardiol* (1988)**11**:1235–44.

98 Berg RA, Otto CW, Kern KB et al, High-dose epinephrine results in greater early mortality after resuscitation from prolonged cardiac arrest in pigs: a prospective, randomized study, *Crit Care Med* (1994)**22**:282–90.

99 Hornchen U, Lussi C, Schuttler J, Potential risks of high-dose epinephrine for resuscitation from ventricular fibrillation in a porcine model, *J Cardiothorac Vasc Anesth* (1993)**7**:184–7.

100 Callaham M, Barton CW, Kayser S, Potential complications of high-dose epinephrine therapy in patients resuscitated from cardiac arrest, *JAMA* (1991)**265**:1117–22.

101 Spear JF, Moore EN, Gerstenblith G, Effect of lidocaine on the ventricular fibrillation threshold in the dog during acute ischemia and premature ventricular contractions, *Circulation* (1972)**46**:65–73.

102 Babbs CF, Yim GK, Whistler SJ, Tacker WA, Geddes LA, Elevation of ventricular defibrillation threshold in dogs by antiarrhythmic drugs, *Am Heart J* (1979)**98**:345–50.

103 Chow MSS, Kluger J, Lawrence R, Fieldman A, The effect of lidocaine and bretylium on the defibrillation threshold during cardiac arrest and cardiopulmonary resuscitation, *Proc Soc Exp Biol Med* (1986)**182**:63–7.

104 Dorian P, Fain ES, Davy JM, Winkle RA, Lidocaine causes a reversible, concentration-dependent increase in defibrillation energy requirements, *J Am Coll Cardiol* (1986) **8**:327–32.

105 Echt DS, Black JN, Barbey JT, Coxe DR, Cato E, Evaluation of antiarrhythmic drugs on defibrillation energy requirements in dogs. Sodium channel block and action potential prolongation, *Circulation* (1989)**79**:1106–17.

106 Iyer SS, Monje E, Ruffy R, Comparative studies on defibrillation energy requirements in the dog, *Proc Assoc Adv Med Instrum* (1989)**24**:45 (abstr).

107 Echt DS, Lee JT, Roden DM et al, Effects of lidocaine on defibrillation energy requirements in patients, *Circulation* (1989)**80**:II-224 (abstr).

108 Jones DL, Klein GJ, Guiraudon GM, Yee R, Brown JE, Sharma AD, Effects of lidocaine and verapamil on defibrillation in humans, *J Electrocardiol* (1991)**24**:299–305.

109 Kerber RE, Pandian NG, Jensen SR et al, Effect of lidocaine and bretylium on energy requirements for transthoracic defibrillation: experimental studies, *J Am Coll Cardiol* (1986)**7**:397–405.

110 Natale A, Jones DL, Kim YH, Klein GJ, Effects of lidocaine on defibrillation threshold in the pig: evidence of anesthesia related increase, *PACE* (1991)**14**:1239–44.

111 Kerber RE, Jensen SR, Gascho JA, Grayzel J, Hoyt R, Kennedy J, Determinants of defibrillation: prospective analysis of 183 patients, *Am J Cardiol* (1983)**52**:739–45.

112 Lake CL, Kron IL, Mentzer RM, Crampton RS, Lidocaine enhances intraoperative ventricular defibrillation, *Anesth Analg* (1986)**65**:337–40.

113 Weaver WD, Fahrenbruch CE, Johnson DD, Hallstrom AP, Cobb LA, Copass MK, Effect of epinephrine and lidocaine therapy on outcome after cardiac arrest due to ventricular fibrillation, *Circulation* (1990)**82**:2027–34.

114 Adgey AA, Cardiopulmonary resuscitation. Guidelines should be reconsidered, *Br Med J* (1993)**307**:626–7.

115 Cingolani HE, Faulkner SL, Mattiazzi AR, Bender HW, Graham TP Jr, Depression of human myocardial contractility with 'respiratory' and 'metabolic' acidosis, *Surgery* (1975)**77**:427–32.

116 Orchard CH, Kentish JC, Effects of changes of pH on the contractile function of cardiac muscle, *Am J Physiol* (1990)**258**:C967–81.

117 Andersen MN, Border JR, Mouritzen CV, Acidosis, catecholamines, and cardiovascular dynamics: when does acidosis require correction? *Ann Surg* (1967)**166**:344–56.

118 Rogers RM, Spear JF, Moore EN, Horowitz LH, Sonne JE, Vulnerability of canine ventricle to fibrillation during hypoxia and respiratory acidosis, *Chest* (1973)**63**:986–94.

119 Gerst PH, Fleming WH, Malm JR, Increased susceptibility of the heart to ventricular fibrillation during metabolic acidosis, *Circ Research* (1966)**19**:63–70.

120 Sing RF, Branas CA, Sing RF, Bicarbonate therapy in the treatment of lactic acidosis: medicine or toxin? *J Am Osteopath Assoc* (1995)**95**:52–7.

121 Mattar JA, Weil MH, Shubin H, Stein L, Cardiac arrest in the critically ill. II. Hyperosmolal states following cardiac arrest, *Am J Med* (1974)**56**:162–8.

122 Jaffe AS, New and old paradoxes. Acidosis and cardiopulmonary resuscitation, *Circulation* (1989)**80**:1079–83.

123 Bishop RL, Weisfeldt ML, Sodium bicarbonate administration during cardiac arrest. Effect on arterial pH, PCO2, and osmolality, *JAMA* (1976)**235**:506–9.

124 Eleff SM, Sugimoto H, Shaffner DH, Traystman RJ, Koehler RC, Acidemia and brain pH during prolonged cardiopulmonary resuscitation in dogs, *Stroke* (1995)**26**: 1028–34.

125 Landow L, Visner MS, Does NaHCO₃ exacerbate myocardial acidosis? *J Cardiothorac Vasc Anesth* (1993)**7**:340–51.

126 Gazmuri RJ, von Planta M, Weil MH, Rackow EC, Cardiac effects of carbon dioxide-consuming and carbon dioxide generating buffers during cardiopulmonary resuscitation, *J Am Coll Cardiol* (1990)**15**:482–90.

127 Huseby JS, Gumprecht DG, Hemodynamic effects of rapid bolus hypertonic sodium bicarbonate, *Chest* (1981)**79**:552–4.

128 Kozeny GA, Murdock DK, Euler DE et al, *In vivo* effects of acute changes in osmolality and sodium concentration on myocardial contractility, *Am Heart J* (1985)**109**:290–6.

129 Agarwal JB, Baile EM, Palmer WH, Reflex systemic hypotension due to hypertonic solutions in pulmonary circulation, *J Appl Physiol* (1969)**27**:251–5.

130 Kette F, Weil MH, Gazmuri RJ, Buffer solutions may compromise cardiac resuscitation by reducing coronary perfusion pressure, *JAMA* (1991)**266**:2121–6.

131 Bleske BE, Rice TL, Warren EW, De Las Alas VR, Tait AR, Knight PR, The effect of sodium bicarbonate administration on the vasopressor effect of high-dose epinephrine during cardiopulmonary resuscitation in swine, *Am J Emerg Med* (1993)**11**:439–43.

132 Aufderheide TP, Martin DR, Olson DW et al, Prehospital bicarbonate use in cardiac arrest: a 3-year experience, *Am J Emerg Med* (1992)**10**:4–7.

133 Dybvik T, Strand T, Steen PA, Buffer therapy during out-of-hospital cardiopulmonary resuscitation, *Resuscitation* (1995)**29**:89–95.

134 Koster RW, Correction of acidosis during cardio-pulmonary resuscitation [editorial], *Resuscitation* (1995)**29**:87–8.

135 Standards and guidelines for cardiopulmonary resuscitation (CPR) and emergency cardiac care (ECC), *JAMA* (1986)**255**:2905–89.

136 Koster R, Carli P, Acid-base management. A statement for the Advanced Life Support Working Party of the European Resuscitation Council, *Resuscitation* (1992)**24**:143–6.

137 Safar P, Cerebral resuscitation after cardiac arrest: a review, *Circulation* (1986)**74 (Suppl IV)**:138–53.

138 Bleyaert AL, Nemoto EM, Safar P et al, Thiopental amelioration of brain damage after global ischemia in monkeys, *Anesthesiology* (1978)**49**:390–8.

139 Brain Resuscitation Clinical Trial I Study Group, Randomised clinical study of thiopental loading in comatose survivors of cardiac arrest, *N Engl J Med* (1986)**314**:397–403.

140 Allen GS, Ahn HS, Preziosi TJ et al, Cerebral arterial spasm—a controlled trial of nimodipine in patients with subarachnoid haemorrhage, *N Engl J Med* (1983)**308**:619–24.

141 Kaste M, Fogelholm R, Erila T et al, A randomized, double-blind, placebo-controlled trial of nimodipine in acute ischemic hemispheric stroke, *Stroke* (1994)**25**:1348–53.

142 Roine RO, Kaste M, Kinnunen A, Nikki P, Sarna S, Kajaste S, Nimodipine after resuscitation from out-of-hospital ventricular fibrillation. A placebo-controlled, double-blind, randomized trial, *JAMA* (1990)**264**:3171–7.

143 Brain Resuscitation Clinical Trial II Study Group, A randomised clinical study of a calcium-entry blocker (lidoflazine) in the treatment of comatose survivors of cardiac arrest, *N Engl J Med* (1991)**324**:1225–31.

144 Jastremski M, Sutton-Tyrrell K, Vaagenes P et al, Glucocorticoid treatment does not improve neurological recovery following cardiac arrest. Brain Resuscitation Clinical Trial I Study Group, *JAMA* (1989)**262**:3427–30.

16

Cardiac risks and general surgery

Douglas Chamberlain

Introduction

Cardiac risk should be a matter of prime concern to all who have an interest in general surgery, whether they be surgeons, anaesthetists, physicians with an advisory role, or the patients themselves. The facts are persuasive. In England and Wales, approximately 3.5 million surgical operations are undertaken each year.[1] The total morbidity is not known, but more than 20 000 patients die in the perioperative period.[1] In the USA, cardiac morbidity is known to be the leading cause of death.[2] This is likely to be true in Britain too, although no definitive prospective studies have been carried out. However, one recent series has underscored the risk in a subset of patients: it showed that myocardial infarction occurred in 6.3% of patients undergoing abdominal aortic surgery.[3] The incidence of coronary events tends to be underestimated in clinical practice, because a high proportion are silent[4,5] and can be detected only by electrocardiography or specific enzyme testing.[6] Hazards are greatest postoperatively in the first few days,[5] but increased risk continues in the longer term, especially — but not exclusively — in those who suffer a postoperative ischaemic episode. In one recent study, patients surviving a postoperative myocardial infarction had a 28-fold increase in the rate of subsequent cardiac complications within 6 months of surgery, a 15-fold increase within 1 year, and a 14-fold increase within 2 years.[7]

Potential risks to patients

Healthy patients are hardly at risk when undergoing most surgical procedures, but those who are vulnerable face protean challenges. These relate both to the intraoperative and postoperative phases. Heart rate usually increases and blood pressure may fall. Changes in body temperature, endothelial function, and the neurohormonal milieu—in particular increased circulating catecholamine concentrations—not only further increase metabolic demand but collectively may also affect coronary flow adversely at a time when augmentation is needed. Coronary constriction may occur from visceral reflexes.[8,9] Moreover, chest and abdominal incisions may influence respiratory efficiency and biochemical disturbances may reduce the oxygen-carrying power of the blood. The potential result of these perturbations is myocardial ischaemia.

Concern about induced ischaemia is not a theoretical concept but a hazard of proven importance. The special risks to patients with coronary artery disease were well established by 1961[10,11] and have been documented repeatedly since then. Taped monitoring demonstrated electrocardiographic changes reflecting the potential hazard from perioperative ischaemia in 1989,[4,12] but observations were limited and made in small specialized groups. Subsequently, an elegant study was reported by the Perioperative Ischemia Research Group who undertook continuous electrocardiographic monitoring before, during, and after surgery in 100 patients with, or at risk of, coronary artery disease who were undergoing noncardiac operations.[2] The frequency and severity of ischaemic ST segment depression was observed throughout the perioperative period, as would be expected in any group with coronary disease who are thereby vulnerable to silent ischaemia,[13] but it was particularly prominent postoperatively: no less than 187 ischaemic periods were observed in 42 of the patients. Some 94% of these episodes were silent, and most occurred without any change in heart rate or blood pressure, suggesting that increased metabolic demand may not be the principal culprit. Importantly, 11 of the 13 subjects who subsequently had an adverse cardiac outcome had demonstrated electrocardiographic evidence of postoperative ischaemia. The authors attributed the absence of special risk during (as opposed to after) the operations to the substantial advances made over the last decade in intraoperative cardiovascular monitoring and therapy, as well as to improved anaesthetic technique. The observation made by Chamberlain and Edmonds-Seal over 30 years ago[14] — that postoperative electrocardiographic deterioration correlated with the duration of major falls in blood pressure during surgery — may no longer have relevance. These days most patients are fit for surgery under general anaesthesia, but many are not fit for the postoperative period.

Myocardial ischaemia is not the only hazard faced by vulnerable patients. Changes in blood coagulation, direct toxic effects of anaesthetics, other adjuvant agents during surgery (such as bladder wash-outs in relation to prostatectomy[15]), and major intravascular or intercompartmental fluid shifts may affect both patients with coronary disease and those with valvar and other cardiac disorders of functional importance. With such a medley of risk one may wonder how vulnerable patients can escape without complications: yet most do escape. For the cardiologist and others charged with making assessments, the difficulty lies in predicting with reasonable accuracy who is likely to do so and who might not.

Role of assessment

Assessment of operative risk is undertaken with several possible objectives and outcomes. An important task, sometimes calling for careful judgement, is to decide how far risk may be reduced by additional investigation and treatment preoperatively, and whether or not any consequent delay can be justified. With or without changes in general management, any of several conclusions or actions may be appropriate. Risk may be judged prohibitive so that surgery should not take place; risk may be acceptable to some patients yet not to others, so that careful discussion is warranted before a decision is taken; in other cases that will proceed, special precautions may be advised for the periods during or after surgery; and in some cases risk may be small, so that reassurance is all that is needed. Any decision to advise against surgery demands careful consideration of the penalty to the patient in terms of impaired quality of life: operations are unlikely to have been suggested without good reason. A balanced view can sometimes be reached only after discussion with both the patient and the surgeon or anaesthetist. The point is worth stressing: in the current hospital environment discussions with colleagues are not always easy to arrange at short notice, but consultation in difficult cases should be accorded the priority it deserves.

Methods of assessment

Although systematic methods for judging operative risk had been in use since 1961,[16] the landmark paper offering a comprehensive and effective methodology for preoperative assessment of patients was published in 1977 by Goldman and colleagues.[17] It was based on a prospective study of 1001 patients over 40 years of age, and was designed to determine by multivariate discriminant analysis the preoperative factors that might affect the development of cardiac complications after major noncardiac operations. Nine independent significant correlates of life-threatening or fatal complications were identified. Each was given a weighting using a system of points (up to 11). The maximum adverse score was 53. A risk index was grouped into four classes with ascending order of risk: class I comprised patients with 0–5 points, class II those with 6–12 points, class III those with 13–25 points, and class IV those with more than 26 points. In the original study, 10 of the 19 postoperative cardiac fatalities occurred in the patients in the highest risk category. The system is still regarded as valid 20 years after publication.

For clinical purposes the Goldman criteria are grouped under five headings (Table 16.1)

The authors recognized that some of their criteria might pose problems for clinicians. For example, definite elevation of the jugular venous pressure was an important indicator of risk, yet the sign can be difficult for non-cardiologists to find.

Therefore, measurement of central venous pressure was suggested as an alternative. The practicality of recognizing a gallop rhythm was not specifically mentioned, but that too can be a difficult physical sign. Because the significance of murmurs may not be straightforward, formal preoperative evaluation was recommended for any murmur that might indicate aortic stenosis. The finding of ventricular premature beats was not based on monitoring of heart rhythm and the authors warned that this factor may loose its discriminatory value

if detected only on out-patient ambulatory recordings. They also accepted that a cohort of only 1001 patients would leave many important prognostic variables inadequately represented so that significance testing could not be performed with validity. The single age criterion of 70 years might now be considered inadequate: major surgery has become commonplace for patients in their 80s and even 90s. But despite these, and other, obvious shortcomings, the risk index was accepted as a useful tool and its value was confirmed by subsequent studies.[18–20]

Inevitably other workers produced modifications of the popular Goldman index, or introduced developments that differed substantially from it. A 1995 review by Mangano and Goldman[21] listed 11 large series relating to surgical risk that were either derived from unselected patients or from patients with some selection criteria of prognostic significance. Inevitably the latter group had higher morbidity and mortality rates than the former. Although selection has some disadvantages in relation to generating an index for a general population, it has advantages too: the increased number of endpoints do add power to analyses, and risk has to be quantified, particularly in patients perceived as being vulnerable.

An important modification of the Goldman index by Detsky et al.[18] was validated on 455 patients representing consecutive referrals to a general medical consultation service: presumably this method of enrollment introduced some measure of bias to higher risk patients. Major cardiac events occurred in 7.9% of the series compared with 5.8% of the Goldman series. Two major modifications were introduced. Additional variables were added, and the scoring system was developed to take greater account of the hazards inherent in the proposed surgery. The additions were plausible as markers of risk: myocardial infarction at any time

1. **Those based on the history**
   age >70 years (5)
   myocardial infarction in the previous 6 months (10)
2. **Those based on the physical examination**
   a third heart sound gallop rhythm or raised jugular venous pressure (11)
   important valvular aortic stenosis (3)
3. **Those based on the electrocardiogram**
   rhythm other than sinus or with only premature atrial contractions (7)
   more than five ventricular premature beats per minute documented at any time before operation (7)
4. **Those based upon the patient's general status**
   Po_2 <60 or Pco_2 >50 mmHg
   potassium <3.0 mEq/L or bicarbonate <20 mEq/L
   blood urea nitrogen >50 mg/dl or creatinine >3.0 mg/dl
   (Note that these are not SI units, and confusion is possible especially with the tests of renal function.)
   abnormal hepatic enzymes
   signs of chronic liver disease or patient bed-ridden from noncardiac causes (3)
5. **Those based on the type of surgery that is proposed**
   intraperitoneal, intrathoracic, or aortic operation (3)
   emergency operations (4)

Table 16.1
The weighted risk score is given in brackets after each factor.

(but with a lower risk score than for recent infarction), angina of more than class 3 of the Canadian Cardiovascular Society, and pulmonary oedema. In addition, criteria were set out that might help the recognition of critical aortic stenosis: if recognized as such, its weighting was to be markedly increased. Risk using the Detsky modifications is calculated as a ratio, with 10

taken as the average risk for any one designated procedure. The 'pre-test' possibility of a major complication is taken as the overall risk of the operation in the specific institution where it is to be carried out: a figure not always readily available. The patient's score is then added to the computation using a nomogram. The risk ratio is read as an intercept between two vertical lines that represent the intrinsic surgical hazard on the one hand and the patient's adverse score on the other.

The Detsky system introduced greater precision into risk assessment, but the authors stressed the limitation inherent in models of this type. Some serious conditions would not have been represented in the original series and would therefore attract no score, and other factors may be more easily recognized by clinical acumen than by objective scoring systems. 'The multifactorial index is merely a model or starting point for clinicians who should not hesitate to make [such] a revision in appropriate circumstances.' This is an important statement for any clinician using a risk index.

The Goldman and Detsky indexes are necessarily somewhat complex. They seek to identify vulnerability arising from any condition within, or acting on the heart that may precipitate myocardial infarction, pulmonary oedema, malignant arrhythmias, or cardiac death. However, simplicity has merit in clinical practice and will always be seen as a worthwhile objective. Thus, in 1993, Ashton and colleagues[22] reasoned that coronary disease is the most powerful risk factor for myocardial infarction and that other adverse influences may not be numerically important in this regard. Their study was also based on the premise that the likelihood of myocardial infarction can be treated as a surrogate for overall cardiac morbidity and mortality. The point could also be made that other cardiac and general conditions that introduce hazard are usually very obvious and hardly require a sophisticated method of risk quantification. They therefore constructed a simple stratification for 1487 male patients over the age of 40 years who had major elective or urgent noncardiac surgery. The high-risk stratum comprised patients with strong evidence of coronary disease based on history, electrocardiography, or angiography; the authors believed that the prevalence of coronary disease in this group must be close to 100%. The intermediate-risk stratum had no evidence of coronary disease but had overt atherosclerotic disease elsewhere (or had undiagnosed atypical chest pain); the estimated prevalence of coronary disease was 30–70%. The low-risk stratum had no overt clinical manifestation of atherosclerotic disease but had recognized and quantifiable risk factors, with an expected prevalence of coronary disease in the range 5–30%. A negligible risk stratum comprising nearly half the total number of patients made up the remainder; the prevalence of coronary disease was believed to be close to zero. Although two-thirds of the patients were evaluated only by chart review, with the possibility of underdiagnosis, this simple approach worked well. The incidence of postoperative infarction in the high, intermediate, and low-risk strata was 4.1%, 0.8%, and 0% respectively (ECG evidence was not available in the negligible-risk stratum). Considering all four strata, the risk of cardiac death was, respectively, 2.3%, 0.4% (one patient), 0.4% (one patient), and 0%. A gradation was also found for total death: 4.1%, 3.5%, 3.1%, 1.2%. On this basis, expensive testing or ancillary treatment seems not to be indicated in the absence of overt atherosclerotic disease.

Clearly other factors should be taken into account despite the value of simple stratification based on the presence or absence of atherosclerotic disease. The three that were shown in this study to have predictive value were: age

over 75 years, the presence of heart failure, and a planned vascular procedure—all familiar indicators of risk identified in earlier studies. Fifteen years of painstaking observation have left clinicians with relatively simple concepts: coronary events pose the greatest threat in terms of cardiac risks, the most powerful predictor is overt atherosclerotic disease, and within this population the very elderly, those with heart failure, and patients undergoing vascular surgery face the greatest risk. This might have been, and doubtless was predicted, but a powerful base of evidence to support clinical judgement is welcome.

Patients undergoing vascular surgery

That patients in need of vascular surgery face higher than average risk is well documented, well recognized, and well understood. The incidence of major cardiovascular complications has ranged from 5% to 40%.[23] Atherosclerosis is rarely confined to one vascular territory. Both aortic and peripheral vascular disease are markers for the presence of coronary disease and also indicators that it may be severe. An angiographic study from the Cleveland Clinic[24] of patients awaiting elective abdominal aortic surgery or aorto-iliac reconstruction showed that 60% of patients had important coronary disease, and that in 30% of them it was judged to be severe. A later publication from the same centre[25] based on 1224 patients who had had coronary angiograms within 6 months of vascular surgery showed that the number of significant lesions (>30% obstruction) provided the best correlation with subsequent myocardial infarction or death. But other important correlates were preoperative bypass surgery, collaterals beyond a total coronary occlusion, the number of diseased vessels, the number of irregular segments, and the number of lesions with at least 50% and 70% obstruction. That the severity and extent of coronary disease predict risk is hardly a surprising finding, but clinical science often torments its practitioners with paradoxes. Here at least, the clinician can feel he or she understands the problem: coronary disease is bad, and bad coronary disease is worse.

The patient facing vascular surgery faces two related problems in addition to the probability of having coronary disease. First, vulnerability to myocardial ischaemia is less likely to be overt than it is in other patients with coronary disease of similar extent who are awaiting general surgery. Lack of mobility in severely arteriopathic patients, in particular those with claudication or cerebrovascular disorders, frequently masks the presence or severity of angina. Criteria other than the history may be needed for adequate judgement of risk. Secondly, the most commonly used method for assessing the functional importance of impaired coronary reserve—simple treadmill testing—is usually impractical, so that other more complex methods may be required.

Investigations to identify and quantify coronary disease
Routine preoperative assessment

All patients over the age of 40 years awaiting surgery that has high intrinsic risk (vascular, chest, or abdominal operations) should have an electrocardiogram and a chest radiograph if these investigations have not been performed within the previous 6 months (and of course they should be undertaken in any case if there is any hint of clinical instability). Results may be helpful if they are markedly abnormal but they provide insufficient evidence to judge that risk is low.

Effort tests

The principal aims of effort tests are to measure functional capacity, to identify and possibly to localize myocardial ischaemia, and to test the stability of cardiac rhythm when the heart is stressed. Poor functional capacity, which has disparate causes, is a powerful prognostic tool.[26] Individuals who can complete three stages of the Bruce protocol are at low risk, and (surgery apart) have an early annual mortality of less than 1% per year.[27] Although ST segment changes alone have not been uniformly helpful in predicting postoperative risk,[28] McPhail and colleagues[29] found that seven of 21 vascular patients with ischaemic changes and impaired effort tolerance had serious postoperative cardiac complications. In general, effort tolerance seems more important than ST segment changes. A routine preoperative effort tolerance test may be superfluous for a patient who can walk two average blocks at normal pace without symptoms.[23] Indeed, it may be counterproductive. Even pronounced ST segment depression in symptomless individuals has low specificity;[30] a spurious change will at best delay appropriate care for a patient awaiting urgent surgery. Moreover, many of the vascular patients needing functional stratification in the absence of a diagnostic history will be incapable of undertaking a treadmill test. In summary, effort tests should be reserved for patients with vascular disease whose effort tolerance and symptomatology are in doubt, yet who are capable of walking adequately on a treadmill. A few patients who have not previously been assessed cardiologically may have additional indications not related to impending surgery.

Nuclear cardiology

Simple gated-pool scanning has been recommended as a screening test for risk assessment, at least in preparation for abdominal aortic surgery.[31] But wider experience has not confirmed any special value for the investigation in this context[32] and it is doubtful whether it can add appreciably to careful clinical evaluation.[21] However, dipyridamole thallium scans have been well validated for their predictive value in this context, at least in selected patients. An important report from a task force of the American College of Cardiology and the American Heart Association[33] on guidelines for perioperative cardiovascular evaluation for noncardiac surgery cites 23 of the major articles relating to the use of dipyridamole-thallium images for preoperative assessment of cardiac risk. The negative predictive value of the normal scans is high at approximately 99% for myocardial infarction and/or death. The positive predictive value has ranged from 4% to 20% in the larger studies. The scoring of scan abnormalities can improve the value of dipyridamole-thallium scans for risk assessment.[34,35] However, as with all tests, positive predictive value has become lower as dipyridamole-thallium scanning has been more widely used (which influences the pretest probability of disease). In addition, for patients who are elderly or who have definite coronary disease, this expensive investigation has little or no additional role as a predictor of outcome.[36]

Echocardiography

While echocardiography and Doppler studies are of value for preoperative assessment of patients with valvar and myocardial problems — especially for quantifying the severity of aortic stenosis — there is no evidence that resting transthoracic or transoesphageal echocardiography can add appreciably to clinical evaluation for those with coronary disease. Exercise echocardiography or, more practically, dobutamine echocardiography offers more

potential: the test can assess not only left ventricular function but also vulnerability to myocardial ischaemia indicated by the appearance or worsening of all wall motion abnormalities. In their recent report, the American task force[33] listed six relevant studies, mostly in relation to patients undergoing peripheral vascular surgery. In these, the negative predictive value ranged from 93% to 100% and the positive predictive value ranged from 7% to 23% for myocardial infarction or death. The published evidence is still small compared with dipyridamole-thallium testing, but wall motion abnormality with low infusion rates seems especially important.[33] The study of Poldermans and colleagues[37] was of special value in that it was relatively large, prospective, blinded, and specifically addressed to patients with peripheral vascular disease. All 15 postoperative complications occurred in the 35 individuals who showed new or worsening wall abnormalities. The two techniques of dipyridamole-thallium scanning and dobutamine echocardiography were reviewed in a recent meta-analysis.[38] The prognostic value was comparable between the techniques but, inevitably, the accuracy varied with coronary artery prevalence. Preference for one or the other at present may depend on local experience and expertise. In the presence of left bundle branch block, thallium scanning with a vasodilator is more specific than thallium scanning with exercise or dobutamine,[39] but the comparison did not extend to dobutamine echocardiography.

Coronary angiography

This provides, as always, a slightly imperfect gold standard for investigating the presence and severity of coronary disease. Severity and extent of disease correlate well with risk, but in the probabilistic arena of risk assessment this can never be translated into certainty for an individual patient. Disease that is impressive angiographically may be stable and sometimes surprisingly unimportant functionally, collaterals may not provide the safety that an observer may expect,[25] and the plaques that rupture and cause occlusion are often angiographically unimpressive. Nevertheless angiographic severity does, in general, correlate well with risk, and patients with coronary arteries that are known to be normal or near normal will cause little concern. But the investigation is needed preoperatively only for patients who require the test for conventional indications. This does occur: many patients come forward for vascular surgery who have not previously been investigated for coronary disease, either because symptoms were masked or because referral was overlooked or unwanted. Angiography is not usually appropriate simply for preoperative risk assessment.

Assessment of cardiac risks

This topic has attracted a large literature, a little controversy, and some confusion. No guidelines can provide optimal advice for individual patients. The assessment of cardiac risk for noncardiac surgery will continue to rely heavily on clinical judgement. Formal risk indices such as that of Goldman et al.[17] or Detsky et al.[18] still have a role, although clinicians who are familiar with them may learn to be less dependent on rigid scoring systems. However, the studies reported in the past two decades have provided many guiding principles. The experienced physician will first give consideration to the nature of the surgical procedure that is planned. The recent American task force[33] stratified surgical procedures into three simple groups. Examples of those intrinsically carrying high risk (often in excess of 5% mortality overall) were emergency procedures especially in the elderly, aortic and other major vascular operations, peripheral vas-

cular surgery, and anticipated long procedures associated with fluid shifts and/or blood loss. The intermediate-risk group (mortality of 1–5% overall) comprised surgery on the head and neck including carotid endarterectomy, intraperitoneal and intrathoracic procedures, orthopaedic operations, and prostatic surgery. The low-risk group (average risk considered less than 1%) were endoscopic procedures, superficial operations, cataract surgery, and breast operations. The last group will not involve major decisions because even high-risk patients should expect a reasonable degree of safety. It is for the high and intermediate surgical risk groups that patient characteristics become an important determinant of serious postoperative complications.

For elective procedures the likelihood of unstable coronary disease, current heart failure, critical aortic stenosis, or malignant arrhythmias will usually warrant postponement, modification of the treatment plan, or cancellation of surgery. Clinically overt but stable coronary disease and mildly symptomatic valvar or myocardial disease will materially increase the likelihood of complications, but clinicians should remember that average surgical risks are derived from the whole spectrum from high to low. When severely symptomatic or very elderly patients are excluded, the hazard ratio for the remainder (in comparison with the average) is likely to be small. However, when stable coronary symptoms are obtrusive, patients may well face risks that are twice or more that of the average patient and such odds may or may not be acceptable. The special problems associated with vascular disease must be remembered: information on functional status may not be available or may be inaccurate. In these instances, as well as in intermediate-risk patients, where decision can be difficult, other ancillary investigations may be helpful. Formal effort testing, dipyridamole-thallium scanning, or dobutamine echocardiography may be used to place the patient within a segment of the prognostic spectrum that ranges at worst from that of the unstable ischaemic subject, to the best that might be anticipated in the presence of stable asymptomatic coronary disease — implying no more than average risk. Complex investigations should not be performed as a matter of routine, even if risk assessment is incomplete without them: the physician must always consider whether or not a management policy might be changed as a result of the findings. Many patients can be assessed as having low risk, for example those without clinically apparent coronary disease or other major heart problems. For such patients simple electrocardiography and chest radiography are, at most, the only investigations needed, and reassurance can be given.

Unnecessary investigations should be avoided, not only because of needless expense but also because results may mislead or delay important treatment. Other purposes of assessment should not be forgotten. Preoperative treatment may improve the prognosis (prophylactic antibiotics should not be forgotten if indicated), special procedures or precautions may need to be arranged, and appropriate preparation for hazards that are inevitable should be discussed fully with patients and relatives for this can mitigate subsequent resentment or grief.

Putting it together

Both risk inherent in the surgery and the vulnerability of the patient must be considered. While formal scoring systems[17,18] are useful and have contributed much to our knowledge, adequate data are never available to translate figures derived from them into a precise individual operative risk. A simple scheme can serve as a model suitable for most clinical assessments, and may be more practical. Based on many of the studies reviewed above, the following approach will resemble that followed, consciously or not, by many clinicians. However, the reader is reminded that all models must be interpreted for individual patients in the light of special circumstances and clinical judgement.

Inherent risk is high in major vascular surgery, operations that are of long duration, procedures with anticipated fluid imbalance, and emergency surgery in elderly patients. It is intermediate in carotid surgery, intraperitoneal surgery, intrathoracic surgery, major orthopaedic surgery, and prostate surgery. It is low for endoscopies, superficial surgery, cataract surgery, and breast operations.

Patients can be characterized. They may have prohibitive, high, intermediate, or low risk. The interaction of the two factors — together with the importance of the procedure — determines whether or not the risk is acceptable (Table 16.2).

Hazardous procedures are not necessarily contraindicated, but the balance of risk and potential benefit should be carefully weighed. Some risk factors, such as smoking and the presence of diabetes, carry their own penalty in terms of complications and should be considered in any assessment.

Conclusions

There are implications to cardiac risk in relation to general surgery apart from assessment. Perhaps more attention should be paid to postoperative care, aimed especially at preventing silent ischaemia, although possible strategies have not been adequately investigated. Risk from postoperative ischaemia may have delayed effects: vulnerable patients who survive major operative procedures apparently without adverse sequelae suffer a relatively high attrition rate even after hospital discharge, and the per-

Prohibitive-risk patients, e.g.

unstable coronary disease	treat as possible to improve risk
very recent myocardial infarction	delay or cancel surgery if possible
current left heart failure	consider only if life-saving
critical aortic stenosis	
malignant arrhythmias	

High-risk patients, e.g.

overt stable coronary disease	high-risk surgery hazardous
vascular disease, poor effort tolerance	intermediate-risk surgery hazardous
vascular disease, thallium redistribution	low-risk surgery acceptable
vascular disease, echocardiographic wall abnormality new or worse with dobutamine	
age over 75 years	
any recent heart failure	
hypoxia, hypercapnia	
important biochemical instability	

Intermediate-risk patients, e.g.

atherosclerosis but not high risk	high-risk surgery hazardous
other valvular and myocardial disease	intermediate-risk surgery acceptable
arrhythmias, important conduction defects	low-risk surgery acceptable

Low-risk patients, e.g.

those with none of the above	high-risk surgery acceptable
	intermediate-risk surgery acceptable
	low-risk surgery acceptable

Table 16.2
Guidelines to determine acceptable risk. For high, intermediate, and low risk surgery, see text on page 309.

iod of increased risk continues for a year or more. Those who do survive postoperative ischaemic complications may warrant subsequent investigation for they have declared their vulnerability.[7] The opportunity for targeted prevention is usually overlooked by cardiologists at the present time.

If I had . . .

If I had any overt cardiac risk and needed general surgery, I would expect a clinical assessment that would include a careful history, especially in relation to my effort tolerance and past history, and also a competent physical examination. I would want a chest radiograph and an electrocardiogram. If I had vascular disease that limited my effort tolerance I would like an additional special investigation, such as a dipyridamole thallium scan or a dobutamine (or exercise) echocardiogram. Above all, I would hope to be advised by a caring, experienced, and wise clinician who would take into account the quality of my life with or without the surgery that was proposed. I would then follow the advice that I was given.

References

1   Campling EA, Devlin HB, Lunn JN, The report of the National Confidential Enquiry into Perioperative Deaths 1993/1994 (NCEPOD).

2   Mangano DT, Hollenberg M, Fegert G et al, and the Study of Perioperative Ischemia (SPI) Research Group, Perioperative myocardial ischemia in patients undergoing noncardiac surgery — I. Incidence and severity during the 4 day perioperative period, *J Am Coll Cardiol* (1991)**17**:843–50.

3   Kalra M, Charlesworth D, Morris JA, Al-Khaffaf H, Myocardial infarction after reconstruction of the abdominal aorta, *Br J Surg* (1993)**80**:28–33.

4   Ouyang P, Gerstenblith G, Furman WR, Golueke PJ, Gottlieb SO, Frequency and significance of early postoperative silent myocardial ischemia in patients having peripheral vascular surgery, *Am J Cardiol* (1989)**64**:1113–16.

5   Mangano DT, Wong MG, London MJ, Tubau LF, Rapp JA and the Study of Perioperative Ischemia (SPI) Research Group, Perioperative myocardial ischemia in patients undergoing noncardiac surgery — II. Incidence and severity during the 1st week after surgery, *J Am Coll Cardiol* (1991)**17**:851–71.

6   Lee TH, Thomas EJ, Ludwig LE et al, Troponin T as a marker for myocardial ischemia in patients undergoing major noncardiac surgery, *Am J Cardiol* (1996)**77**:1031–6.

7   Mangano DT, Browner WS, Hollenberg M, Li J, Tateo MS, for the Study of Perioperative Ischemia Research Group, Long-term cardiac prognosis following noncardiac surgery, *JAMA* (1992)**268**:233–9.

8   Gilbert NC, LeRoy GV, Fenn GK, The effect of distension of abdominal viscera on the blood flow in the circumflex branch of the left coronary artery of the dog, *Am Heart J* (1940)**20**:519–24.

9   Chauhan A, Mullins PA, Taylor GED, Petch MC, Schofield PM, Cardioesophageal reflex; a mechanism for 'linked angina' in patients with angiographically proven coronary artery disease, *J Am Coll Cardiol* (1996)**27**:1621–8.

10 Nachlas MM, Abrams SJ, Goldberg MM, The influence of arteriosclerotic heart disease on surgical risk, *Am J Surg* (1961)**101**:447–55.

11 Driscoll AC, Hobika JH, Etsten BE, Proger S, Clinically unrecognized myocardial infarction following surgery, *N Engl J Med* (1961)**264**:633–9.

12 Raby KE, Goldman L, Creager MA et al, Correlation between preoperative ischemia and major cardiac events after peripheral vascular surgery, *N Engl J Med* (1989)**321**:1296–300.

13 Stern S, Tavoni D, Early detection of silent ischaemic heart disease by 24-hour electrocardiographic monitoring of active subjects, *Br Heart J* (1974)**36**:481–6.

14 Chamberlain DA, Edmonds-Seal J, Effects of surgery under general anaesthesia on the electrocardiogram in ischaemic heart disease and hypertension, *Br Med J* (1964)**ii**:784–7.

15 Editorial, Monitoring TURP, *Lancet* (1991)**338**:606–7.

16 Dripps RD, Lamont A, Eckenhoff JE, The role of anaesthesia in surgical mortality, *JAMA* (1961)**178**:261–6.

17 Goldman L, Caldera DL, Nussbaum SR et al, Multifactorial index of cardiac risk in noncardiac surgical procedures, *N Engl J Med* (1977)**297**:845–50.

18 Detsky AS, Abrams HB, Forbath N, Scott JG, Hilliard JR, Cardiac assessment of patients undergoing noncardiac surgery: a multifactorial clinical risk index, *Arch Intern Med* (1986)**146**:2131–4.

19 Zeldin RA, Math B, Assessing cardiac risk in patients who undergo noncardiac surgical procedures, *Can J Surg* (1984)**27**:402–4.

20 Jeffrey CC, Kunsman J, Cullen DJ, Brewster DC, A prospective evaluation of cardiac risk index, *Anesthesiology* (1983)**58**:462–4.

21 Mangano DT, Goldman L, Preoperative assessment of patients with known or suspected

coronary disease, *N Engl J Med* (1995) **333**:1750–6.

22 Ashton CM, Petersen NJ, Wray NP et al, The incidence of perioperative myocardial infarction in men undergoing noncardiac surgery, *Ann Intern Med* (1993)**118**:504–10.

23 Wong T, Detsky AS, Preoperative cardiac risk assessment for patients having peripheral vascular surgery, *Ann Intern Med* (1992)**116**:743–53.

24 Hertzer NR, Beven EG, Young JR et al, Coronary artery disease in peripheral vascular patients. A classification of 1000 coronary angiograms and results of surgical management, *Ann Surg* (1984)**199**:223–33.

25 Ellis SG, Hertzer NR, Young JR, Brener S, Angiographic correlates of cardiac death and myocardial infarction complicating major non-thoracic vascular surgery, *Am J Cardiol* (1996)**77**:1126–8.

26 Morris CK, Ueshima K, Kawaguchi T, Hideg A, Froelicher VF, The prognostic value of exercise capacity: a review of the literature, *Am Heart J* (1991)**122**:1423–31.

27 Weiner DA, Ryan TJ, McCabe CH et al, Prognostic importance of a clinical profile and exercise test in medically treated patients with coronary artery disease, *J Am Coll Cardiol* (1984)**3**:772–9.

28 Carliner NH, Fisher ML, Plotnick GD et al, Routine preoperative exercise testing in patients undergoing major noncardiac surgery, *Am J Cardiol* (1985)**56**:51–8.

29 McPhail N, Calvin JE, Shariatmadar A, Barber GG, Scobie TK, The use of preoperative exercise testing to predict cardiac complications after arterial reconstruction, *J Vasc Surg* (1988)**7**:60–8.

30 Froelicher VF, Yanowitz FG, Thompson AJ, Lancaster MC, The correlation of coronary angiography and the electrocardiographic response to maximal treadmill test in 76 asymptomatic men, *Circulation* (1973)**48**:597–604.

31 Pasternack PF, Imparato AM, Bear G et al, The value of radionuclide angiography as a predictor of perioperative myocardial infarction in patients undergoing abdominal aortic aneurysm resection, *J Vasc Surg* (1984)**1**:320–5.

32 Kazmers A, Cerqueira MD, Zierler RE, Perioperative and late outcome in patients with left ventricular ejection fraction of 35% or less who require major vascular surgery, *J Vasc Surg* (1988)**8**:307–15.

33 ACC/AHA Task Force Report, Guidelines for perioperative cardiovascular evaluation for noncardiac surgery, *J Am Coll Cardiol* (1996)**27**:910–48.

34 Brown KA, Rowen M, Extent of jeopardized viable myocardium determined by myocardial perfusion imaging best predicts perioperative cardiac events in patients undergoing noncardiac surgery, *J Am Coll Cardiol* (1993)**21**:325–30.

35 Lette J, Waters D, Cerino M, Picard M, Champagne P, Lapointe J, Preoperative coronary artery disease risk stratification based on dipyridamole imaging and a simple three-step, three-segment model for patients undergoing noncardiac vascular surgery or major general surgery, *Am J Cardiol* (1992)**69**:1553–58.

36 Baron J-F, Mundler O, Bertrand M et al, Dipyridamole-thallium scintigraphy and gated radionuclide angiography to assess cardiac risk before abdominal aortic surgery, *N Engl J Med* (1994)**330**:663–9.

37 Poldermans D, Fioretti PM, Forster T, Dobutamine stress echocardiography for assessment of perioperative cardiac risk in patients undergoing major vascular surgery, *Circulation* (1993)**87**:1506–12.

38 Shaw LJ, Eagle KA, Gersh BJ, Miller DD, Meta-analysis of intravenous dipyridamole-thallium-201 imaging (1985 to 1994) and dobutamine echocardiography (1991 to 1994) for risk stratification before vascular surgery, *J Am Coll Cardiol* (1996)**27**:787–98.

39 O'Keefe JH, Bateman TM, Barnhart CS, Adenosine thallium-201 is superior to exercise thallium-201 for detecting coronary artery disease in patients with left bundle branch block, *J Am Coll Cardiol* (1993)**21**:1332–8.

17

Myocarditis

Howard Why and Peter Richardson

Introduction

The practical problem of myocarditis in a clinical setting is first and foremost one of diagnosis. The task of distinguishing patients with this condition from those with more common causes of cardiac failure and arrhythmias is not an easy one. Whilst a number of features may suggest myocarditis, in practical terms the precise diagnosis cannot be made without full investigation, including coronary arteriography and endomyocardial biopsy. This information has important implications for the management and prognosis of the patient, including the final decision as to whether cardiac transplantation may be the only treatment option.

Definitions

Any condition producing infiltration of the myocardium with inflammatory cells may be termed a myocarditis. The histological changes are often widespread and involve the endocardium and pericardium, giving rise to the expressions myopericarditis and pancarditis, both of which imply active involvement of the myocardium in the inflammatory process. Whilst in many cases the myocardium is globally affected, focal forms may also exist in which changes are limited to a discrete portion of the myocardium.

Pathological definition of myocarditis

As recently as the 1950s, no precise clinical or pathological criteria were established for the diagnosis of myocarditis. The development of safe and effective methods of transvascular endomyocardial biopsy allowed cardiac tissue to be obtained *in vivo* for histological examination,[1–3] thus necessitating the development of histopathological criteria for diagnosis.

A more precise pathological definition of myocarditis was put forward, requiring the demonstration of myocyte necrosis and myocardial infiltration with inflammatory cells.[4] Based upon this proposal, myocarditis was defined in 1984 by an international panel of pathologists as 'a process characterized by an inflammatory infiltrate of the myocardium with necrosis and/or degeneration of adjacent myocytes not typical of the ischaemic damage associated with coronary disease'. Strict histological guidelines for diagnosis were laid down in what are now universally called the Dallas criteria.[5] As the changes are often focal, examination of multiple endomyocardial biopsy samples is often required for the diagnosis to be made or refuted.[6]

Acute myocarditis is diagnosed only when the presence of acute inflammatory cells in close proximity to the myocardial fibres is associated with myocyte necrosis, vacuolization or disruption.[5] An infiltrate seen in the absence of myocyte damage, or a sparse infiltrate not in direct contact with the myocyte suggests a resolving or healing myocarditis. Subsequent complete resolution of the inflammatory infiltrate with a variable degree of interstitial fibrous replacement, endocardial thickening, myocyte attenuation and nuclear hypertrophy indicate a resolved or healed myocarditis. The latter changes are nonspecific and are indistinguishable from those seen in dilated cardiomyopathy (DCM).[7] An unequivocal diagnosis of resolving or resolved myocarditis, therefore, can be made only if acute myocarditis has previously been demonstrated on biopsy.

WHO/ISFC classification of cardiomyopathies — dilated cardiomyopathy

To introduce some uniformity into the nomenclature of heart muscle diseases, the World Health Organization (WHO) and International Society and Federation of Cardiology (ISFC) commissioned a task force of cardiologists and cardiac pathologists to discuss the subject. They broadly adopted the classification that Goodwin and Oakley made a decade earlier,[8] defining the cardiomyopathies as 'heart muscle diseases of unknown cause'. Dilated cardiomyopathy was described as follows:

> The condition is recognised by dilatation of the left or right ventricle, or both ventricles. Dilatation often becomes severe and is invariably accompanied by hypertrophy. Systolic ventricular function is impaired. Congestive heart failure may or may not supervene. Presentation with disturbances of ventricular or atrial rhythm is common and death may occur at any stage.[9]

The classification has recently been revised and it is now accepted that dilated cardiomyopathy may be idiopathic or associated with an underlying cause, for example familial/genetic, viral and/or immune, or alcoholic/toxic. Myocarditis, which may also have a viral pathogenesis, has been termed an inflammatory cardiomyopathy when associated with myocardial dysfunction.[10]

Aetiology

Myocarditis may be idiopathic or secondary to a variety of infectious and noninfectious agents (Table 17.1), but is caused most frequently by viral infection. Many viruses are associated with myocarditis in humans (Table 17.2). Probably the most frequently encountered of these are the enteroviruses, a ubiquitous group of single-stranded RNA viruses,[11] some of which show tropism for cardiac and skeletal muscle. The pre-eminence of the enteroviruses in causing myocarditis may be challenged in the future, however, by the ever-increasing number of patients affected by the human immunodeficiency virus.[12] This agent also appears to have a predilection for heart muscle and myocarditis is found in up to 50% of postmortem studies performed on HIV-infected patients.[13] Others have suggested, however, that the cardiac muscle damage observed in such patients is largely due to either immune mechanisms or infection with opportunistic pathogens such as *Toxoplasma* species and cytomegalovirus.

Besides viruses, almost any other infective agent may involve the myocardium to produce a myocarditis. In recent years the increasing use of immunosuppressive agents has increased the likelihood of opportunistic infection, particularly by fungi such as *Candida, Aspergillus, Cryptococcus, Coccidiodis* and *Toxoplasma* species. Lyme disease, a systemic illness caused by infection with the spirochaete *Borrelia burgdorferi*, has been recently identified as disease that may also preferentially strike the heart, mimicking viral myocarditis.[14] The cardiac

- **Idiopathic**
- **Infectious**
  Viral
  Bacterial
  Rickettsial
  Protozoal
  Metazoal
- **Immune-mediated**
  Postinfectious
  Transplant rejection
  Peripartum (?) — the mechanism of this
  illness remains unclear
- **Toxic**
  Alcohol
  Drugs
  Heavy metals
  Poisons
  Anaesthetic agents
- **Endocrine**
  Thyrotoxicosis
  Cushing's syndrome
  Catecholamines (phaeochromocytoma)
  Carcinoid syndrome
- **Granulomatous**
  Sarcoidosis
- **Multisystem disorders**
  Systemic lupus
  Polymyositis
  Rheumatoid
  Churg–Strauss syndrome
- **Physical agents**
  Ionizing radiation
  Electric shock

Table 17.1
Causes of myocarditis. Most are rare and the great majority of cases are infectious, mainly viral in origin.

Group	Virus	Genomic material
Enteroviruses	Coxsackie A virus	RNA
	Coxsackie B virus	RNA
	Echovirus	RNA
	Poliovirus	RNA
Orthomyxovirus	Influenza A and B viruses	RNA
Paramyxovirus	Mumps virus	RNA
	Rubeola (measles) virus	RNA
Togavirus	Rubella virus	RNA
Herpesvirus	Cytomegalovirus	DNA
	Epstein–Barr virus	DNA
	Varicella–zoster virus	DNA
	Herpes simplex virus	DNA
Adenovirus	Adenovirus	DNA
Retrovirus	Human immunodeficiency virus	DNA

Table 17.2
Viruses commonly associated with myocarditis in humans.

phase of the infection is characterized by reversible conduction defects but dilated heart muscle in the presence of Lyme disease has been reported.[15] In South America, trypanosomiasis (Chagas' disease) may affect the heart muscle producing a myocarditis. Clinically, three phases are recognized. The acute phase produces systemic symptoms with fever, lymphadenopathy and skin rash associated with nonspecific ECG changes. Serological testing remains positive during a latent phase lasting up to 20 years. The final chronic phase is characterized initially by rhythm disturbances followed by cardiomegaly and congestive cardiac failure.[16]

In the absence of infection, probably the most commonly encountered form of myocarditis is that caused by drugs, most notably the anthracylines such as adriamycin. These can induce an irreversible heart muscle disease with myocytolysis. Both echocardiography and endomyocardial biopsy have been used to monitor patients during treatment with these agents.[17,18] The latter is especially useful as characteristic lesions are observed in the myocytes with myofibrillar loss and sarcotubular dilatation.[17]

Other rarer causes of drug-induced heart muscle disease include the amphetamines, cocaine, inhaled volatile agents including carbon tetrachloride, phenothiazines, antidepressants and lithium carbonate. Toxic agents that have been identified include cobalt (once used as a frothing agent in beer), ionising irradition and other heavy metals.

Clinical features

Incidence and presentation

The diagnosis of viral myocarditis is usually suggested by a history of previous viral-like illness, electrocardiographic changes, a change in heart size on the chest X-ray and a four-fold rise in the appropriate viral titres. There are major difficulties, however, if this approach is relied upon for diagnosis. Many patients confuse the initial shortness of breath of impending pulmonary oedema with the symptoms of viral infection. Furthermore, as presentation is often delayed until there is established myocardial dysfunction, antibody titres have already risen to peak values. These factors have led to rather imprecise data on incidence of myocarditis in the published literature predating the introduction of histological criteria for diagnosis.

Attempts to quantify the number of patients with myocarditis are further confounded by the very variable clinical severity of the condition itself. Up to 5% of patients may be asymptomatic and evidence of myocarditis may be found only at post mortem following sudden accidental death.[19,20] The incidence of biopsy-proven myocarditis in patients with 'primary' atrial fibrillation was approximately 20%[21] whilst unsuspected myocarditis has been detected in up to 17% of patients presenting with life-threatening arrhythmias.[22,23] Myocarditis may be found in up to 20% of children who die suddenly.[20,24] In some patients the systemic illness may overshadow the cardiovascular features, which may be as mild as a sinus tachycardia out of proportion to the pyrexia. In such cases the diagnosis is easily overlooked.[25,26]

The typical presenting features include a systemic pyrexial illness accompanied by nonspecific ECG changes, cardiomegaly and regional or global cardiac dysfunction with a variable degree of cardiac failure. A diagnosis of myocarditis has often been based upon the finding of ECG abnormalities in the course of a viral illness. Such changes occur in up to 40% of viral infections,[27] however, and may be induced not by myocardial involvement but by other coincident processes, for example tachycardia, hypoxia and electrolyte disturbances. The true incidence of cardiac involvement in viral illness is unknown, but it has been estimated that at least 5% of a virus-infected population experience some cardiovascular symptoms.[28,29] Higher percentages may be encountered during epidemics and coxsackie B virus myocarditis is particularly common during the neonatal period, late childhood and adolescence.[11] Information from the World Health Organization Global Surveillance of Virus Diseases programme between 1975 and 1985 indicates that cardiovascular symptoms and signs occurred in 3.5% of patients affected by the six coxsackie B serotypes and around 1% of patients with coxsackie A virus infections. Overall, enterovirus infections accounted for 30% of over 280 000 cases of viral illness reported but 67% of patients experiencing cardiovascular sequelae.

Viral myocarditis may have a seasonal distribution depending upon the infectious agent involved. The enteroviruses are more prevalent in summer and autumn,[28] whilst influenza infections are largely confined to the winter months.[11] Viral myocarditis due to the coxsackie viruses is more common among men than women by a factor of 2:1.[29–31] Whether the same is true for other viruses is unknown.

The absolute incidence of enteroviral myocarditis remains unclear. In 1967, 860 deaths were attributed to myocarditis in the USA, an incidence of 0.4 per 100 000 population.[32] Since conservative estimates are that at least 90% of patients recover fully,[33] the minimum incidence is of the order of 4 cases per 100 000 population per annum. In view of the frequency of myocarditis at autopsy in sudden death (see above), it is likely that this is a gross underestimate.

Examination

Myocarditis produces no specific clinical features. In those patients who have been in long-standing cardiac failure, cachexia may be present. Pyrexia is a feature of the acute phase of the illness. Cardiovascular examination may reveal a sinus tachycardia, atrial fibrillation or ventricular ectopic activity. When marked impairment of cardiac function is present, there may be hypotension with systolic pressure <100 mmHg. The heart is frequently enlarged and third and fourth heart sounds may be audible, producing a gallop rhythm. Functional mitral and tricuspid regurgitation may result from the ventricular dilatation. If the pericardium is involved, a pericardial friction rub may be detected. In the most severe cases, biventricular cardiac failure may be manifested with pleural effusions, and sacral and peripheral oedema, as well as hepatomegaly and ascites. In this latter presentation, the differential diagnosis should include both restrictive and constrictive disease of the myopericardium. Thrombus may form in the dilated, hypocontractile cardiac chambers and both pulmonary and systemic embolization may also occur, the risk of which is enhanced when atrial fibrillation is present.

Noninvasive investigations

The clinical investigation of the patient with myocarditis requires the full use of both noninvasive and invasive cardiological techniques as well as routine and more complex laboratory investigations.

Electrocardiography

In myocarditis or dilated cardiomyopathy the involvement of the myocardium by the inflammatory process is usually diffuse, but in some patients it may be focal. Therefore, the electrocardiographic effects of myocarditis depend upon both the extent and sites of inflammatory cell infiltrate. It will be readily appreciated that a small single lesion involving the conducting system may produce serious consequences[34] while diffuse disease within, for example, the posterior left ventricular wall, might produce little electrocardiographic alteration.

In myocarditis the electrocardiographic abnormalities are largely transient but are a common manifestation of myocardial involvement. The changes may mimic ischaemia, the most commonly encountered abnormalities being ST segment and T wave changes, atrioventricular arrhythmias, and atrioventricular and interventricular conduction defects.[26]

In a study by Kitura and Morita,[35] those patients with third degree AV block had the worst prognosis. Atrial fibrillation, when present, was frequently long-standing. In a further study of 20 patients with biopsy-proven myocarditis followed for 10 years, the electrocardiogram returned to normal in only two patients. The remainder showed persistent changes including interventricular conduction disturbance. Three patients required permanent pacemakers. In this series, three of the patients progressed from myocarditis to DCM.[36] The use of 24-hour Holter monitoring allows better documentation of paroxysmal arrhythmias which are of either atrial or ventricular origin.

The examination of myocardial tissue obtained by endomyocardial biopsy may allow the origin of cardiac arrhythmias to be confirmed as postmyocarditic. Strain et al. studied 18 patients with ventricular tachycardia or fibrillation with structurally normal hearts.[22] None of those patients was found to have significant coronary arterial lesions or impairment of left ventricular function at cardiac catheterization. Right ventricular biopsy, however, revealed histological abnormalities in 16 of 18

patients (89%). Nine of these (50%) had histological changes of nonspecific cardiomyopathy, while three (17%) were diagnosed with subacute inflammatory myocarditis.

X-ray examination

Routine chest radiography is mandatory. The diagnosis may be suspected because of unexplained cardiomegaly with or without the X-ray appearances of left ventricular failure. A pericardial effusion may be associated with myopericarditis and thus cardiac enlargement may not be solely due to underlying ventricular dilatation. The accumulation of pericardial fluid produces a rapid increase in heart size. Similarly, when spontaneous improvement in ventricular function occurs there may be a dramatic decrease in cardiothoracic ratio.

Echocardiography

Probably the most useful noninvasive investigation in patients with suspected myocarditis or cardiomyopathy is transthoracic echocardiography. This not only allows visualization of the myocardium and pericardium but also provides a simple and relatively accurate noninvasive means of assessing systolic cardiac function. In pericarditis, the presence and extent of any pericardial effusion may be assessed and the severity of cardiac tamponade estimated. In the same way, signs of constriction/restriction are readily identified with alterations in the transmitral filling pattern and dilatation of the inferior vena cava.

Echocardiography allows accurate measurement of the left ventricular dimensions and exclusion of any intrinsic valvar heart disease together with an assessment of the extent of any functional valve regurgitation. Estimates of pulmonary artery pressure for the identification of pulmonary hypertension can be made where tricuspid regurgitation is found.

Intracardiac thrombus may be visualized by transthoracic echocardiography, especially when the clot is in the left ventricle. The discrimination of left atrial thrombus remains poor but the use of transoesophageal echocardiography provides excellent data in this regard. Specific heart muscle disease, particularly amyloid, can usually be differentiated and atrial myxomas excluded. Confirmation of the suspected diagnosis of amyloid heart disease requires endomyocardial biopsy. In view of the diagnostic information that can be obtained by echocardiography, this investigation should be performed prior to any invasive studies. Furthermore, echocardiography is invaluable for the serial noninvasive assessment of left ventricular function and pulmonary artery pressures. The one major limitation of the technique is that definition of the anatomy of the coronary arterial tree is not currently possible.

In patients with diffuse myocardial involvement from myocarditis, the typical echocardiographic findings are a globally dilated left ventricular cavity with reduced systolic contraction. The left ventricle may be markedly dilated with an increase in both end-systolic and end-diastolic dimensions. In those patients with more focal disease, however, the only clues to the diagnosis may be segmental wall motion abnormalities. In such circumstances the left ventricular size may be normal or only minimally dilated. Occasionally there may be a localized ventricular aneurysm. These changes may be identical to those seen in coronary arterial disease and therefore arteriography remains mandatory to be certain of the origin of the myocardial disease. Intracavity thrombus can also be detected by echocardiography. This may be present either in the form of a discrete pedunculated lesion, or more frequently as thrombus adherent to the intracavity wall.

Echocardiography is a sensitive means of detecting pericardial effusions. The presence of even small effusions is of diagnostic value as they may signify an inflammatory process. The combination of 2D imaging and mitral inflow Doppler studies allows the detection of haemodynamic compromise and cardiac tamponade. In addition, some degree of pericardial thickening can occasionally be seen, but the possible differential diagnosis of pericardial infiltration by a tumour such as lymphoma or metastatic carcinoma must be borne in mind.

Radionuclide scanning

Radionuclide techniques can be used in the detection of myocarditis. Imaging with gallium-67 has been used to predict myocardial inflammation in patients with suspected DCM and the findings were then correlated with the endomyocardial biopsy diagnosis.[37] Monoclonal antimyosin antibodies labelled with indium-111 have shown some promise in the detection of acute myocyte necrosis in patients with suspected myocarditis with left ventricular dilatation.[38,39] Initial studies using this technique have shown a specificity of 58% and a sensitivity of 100%. Positive uptake of this radiolabelled antibody in the myocardium of patients with DCM indicates the possibility of an ongoing process of active myocyte damage. As yet, these changes have not been correlated with the myocardial histology. Gated radionuclide ventriculography can be used to assess left ventricular function and provides a method for the serial assessment of ejection fraction following an initial histological diagnosis of acute myocarditis.

Invasive investigation

In the assessment of a patient with suspected myocarditis or DCM, selective coronary arteriography is essential as a globally dilated, poorly contracting left ventricle may result from occult coronary artery disease.[40] The findings of LV ejection fraction below 40% and elevated pressures are indicators of an adverse prognosis.

Endomyocardial biopsy

The technique of endomyocardial biopsy pioneered by Konno and Sakakibara in 1962[1] has been modified subsequently with the development of a percutaneous method of bioptome introduction using a long sheath and an adapted biopsy forceps.[41] This technique is usually employed from the femoral approach and may form part of the routine diagnostic cardiac catheterization procedure in a patient with suspected myocarditis. This approach allows biopsy of either ventricle. Alternatively, the right ventricle may be approached using a short sheath and steerable forceps inserted via a percutaneous puncture of the jugular or subclavian vein.[42] Clinically, the value of endomyocardial biopsy has been the histopathological confirmation of suspected myocarditis or specific heart muscle disease, as well as serial biopsy for the detection of rejection in the transplanted heart. The incidence of histologically proven myocarditis in large series of patients with heart muscle disease has varied widely from 3% to 63%,[43–45] depending greatly on patient presentation and case selection. In the analysis of a large series of patients, our own experience is that myocarditis is present in approximately 4.5%[46] of all forms of dilated heart muscle disease and in 19% of those with acute cardiac dilatation which has occurred within the last 9 months.[43]

As well as allowing histological confirmation of typical lymphocytic myocarditis, endomyocardial biopsy also provides the opportunity to diagnose and exclude rarer forms of heart muscle disease, for example giant cell myocarditis.[47] This form has a poor prognosis. In one follow-up series only 20% of patients with giant cell myocarditis survived compared with 70% of patients with the lymphocytic type, and giant cell myocarditis was more likely to be associated with ventricular arrhythmias. Sarcoidosis can be differentiated from giant cell myocarditis on endomyocardial biopsy,[48] and, importantly, may respond to immunosuppressive therapy.[49]

Laboratory investigations

Laboratory investigations form part of the routine assessment of patients with suspected myocarditis although most are not, by themselves, diagnostic. Routine screening may include haematological and biochemical parameters, sedimentation rate, C-reactive protein and protein electrophoresis. Evidence of infection or inflammation may be sought by blood, urine and CSF cultures and virological screening may be performed as detailed below. Autoantibody screening, including antinuclear antibodies and anti-DNA antibodies, may be positive in connective tissue disorders. A variety of other autoantibodies have been described in myocarditis but, as yet, these have found no routine clinical application.[50]

Virological investigations

Many viruses are associated with myocarditis in humans (see Table 17.2). Among the most frequently encountered are the enteroviruses,[11] which show tropism for cardiac and skeletal muscle. In animal models myocarditis can be produced regularly by innoculation with enteroviruses. Over 70 serotypes are known to infect humans and these include the coxsackie A viruses, coxsackie B viruses, polioviruses and echoviruses (along with a number of newly isolated enteroviruses). They are usually transmitted by the faecal–oral route, although in conditions of good hygiene respiratory transmission may be important. Enterovirus infections are frequently asymptomatic. However, noncardiac manifestations of infection range from a mild febrile illness, with or without myalgia, to an aseptic meningitis or even a fulminating multisytem infection.

Lerner and Wilson described criteria suggesting a viral aetiology for myocarditis in 1973.[51] These were:

- isolation of live virus from myocardial tissue, or
- a four-fold or greater rise in specific neutralizing antibody titres between acute and convalescent sera.

It remains possible, however, that isolation of a virus or demonstration of an antibody response may be a coincidental finding as the enteroviruses are ubiquitous in nature.[52] Attempts to culture virus from myocardial tissue, particularly from endomyocardial biopsies, have been almost universally unsuccessful. In a review of the literature in 1977, Grist identified only 17 cases of virus isolation from the myocardium.[53] In practice, routine virological screening should include paired sera for neutralizing antibodies.

The development of molecular biological techniques using initially group-specific molecular hybridization probes[54,55] and more recently the polymerase chain reaction (PCR) for gene amplification,[56] has allowed the identification of viral nuclear material (RNA in the case of enteroviruses) in tissue obtained by endomyocardial biopsy. These methods now provide compelling evidence of the presence of enterovirus within the myocardium of patients with all stages of myocarditis and DCM.

The frequency of enterovirus RNA detection by these techniques varies according to the clinical presentation of the patients tested and the precise methodology employed. Using a technique of *in situ* hybridization, Kandolf et al. demonstrated virus not only in those patients with histological evidence of acute myocarditis, but also within apparently normal areas of myocardium. Replicating enterovirus RNA was found to be present in 23 out of 95 (24%) patients with clinically diagnosed myocarditis, including 10 out of 33 (30%) patients with DCM of recent onset. All the 53 patients in a pathological control group with other specific heart muscle diseases not consistent with a primary viral aetiology (for example ischaemic, hypertrophic and metabolic cardiomyopathy) were negative when their myocardial tissue was examined.[57] Enterovirus sequences have also been detected in 30% of biopsy samples taken from the explanted hearts of patients undergoing cardiac transplantation for end-stage DCM. In contrast, virus sequences were detected in the hearts of only 5% of patients with end-stage coronary disease.[58]

The polymerase chain reaction (PCR) for gene amplification has provided a sensitive and specific method for the detection of virus in small tissue samples where low copy numbers of the viral genome may be present. There have been conflicting results, however, from different centres using PCR.[59–61] Despite the wide variation in reported enteroviral RNA PCR detection rates, increasing familiarity and experience with the technique and its potential pitfalls have led to some semblance of consistency in the results of more recent series.[61–64] The overall enterovirus RNA detection rate for these studies has been 30% in patients with myocarditis or DCM compared with approximately 2% in control subjects. The study of Martin et al.[64] deserves special mention as RNAs for adenovirus and herpes simplex virus were also identified in a large proportion of patients. Importantly, no patient tested positive for the RNA of more than one virus group and again, all control samples were negative.

It is clear that the results of PCR studies are now appearing very similar to those from nucleic acid hybridization. Enteroviral RNA sequences may be detected in the myocardium in 20–50% of patients with myocarditis or DCM. Not surprisingly, higher detection rates seem to be found in samples from patients with acute myocarditis but a significant proportion of patients with end-stage DCM still have detectable enteroviral RNA sequences in the myocardium at the time of cardiac transplantation. The detection of enteroviral RNA in myocardial tissue from patients without these two conditions is a rarity.

The association of myocarditis with dilated cardiomyopathy

As the histological appearances of the healed phase of myocarditis are indistinguishable from those in DCM, many researchers have suggested that some, if not all cases of DCM may result from a previous myocarditis. Considerable weight is lent to this theory by studies of clinical and histological disease progression, and virological studies demonstrating evidence of previous viral infection in DCM.

Clinical studies of disease progression

A number of follow-up studies of enteroviral myocarditis have reported persistent or relapsing cardiac dysfunction, with a variable proportion of patients developing a clinical condition indistinguishable from DCM. As early as 1965, Levander-Lindgren re-evaluated the status of 174 patients with clinically diagnosed myocarditis with a mean follow-up period of 7 years. He identified 86 patients in whom the original illness was either idiopathic or associated with a nonstreptococcal infection. Three patients had died cardiac deaths at an interval from their original illness. Cardiac symptoms persisted in 38 patients (44%) with residual ECG abnormalities in 25 cases (29%). Seven patients had radiological evidence of cardiomegaly.[65]

Bengtsson and Lamberger recorded persistent cardiac symptoms and abnormalities in 30% of 90 patients examined 5 years after an episode of presumptive acute myocarditis,[66] while Sainani observed persistent signs of heart failure and ECG abnormalities in 5 out of 22 patients with proven coxsackie virus myocarditis. Even in those who recovered, this was delayed for several months in some cases.[30] Smith reported a series of 42 adults with coxsackie virus B myopericarditis: 82% made a complete clinical recovery, although in 12 patients recovery was delayed for 3 months or longer. The disease process recurred in seven patients and was fatal in two of these. Persistent electrocardiographic abnormalities occurred in six patients for a period of up to 6 years and three had residual cardiomegaly indistinguishable from DCM.[31]

Levi and Proto originally reported 22 cases of coxsackie virus heart disease in 1971 with the diagnosis based upon a four-fold or greater rise in antibody titres or isolation of coxsackie virus.[67] In a follow-up study to look for the development of DCM, 11 patients were excluded because of the presence of other potentially confounding factors (hypertension, diabetes or excessive alcohol intake). One patient had died during the initial illness. The remaining 10 patients were followed up for between 4 and 6 years, along with 10 age- and sex-matched control subjects.[68] At follow-up, three out of 10 patients had abnormal systolic cardiac function consistent with DCM.

In a further study, the same authors followed a group of 68 patients with a clinical diagnosis of viral myocarditis for up to 15 years.[69] The patients were divided into two groups on the basis of their original serology. Of 42 patients with positive coxsackie virus serology (four-fold or greater rise in complement fixing antibodies) 10 had died at follow-up — three from myocarditis and seven from dilated cardiomyopathy or its complications. No patients with negative coxsackie virus serology died. A number of patients were also examined clinically at follow-up. Over half of the coxsackie-positive group had persistent ECG abnormalities: ECGs in the negative serology group were all normal.

Histological studies of disease progression

Several studies report patients with acute myocarditis followed up by clinical assessment and serial endomyocardial biopsy studies. Billingham and Tazelaar[70] performed sequential endomyocardial biopsies on 20 patients with myocarditis. The interval between biopsies ranged from 1 to 12 months. In eight cases (40%) the morphological changes were those of dilated cardiomyopathy. Of these eight patients, two died, three proceeded to orthotopic cardiac transplantation and three remained on medical therapy with stable symptoms of heart failure.

Quigley et al.[71] studied 23 patients with biopsy-proven acute myocarditis over a 5-year period. The cardiac histology was evaluated sequentially in 14 patients, seven of whom developed changes compatible with a diagnosis of dilated cardiomyopathy. In all seven cases, this histological progression was accompanied by evidence of left ventricular dysfunction. Two of these patients died during the follow-up period. A further five patients who did not undergo repeat endomyocardial biopsy also developed the classical clinical features of dilated cardiomyopathy. Two of these patients also died during follow-up, the histological findings at autopsy being consistent with dilated cardiomyopathy. In an earlier study by the same group,[72] a similar progression was seen in two out of 12 patients treated with immunosuppression for acute myocarditis.

Virological studies in dilated cardiomyopathy

Several authors have examined patients with dilated cardiomyopathy for serological evidence of previous enteroviral infection. Kawai found a statistically higher percentage of patients with dilated cardiomyopathy than normal controls had elevated antibody titres to coxsackie B viruses and herpes viruses.[73] Cambridge and colleagues studied 50 patients with dilated cardiomyopathy for evidence of previous coxsackie B virus infection and compared these with age- and sex-matched controls who had been admitted to hospital for investigation of other cardiac diseases.[74] High coxsackie B virus neutralization titres (>1024) were significantly more frequent among patients with dilated cardiomyopathy (15 out of 50 in the cardiomyopathy group versus one out of 50 controls) and these titres were associated with a short history of symptoms (<1 year) and also with a febrile illness at the onset. Of the 18 patients in this series that underwent biopsy, none showed evidence of myocarditis, including the 12 patients in whom the viral titres were raised. It was not possible to culture coxsackie virus from any of the endomyocardial biopsy samples in this series.

Morgan-Capner studied 54 patients with either dilated cardiomyopathy or histological changes of a healing myocarditic process.[52] Eleven of these patients had elevated coxsackie

B virus neutralization titres compared with only two out of 40 controls, a similar finding to that of Cambridge et al.[74] Muir looked for evidence of enterovirus infection in patients with dilated cardiomyopathy using an immunoassay for enterovirus-specific IgM.[75] This would normally be expected to decline within 6 months of infection. Positive assays were found in patients before, and up to 4 years after cardiac transplantation in 28 out of 86 (33%) patients compared with only 12% of controls. The authors concluded that this provided evidence not only of an association between enterovirus infection and dilated cardiomyopathy but also of the establishment of persistent enterovirus infection in these patients.

Possibly the best evidence for enteroviral involvement in both acute myocarditis and dilated cardiomyopathy comes from molecular biological studies using nucleic acid hybridization and PCR techniques to search for evidence of enterovirus infection in myocardial tissue. Tissue obtained from animals with experimentally produced myocarditis has been studied extensively, along with heart muscle obtained from patients with all stages of myocarditis and dilated cardiomyopathy. Human samples obtained by endomyocardial biopsy, from the explanted hearts of transplant recipients and postmortem specimens (including formalin-fixed tissue) have all been examined. The results of several of these studies have already been discussed above in relation to myocarditis but many examined mixed populations of patients with all stages of heart muscle disease. The results are summarized in Tables 17.3 and 17.4.

Author	Tissue source	Method	Heart muscle disease	Controls	Comments
Bowles (1986)[55]	Biopsy	SB	9/17 (53%)	0/4 (0%)	Mixed group of myocarditis and DCM
Easton (1988)[76]	Post mortem	IS	6/13 (43%)	0/5 (0%)	Histologically proven myocarditis with evidence of coxsackie virus infection
Bowles (1989)[58]	TP	SB	6/21 (29%)	1/19 (5%)	End-stage disease (at transplantation)
Kandolf (1990)[57]	Biopsy/TP	IS	31/143 (22%)	0/53 (0%)	Mixed group from acute myocarditis to end-stage at transplantation
Hilton (1993)[77]	Post mortem	IS	2/10 (20%)	0/10 (0%)	Parallel study with PCR on same samples (see Table 17.4)

Table 17.3
Molecular hybridization studies for the detection of enterovirus RNA in human cardiac tissue. Figures represent number of subjects in whom enteroviral RNA was detected/total number of subjects tested. Control samples were human cardiac tissue from pathologically normal hearts or heart muscle diseases of known origin.
Abbreviations: Biopsy=endomyocardial biopsy, TP=explanted tissue during cardiac transplantation, SB=slot-blot hybridization, IS=in-situ hybridization.

Author	Tissue source	Acute myocarditis	Dilated cardiomyopathy	Controls
Jin (1990)[78]	EMB	* 2/4 (50%)	3/28 (11%)	0/20 (0%)
Weiss (1991)[79]	EMB EXP	1/5 (20%)	0/11 (0%)	0/21 (0%)
Chiang (1992)[80]	EXP	–	3/4 (75%)	0/6 (0%)
Grasso (1992)[81]	EXP	–	0/21 (0%)	0/20 (0%)
Keeling (1992)[82]	EMB PM	* 0/2 (0%)	6/48 (13%)	13/75 (17%)
Koide (1992)[83]	EMB	6/12 (50%)	5/22 (23%)	0/9 (0%)
Petitjean (1992)[84]	EMB	3/10 (30%)	30/45 (67%)	9/23 (39%)
Weiss (1992)[85]	EXP	–	5/11 (45%)	9/24 (38%)
Zoll (1992)[86]	EMB	–	1/5 (20%)	0/8 (0%)
Hilton (1993)[77]	PM	2/10 (20%)	–	0/10 (0%)
Katsuragi (1993)[87]	PM	0/3 (0%)	3/9 (33%)	1/10 (10%)
Liljeqvist (1993)[59]	EMB	–	0/35 (0%)	0/15 (0%)
Severini (1993)[60]	EMB	1/1 (100%)	1/10 (10%)	All negative
Schwaiger (1993)[61]	EMB	–	6/19 (32%)	0/21 (0%)
Kämmerer (1994)[63]	EMB	–	10/47 (21%)	2/70 (3%)
†Martin (1994)[64]	EMB EXP PM	* 6/18 (33%) * [5/18 (28%) AV]	1/16 (6%) [9/16 (56%) AV] [2/16 (13%) HSV]	0/17 (0%)
Satoh (1994)[62]	EMB	–	17/35 (49%)	0/10 (0%)

Table 17.4

PCR studies which have examined the incidence of detection of enterovirus RNA sequences in human myocardial tissue. Figures given are for number of subjects in whom enteroviral RNA was detected/total number of subjects tested except (†) where figures also given for adenovirus and herpes simplex virus. The figures in the column for acute myocarditis refer only to patients in whom the diagnosis was confirmed histologically in the studies marked (*). All other patients are included in the dilated cardiomyopathy column. Abbreviations: EMB endomyocardial biopsy, PM post mortem, EXP explanted tissue during cardiac transplantation, AV adenovirus, HSV herpes simplex virus.

Treatment

Myocarditis may present as clinically suspected inflammatory myocarditis, unexplained cardiac failure, or unexplained cardiac arrhythmias. To decide the optimal therapy, identification of inflammatory myocardial changes by biopsy is essential because in our experience, presence of inflammation indicates the possibility of spontaneous improvement in left ventricular function and/or resolution of arrhythmias in around 50% of patients. In those patients in whom the myocardial changes are consistent with dilated cardiomyopathy, spontaneous improvement is unlikely unless a precipitating cause such as alcohol misuse, drug exposure or pregnancy is identifiable.

Heart failure

The mainstay of therapy of myocarditis is the symptomatic treatment of heart failure. This may include bed rest and restriction of salt intake but pharmacological terms encompasses the prescription of diuretics, ACE inhibitors, vasodilators, digoxin (even in patients with sinus rhythm) and the consideration of beta blockade.[88–91] In the acute phase intravenous inotropic support may be required and the use of intra-aortic balloon counterpulsation may be needed as a bridge to cardiac transplantation.

Thromboembolic complications may result from clot formation in any cardiac chamber and therefore anticoagulation should be considered in all patients with atrial fibrillation and those in sinus rhythm with significant impairment of ventricular function. In many of the latter patients, thrombus may be visible on echocardiography.

Arrhythmias

As previously discussed, both supraventricular and ventricular arrhythmias are common in patients with myocarditis. Atrial fibrillation and supraventricular tachycardias can contribute significantly to the severity of cardiac failure in spite of conventional antifailure treatment while ventricular arrhythmias are of prognostic importance. Although digoxin may play a part in controlling the ventricular response rate in atrial fibrillation and exert a positive inotropic effect, when combined with diuretic treatment it may be proarrhythmic if hypokalaemia is present. Similarly, digitalis toxicity may a problem in patients with a degree of renal impairment. Recent studies suggest that amiodarone may have long-term benefit on ventricular function over and above its excellent antiarrhythmic profile. For this reason it might be considered the antiarrhythmic agent of choice in such patients.

Specific therapy

In spite of the increasing body of evidence implicating a viral/immune pathogenesis for myocarditis, to date there is no specific antiviral therapy, nor is the routine use of immunosuppressive agents advised. The recent Myocarditis Treatment Trial[92] did not show a significant benefit from prednisolone and cyclosporin, either alone or in combination, when compared with conventional medical treatment. Several small clinical studies have reported improvement in cardiac function in some patients with biopsy-proven myocarditis when treated with immunosuppression and therefore it can be considered in patients with acute histological changes of myocarditis and deteriorating ventricular function when transplantion is unavailable.

Transplantation

Cardiac transplantation is now established as a viable therapeutic option in patients for whom conventional medical therapy has failed. Its major limitation lies in the current shortage of suitable donor hearts. Analysis of the data from the USA cardiac transplantation registry suggests that the outcome in patients with acute myocarditis is less satisfactory than in individuals with dilated cardiomyopathy. Such patients may have little other option, however, if they are to survive. In the future, the development of reliable artificial hearts may render transplantation obsolete or at least provide a window for recovery for patients with fulminant acute myocarditis.

Conclusions

Myocarditis is an important part of the differential diagnosis of any patient presenting with unexplained heart failure, and particularly a clinical diagnosis of dilated cardiomyopathy. When coronary artery disease has been excluded, only endomyocardial biopsy and histological examination of the myocardial tissue will provide an accurate diagnosis. In our experience, this has important implications for the patient's prognosis and the potential for recovery of left ventricular function. This, in turn, may influence the need for eventual cardiac transplantation.

From the medical point of view, no specific therapy has emerged at present. Pharmacological management is identical to that of heart failure from any cause, although specific therapies may be directed against complications such as cardiac arrhythmias and thromboembolic disease.

If I had...

If I presented with a history of 'flu-like' illness associated with an arrhythmia, an abnormal ECG or cardiac enlargement on chest X-ray, then I would first wish to have my ventricular function assessed by echocardiography. In the event of it showing minor dilatation, modest impairment of left ventricular function or a segmental wall motion abnormality suggesting a focal myocarditis, I would be content to be observed without therapy and for the examination to be repeated in 2–3 months.

If I presented in similar circumstances but with symptomatic heart failure and the echocardiogram demonstrated an ejection fraction of 40% or less, then I would accept the need for full invasive assessment including coronary angiography and endomyocardial biopsy. I do not believe that the data support the use of immunosuppression but, if necessary, I would wish to be assessed for cardiac transplantation.

References

1   Sakakibara S, Konno S, Endomyocardial biopsy, *Jpn Heart J* (1962)**3**:537–43.

2   Richardson PJ, King's endomyocardial bioptome, *Lancet* (1974)**i**:660–1.

3   Caves PK, Schulz WP, Dong E Jr, Stinson EB, Schumway NE, A new instrument for transvenous cardiac biopsy, *Am J Cardiol* (1974)**33**:264–7.

4   Olsen EGJ, Myocarditis — a case of mistaken identity? *Br Heart J* (1983)**50**:303–11.

5   Aretz HT, Billingham ME, Edwards WD et al, Myocarditis: a histopathologic definition and classification, *Am J Cardiovasc Pathol* (1986)**1**:3–14.

6   Baandrup U, Florio RA, Olsen EGJ, Do endomyocardial biopsies represent the morphology of the rest of the myocardium? *Eur Heart J* (1982)**3**:171–8.

7   Olsen EGJ, Histomorphologic relation between myocarditis and dilated cardiomyopathy. In: Bolte H-D, ed. *Viral heart disease* (Springer Verlag: Berlin, 1984) 5–12.

8   Goodwin JF, Oakley CM, The cardiomyopathies [editorial], *Br Heart J* (1972)**34**:545–52.

9   WHO/ISFC Task Force, Report of the International Society and Federation of Cardiology/World Health Organization. Task force on the definition and classification of cardiomyopathies, *Br Heart J* (1980)**44**:672–3.

10 Richardson P, McKenna W, Bristow M et al, Report of the 1995 World Health Organisation/International Society and Federation of Cardiology Task Force on the Definition and Classification of Cardiomyopathies, *Circulation* (1996)**93**:841–2.

11 Woodruff JF, Viral myocarditis: a review, *Am J Pathol* (1980)**101**:427–79.

12 Baroldi G, Corallo S, Moroni M et al, Focal lymphocytic myocarditis in acquired immunodeficiency syndrome (AIDS): a correlative morphologic and clinical study in 26 consecutive fatal cases, *J Am Coll Cardiol* (1988)**12**:463–9.

13 Anderson DW, Virmani R, Reilly JM et al, Prevalent myocarditis at necropsy in the acquired immunodeficiency syndrome, *J Am Coll Cardiol* (1988)**11**:792–9.

14 Klein J, Stanek G, Bittner R et al, Lyme borreliosis as a cause of myocarditis and heart muscle disease, *Eur Heart J* (1991)**12(suppl D)**:73–5.

15 Stanek G, Klein J, Bittner R, Glogar D, Isolation of *Borrelia burgdorferi* from the myocardium of a patient with longstanding cardiomyopathy, *N Engl J Med* (1990)**322**:349–52.

16 Puigbo JJ, Valecillos R, Hirschhaut E et al, Diagnosis of Chagas' cardiomyopathy. Non-invasive techniques, *Postgrad Med J* (1977)**53**:527.

17 Bristow MR, Mason JW, Billingham ME, Daniels JR, Dose-effect and structure-function relationships in doxorubicin cardiomyopathy, *Am Heart J* (1981)**102**:709–18.

18 Mason JW, Bristow MR, Billingham ME, Daniels JR, Invasive and non-invasive methods of assessing adriamycin cardiotoxic effects in man: superiority of histopathologic assessment using endomyocardial biopsy, *Cancer Treat Rep* (1978)**62**:857–64.

19 Stevens PJ, Underwood-Ground KE, Occurrence and significance of myocarditis in trauma, *Aerospace Med* (1970)**47**:776–80.

20 Bandt CM, Staley NA, Noren GR, Acute viral myocarditis: clinical and histologic changes, *Minn Med* (1979)**62**:234–7.

21 Frustaci A, Caldarulo M, Buffon A, Bellocci F, Fenici R, Melina D, Cardiac biopsy in patients with 'primary' atrial fibrillation. Histologic evidence of occult myocardial diseases, *Chest* (1991)**100**:303–6.

22 Strain J, Grose R, Factor S, Fisher J, Results of endomyocardial biopsy in patients with spontaneous ventricular tachycardia without apparent structural disease, *Circulation* (1983)**68**:1171–81.

23 Vignola P, Kazutara A, Pauls S *et al.* Lymphocytic myocarditis presenting as unexplained ventricular tachycardia: diagnosis

with endomyocardial biopsy and response to immunosuppression, *J Am Coll Cardiol* (1984)**4**: 812–19.

24 Okuni M, Yamada T, Mochizuki S, Sakurai I, Studies on myocarditis in childhood with special reference to the possible role of immunological process and the thymus in the chronicity of the disease, *Jpn Circ J* (1975)**39**:463–70.

25 Fuster V, Gersh BJ, Giuliani ER, Tajik AJ, Brandenburg RO, Frye RL, The natural history of idiopathic dilated cardiomyopathy, *Am J Cardiol* (1981)**47**:525–31.

26 Reyes MP, Lerner AM, Coxsackie myocarditis — with special reference to acute and clinical effects, *Prog Cardiovasc Dis* (1985)**27**:373–94.

27 Fish M, Barton HR, Heart involvement in infectious mononucleosis, *Arch Intern Med* (1958)**101**:636–44.

28 Public Health Laboratory Service, Coxsackie B5 virus infections in 1965, *Br Med J* (1967)**4**:575–7.

29 Grist NR, Bell EJ, Coxsackie viruses and the heart, *Am Heart J* (1969)**77**:295–300.

30 Sainani GS, Krompotic E, Slodki SJ, Adult heart disease due to coxsackie virus B infection, *Medicine* (1968)**47**:133.

31 Smith WG, Coxsackie B myopericarditis in adults, *Am Heart J* (1970)**80**:34–46.

32 *Vital statistics of the United States 1967: Vol II. Mortality. Part A.* (US Department of Health, Education and Welfare, Public Health Service: Washington, DC, 1969).

33 Peters NS, Poole-Wilson PA, Myocarditis — continuing clinical and pathologic confusion, *Am Heart J* (1991)**121**:942–7.

34 James TN, Schlant RC, Marshall TK, Randomly distributed focal myocardial lesions causing destruction of the His bundle or a narrow origin left bundle branch, *Circulation* (1978)**57**:816.

35 Kitaura Y, Morita H, Secondary myocardial disease, virus myocarditis and cardiomyopathy, *Jpn Circ J* (1979)**43**:1017–31.

36 Sekiguchi M, Hiroe M, Kaneko M, Kusakase K, Natural history of 20 patients with biopsy proven acute mycarditis—10 year follow up, *Circulation* (1985)**72**(suppl 3):109.

37 O'Connell JB, Henlan RE, Robinson JA, Subramaman R, Scanlon PJ, Gunner RM, Gallium-67 imaging in patients with dilated cardiomyopathy and biopsy proven myocarditis, *Circulation* (1984)**70**:58–62.

38 Yasuda TS, Palacios IF, Dec W et al, Indium-111 monoclonal antimyosin antibody imaging in the diagnosis of acute myocarditis, *Circulation* (1987)**76**:306–11.

39 Rezkella S, Khoner RA, Khaw BA et al, Detection of experimental myocarditis by monoclonal antimyosin antibody FAB fragments, *Am Heart J* (1989)**117**:391–5.

40 Raftery EB, Banks DC, Oram S, Occlusive disease of the coronary arteries presenting as pacing congestive cardiomyopathy, *Lancet* (1969)**ii**:1147–450.

41 Richardson PJ, Endomyocardial biopsy: technique and evaluation of a new disposable forceps and catheter sheath system. In: Bolte H-D, ed. *Viral heart disease* (Springer Verlag: Berlin, 1983)173–6.

42 Caves PK, Stinson EB, Billingham ME, Shumway NE, Serial transvenous biopsy of the transplanted human heart. Improved management of acute rejection episodes, *Lancet* (1974)**i**:821–6.

43 Maisch B, The use of myocardial biopsy in heart failure, *Eur Heart J* (1988)**9**(suppl H): 59–71.

44 Zee Cheng CS, Tsai CC, Palmer DC, Codd JE, Pennington DC, Williams CA, High incidence of myocarditis diagnosed by endomyocardial biopsy in patients with idiopathic congestive cardiomyopathy, *J Am Coll Cardiol* (1984)**3**: 63–70.

45 Dec GW, Palacios IF, Fallon JT et al, Active myocarditis in the spectrum of acute dilated cardiomyopathies — clinical features, histologic correlates and clinical outcome, *N Engl J Med* (1985)**312**:885–90.

46 Baandrup U, Florio BA, Rehalin M, Richardson PJ, Olsen EGJ, Critical analysis of endomyocardial biopsies from patients with suspected cardiomyopathy. II. Comparison of histology and clinical/haemodynamic information, *Br Heart J* (1981)**45**:487–93.

47 Davidoff R, Palacios E, Southern J, Fallon JT, Newell J, Dec W, Giant cell and lymphocytic myocarditis — comparison of clinical factors and long term outcome, *Circulation* (1991)**83**: 953–61.

48 Johanssen A, Isolated myocarditis versus myocardial sarcoidosis, *Acta Pathol Microbiol Scand* (1967)**67**:15–26.

49 Lorell B, Alderman EL, Mason JW, Cardiac sarcoidosis: diagnosis with endomyocardial biopsy and treatment with corticosteroids, *Am J Cardiol* (1978)**42**:143–6.

50 Richardson PJ, Why HJF, Maisch B, Myocarditis, myopericarditis and dilated cardiomyopathy. In: Julian D, Camm AJ, Fox KM, Hall RJC, Poole-Wilson PA, eds. *Diseases of the heart* (WB Saunders: London, 1996)489–505.

51 Lerner AM, Wilson FM, Virus myocardiopathy, *Prog Med Virol* (1973)**15**:63–91.

52 Morgan-Capner P, Richardson PJ, McSorley C, Daly K, Pattison JR, Virus investigations in heart muscle disease. In: Bolte H-D, ed. *Viral heart disease* (Springer Verlag: Berlin, 1984)99–115.

53 Grist NR, Coxsackie virus infections of the heart. In: Waterson AP, ed. *Recent advances in clinical virology. Vol 1.* (Churchill Livingstone: Edinburgh, 1977)141.

54 Kandolf R, Hofschneider PH, Molecular cloning of the genome of a cardiotropic coxsackie B3 virus: full length reverse-transcribed recombinant cDNA generates infectious virus in mammalian cells, *Proc Natl Acad Sci USA* (1985)**82**:4818–22.

55 Bowles NE, Richardson PJ, Olsen EGJ, Archard LC, Detection of coxsackie-B-virus-specific RNA sequences in myocardial biopsy samples from patients with myocarditis and dilated cardiomyopathy, *Lancet* (1986)**i**:1120–23.

56 Saiki RK, Gelfand DH, Stoffel S et al, Primer-directed enzymatic amplification of DNA with a thermostable DNA polymerase, *Science* (1988)**239**:487–91.

57 Kandolf R, Canu A, Klinger K et al, Molecular studies in enteroviral heart diseases. In: Brinton MA, Henry FX, eds. *New aspects of positive-strand RNA viruses* (American Society for Microbiology: Washington, 1990)340–8.

58 Bowles NE, Rose ML, Taylor P et al, End-stage dilated cardiomyopathy: persistence of enterovirus RNA in myocardium at cardiac transplantation and lack of immune response, *Circulation* (1989)**80**:1128–36.

59 Liljeqvist J-Å, Bergström T, Holmström S et al, Failure to demonstrate enterovirus aetiology in Swedish patients with dilated cardiomyopathy, *J Med Virol* (1993)**39**:6–10.

60 Severini GM, Mestroni L, Falaschi A, Camerini F, Giacca M, Nested polymerase chain reaction for high-sensitivity detection of enteroviral RNA in biological samples, *J Clin Microbiol* (1993)**31**:1345–9.

61 Schwaiger A, Umlauft F, Weyrer K et al, Detection of enteroviral ribonucleic acid in myocardial biopsies from patients with idiopathic dilated cardiomyopathy by polymerase chain reaction, *Am Heart J* (1993)**126**:406–10.

62 Satoh M, Tamura G, Segawa I, Hiramori K, Satodate R, Enteroviral RNA in dilated cardiomyopathy, *Eur Heart J* (1994)**15**:934–9.

63 Kämmerer U, Kunkel B, Korn K, Nested PCR for specific detection and rapid identification of human picornaviruses, *J Clin Microbiol* (1994)**32**:285–91.

64 Martin AB, Webber S, Fricker FJ et al, Acute myocarditis. Rapid diagnosis by PCR in children, *Circulation* (1994)**90**:330-9.

65 Levander-Lindgren M, Studies in myocarditis. IV. Late prognosis, *Cardiologia* (1965)**47**:209.

66 Bengtsson E, Lamberger B, Five years follow-up study of cases suggestive of acute myocarditis, *Am Heart J* (1966)**72**:751–63.

67 Levi GF, Proto C, Coxsackie virus heart disease, *Lancet* (1971)**i**:298.

68 Levi CF, Proto C, Quadri A, Ratti S, Coxsackie virus heart disease and cardiomyopathy, *Am Heart J* (1977)**93**:419–21.

69 Levi G, Scalvini S, Volterrani M, Marangoni S, Arosio G, Quadri A, Coxsackie virus heart disease: 15 years after, *Eur Heart J* (1987)**8**(**suppl J**):1303–7.

70 Billingham ME, Tazelaar HD, The morphological progression of viral myocarditis, *Postgrad Med J* (1986)**62**:581–4.

71 Quigley PJ, Richardson PJ, Meaney BT et al, Long-term follow-up of acute myocarditis. Correlation of ventricular function and outcome, *Eur Heart J* (1987)**8**(**suppl J**):39–42.

72 Daly K, Richardson PJ, Olsen EGJ et al, Acute myocarditis: role of histological and virological examination in the diagnosis and assessment of immunosuppressive treatment, *Br Heart J* (1984)**51**:30–5.

73 Kawai C, Idiopathic cardiomyopathy. A study on the infectious-immune theory as the cause of the disease, *Jpn Circ J* (1971)**35**:765–70.

74 Cambridge G, MacArthur CGC, Waterson AP, Goodwin JF, Oakley CM, Antibodies to cox-sackie B viruses in primary congestive cardio-myopathy, *Br Heart J* (1979)**41**:692–6.

75 Muir P, Tilzey AJ, English TAH, Nicholson F, Signey M, Banatvala JE, Chronic relapsing peri-carditis and dilated cardiomyopathy: serologi-cal evidence of persistent enterovirus infection, *Lancet* (1989)**i**:804–7.

76 Easton AJ, Eglin RP, The detection of coxsack-ievirus RNA in cardiac tissue by *in situ* hybri-dization, *J Gen Virol* (1988)**69**:285–91.

77 Hilton DA, Variend S, Pringle JH, Demonstration of Coxsackie virus RNA in for-malin-fixed tissue sections from childhood myocarditis cases by *in situ* hybridisation and the polymerase chain reaction, *J Pathol* (1993)**170**:45–51.

78 Jin O, Sole MJ, Butany JW et al, Detection of enterovirus RNA in myocardial biopsies from patients with myocarditis and cardiomyopathy using gene amplification by polymerase chain reaction, *Circulation* (1990)**82**:8–16.

79 Weiss LM, Movahed LA, Billingham ME, Cleary ML, Detection of coxsackievirus B3 RNA in myocardial tissues by the polymerase chain reaction, *Am J Pathol* (1991)**138**:497–503.

80 Chiang FT, Lin LI, Tseng YZ et al, Detection of enterovirus RNA in patients with idiopathic dilated cardiomyopathy by polymerase chain reaction, *J Formosan Med Assoc* (1992)**91**:569–74.

81 Grasso M, Arbustini E, Silini E et al, Search for coxsackievirus B3 RNA in idiopathic dilated cardiomyopathy using gene amplification by polymerase chain reaction, *Am J Cardiol* (1992)**69**:658–64.

82 Keeling PJ, Jeffery S, Caforio AL et al, Similar prevalence of enteroviral genome within the myocardium from patients with idiopathic dilated cardiomyopathy and controls by the polymerase chain reaction, *Br Heart J* (1992)**68**:554–9.

83 Koide H, Kitaura Y, Deguchi H, Ukimura A, Kawamura K, Hirai K, Genomic detection of enteroviruses in the myocardium—studies on animal hearts with coxsackievirus B3 myocar-ditis and endomyocardial biopsies from patients with myocarditis and dilated cardio-myopathy, *Jpn Circ J* (1992)**56**:1081–93.

84 Petitjean J, Kopecka H, Freymuth F et al, Detection of enteroviruses in endomyocardial biopsy by molecular approach, *J Med Virol* (1992)**37**:76–82.

85 Weiss LM, Liu XF, Chang KL, Billingham ME, Detection of enteroviral RNA in idiopathic dilated cardiomyopathy and other human car-diac tissues, *J Clin Invest* (1992)**90**:156–9.

86 Zoll GJ, Melchers WJG, Kopecka H, Jambroes G, van der Poel HJA, Galama JMD, General primer-mediated polymerase chain reaction for detection of enteroviruses: application for diagnostic routine and persistent infections, *J Clin Microbiol* (1992)**30**:160–5.

87 Katsuragi M, Yutani C, Mukai T et al, Detection of enteroviral genome and its signifi-cance in cardiomyopathy, *Cardiology* (1993) **83**:4–13.

88 Waagstein F, Hjalmarson A, Varnauskas E, Wallentin I, Effect of chronic β-adrenergic receptor blockade in congestive cardio-myopathy, *Br Heart J* (1975)**37**:1022–36.

89 Bristow MR, Ginsburg R, Minobe W et al, Decreased catecholamine sensitivity and β-adre-nergic-receptor density in failing human hearts, *N Engl J Med* (1982)**307**:205–11.

90 Waagstein F, Bristow MR, Swedberg K et al, Beneficial effects of metoprolol in idiopathic dilated cardiomyopathy, *Lancet* (1993)**342**:1441–6.

91 Packer M, Bristow MR, Cohn JN et al, The effect of carvedilol on morbidity and mortality in patients with chronic heart failure, *N Engl J Med* (1996)**334**:1349–55.

92 Mason JW, O'Connell JB, Herskowitz A et al, A clinical trial of immunosuppressive therapy for myocarditis, The Myocarditis Treatment Trial Investigators, *N Engl J Med* (1995)**333**:269–75.

18

Gene therapy

Claire M Dollery and Michael Marber

Background

Gene therapy is the introduction of foreign genetic material (usually DNA) into somatic cells to modify their genetic content and achieve a therapeutic endpoint. The term gene therapy may encompass diverse aims, from the replacement of an absent or defective gene to facilitate cell function, to the transfer of a gene with a cytotoxic product to cause cell death. Gene therapy has developed rapidly since the technology to transfer and express genes has improved, in parallel with the discovery of new genes which have therapeutic potential. While initial studies used marker genes to assess the safety and efficiency of gene transfer and expression, there are now more than 100 clinical protocols for human gene therapy approved in the USA.[1]

The first clinical demonstration of effective gene transfer was carried out in 1989 when tumour infiltrating lymphocytes were removed from cancer patients, genetically marked (by transfer of a gene for neomycin resistance) and then returned to the patient, in whom they could later be detected.[2] The next step was to use these techniques to modify disease states. Patients with adenosine deaminase deficient severe combined immunodeficiency disease (SCID) were the subjects of a study which successfully modified their lymphocytes *ex vivo*. The gene for adenosine deaminase was transferred to the subjects' lymphocytes *in vitro* and they were then reintroduced into the patients with a measurable but temporary clinical improvement.[3] Of more relevance to cardiovascular disease, a clinical trial of *ex vivo* gene therapy has successfully modified the lipid profile of a patient with familial hypercholesterolaemia.[4] Furthermore, intra-arterial administration of the gene encoding vascular endothelial growth factor (VEGF), an angiogenic factor, is being evaluated in severe peripheral vascular disease with encouraging initial results.[5]

There are many potential uses for gene therapy in cardiovascular disease but experience from other fields suggests that some caution is required. Cystic fibrosis is one of the diseases which has been most actively targeted for gene therapy, with two major trials employing adenoviral liposome-mediated transfer of the gene encoding the cystic fibrosis transmembrane regulator.[6] These trials have confirmed that human gene transfer is possible but have been unable to demonstrate clinical improvement or prolonged gene expression. Despite this, some patients experienced side effects. This highlights the difference between successful gene transfer and effective gene therapy. The latter requires not only efficient gene transfer but also transcription of enough foreign DNA to correct a functional defect while provoking a minimal immune response.[6]

To justify the complexity of genetic therapy approaches to human disease, it is necessary to consider both obstacles to, and targets for, gene transfer.

Gene therapy for single gene disorders

Gene therapy can be used to treat single gene disorders such as Duchenne muscular dystrophy[7] or familial hypercholesterolaemia (FH)[8] where the aim is to correct the patient's genetic defect and phenotype. For example, in FH the gene encoding the low-density lipoprotein receptor could be transferred to normalize the patient's lipid metabolism. The defect is well characterized, the corrective gene is sequenced and therefore the necessary information is available to the gene therapist. The limiting factors are the ability to transfer this gene to some or all of the patient's cells, ensuring robust expression of the gene, and maintaining prolonged gene expression without toxicity.

Gene therapy is not necessarily appropriate to all single gene disorders. Recent research into the molecular genetics of hypertrophic cardiomyopathy has enhanced our understanding and led to genetic counselling.[9] This disorder follows a dominant inheritance pattern and there is therefore both a normal and an abnormal copy of the relevant contractile protein gene. The phenotype is the result of an interaction of the normal with the abnormal contractile protein. Providing further copies of the normal gene via genetic transfer approaches is unlikely to ameliorate the disease. In addition, all current gene therapy strategies involve augmentation of the existing genetic code with no techniques available to remove or modify the human genome *in situ*. Gene therapy is perhaps more likely to find an application in common polygenic disorders such as atherosclerosis. This may not necessarily involve altering the underlying pathological process, which could be irreversible and resistant to gene transfer. It is more likely that the expression of gene products more akin to the physiological antagonists of traditional pharmacology will prove fruitful. For example, the current clinical trial of intra-arterial application of plasma DNA encoding the angiogenic factor VEGF to the severely ischaemic lower limb, aims to induce angiogenesis and therefore relieve pain and ulceration without an antiatherosclerotic effect.[5]

Principles of gene transfer

Gene transfer systems aim to improve on existing therapies whether these are pharmacological or involve the administration of a recombinant protein produced in a laboratory. The first step in gene therapy is identifying the gene to be inserted; once this is accomplished, the gene of interest can be extracted from cells. The DNA must be recombined into a form which is likely to be expressed in the target cell, and to this end a number of different techniques have been developed to transport the DNA; these transport systems are called vectors. The entry of the DNA into the target cell is governed by the efficiency of delivery of the gene to the target cell, the physical properties   of the vector and the time of exposure to the target.

The vector carrying the DNA must first attach to and then cross the cell membrane, traverse the cytoplasm evading lysosomal digestion, and enter the nucleus where initiation of transcription of the DNA strand takes place. Current vectors used to aid DNA transport include those that make use of naturally occurring systems which insert foreign DNA into cells in disease states, that is the viral vectors and man-made transfer systems such as the cationic liposomes (Figure 18.1). The adenovirus, for example, has a specific receptor which enables entry into the cell and viral coat proteins which disrupt the intracellular host defences that normally cause destruction of the viral DNA and the gene of interest. Liposomes fuse with the cell membrane and release sufficient DNA into the cytoplasm so that even without a protective

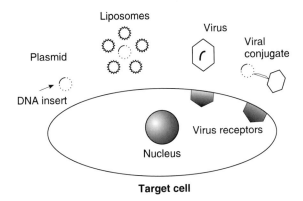

Figure 18.1
Gene delivery vectors.

transfer mechanism, ample DNA reaches the nucleus. All viral vectors used in gene therapy have been rendered replication deficient so that they can infect the host cell but cannot then replicate. This is accomplished by cutting specific genes out of the viruses which are essential for their replication. The replication-deficient vector is then grown in cells which have been modified to express the deficient genes, i.e. they are complementary to the deleted virus. This allows large amounts of the vector to be produced but once it is separated from the complementing cells, it can no longer replicate.

Once DNA reaches the nucleus, it is transcribed only if it has the appropriate initiation signals. In addition, the gene of interest can be combined with a powerful promoter so that a therapeutic effect may be achieved with lesser amounts of the vector, with a consequent reduction in toxicity. Tissue-specific promoters are also being investigated, for example an actin promoter when targeting smooth muscle cells, but these often achieve specificity at the expense of efficiency. The duration of expression of a gene may also determine its uses in gene therapy. This is often governed by the vector used to administer it. Genes delivered using liposomes or adenoviruses do not integrate into the host genome and therefore have a limited lifespan, while retrovirally administered genes are inserted into the genome and are, in theory, limited only by the life of the infected cell or its progeny. These differences raise a number of safety and practical issues. For example, while there is little advantage to the patient with familial hypercholesterolaemia in transiently augmenting LDL receptor levels, a patient undergoing angioplasty requires only short-term expression to prevent initiation of the re-stenotic process.

The viral vectors

The retroviruses

Retroviruses were the first viral vectors used in vascular gene transfer.[10–13] Retroviruses can integrate only into the genome of dividing cells. This makes them unsuitable for use in cardiac myocytes which are terminally differentiated, and limits their use in smooth muscle cells (*in vivo*). They are capable of stable gene expression but are hampered by their low efficiency of gene transfer. As few as 100 cells may be transduced in a 2 cm arterial segment.[14] The DNA transferred by this method is integrated into the host genome, increasing the duration of the gene expression (for example, 12 months in the rat carotid artery).[15] However, there is no external control of the genomic site into which the DNA is inserted, raising the theoretical risk of insertional mutagenesis where a native gene may be disrupted or separated from its normal control elements. Hence abnormal cell growth and malignancy may result.[16] In common with all viral vectors there is also the potential risk of the virus reacquiring its replication ability by, for example, recombining with endogenous human retroviral sequences. The predilection of retroviruses for dividing cells has resulted in most of their use being *ex vivo*, for example they have been used *ex vivo* to modify hepatocytes which are then reintroduced to express the LDL receptor.[4] This technique has been used to treat a woman with familial hypercholesterolaemia. Retroviruses have also been used to improve the performance of bioprostheses such as vascular grafts and stents.[17] Whilst there is still interest in using retroviruses for *ex vivo* gene transfer, other vectors have now been developed in an attempt to overcome some of their disadvantages.

The adenoviruses

Adenoviruses are the most widely used viral vectors in vascular biology. The adenovirus genome is very well characterized and is relatively easy to manipulate. This has led to the development of a number of different adenoviral vectors which have been made replication-incompetent by removal of essential genes.[18] Adenoviruses deleted in this way can accommodate the insertion of relatively large genes (8.3 kilobases) and high titre viral stocks can be grown readily in the laboratory.[19] They also are efficient at infecting many different cell types in many species, which has facilitated their development. An important advantage over the retroviruses is their ability to infect quiescent nondividing cells (Figure 18.2). They are highly efficient in transferring genes due to their cell surface receptor and endosomal disrupter. Their efficiency is superior to retroviruses and liposomes in normal, uninjured and atherosclerotic blood vessels (Figure 18.3).[20–23] Adenoviruses also have a safety advantage over retroviral vectors in that they do not insert their DNA into the host chromosomes and while this reduces their duration of action, it reduces the chances of insertional mutagenesis. Insertion of viral genes into the host genome can occur but is very rare.[24]

Use of live adenoviruses as vaccines over some years has not revealed an increased frequency of malignancy and is safe even in immunocompromised subjects.[25] The principal problem with adenoviruses is their ability to provoke a humoural and cellular immune response, which may result in destruction of the infected cell (Figure 18.4). This limits expression of the transferred gene. In addition, they cause production of circulating neutralizing antibodies which prevent successful repeat administrations.[26] Both these problems are likely to have afflicted the early adenovirus clinical trials, such as those in cystic fibrosis.[6, 27] To date, the most widely used vectors have been the so-called first-generation adenoviruses which have E1A and E1B genes deleted to prevent replication. Now, however, further research is being concentrated on second- and third-generation vectors. These newer vectors are rendered even more severely genetically deficient by deletion of viral genes such as those encoding the adenoviral DNA polymerase or the DNA binding protein.[28,29] These deletions further limit transcription of antigenic structural virion protein, ultimately minimizing the inflammatory response and improving the duration of transgene expression.[29]

Other viral vectors

A number of other viruses are now being investigated for use in gene therapy. Herpes viruses have been used in the cardiovascular system in experimental animals and adeno-associated virus has been approved for clinical trials but has not been used extensively in the heart or the vasculature.

Herpes virus vectors were originally developed to target the nervous system, where they are able to remain latent for long periods.[30] Herpes simplex 1 vectors can be divided into two types: disabled viruses and defective viruses

A

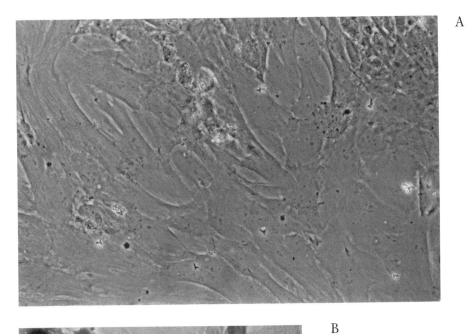

B

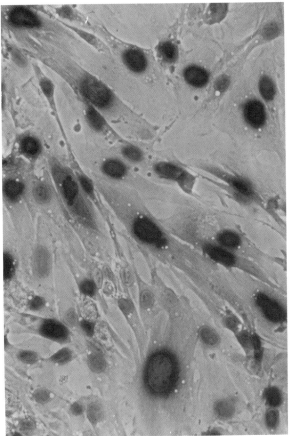

Figure 18.2
Adenovirus-mediated transgene expression in rat aortic vascular smooth muscle cells (VSMC). Uninfected VSMCs (A) or VSMCs infected with a nuclear localized beta galactosidase adenoviral vector (B) were fixed and stained with X-gal. The nuclear dark blue colouration is secondary to the presence of a bacterial form of the enzyme, β-galactosidase. Where present, this enzyme splits a chromogen substrate (X-gal) to cause colour conversion from yellow to blue. (C Dollery, unpublished data.)

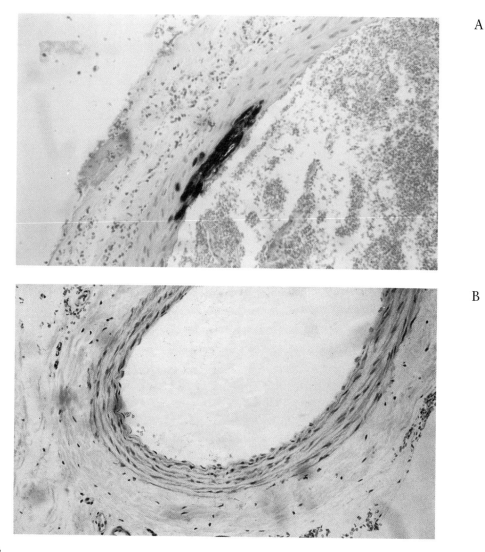

Figure 18.3

In vivo *gene delivery to the rat carotid artery. 1 x 10⁹ plaque-forming units of adenovirus (encoding β-galactosidase) was instilled into an isolated segment of the left carotid artery (A) immediately following balloon injury. The right carotid artery, which was not injured or exposed to virus, was used as a control (B). Both arteries were fixed and stained with X-gal 2 days later. The dark blue discoloration indicates successful* in vivo *gene transfer to the arterial wall. (C Dollery, unpublished data.)*

or amplicons. The former have genes deleted to make them unable to replicate (either in all cells or in neurons) and are grown on complementing cell lines. The latter are short sequences of the HSV genome encoding replication and packaging signalling sequences but little else. They cannot replicate unless a helper virus is present. Disabled HSV vectors have been used

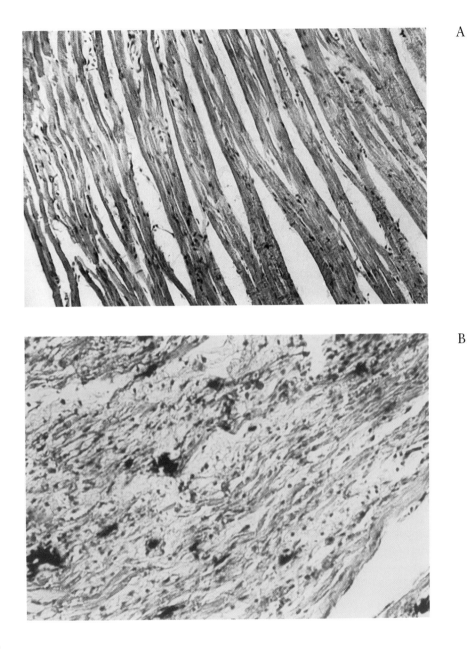

A

B

Figure 18.4
Inflammatory response associated with adenovirus mediated gene tranfer in vivo *in the rabbit by intracoronary injection. The appearances of the right ventricular and left ventricular myocardium 3 days after right coronary artery injection of 1 x 10^{11} plaque-forming units of a replication-defective adenovirus serotype 5. These haemotoxylin and eosin stained specimens were prepared from the left and right ventricular free walls of the heart depicted in Figure 18.6. (A) Near normal appearance of the myocardium from the left ventricular free wall. (B) In contrast, the myocardium from the right ventricular free wall is grossly disorganized with myocytolysis and an inflammatory infiltrate. Changes occur both close to and at a distance from islands of X-gal staining. (M Marber, unpublished data.)*

to express a marker gene in cardiac myocytes in culture and *in vivo*. However, they show poor results in smooth muscle cells with little gene expression and significant toxicity.[31] Amplicon vectors encoding VEGF have been used *ex vivo* to infect fibroblasts in cultures. Infected cells were reimplanted *in vivo*, where they elicited a brisk angiogenic response.[32]

The human parvovirus adeno-associated virus (AAV) resembles the herpes amplicon in that it is incapable of replicating without a helper virus.[33] However, it has some advantages in that the helper virus can be killed by heat while AAV is resistant. When a cell is infected with AAV the viral DNA and any accompanying gene is inserted into the host genome but, unlike the retroviruses, this occurs at a specific site on chromosome 19 with a reduced risk of insertional mutagenesis. This virus can infect nondividing cells of many different types but efficiency is limited. AAV has been hampered by low efficiency and an inability to manufacture high titre viral stocks.

The nonviral vectors
Plasmid expression vectors

Plasmid expression vectors are the lowest common denominators of gene therapy, containing only the gene of interest and the minimal genetic material necessary to control transgene expression. They are made by inserting a gene into a bacterial plasmid. These plasmids are circular pieces of DNA containing regulatory sequences that enhance gene transcription in eukaryotic cells and can be grown in bacteria. The disadvantage of the system is that DNA carries a negative charge, making it difficult to cross the lipid bilayer and therefore hampering entry into the cell. The advantage is that isolated plasmids do not have a complicated vector system attached to them, which may cause toxicity in

its own right. These simple but inefficient vectors have been chosen to deliver VEGF for the current clinical trials of angiogenesis and restenosis in peripheral vascular disease.[5]

Cationic liposomes

Cationic liposomes were designed to increase the efficiency of plasmid DNA transfer without altering the safety profile. The lipid solution is mixed with the plasmid DNA and forms a lipid bilayer around it. The resultant liposome is then able to adhere to and fuse with the cell membrane, causing release of DNA into the cell cytoplasm. A large proportion of the DNA will be removed by endosomal breakdown before reaching the nucleus. It has been estimated that only one in every 1000 plasmids presented to the cell by liposomes will reach the nucleus.[34] Liposomes have the advantage that they are quite efficient for gene delivery but cannot be targeted except by their anatomical distribution, and may show overall gene expression levels as low as 0.1–1%.[35] In common with the adenoviruses, they express genes only transiently and are not known to be associated with insertional mutagenesis. There is no size constraint on the amount of DNA that can be incorporated into liposomes and they will enter both quiescent and dividing cells. Their safety profile *in vivo* is excellent and work continues to perfect liposomal lipid content to increase the efficiency of overall gene expression.

Viral conjugates

The viral conjugate vectors have been engineered to possess many of the advantages of viruses while avoiding their toxic effects. The most successful conjugate to be used in the cardiovascular system at present is the combination of Sendai virus (haemagglutinating virus of Japan) and liposomes, in which the virus is inactivated with ultraviolet irradiation and then combined with a liposome containing a plasmid.[36] The resultant conjugate can avoid the toxicity of a complete viral particle but yet uses components of the inactivated virus with greater efficiency. This technique has been used to transfer genes of the renin–angiotensin system and nitric oxide (NO) synthase in animal models of vascular disease. Conjugates have also been made which incorporate defective adenoviral particles to facilitate cell entry and nuclear transfer. In this system, plasma DNA is polylysine linked to defective or irradiated particles that contain adenoviral capsid but no functional DNA. This system has been assessed in vein graft models[37] and has the advantage that since only the adenoviral coat protein is required, there is no constraint on the size of the gene transferred and no toxicity related to the adenoviral genome.

Delivery devices

The design and development of the vectors discussed above are aimed at maximizing gene transfer and expression. Parallel evolution has occurred in the physical methods of gene delivery. Delivery devices have been tailored to the intended target tissue for gene therapy. To target the myocardium, an injection of the vector into the coronary artery is appropriate and sufficient. This will not result in gene transfer to the coronary arteries since the vector is rapidly washed downstream into the capillaries, and hence there is only a transient exposure to the vessel wall. Interrupting flow in an artery prolongs the time available for gene transfer but in the coronary arteries this will cause ischaemia or infarction.

The large number of coronary angioplasties performed, and the continued problems with restenosis, has caused most research in this area to concentrate on delivery devices applicable to the coronary circulation, although designs are coincidentally also suitable for peripheral vascular applications. The main types of delivery device under evaluation are summarized in Figure 18.5. They are most conveniently divided into diffusion systems, pressure systems and other physical methods. The features of these devices tend to dictate their efficiency in transducing the different layers of the arterial wall and the degree of damage they may cause.

Diffusion devices

The double balloon catheter
The first local delivery device used for gene transfer was the double balloon catheter, a percutaneous equivalent of the lumenal dwell techniques used in surgical animal models. When the two balloons are inflated, low pressure can be applied to the isolated space. This enhances uptake of the infusate into the tissues. The double balloon catheter has been validated *in vivo* with both adenoviral and liposomal vectors in normal, injured, and atherosclerotic vessels.[35,38] It has the advantage of allowing prolonged exposure to the vector, which enhances the efficiency of gene delivery. In addition, relatively little injury occurs because of the low pressures employed. Unfortunately, these catheters have no distal perfusion capabilities, preventing prolonged inflations in coronary arteries. Concern has also been expressed that the relatively long distance between balloons may allow significant leakage of vector into arterial side branches and that the balloons may cause vascular injury.

The multichamber balloon
This device was designed to provide a low pressure diffusion system in combination with

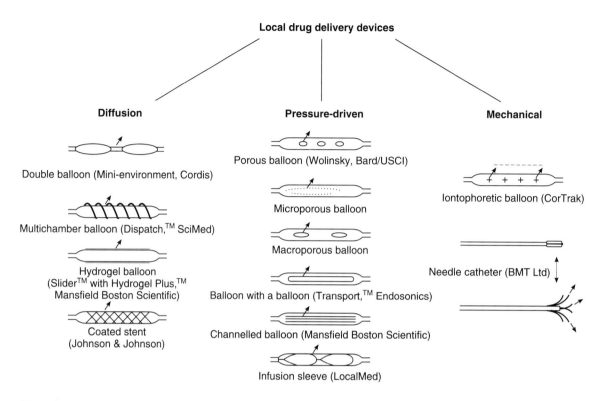

Local drug delivery devices

Diffusion

Double balloon (Mini-environment, Cordis)

Multichamber balloon (Dispatch,™ SciMed)

Hydrogel balloon
(Slider™ with Hydrogel Plus,™
Mansfield Boston Scientific)

Coated stent
(Johnson & Johnson)

Pressure-driven

Porous balloon (Wolinsky, Bard/USCI)

Microporous balloon

Macroporous balloon

Balloon with a balloon (Transport,™ Endosonics)

Channelled balloon (Mansfield Boston Scientific)

Infusion sleeve (LocalMed)

Mechanical

Iontophoretic balloon (CorTrak)

Needle catheter (BMT Ltd)

Figure 18.5
Types of delivery device. Reproduced with permission from Hofling B, Huehns TY, Clinical perspective, intravascular local drug delivery after angioplasty, Eur Heart J (1995)**16:**437–40.

a perfusion catheter. The catheter achieves these aims and can deliver drug to the endothelium, subendothelium and adventitia. In common with the double balloon catheter, vector can be lost into side branches and there is an additional risk of the coils causing occlusion and ischaemia if they are inadvertently positioned over a side branch. The catheter also causes a characteristic 'zebra' distribution of infusate since cells beneath the coils are not exposed to the infusate. Theoretically this may result in a 'zebra' pattern of restenosis unless the inserted gene has a bystander effect (for example, a secreted protein). This multichamber balloon has been used clinically for local thrombolysis[39] and is currently being evalu-

ated in animal models as a gene delivery device.

The hydrogel balloon
The hydrogel balloon is the only gene delivery device currently used in clinical trials.[5] This catheter is a standard angioplasty balloon (without a perfusion lumen) coated with a hydrophilic polymer which adsorbs aqueous solutions which may contain conventional drug or DNA. Once the gel dries, the balloon is introduced into the patient within a protective sheath. The sheath is then withdrawn at the delivery site and the balloon is inflated. This presses the hydrogel coating into the artery, achieving transfer to the medial and adventitial

layers. The degree of injury and, to some extent, the distribution of vector is related to the inflation pressures used. Significant wash-out of the coating of the balloon has been documented (up to 65%)[40] and although this is minimized by use of a sheath, the time from sheath removal to inflation must be minimized. There are also limitations to the amount of vehicle that can be applied to the balloon.

Coated stents have also been employed in gene transfer, for example stents have been seeded with retrovirally transduced endothelial cells.[17]

Pressure-driven devices

The pressure-driven devices all depend upon the forcing of the vector into the arterial wall by pressure. The systems have been used successfully in animal models to transfer genes to normal and atherosclerotic arteries, and are more successful than most other devices at gene transfer to the media.[23] The efficiency of delivery depends on the pressure, pore size, and fit of the balloon to the artery. There is an inverse relation between wash-out and transfer of the vector, with the latter often accompanied by severe vascular injury and dissection at the pore sites due to a traumatic jet effect. The balloon within a balloon catheter seeks to overcome these problems by separating the pressure in the drug delivery lumen from the pressure in the angioplasty balloon inflation lumen. Fluorescent antisense oligonucleotides in the intima, adjacent media and adventitia (but not the interposing media) are seen when this device is used in explanted hearts from transplant recipients.[41] This catheter, approved for clinical use, is being evaluated for local thrombolytic agent delivery.

The multichannel balloon, similar in principle, employs multiple instead of a single balloon channel. It has been used to deliver adenovirus to atherosclerotic vessels in a rabbit model.[22] The infusion sleeve is designed to be able to infuse vector proximal, around, or distal to the angioplasty balloon. The device is also in clinical trial for local thrombolysis but has not, as yet, been used for gene transfer.

Mechanical devices

The iontophoresis catheter is intended to improve on the efficiency of passive diffusion transfer efficiency without causing the damage to the vessel wall that is associated with pressure-driven devices. The principle employed is vector entry into cells using an electric field as the driving energy. Delivery is optimal when very small charged molecules are transferred but iontophoresis has been used to transfer DNA plasmids effectively.[42] The system has good penetration of all layers of the arterial wall but may not be suited to all vectors. Perfusion cannot be maintained with the currently available catheters.

The needle injection catheter aims to deliver substances preferentially to the adventitia. This layer is being increasingly recognized as the site of the early events in restenotic process. The device causes little local trauma but may deliver vector to adjacent tissues. Although being investigated with retroviral vectors, it has not been used for gene transfer to date.

Antisense oligonucleotides

The use of antisense oligonucleotides to suppress expression of target genes has attracted both interest and controversy in recent years. The principle of antisense therapy is to introduce a short length of single-stranded DNA into a cell which is complementary to the mRNA of a particular gene. The antisense oligonucleotide will then bind to the mRNA and prevent translation. This approach is inefficient and can be used only to target genes that produce mRNA at a relatively low abundance. It has a limited duration of action as the antisense molecules are subject to enzyme digestion. (They must be made relatively resistant to digestion by chemical modification of their backbone.) In theory, at least, antisense is a highly specific and readily localized therapy in which the design of new 'drugs' (that is, new oligonucleotides) is straightforward and fast. The successes in the antisense literature have used oligonucleotides to target cellular proliferation postangioplasty. In particular antisense to *c-myb*, *c-myc*, the proliferating cell nuclear antigen, the cdc-2 kinase and the cdk-2 kinase have suppressed neointimal formation in the rat carotid model of balloon angioplasty.[43] This effect of antisense *c-myc* has also been shown in porcine coronary arteries and a clinical trial of antisense in coronary angioplasty has been planned.

Recent doubts about antisense use have occurred with increasing realization that we do not fully understand the underlying mechanisms. There are questions regarding the specificity of antisense oligonucleotides and reproducibility of results. These may reflect problems with delivery. Some of the possible mechanisms of action include the following:

- Formation of a duplex with target mRNA which causes steric interference, preventing binding to the ribosome and therefore translation;
- Induction of mRNA cleavage by the nucleotide breakdown enzyme RNase H;
- Oligonucleotides entering the nucleus, binding to mRNA and preventing transport into the cytoplasm. The specificity of oligonucleotides is based on the ability of the purine and pyrimidine subunits of the genome to bind only in A-T and C-G combinations. The oligonucleotide used must therefore be long enough (contain enough bases) to hybridize

uniquely to the intended mRNA. Unfortunately there are many sequences that are common to numerous mRNAs, and therefore unique sequences must be found and targeted. In addition, minor mismatches do not inhibit formation of a duplex and RNase H can be induced by as few as four matched bases. Elongating the oligonucleotide simply enhances the probability of binding to common sequences in other mRNAs.

There are other biological effects that may occur independently of specific binding. For example, RNA duplexes can induce interferon synthesis and activate adenylate cyclase. Nonspecific effects on cell proliferation are seen if four guanosine residues are present within an oligonucleotide.[44] As well as these RNA duplex interactions, oligonucleotides may also bind to intracellular proteins and alter their functions.

These problems have complicated antisense research study design, with up to six controls needed to prove that a true antisense mechanism is responsible for any changes seen.[43] These problems have currently tempered enthusiasm for taking antisense methods into clinical trials.

Gene transfer for hypercholesterolaemia/ atherosclerosis

Familial hypercholesterolaemia is one of the few instances in which gene transfer strategies have been successful in modifying the phenotype of an autosomal dominant disease. *Ex vivo* gene transfer was originally studied in the Watanabe rabbit using retroviral vectors expressing the human LDL receptor to transfect hepatocytes *ex vivo*; stable long-term improvement in cholesterol levels resulted.[45] Human trials were then based on a similar protocol, in which the left lateral segment of the liver was removed surgically and the resultant tissue enzymatically digested and cultured. The retroviral vector expressing the LDL receptor was then used to infect the cells and the resultant cells were infused into the patient's portal vein. Stable engraftment of these cells was detected at 4 months on liver biopsy and an improvement in LDL/HDL ratio from 10/13 before gene therapy to 5/8 after gene therapy persisted up to 18 months after the treatment.[8] Other groups have targeted the same disease with adenoviral vectors expressing the LDL receptor. These have the advantage that adenoviruses are highly efficient at infecting hepatic tissue but they are limited by their brief duration of expression. In a rabbit model using this system, plasma cholesterol was reduced from a mean of 825.5 mg/dl to 247.3 mg/dl and LDL levels dropped dramatically, with a 300–400% increase in HDL.[46] In a further experiment, knock-out mice lacking the LDL receptor were given this vector into a peripheral vein and the hypercholesterolaemia was corrected within 4 days.[47] A different approach to the manipulation of lipid metabolism has been the use of an adenoviral vector encoding apolipoprotein A-1 in normal mice, which produced a transient increase in both total cholesterol and, more importantly, HDL cholesterol.[48]

Gene transfer for angioplasty restenosis

Gene transfer strategies in the treatment of restenosis have grown out of the work described above which established the principle of direct *in vivo* gene transfer. Current results suggest that adenoviral vectors are the most efficient gene transfer vectors, (10-fold to 100-fold better than liposomes) while liposomes are the safest.[23] The most efficient gene delivery devices for smooth muscle cells in the media of an artery are also those that cause the most injury to the artery but multiple strategies are being adopted to over come this. There are also differences in susceptibility to gene transfer between normal and atherosclerotic arteries and between injured and uninjured arteries. In general, regardless of the vector used, it is easier, although not essential, to transfer genes to actively dividing cells such as smooth muscle cells after arterial injury.[49] Atherosclerotic vessels are relatively resistant to gene transfer unless this is accompanied by balloon injury.[22] The first demonstrations of actual modification of the *in vivo* function of cells in the arterial wall involved the use of retroviral vectors to transfer HLA-B7 and liposomes to transfer transforming growth factor β1 (TGF β1), platelet derived growth factor B (PDGF B), and fibroblast growth factor 1 (FGF 1).[10–12,50]

The trigger event in angioplasty restenosis is the procedural insult, which then gives rise to a cascade of endothelial denudation, growth factor release, smooth muscle cell migration and proliferation, extracellular matrix deposition and finally re-endothelialization. The relative contributions of fibrocellular intimal hyperplasia and vascular remodelling continue to be debated, with information accumulating from clinical studies using intravascular ultrasound and research into the role of the adventitia in the restenotic process.[51,52] However, there seems little doubt that cell proliferation has some role to play and this has led several groups to target the common pathways of cell cycle regulation and DNA replication.[53–55]

Gene transfer to inhibit cell proliferation

Guzman et al. used cytotoxic gene transfer to kill all proliferating cells expressing the transgene. They incorporated the gene for herpes simplex thymidine kinase (HSV-tk) in an adenoviral vector and delivered the gene to rat carotid arteries, porcine iliofemoral arteries and rabbit hyperlipidaemic arteries.[53–55] The animals were then given ganciclovir systemically, which is harmless unless phosphorylated by HSV-tk. However, the phosphorylation product is incorporated into the DNA of replicating cells and causes DNA chain termination and cell death. The phosphorylation product is able to diffuse into adjacent dividing cells, producing a bystander effect which improves the efficiency of this approach. In all the species tested, neointimal formation was limited by gene transfer, by 50–87% in porcine and by 39–61% in atherosclerotic rabbit iliofemoral arteries.

A number of cytostatic approaches to inhibiting cell proliferation have been used, employing both gene transfer and antisense approaches. The antisense targeting of c-myc and c-myb have already been discussed. Chang et al. investigated the retinoblastoma (Rb) gene product to inhibit cell proliferation.[56] This protein is usually phosphorylated in dividing cells while the active nonphosphorylated form of the protein binds to cellular transcription factors, arresting the cell cycle. The gene for a constitutively active nonphosphorylatable form of the Rb gene product was incorporated into an adenoviral vector and, using the double balloon catheter, administered to porcine iliofemoral arteries immediately after angioplasty. This significantly reduced SMC proliferation and reduced neointimal hyperplasia by 40–50%. The same group, using an adenoviral vector, has subsequently overexpressed p21, which is an inhibitor of cyclin/cyclin-dependent kinase. The cyclin/cyclin-dependent kinase complex is thought to be essential for the phosphorylation of the Rb gene product and therefore its inhibition will cause cell cycle arrest. The p21 protein

also binds to PCNA to inhibit cell cycle progression. Transfer of the gene encoding p21 after balloon injury in the rat carotid model inhibited neointimal formation by 46%. Diverse methods, from antisense to both cytotoxic and cytostatic gene transfer strategies, have all managed to achieve similar degrees of inhibition of restenosis. An interesting new manipulation of the molecular biology of the vasculature has been the use of a DNA decoy. Morishita et al. have investigated inhibiting the transcription factor E2F by introducing double-stranded DNA containing the E2F binding site, which can then decoy E2F and prevent it interacting with other genes.[57] E2F is pivotal in the activation of genes such as c-myc, cdc2, and the gene encoding PCNA. A conjugate of haemagglutinating virus of Japan and liposomes (HVJ-liposome complex) has been used to introduce the double-stranded DNA into injured rat carotid arteries. Mean intimal/medial ratio was reduced from 1.12 to 0.29 and the effect was maintained 8 weeks after the single administration. This technique has drawn on our knowledge of transfer of single-stranded antisense oligonucleotides and gene transfer vector developments, but unlike the other gene transfer experiments discussed here, there is no intention of the DNA encoding an mRNA and producing a protein product; the DNA itself is now the drug.

Gene transfer to prevent thrombosis

An alternative strategy has been to target local thrombotic mechanisms. The gene encoding human cyclo-oxygenase 1 has been incorporated in a first-generation adenoviral vector and instilled into previously injured porcine carotid arteries in order to increase prostacyclin synthesis and thus reduce thrombosis.[58] Recombinant hirudin, a highly potent and specific inhibitor of thrombin, has also been transferred into cells and into injured rat carotid arteries using an adenoviral vector. Increased hirudin production was seen in the arteries and a 35% reduction in neointimal formation was detected.[59] This may reflect the known ability of thrombin to cause VSMC migration and proliferation via the release of growth factors from the extracellular matrix. These approaches, which appear to target thrombosis, in fact have multiple effects on the arterial wall.

Gene transfer to restore endothelial function

Both accelerating the re-endothelialization of the vessel after balloon injury and restoring its function by replacing nitric oxide have been used to ameliorate restenosis. VEGF is a potent and specific mitogen for endothelial cells. The recombinant VEGF protein has been applied to rat carotid arteries after injury and has been shown to reduce neointimal formation and accelerate the restoration of endothelial continuity.[60] However, transfer of the gene encoding VEGF has not been used in this setting but the results obtained in the rat model have contributed to the gene transfer work, with VEGF currently being applied to peripheral vascular disease both in angiogenesis and restenosis.[5,61] Restenosis is likely to be triggered by the early release of mitogens and chemotactic factors after endothelial denudation. It has been suggested that under normal conditions, the endothelium may supply inhibitory factors to keep this process in check. The ability of nitric oxide (NO) to inhibit platelet aggregation and VSMC migration and proliferation *in vitro* implicates it in this process. The first demonstration of ability to transfer genes with potential therapeutic use to the vasculature used the HVJ-liposome complex of the gene for endothelial cell nitric oxide synthase (ecNOS) to over-express nitric oxide synthase and hence nitric oxide after balloon injury in the rat.[62] The investigators were able to demonstrate restored NO production and vascular reactivity, in addition to a 70% reduction in neointimal formation.

Both antisense and gene transfer techniques have been used with success to suppress neointimal formation in animal models of angioplasty restenosis in normal and atherosclerotic vessels. After the failure of pharmacological agents such as ACE inhibitors to alter restenosis in man, despite favourable results in small animals, more groups are now testing gene transfer methods in porcine peripheral and coronary models. At present, no one gene or antisense molecule has been shown to be superior to another and apart from marker gene studies comparing vectors or delivery devices, there is a paucity of comparative data. Exciting work continues in this field, such as the recent E2F decoy study, but it seems possible that a combination of several strategies may be needed to overcome the considerable biological redundancy in the restenotic cascade.

Gene transfer for vein grafts and bioprostheses

Veins and bioprostheses are an attractive prospect for gene transfer because the physical problems of accessing the target tissue are greatly reduced by pretreating a stent or graft or by administering a vector to a vein when it is harvested intraoperatively. The genes encoding β-galactosidase and vascular cell adhesion molecule-1 (VCAM-1) have been transferred successfully to veins after harvest. The gene products were then detectable 3 days after the vein had been interposed as a vascular graft in the porcine carotid artery.[63] Antisense to the cell cycle regulators PCNA and cdc-2 kinase, already discussed in relation to restenosis, have been delivered to veins using HVJ-liposome complexes in a rabbit model. This resulted in a substantial decrease in neointimal formation in the antisense vein grafts versus controls but a compensatory medial hypertrophy occurred. The authors have suggested that this may have conferred a more arterial phenotype on the grafts and was shown to render them relatively resistant to diet-induced atherosclerosis.[64] The possibility of genetically engineering stents or grafts has also been investigated, although the former is hampered by the tendency for the lumenal coating to be removed during stent implantation. Retroviral vectors have been used to transfer tissue type plasminogen activator (TPA) and urokinase plasminogen activator (UPA) to endothelial cells in culture, which have then been seeded into grafts. Dichek et al. were able to show enhanced local antithrombotic activity in a baboon model but investigated only very short-term expression.[65] However, Dunn et al. have found that gene expression declines progressively as vein grafts are exposed to flow due to loss of endothelial cells from the graft.[66] This was marked in TPA-expressing grafts, possibly due to excessive plasmin causing matrix breakdown and detachment. This highlights another problem encountered in gene transfer. Although the encoded protein may be seemingly benign, its overexpression may result in nonphysiological concentrations which disrupt homeostasis with unwanted results.

Arterial gene therapy for peripheral vascular disease

A number of the studies already mentioned have assessed gene transfer or antisense strategies in the iliac or femoral arteries in animal models. In general, however, these studies have used the peripheral arteries as convenient models for coronary disease and not targeted the peripheral vasculature specifically. It is the peripheral vascular system which has given rise to the first clinical cardiovascular trial of gene transfer. Isner et al. have investigated the ability of VEGF to induce angiogenesis in ischaemic limbs. This was originally studied in rabbits whose hind limb had been rendered ischaemic by the removal of the femoral artery. A plasmid encoding VEGF was then applied to the iliac artery using a hydrogel balloon catheter. VEGF mRNA was detected at the site by reverse transcriptase polymerase chain reaction. More importantly, an angiogenic response was seen in the hind limb using serial angiography and treated animals had better calf blood pressure ratio than the controls.[67] This study forms the basis for the clinical trial which has the principal objective of documenting the safety of intra-arterial administration of a plasmid vector encoding VEGF.[5] The secondary objectives are to determine the bioactivity of the transferred gene product by examining the effect on rest pain and ulceration, and to document the anatomical and physiological extent of angiogenesis. The patients admitted to the trial have end-stage vascular disease not amenable to surgical or other established intervention. Entry criteria include rest pain and nonhealing ischaemic ulcers. The patients are therefore suffering severe disease which, while it is the most difficult to treat, may be also the most amenable to angiogenesis. They are unlikely to undergo regression of disease with time, as is seen in the milder peripheral vasculopaths (particularly if they can stop smoking and start walking). The protocol will recruit 22 patients who will (in pairs) receive escalating doses of DNA from 100µg to 4000µg. Angiogenesis will be assessed by the primary clinical end-points of resolution of rest pain and decreasing analgesic requirement and healing ulcers. In addition, ankle brachial index of peripheral vascular resistance, magnetic resonance angiography, diagnostic angiography, and intravascular Doppler flow will be measured. The VEGF plasmid will be delivered to a normal segment of profunda femoral artery to optimize transfer efficiency using the hydrogel balloon. The investigators then anticipate that the transduced cells expressing VEGF will secrete it into the arterial circulation downstream of the delivery site, causing angiogenesis. It is not anticipated that the gene will be expressed for the length of the trial but that an angiogenic process will be initiated which will improve the peripheral circulation in the long term. One of the obvious concerns is that this hypothesis involves a semi-systemic effect of secreted VEGF and therefore an angiogenic response might occur in other regions, for example at the site of an occult tumour. All the patients are screened for malignancy before acceptance into the trial and this will be an important safety consideration when the results are available. The trial does not include a control group. It was decided that it was unethical to manipulate the vasculature of a patient with critical limb ischaemia to deliver a placebo plasmid to a normal area of artery without any intention to perform angioplasty on the vessel or improve flow. Preliminary reports from the trial appear encouraging with evidence of an angiogenic response without major side effects but failure to modify the long-term natural history of the disease at the current dosage.[68] The full results are eagerly awaited.

The same plasmid vector and delivery system is now being used to target restenosis in the superficial femoral artery where , similar to coronary angioplasty, there is a 90% angiographic initial success but 60% of the patients develop restenosis.[61] Three groups of 20, 15 and 15 patients will be studied with 1000µg, 2000µg, and 4000µg being used in each successive group. The primary objective is to determine safety of gene transfer and the secondary objective is to assess the bioactivity of the therapy to inhibit restenosis. The criteria for restenosis will include clinical history, ankle/brachial index, colour flow duplex sonography, exercise testing, digital angiography, and intravascular ultrasound. No control group receiving angioplasty only has been included. Necropsy or amputation specimens will be analysed by RT-PCR for evidence of gene transfer but the initial protocol does not involve moitoring serum VEGF levels.

Gene transfer for ischaemic heart disease

The most logical approach to the treatment of ischaemic heart disease would be to prevent the formation of coronary atherosclerosis or reverse the atherosclerotic process once it had become established. Although the likelihood of ischaemic heart disease can be reduced by risk factor modification, the majority of individuals with ischaemic heart disease do not have sufficiently abnormal premorbid risk factors.[69-71] Similarly, in patients with established ischaemic heart disease correction of more moderate risk factors may prevent reinfarction[70,71] but, since plaque regression is minimal,[71] there is little evidence of reversion of the atherosclerotic process. In addition, the first symptom of ischaemic heart disease is frequently acute myocardial infarction. This results in irreversible myocyte loss which leads to progressive left ventricular dysfunction and heart failure in approximately 30% of survivors of anterior infarction.[72] In view of these limitations of conventional medical therapies, it could be argued that there is a need for powerful strategies that influence the natural history of ischaemic heart disease by altering the underlying pathobiology. However, in contrast to the first part of this chapter, amelioration of ischaemic heart disease requires gene transfer to the myocardium rather than the arterial wall.

Gene transfer to the myocardium is in its infancy and at present is performed only in animal models. As may be expected from work in restenosis, selective injection of the left and right coronary arteries of the rabbit with a replication-deficient type 5 adenovirus (Ad5) and liposome–DNA complexes coding for β-galactosidase (β-gal) results in gene expression in the distribution of the injected coronary artery at 5 days (Figure 18.6). The major drawback of intracoronary injection of adenovirus is an intense myocardial inflammatory infiltrate associated with myocardial necrosis (*see* Figure 18.4).

An advantage of intracoronary injection is the possibility of localizing the delivery vector to the ischaemic tissue. Although this is theoretically possible, there are a number of practical difficulties. Ischaemia may be patchy, and this would be a particular problem with small vessel disease. It is unlikely that there would be complete first pass myocardial clearance of vector. Therefore some spillover of vector into the pulmonary and systemic circulation would inevitably result in distant and inappropriate transgene expression. An elegant approach to overcome these difficulties would be to incorporate response elements within the transgenic promoter that would sense and respond to the ischaemic environment.

The gene for erythropoeitin, certain glycolytic enzymes and vascular endothelial growth factor contain sequences of DNA within their promoters and enhancers that confer hypoxic inducibility.[73,74] These DNA sequences, or elements, bind a factor that ensures transcriptional activation under the appropriate physiological circumstances.[75] When incorporated within a transgene, these elements may be able to ensure that gene expression is appropriately localized

to ischaemic tissue. Preliminary evidence of targeting gene expression to ischaemic rat myocardium suggests this is the case.[76]

Therapeutic targets for gene transfer

Angiogenesis to attenuate ischaemia

Basic fibroblast growth factor (bFGF) is a peptide that is widely distributed and known to stimulate the proliferation and migration *in vitro* of the three principal vascular cell types — endothelial cells, fibroblasts and smooth muscle cells — responsible for collateral growth *in vivo*.[77,78] Until recently, only the effects of exogenous recombinant bFGF have been examined. An alternative approach is to induce lasting collaterals by increasing the synthesis of bFGF within the heart by transferring the encoding gene. There are advantages to such an approach since the endothelial barrier and short intravascular half-life severely limit the activity of intra-arterial bFGF.[79] In addition, local secretion would ensure that trophic response is limited to the myocardium and would avoid the need for repeated infusions to maintain collateral patency.

These considerations have prompted Giordano et al.[80] to examine the angiogenic potential of an adenoviral vector encoding a secreted fibroblast growth factor, FGF-5. The model used was the pig ameriod constrictor model. In this model, a slow epicardial constriction of the circumflex coronary artery results in total occlusion over a period of 10 days. The circumflex bed has no significant infarction but is rendered critically ischaemic with an absent flow reserve, 38 days after ameriod placement animals were paced, while regional function was assessed echocardiographically and blood

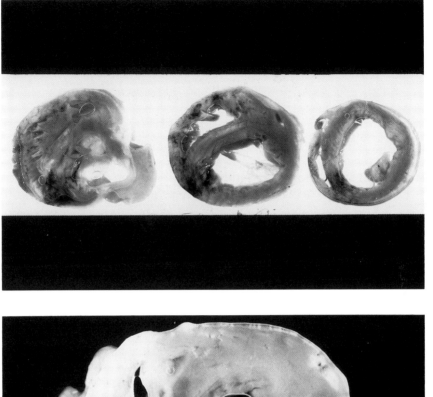

A

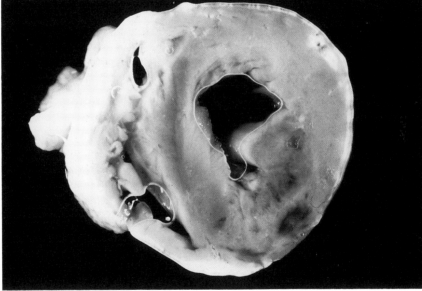

B

Figure 18.6
The appearances of rabbit myocardium 3 days after intracoronary injection of a type 5 adenovirus or DNA-liposome complexes coding for β-galactosidase. (A) These samples were prepared after right coronary artery injection of 1 x 10¹¹ plaque-forming units of adenovirus. (B) This sample was prepared after lateral circumflex injection of 200μg of DNA complexed to cationic liposomes. The blue discoloration is secondary to the presence of a bacterial form of β-galactosidase. Hence, the intracoronary injection of both adenovirus and liposome DNA complexes is capable of mediating myocardial gene transfer and expression. (M Marber, unpublished data.)

flow was measured with the use of micro-spheres. The following day, 4×10^{11} adeno-virus particles were injected down left and right coronary arteries. The adenovirus encoded either FGF-5 or a β-gal reporter gene. Twelve weeks after injection, only those pigs injected with the FGF-5 virus had improved myocardial blood flow and function during pacing.[80] In addition these pigs had a higher density of small myocardial vessels on histology and enhanced echocardiographic contrast within the circumflex bed following left atrial injec-tion.[80] Suprisingly, these authors found little evidence of viral genome or transgene in distant organs. The authors ascribed this to occlusive engagement of the coronary ostia during virus delivery.

Proteins that enhance myocardial resistance to ischaemia

An alternative approach to limit ischaemic myo-cardial damage would be to increase the inher-ent resistance of the myocardium. A family of proteins known as heat shock or stress proteins attenuate cell injury following denaturing stres-ses such as heat,[81] and are also capable of rena-turing and returning protein function in vitro.[81] The hypothesis was formulated that stress pro-teins may be capable of protecting cells, includ-ing myocytes, from ischaemic injury.[81] This hypothesis was supported by the initial studies of Currie et al. which suggested that myocardial stress proteins, elevated by whole body heat stress, may protect the rat heart from ischaemic injury.[82] Subsequent studies by independent investigators, including ourselves, have now confirmed these observations in other species and models of myocardial ischaemic injury.[83,84] Thus far transfer of the gene for hsp70i has been undertaken only in adult rat cardiocytes

in culture. An adenoviral vector was used to transfer the gene and preliminary evidence sug-gests that this strategy is able to attenuate ischaemic injury.[85]

There is also interest in using gene transfer to mimic ischaemic preconditioning to protect the myocardium. Ischaemic preconditioning describes the resistance to ischaemic injury that follows brief periods of myocardial ischae-mia.[86] The brief ischaemic trigger delays the onset and slows the rate of myocardial necrosis occurring in response to subsequent prolonged ischaemia.[86] The resulting level of protection is profound, with a typical four-fold reduction in the volume of myocardial infarction.[86] Unfortunately, the benefit of ischaemic precon-ditioning is short-lived and disappears when the interval between the short ischaemic trigger and the subsequent prolonged ischaemia is greater than 60 minutes.[87] Considerable evi-dence suggests that the translocation and acti-vation of the n-protein kinase C-ε (nPKC-ε) and nPKC-δ isotypes play a central role in the preconditioning process,[88] a finding consis-tent with the previously reported predomi-nance of these isotypes in cardiac myocytes.[89] Mutant PKC isotypes are available that have been rendered constitutively active by small deletions or single amino acid substitutions and are under investigation by several groups.[90] An adenoviral conjugate has been used successfully to transfer PKC-δ to cardio-cytes but functional studies are awaited.[91]

A major drawback of the strategies described in this and the previous sections is the need to administer therapy before acute myocardial infarction, since infarct limitation will occur only with the prior formation of adequate amounts of myocardial cytoprotective protein or collaterals. Clearly it is not practicable to anticipate acute myocardial infarction.

Postinfarction manipulation of scar and myocardium to prevent heart failure

The factors that influence postinfarction remodelling are not well understood. However, interventions at this point are attractive since they do not rely on early patient presentation and are therefore likely to be widely applicable.[92] After infarction an increase in contractility occurs within the noninfarcted segments to maintain stroke volume. The increased wall stress and haemodynamic load result in compensatory hypertrophy of the remaining myocardium. In a significant proportion of individuals with large areas of infarction the hypertrophy fails fully to compensate and is associated with abnormalities of relaxation and progressive left ventricular dilatation. The abnormalities in relaxation are coincident with a down-regulation of sarcoplasmic reticulum Ca^{2+}-ATPase protein (SERCA-2).[93] This protein is responsible for the clearance of cytosolic calcium during systole and therefore indirectly for the normal relaxation of the heart. The gene for SERCA-2 has been incorporated into an adenoviral vector and transferred to adult cardiocytes in culture.[94] This strategy is associated with an acceleration of cytosolic calcium clearance at end-systole and a more speedy relaxation of myocyte contraction.[94] As yet, this strategy has not been examined *in vivo*.

Perhaps the most powerful postinfarction manipulation would be to convert fibroblasts to myocytes within the healing zone of infarction. Although this sounds ambitious, there is preliminary evidence to suggest conversion is possible by the expression of myogenic determination factor (Myo-D) or the $5'$ untranslated mRNA of muscle-specific genes.[95]

If I had . . .

If I had the opportunity to participate in a gene therapy clinical trial I would want to have explored all possible alternatives and have been fully informed of likely efficacy and toxicity. I would have to accept that human gene therapy is an experimental treatment and that the choice being offered is quite different from that, say, of patients recruited to one limb or another of the ISIS or RITA trials. I would consider participating in a trial at this early stage

Vector	Gene transfer efficiency	Duration of expression	Safety	Insertional mutagenesis risk	Clinical trials approved
Retrovirus	+	+++	++	++	93
Adenovirus	+++	++	++	+	18
Liposomes	++	++	+++	+	16
Plasmids	+	++	+++	+	5

Table 18.1
Relative advantages and disadvantages of gene therapy vectors.

only if I felt that I had exhausted conventional therapy and had a very poor prognosis. In taking this somewhat cautious attitude I would also acknowledge that it is only by trials of this kind that medicine has progressed. I would be confident that the preliminary reports of trials of the use of VEGF in peripheral vascular disease suggest that I may stand to gain significantly but I would keep a wary eye on the results of my assessments. I would also watch for new generations of adenoviruses and disabled conjugate vectors, expecting them to have improved safety profiles and significantly greater efficiency.

In summary, the future is bright but presently I would be extremely cautious and if possible wait for the inevitable evolution of this embryonic field.

Glossary

Amplicon: A vector containing very short sequences of viral genome encoding essential functions that allow replication and packaging when a helper virus is present.

Antisense oligonucleotides: A single strand of DNA (or RNA) which is complementary to an RNA sense strand and will therefore bind to it preventing translation.

Cytostatic: Arrests the cell cycle preventing further division.

Cytoxic: Directly lethal to the cell.

Gene therapy: The introduction of foreign genetic material (usually DNA) into somatic cells in order to modify their genetic content and achieve a therapeutic end point.

Insertional mutagenesis: Disruption of a gene or separation of the gene from its normal control resulting in alteration of the gene product or its quantty.

Marker gene or reporter gene: A gene whose produce can be identified easily and is not usually present in the target cell, thus allowing assessment of gene expression with relative ease.

Phentotype: The characteristics of a cell or an organism that are determined by the interaction of genetic make-up and environment.

Plasmids: Circular strands of DNA that replicate in bacteria and which can be modified to express genes in mammalian cells.

Promoter: The region of a gene that binds RNA polymerase and initiates gene transcription. A promoter may be constitutively active in all cells, have cell type-specific activity, or be inducible, i.e. be switched on by the appropriate trigger.

Transcription: The synthesis of mRNA from a DNA template by RNA polymerase.

Transgene: The gene which has been transferred to a new cell.

Translation: The synthesis of proteins from mRNA by ribosomes.

Vectors: An autonomously replicating unit of DNA into which genes can be inserted and then introduced into target cells.

References

1 Human gene marker/therapy clinical protocols. *Hum Gene Ther* (1996)**7**:2287–313.

2 Rosenberg SA, Aebersold P, Cornetta-K et al, Gene transfer into humans — immunotherapy of patients with advanced melanoma, using tumor-infiltrating lymphocytes modified by retroviral gene transduction, *N Engl J Med* (1990)**323**:570–8.

3 Blaese RM, Culver KW, Miller-AD et al, T lymphocyte-directed gene therapy for ADA- SCID: initial trial results after 4 years, *Science* (1995)**270**:475–80.

4 Grossman M, Raper SE; Kozarsky-K et al, Successful *ex vivo* gene therapy directed to liver in a patient with familial hypercholesterolaemia, *Nat Genet* (1994)**6**:335–41.

5 Isner JM, Walsh K, Symes J et al, Arterial gene therapy for therapeutic angiogenesis in patients with peripheral arterial disease, *Circulation* (1995)**91**:2687–92.

6 Knowles MR, Hohneker KW, Zhou Z et al, A controlled study of adenoviral-vector-mediated gene transfer in the nasal epithelium of patients with cystic fibrosis, *N Engl J Med* (1995)**333**: 823–31.

7 Mendell JR, Kissel JT, Amato AA et al, Myoblast transfer in the treatment of Duchenne's muscular dystrophy, *N Engl J Med* (1995)**333**:832–8.

8 Grossman M, Raper SE, Kozarsky K et al, Successful *ex vivo* gene therapy directed to liver in a patient with familial hypercholesterolaemia, *Nat Genet* (1994)**6**: 335–41.

9 Watkins H, McKenna WJ, Thierfelder L et al, Mutations in the genes for cardiac troponin T and alpha-tropomyosin in hypertrophic cardiomyopathy, *N Engl J Med* (1995)**332**:1058–64.

10 Nabel EG, Yang Z, Liptay S et al. Recombinant platelet-derived growth factor B gene expression in porcine arteries induce intimal hyperplasia *in vivo*, *J Clin Invest* (1993)**91**:1822–9.

11 Nabel EG, Shum L, Pompili VJ et al, Direct transfer of transforming growth factor beta 1 gene into arteries stimulates fibrocellular hyperplasia, *Proc Natl Acad Sci USA* (1993)**90**:10759–63.

12 Nabel EG, Yang ZY, Plautz G et al, Recombinant fibroblast growth factor-1 promotes intimal hyperplasia and angiogenesis in arteries *in vivo*, *Nature* (1993)**362**:844–6.

13 Wilson JM, Birinyi LK, Salomon RN, Libby P, Callow AD, Mulligan RC, Implantation of vascular grafts lined with genetically modified endothelial cells, *Science* (1989)**244**:1344–6.

14 Flugelman MY, Jaklitsch MT, Newman KD, Casscells W, Bratthauer GL, Dichek DA, Low level *in vivo* gene transfer into the arterial wall through a perforated balloon catheter, *Circulation* (1992)**85**:1110–17.

15 Clowes MM, Lynch CM, Miller AD, Miller DG, Osborne WR, Clowes AW, Long-term biological response of injured rat carotid artery seeded with smooth muscle cells expressing retrovirally introduced human genes, *J Clin-Invest* (1994)**93**:644–51.

16 McCormick PJ, Shin HS, Analysis of a nontumorigenic embryonal carcinoma cell line, *Exp Cell Res* (1990)**189**:183–8.

17 Dichek DA, Neville RF, Zwiebel JA, Freeman SM, Leon MB, Anderson WF, Seeding of intravascular stents with genetically engineered endothelial cells, *Circulation* (1989)**80**: 1347–53.

18 Graham FL, Prevec L, Manipulation of adenoviral vectors. In: Murray EJ, ed. *Gene transfer and expression vectors* (Humana: Clifton, NJ, (1991)109–27.

19 Bett AJ, Haddara W, Prevec L, Graham FL, An efficient and flexible system for construction of adenovirus vectors with insertions or deletions in early regions 1 and 3, *Proc Natl Acad Sci USA* (1994)**91**:8802–6.

20 Lemarchand P, Jones M, Yamada I, Crystal RG, *In vivo* gene transfer and expression in normal uninjured blood vessels using replication-deficient recombinant adenovirus vectors, *Circ Res* (1993)**72**:1132–8.

21 Guzman RJ, Lemarchand P, Crystal RG, Epstein SE, Finkel T, Efficient and selective adenovirus-mediated gene transfer into vascular neointima, *Circulation* (1993)**88**:2838–48.

22 Feldman LJ, Steg PG, Zheng LP et al, Low-efficiency of percutaneous adenovirus-mediated arterial gene transfer in the atherosclerotic rabbit, *J Clin Invest* (1995)**95**:2662–71.

23 French BA, Mazur W, Ali NM et al, Percutaneous transluminal *in vivo* gene transfer by recombinant adenovirus in normal porcine coronary arteries, atherosclerotic arteries, and two models of coronary restenosis, *Circulation* (1994)**90**:2402–13.

24 Ali M, Lemoine NR, Ring CJA, The use of DNA viruses as vectors for gene therapy, *Gene Ther* (1994)**1**:367–84.

25 Rhoads JL, Birx DL, Wright DC et al, Safety and immunogenicity of multiple conventional immunizations administered during early HIV infection, *J Acquir Immune Defic Syndr* (1991)**4**:724–31.

26 Wilson JM, Adenoviruses as gene-delivery vehicles [editorial]. *New Engl J Med* (1996)**334**:1185–7.

27 Leiden JM, Gene therapy—promises and pitfalls [editorial], *New Engl J Med* (1995)**333**:871–3.

28 Amalfitano A, Begy CR, Chamberlain JS, Improved adenovirus packaging cell lines to support the growth of replication-defective gene-delivery vectors, *Proc Natl Acad Sci* (1996)**93**:3352–6.

29 Engelhardt JF, Ye X, Doranz B, Wilson JM, Ablation of E2A in recombinant adenoviruses improves transgene persistence and decreases inflammatory response in mouse liver, *Proc Natl Acad Sci* (1994)**91**:6196–200.

30 Coffin RS, Latchman DS, Herpes simplex virus based vectors. In: Latchman DS, ed. *Genetic manipulation of the nervous system* (Academic Press: London 1996) 99–111.

31 Coffin RS, Howard MK, Cumming DVE et al, Gene delivery to the heart *in vivo* and to cardiac myocytes and vascular smooth muscle cells *in vitro* using herpes virus vectors, *Gene Ther* (1996)**3**:560–6.

32 Mesri EA, Federoff HJ, Brownlee M, Expression of vascular endothelial growth factor from a defective herpes simplex virus type 1 amplicon vector induces angiogenesis in mice, *Circ Res* (1995)**76**:161–7.

33 Kotin RM, Prospects for the use of adeno-associated virus as a vector for human gene therapy, *Hum Gene Ther* (1994)**5**:793–801.

34 Crystal RG, The gene as the drug, *Nat Med* (1995)**1**:15–17.

35 Nabel EG, Plautz G, Nabel GJ, Site specific gene expression *in vivo* by direct gene transfer into the arterial wall, *Science* (1990)**249**:1285-8.

36 Morishita R, Gibbons GH, Kaneda Y, Ogihara T, Dzau VJ, Novel and effective gene transfer technique for study of vascular renin angiotensin system, *J Clin Invest* (1993)**91**:2580–5.

37 Kupfer JM, Ruan XM, Liu G, Matloff J, Forrester J, Chaux A, High-efficiency gene transfer to autologous rabbit jugular vein grafts using adenovirus-transferrin/polylysine-DNA complexes, *Hum Gene Ther* (1994)**5**:1437–43.

38 Ohno T, Gordon D, San H et al, Gene therapy for vascular smooth muscle cell proliferation after arterial injury, *Science* (1994)**265**:781–4.

39 Mitchell JF, Fram DB, Azrin MA, Localized intracoronary delivery of urokinase with the channelled balloon: pharmacokinetics of drug delivery and washout, *J Am Coll Cardiol* (1995)**25**:347A (abstr).

40 Mitchel JF, Azrin MA, Fram DB et al, Inhibition of platelet deposition and lysis of intracoronary thrombus during balloon angioplasty using urokinase-coated hydrogel balloons, *Circulation* (1994)**90**:1979–88.

41 Gunn J, Holt C, Shepherd L et al, Local delivery of antisense oligonucleotide via double skinned porous balloon, *Eur Heart J* (1995)**16**:484 (abstr).

42 Pompilli VJ, Srivatsa SS, Jorgenson MA, Direct gene transfer and expression with arterial iontophoretic catheter delivery, *J Am Coll Cardiol* (1995)**25**:996–1011 (abstr).

43 Bennett MR, Schwartz SM, Antisense therapy for angioplasty restenosis. Some critical considerations, *Circulation* (1995)**92**:1981–93.

44 Yaswen P, Stampfer MR, Ghosh K, Cohen JS, Effects of sequence of thioated oligonucleotides on cultured human mammary epithelial cells, *Antisense Res Dev* (1993)**3**:67–77.

45 Chowdhury JR, Grossman M, Gupta S, Chowdhury NR, Baker JR Jr, Wilson JM,

Long-term improvement of hypercholesterolemia after *ex vivo* gene therapy in LDLR-deficient rabbits, *Science* (1991)**254**:1802–5.

46 Li J, Fang B, Eisensmith RC et al, *In vivo* gene therapy for hyperlipidemia: phenotypic correction in Watanabe rabbits by hepatic delivery of the rabbit LDL receptor gene, *J Clin Invest* (1995)**95**:768–73.

47 Ishibashi S, Brown MS, Goldstein JL, Gerard RD, Hammer RE, Herz J, Hypercholesterolemia in low density lipoprotein receptor knockout mice and its reversal by adenovirus-mediated gene delivery, *J Clin Invest* (1993)**92**:883–93.

48 Kopfler WP, Willard M, Betz T, Willard JE, Gerard RD, Meidell RS, Adenovirus-mediated transfer of a gene encoding human apolipoprotein A-I into normal mice increases circulating high-density lipoprotein cholesterol, *Circulation* (1994)**90**:1319–27.

49 Li JJ, Ueno H, Tomita H et al, Adenovirus-mediated arterial gene transfer does not require prior injury for submaximal gene expression, *Gene Ther* (1995)**2**:351–4.

50 Nabel EG, Plautz G, Nabel GJ, Transduction of a foreign histocompatibility gene into the arterial wall induces vasculitis, *Proc Natl Acad Sci USA* (1992)**89**:5157–61.

51 Potkin BN, Keren G, Mintz GS et al, Arterial responses to balloon coronary angioplasty: an intravascular ultrasound study, *J Am Coll Cardiol* (1990)**20**:942–51.

52 Shi Y, Pieniek M, Fard A et al, Adventitial remodeling after coronary arterial injury, *Circulation* (1996)**93**:340–8.

53 Guzman RJ, Hirschowitz EA, Brody SL, Crystal RG, Epstein SE, Finkel T, *In vivo* suppression of injury-induced vascular smooth muscle cell accumulation using adenovirus-mediated transfer of the herpes simplex virus thymidine kinase gene, *Proc Natl Acad Sci USA* (1994)**91**:10732–6.

54 Chang MW, Ohno T, Gordon D et al, Adenovirus-mediated transfer of the herpes simplex virus thymidine kinase gene inhibits vascular smooth muscle cell proliferation and neointima formation following balloon angioplasty of the rat carotid artery, *Mol Med* (1995)**1**:172–81.

55 Simarai RD, San H, Rekhter M, Ohno T, Gordon D, Nabel EG, Regulation of cellular proliferation and intimal formation following balloon injury in atherosclerotic rabbit arteries, *J Clin Invest* (1996) **98**:225–35.

56 Chang MW, Barr E, Seltzer J et al, Cytostatic gene therapy for vascular proliferative disorders with a constitutively active form of the retinoblastoma gene product, *Science* (1995)**267**:518–22.

57 Morishita R, Gibbons GH, Horiuchi M et al, A gene therapy strategy using a transcription factor decoy of the E2F binding site inhibits smooth muscle proliferation *in vivo*, *Proc Natl Acad Sci USA* (1995)**92**:5855–9.

58 Zlodhelyi P, McNatt J, Loose-Mitchell D et al, Prevention of arterial thrombosis by adenovirus-mediated transfer of cyclooxygenase gene, *Circulation* (1996)**93**:10–17.

59 Rade JJ, Schulick AH, Dichek DA, Local adenoviral-mediated expression of recombinant hirudin reduces neointimal formation after arterial injury, *Nat Med* (1996)**2**:293–8.

60 Asahara T, Bauters C, Pastore C et al, Local delivery of vascular endothelial growth factor accelerates reendothelialization and attenuates intimal hyperplasia in balloon-injured rat carotid artery, *Circulation* (1995)**91**:2793–801.

61 Isner JM, Clinical protocol: arterial gene therapy for restenosis, *Hum Gene Ther* (1996)**7**:989–1011.

62 von der Leyen HE, Gibbons GH, Morishita R et al, Gene therapy inhibiting neointimal vascular lesion: *in vivo* transfer of endothelial cell nitric oxide synthase gene, *Proc Natl Acad Sci USA* (1995)**92**:1137–41.

63 Chen SJ, Wilson JM, Muller DW, Adenovirus-mediated gene transfer of soluble vascular cell adhesion molecule to porcine interposition vein grafts, *Circulation* (1994)**89**:1922–8.

64 Mann MJ, Gibbons GH, Kernoff RS et al, Genetic engineering of vein grafts resistant to atherosclerosis, *Proc Natl Acad Sci USA* (1995)**92**:4502–6.

65 Dichek DA, Anderson J, Kelly AB, Hanson SR, Harker LA, Enhanced in vivo antithrombotic effects of endothelial cells expressing recombinant plasminogen activators transduced with retroviral vectors, *Circulation* (1996)**93**:301–9.

66   Dunn PF, Deutsch M, Meinhart J et al, Seeding of vascular grafts with genetically modified endothelial cells: secretion of recombinant TPA results in decreased seeded cell retention *in vitro* and *in vivo*, *Circulation* (1996)**93**: 1439–46.

67   Takeshita S, Tsurumi Y, Couffinahl T et al, Gene tranfer of naked DNA encoding for three isoforms of vascular endothelial growth factor stimulates collateral development *in vivo*, *Lab Invest* (1996)**75**:487–501.

68   Isner JM, Pieczek A, Schainfeld R et al, Clinical evidence of angiogenesis after arterial gene transfer of phVEGF$_{165}$ in patient with ischaemic limb, *Lancet* (1996)**348**:370–4.

69   Sheperd J, Cobbe SM, Ford I et al, Prevention of coronary heart disease with pravastatin in men with hypercholesterolemia, *N Engl J Med* (1995)**333**:1301–7.

70   The Scandinavian Simvastatin Survival Group, Randomised trial of cholesterol lowering in 4444 patients with coronary heart disease; the Scandinavian Simvastatin Survival Study (4S), *Lancet* (1994)**344**:1383–9.

71   Jukema JW, Bruschke AVG, van Boven AJ et al, Effects of lipid lowering by pravastatin on progression and regression of coronary artery disease in symptomatic men with normal to moderately elevated serum cholesterol levels, *Circulation* (1995)**91**:2528–40.

72   ASPIRE Steering Group, A British cardiac survey of the potential for the secondary prevention of coronary disease: ASPIRE (Action on Secondary Prevention through Intervention to Reduce Events), *Heart* (1996)**75**:334–42.

73   Madan A, Curtin PT, A 24-base-pair sequence 3' to the human erythropoietin gene contains a hypoxia-response transcriptional enhancer, *Proc Natl Acad Sci USA* (1993)**90**:3928–32.

74   Liu Y, Cox SR, Morita T, Kourembanas S, Hypoxia regulates vascular endothelial growth factor gene expression in endothelial cells. Identification of a 5' enhancer, *Circ Res* (1995)**77**:638–43.

75   Wang GL, Jiang BH, Rue EA, Semenza GL, Hypoxia-inducible factor 1 is a basic-helix-loop-helix-PAS heterodimer regulated by cellular O_2 tension, *Proc Natl Acad Sci* (1995)**92**:5510–14.

76   Webster KA, Wu X, Prentice H et al, Hypoxia regulated vectors for targeting genes to ischaemic myocardium, *Circulation* (1995)**8**:756 (abstr).

77   Cummins P, Fibroblast and transforming growth factor expression in the cardiac myocyte, *Cardiovasc Res* (1993)**27**:1150–4.

78   Schott RJ, Morrow LA, Growth factors and angiogenesis, *Cardiovasc Res* (1993)**27**: 1155–61.

79   Harada K, Grossman W, Freidman M et al, Basic fibroblast growth factor improves myocardial function in chronically ischemic porcine hearts, *J Clin Invest* (1994)**94**:623–30.

80   Giordano FJ, Ping P, McKirnan MD et al, Intracoronary gene transfer of fibroblast growth factor-5 increases blood flow and contractile function in an ischemic region of the heart, *Nat Med* (1996)**2**:534–9.

81   Yellon DM, Marber MS, HSP70 in myocardial ischaemia, *Experientia* (1994)**50**:1075–84.

82   Currie RW, Karmazyn M, Kloe M, Mailer K, Heat shock response is associated with enhanced postischaemic ventricular recovery, *Circ Res* (1988)**63**:543–9.

83   Marber MS, Latchman DS, Walker JM, Yellon DM, Cardiac stress protein elevation 24 hours after brief ischemia or heat stress is associated with resistance to myocardial infarction, *Circulation* (1993)**88**:1264–74.

84   Marber MS, Walker JM, Latchman DS, Yellon DM, Myocardial protection following whole body heat stress in the rabbit is dependent on metabolic substrate and is related to the amount of the inducible 70 kiloDalton heat stress protein, *J Clin Invest* (1994)**93**:1087–94.

85   Giordano F, Mestril R, Dillmann W, Adenovirus mediated inducible heat shock protein 70 gene transfer protects against simulated ischaemia in a muscle derived cell line, *J Am Coll Cardiol* (1995)**25**:324A (abstr).

86   Murry CE, Jennings RB, Reimer KA, Preconditioning with ischemia: a delay of lethal cell injury in ischemic myocardium, *Circulation* (1986)**74**:1124–36.

87   Marber MS, Walker DM, Yellon DM, Ischaemic preconditioning, *Br Med J* (1994)**308**:1–2.

88   Mitchell MB, Meng X, Ao L, Brown JM, Harken AH, Banerjee A, Preconditioining of

isolated rat heart is mediated by protein kinase C, *Circ Res* (1995)**76**:73–81.

89 Pucéat M, Hilal-Dandan R, Strulovic B, Brunton LL, Heller Brown J, Differential regulation of protein kinase C isoforms in isolated neonatal and adult rat cardiomyocytes, *J Biol Chem* (1994)**269**:16938–44.

90 Decock JBJ, Gillespie-Brown J, Parker PJ, Sugden PH, Fuller SJ, Classical, novel and atypical isoforms of PKC stimulate ANF- and TRE/AP-1-regulated-promoter activity in ventricular cardiomyocytes, *Febs Letts* (1994)**356**:275–8.

91 Kohout TA, O'Brian JJ, Gaa ST, Lederer WJ, Rogers TB, Novel adenovirus component system that transfects cultured cardiac cells with high efficiency, *Circ Res* (1996)**78**:971–7.

92 Marber MS, Brown DL, Kloner RA, The open artery hypothesis. To open or not to open that is the question. Clinical perspectives review, *Eur Heart J* (1996)**17**:505–9.

93 Arai M, Matsui H, Periasamy M, Sarcoplasmic reticulum gene expression in cardiac hypertrophy and heart failure, *Circ Res* (1994)**74**:555–64.

94 Giordano FJ, He H, McDonnough, Hilal-Dandan R, Sayen MR, Dillmann WH, Reconstitution and increased expression of the sarcoplasmic reticulum Ca^{++} ATPase (SERCA2) gene, *Circulation* (1995)**92**:I–756 (abstr).

95 L'Ecuyer TJ, Morriss EM, Schutte BC, Fulton AB, Muscle-specific differentiation induced by expression of the 3' untranslated region of α-striated tropomyosin, *Circulation* (1995)**92**:I–369 (abstr).

19

Heart transplantation in adults and children

Frances L Johnson and John S Schroeder

Introduction

The risk-to-benefit ratio for cardiac transplantation is continually changing with advances in the medical treatment of heart failure, mechanical circulatory devices, and better operative outcomes for conventional operations performed on patients with low ejection fractions. Despite this, cardiac allotransplantation still offers significant prolongation of life and improvement in quality of life to a carefully selected group of patients with irreversible end-stage heart disease, and it remains the standard of therapy for such patients.

History

Experimental orthotopic heart transplantation was performed using canine models in the 1950s and 1960s, during which time considerable advances were made in surgical technique, cardiopulmonary bypass, and organ preservation. Lower and Shumway performed the first such operation leading to complete recovery of the animal in 1959,[1] and later reported the efficacy of immunosuppression and techniques for monitoring cardiac graft rejection using the surface electrocardiogram.[2] This set the stage for the first successful human cardiac transplantation, which was performed in South Africa by Christiaan Barnard on December 12, 1967.[3]

Postoperative results were poor due to infection and graft rejection during the first decade of clinical experience,[4] but results gradually improved through continued clinical investiga-

tion, principally at Stanford University,[5,6] where Norman Shumway pioneered the surgical technique that has remained the standard into the 1990s. The introduction of cyclosporin A as an immunosuppressive agent in 1980 significantly decreased the incidence of acute graft rejection, improved patient survival[7] and ushered in a new era in cardiac transplantation.

Furthermore, this improved survival led to a worldwide expansion of the procedure. The 1996 International Society of Heart and Lung Transplantation (ISHLT) registry reports an average survival of 81% at 1 year and 73% at 3 years for adults transplanted since 1990, and similar survival statistics for children over the age of 5 years.[8] Over 3000 heart transplants are typically performed worldwide each year, approximately 300 of which are performed in children less than 18 years.[9] Waiting lists for cardiac transplantation continue to increase, so the procedure is now limited only by the donor supply.

Synopsis

This chapter reviews the indications for cardiac transplantation and recipient selection, pre-transplant management, mechanical bridges to transplantation, the surgical procedure, and post-transplant patient management. Special consideration is given to controversies in recipient selection, immunosuppressive therapy and potential adverse drug interactions, and the role of the primary-care physician in management of the post-transplant patient.

Indications and selection of candidates

Indications

Heart transplantation is indicated for patients who have irreversible end-stage (New York Heart Association class III to IV) congestive heart failure despite aggressive medical therapy or conventional surgery, and who have an estimated survival of 12 to 24 months. Furthermore, candidates must be free of comorbid conditions which would limit their postoperative survival or rehabilitation. Pediatric criteria are similar, with the caveat that profound growth retardation is an indication even if a patient is well compensated with respect to NYHA functional class symptoms.

The most common etiologies of heart failure requiring transplantation in adults are coronary artery disease and cardiomyopathy.[8] Valvular disease, congenital heart disease, miscellaneous causes, and retransplant combined account for less than 10% of cases (Figure 19.1). In the pediatric population, congenital heart disease accounts for 78% of transplants in the first year of life, but only 30% of cases in the 6–18-year age range. Cardiomyopathy is the second most common etiology in children less than 1 year of age, and this diagnosis predominates thereafter (Figure 19.2).[8]

Patient selection

General approach

Selection criteria vary between transplant centers and undergo continual refinement as experience dictates.[10] Emphasis should be placed on maximizing medical therapy, determining an individual's prognosis, and identifying reversible causes of heart failure. Any absolute or relative contraindications to the procedure should be screened for in a stepwise and cost-effective manner. The flow diagram (Figure 19.3) is an example of our approach to patients referred for transplant evaluation. This approach acknowledges the tendency for a subset of patients to experience significant clinical improvement following appropriate medical therapy[11] or conventional surgery, and defers listing on the active transplant waiting list until the patient's 12–24-month prognosis is clearly better with transplantation than with continued medical therapy.

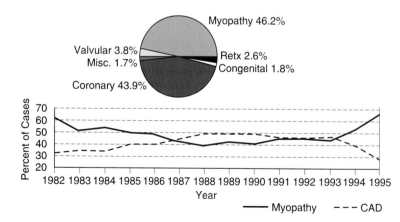

Figure 19.1
Adult heart transplantation indications. Myopathy and coronary artery disease are the major indications for adult heart transplantation, with myopathy recently predominating. All other indications account for less than 10% of adult cases. Reproduced from Hosenpud et al. (1996)[8] with permission from the International Society of Heart and Lung Transplantation.

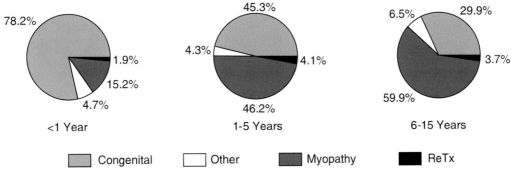

Figure 19.2
Pediatric heart transplantation by age (1982–1995). Congenital heart disease is the major indication for heart transplantation in the first year of life. Myopathy is the second most common indication in the first year and predominates thereafter. All other etiologies combined account for 6–11% of cases. Reproduced from Hosenpud et al. (1996)[8] with permission from the International Society of Heart and Lung Transplantation.

Screening tests

Typical screening tests are outlined in Figure 19.3. Potential recipients should have the etiology of their heart failure and the severity of their cardiac dysfunction defined early in the course of evaluation. A chest radiograph, electrocardiogram, echocardiogram, and stress testing or cardiac catherization should be performed on all referred adult and pediatric patients. Controversy remains over whether all patients should undergo coronary angiography or whether noninvasive testing is sufficient to screen for coronary artery disease and coronary anomalies; therefore clinical judgment is advised. Screening laboratory investigations such as a complete chemistry panel, complete blood count with white cell differential, urinalysis, iron studies, and thyroid function tests will often identify coexistent systemic diseases and/or potentially reversible causes of cardiac dysfunction. The role of endomyocardial biopsy in the diagnosis and treatment of end-stage cardiac disease is limited,[12] although it is the gold standard for identifying acute myocarditis and infiltrative myocardial diseases such as amyloidosis and sarcoidosis. Endomyocardial biopsy should be performed when the history or screening laboratory tests are suggestive of these conditions, and should be strongly considered if symptoms are of less than 6 months' duration and the patient has few risk factors for coronary artery disease.

Following the initiation of optimal medical therapy and the treatment of any underlying reversible causes (lymphocytic myocarditis, sarcoidosis, reversible myocardial ischemia, tachycardia, or ethanol-induced cardiomyopathy), a more detailed assessment of a patient's prognosis is warranted. A patient's maximum oxygen consumption ($VmaxO_2$) is one of the more sensitive predictors of mortality from congestive heart failure in the absence of unstable ischemic syndromes or life-threatening arrhythmias.[13] When a patient's $VmaxO_2$ is less than or equal to 14 ml/kg/min, as determined by standardized bicycle ergometry, the survival benefit of cardiac transplantation begins to exceed that of medical therapy alone.[14,15] At our institution, $VmaxO_2$ testing at 6-month intervals is used as one guide in determining when to place a patient on the active transplant waiting list.

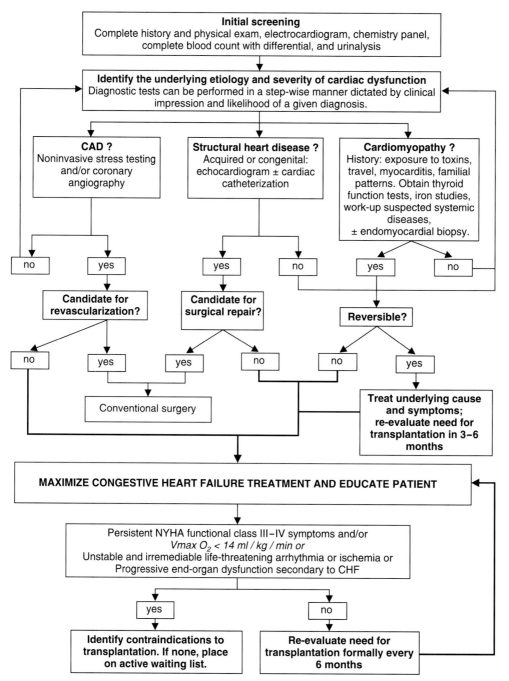

Figure 19.3
Recipient selection and management scheme. Proper selection and management of the cardiac transplant candidate involves identifying the cause of the congestive heart failure, maximizing medical or surgical treatment, and reassessing the patient's clinical stability at regular intervals.

Contraindications

The identification of contraindications is an important aspect of patient selection, but is sometimes difficult due to progressive changes in defining exclusionary criteria. Table 19.1 lists generally accepted absolute contraindications and Table 19.2 relative contraindications to heart transplantation. Some of the more important or controversial exclusion criteria are discussed in more detail below.

Recipient age   For 10 782 cases transplanted in the USA between the years of 1987 and 1994, recipient age was a risk factor for 1-year mortality in both the very young (<5 years) and the old (>60 years).[9,16] The odds ratios for 1-year mortality in these groups were 1.62 (p = <0.001) and 1.73 (p = <0.001), respectively. Other investigators confirm these findings and report that recipients over the age of 60 have a significantly higher number of fatal infections and malignancies than their younger cohorts. These adverse outcomes are somewhat balanced by a lower incidence of acute graft rejection.[17]

Despite this, many programs do not impose strict age limits on candidates, preferring to

- Age >60 years
- Diabetes mellitus without end-organ damage
- Previous mycobacterial or fungal infection
- Distant malignancy
- Moderate irreversible pulmonary hypertension
- Previous cerebrovascular accident
- Active myocardial infiltrative and/or inflammatory disease

Table 19.2
Relative contraindications to cardiac transplantation.

evaluate individuals based upon their 'physiologic age' and other factors which would affect their survival. Older patients can undeniably benefit from the procedure, leading to an ethical dilemma in which physicians are torn between the responsibility of allocating a scarce resource for the greatest good and advocacy for critically ill patients. Some programs have addressed this issue by utilizing marginal

- Moderate to severe renal, pulmonary, hepatic, peripheral vascular, or systemic disease not attributable to CHF
- Diabetes mellitus with end-organ dysfunction
- Active infection
- Recent pulmonary infarction
- Coexisting malignancy
- Severe irreversible pulmonary hypertension
- Active peptic ulcer disease
- Severe obesity
- Severe osteoporosis
- Active or recent substance abuse, including alcohol and tobacco
- Psychiatric disease or mental disability shown to limit the patient's ability to comply with a complex medical regimen

Table 19.1
Contraindications to cardiac transplantation.

donors for the older patient, and acceptable short- and mid-term results have been reported.[18]

Diabetes mellitus Diabetes was previously considered a contraindication to transplantation. However mid- and long-term follow-up of a limited number of these patients shows no difference in 1- and 5-year survival rates post-transplant, incidence of infection, incidence of coronary artery disease, or incidence of renal failure.[19-21] Diabetic patients routinely require more insulin post-transplantation or start insulin if they were previously maintained on oral hypoglycemic agents, presumably due to the effect of prednisone therapy. Diabetics without end-organ complications of their disease may now be considered for transplantation even if they are insulin-dependent, and some centers may even consider patients with end-organ complications on an individual basis. Combined kidney and heart transplantations have been performed in diabetic patients who are excellent candidates in other respects, although the long-term success of this strategy remains unclear.

Infection Active bacterial infection is considered a temporary contraindication to surgery, and a patient should be placed on 'hold' status until resolution of the illness. A possible exception to this is progressive cardiac failure due to refractory endocarditis.[22] Potential recipients should also be screened for chronic infections which could adversely affect post-transplant survival, such as HIV, hepatitis B and C, and tuberculosis.

Recent pulmonary infarction Pulmonary thromboembolism is considered a contraindication due to the increased risk of infection in the involved lung parenchyma during immunosupression.[23] Ordinarily, a matter of months should pass and the chest radiograph should show improvement before accepting or reactivating a patient on the transplant waiting list.

Active peptic ulcer disease Transplantation should not be undertaken in patients with active peptic ulcer disease. The risk of bleeding, gastric perforation, and superimposed viral or fungal infections is unacceptably high as a result of operative anticoagulation, high-dose steroids, and immunosuppressive agents. Resolved peptic ulcer disease is not an absolute contraindication, although screening for occult disease in these patients is advised.

Coexistent or recent malignancy Patients with malignancy are generally not considered candidates, but those with distant malignancies have undergone heart transplantation successfully.[24] Patients who have been free of disease for 5 years or more should be screened for any evidence of recurrence, and then the patient's original diagnosis, staging, and treatment should be reviewed with an oncology consultant to determine the likelihood that the patient is free of malignancy. Age-appropriate cancer screening should be performed on all potential recipients.

Coexistent hepatic, renal, pulmonary, or systemic disease Patients with irreversible, moderate to severe organ dysfunction which is not secondary to severe heart failure are generally excluded. Due to the myriad and often profound effects of severe congestive heart failure, a patient may require repeat evaluation of end-organ function on optimal therapy, including inotropic agents, before this distinction can be made.

A previous history of jaundice or hepatic dysfunction not attributable to heart failure should prompt screening tests to rule out viral hepatitis and cirrhosis. A liver biopsy is indicated if the noninvasive studies are nondiagnostic. Patients with evidence of chronic active hepatitis B or C by serology or polymerase chain reaction are generally not considered candidates, although some programs are cautiously accepting selected individuals.

Renal dysfunction is common among patients referred for transplantation evaluation. A serum creatinine level of 2.0 mg/dl or more, or a creatinine clearance of <50 ml/min is considered grounds for exclusion if heart failure management has been optimized and there is no further improvement following the use of intravenous inotropic agents and renal-dose dopamine. It is our practice to obtain urinalyses for all patients and 24-hour creatinine clearance measurements for patients with serum creatinines greater than 1.4 mg/dl.

Moderate to severe pulmonary disease is also considered an exclusion criterion. Therefore patients with a history of pulmonary disease, tobacco smoking, or amiodarone use should undergo formal pulmonary function testing. Patients with cardiopulmonary failure, such as those with complex congenital heart disease and primary pulmonary hypertension, should be considered for heart-lung transplantation if they are less than 45 years of age. Severe and irreversible pulmonary hypertension markedly increases the risk of acute right ventricular failure in the perioperative period as the normal doner right ventricle attempts to pump against a fixed, elevated pulmonary vascular resistance (PVR). The perioperative incidence of right ventricular failure increases significantly when the PVR increases above 3.0 pulmonary resistance units ([mean pulmonary artery pressure − mean pulmonary capillary wedge pressure]/cardiac output in liters per minute) or the transpulmonary gradient rises above 15 mmHg in the adult population.[5] Most centers would consider an adult with PVR >6 Resistance units, despite hemodynamic maneuvers such as nitroprusside or PGE infusion, to be an unacceptable candidate, and a patient with a PVR of 3 to 6 units would be considered a high-risk candidate.[25,26] Pediatric patients with secondary pulmonary hypertension fare better postoperatively than their adult counterparts, and therefore PVR

values as high as 12 units may be considered acceptable. The pulmonary vascular resistance index (PVR corrected by body surface area) appears to be a more accurate predictive marker of perioperative right heart failure in the pediatric population.[27]

Symptomatic peripheral or cerebrovascular disease is generally considered exclusionary, and some centers consider moderate to severe carotid artery stenosis a contraindication even without symptoms. Other centers have performed transplantations on such patients following surgical revascularization. Carotid ultrasound examination is recommended for patients of advanced age or those with symptomatic atherosclerotic disease at any site. Clinical decisions regarding the listing of any patient with coexistent vascular disease rest on an experienced clinician's judgment of whether or not the disease is severe enough to affect adversely post-transplant survival and rehabilitation.[28,29]

Severe obesity and severe osteoporosis Both these problems will be accelerated considerably by post-transplant medical regimens containing prednisone, and significant disability due to these problems is not uncommon. Morbid obesity (>30% of ideal body weight) increases the risk of post-transplant complications such as diabetes, hypertension, and compression fractures. Obese patients will predictably gain weight after transplantation. However the average total weight gain following transplantation appears to be independent of preoperative obesity.[30]

Active myocardial infiltrative or inflammatory disease Patients with active myocarditis may have a poorer outcome after transplantation than those without active myocarditis.[31] Fortunately, a great many of these patients will improve with supportive therapy and may never need transplantation. An exception to this appears to be giant cell myocarditis, a rare form characterized pathologically by the presence of multinucleated giant cells, and clinically by a rapidly fatal course for the majority of patients, often due to fatal arrhythmias.[32] It remains unclear whether corticosteroids, other immuno-suppressive agents, or antiarrhythmic drugs and devices will improve the prognosis in these patients. At Stanford, they have been success-fully transplanted with good long-term out-comes even though giant cells may recur in the graft. However at least one case of sympto-matic recurrence in an allograft has been reported.[33]

Amyloidosis is an example of an infiltrative disease which commonly recurs in the allo-grafted heart and leads to progressive graft fail-ure.[34] Therefore, heart transplantation for cardiac amyloidosis is not generally recom-mended. Conversely, patients with isolated car-diac sarcoidosis have had good intermediate results with transplantation,[35] and should be considered acceptable candidates as long as there is not active disease affecting other organs.

Active or recent substance abuse Most trans-plant programs consider active substance abuse, including the use of tobacco and alcohol, a con-traindication to transplantation. More than 6 months of demonstrated abstinence and prefer-ably enrollment in a drug or alcohol rehabilita-tion program is preferred.

Psychosocial instability Medical noncompli-ance has a profound effect on graft survi-val,[36,37] so patients should be thoroughly screened for psychiatric disorders, mental dis-ability, and/or social factors which would adversely affect compliance. Evaluation by a trained psychiatrist or behavioral psychologist and a social worker can be helpful in identifying patients who may be unwilling or unable to comply with a complicated post-transplantation treatment regimen. This evaluation also allows the medical team to identify what additional social or financial support may be needed, espe-cially in the case of pediatric patients.

HLA-typing and alloantibody screening

Prospective HLA matching between the donor and recipient in heart transplantation is not done because it increases donor ischemia time. Although academic centers have maintained records regarding HLA compatibility and have shown a correlation between the degree of HLA matching and outcome,[38–40] many transplant centers no longer perform recipient tissue typing in the interest of cost containment.

In contrast, a panel of reactive antibodies (PRA) should be performed for all potential recipients. Unlike HLA antigen matching, this serological cross-match determines whether a potential recipient has preformed antibodies against a wide panel of donor antigens. The assay is reported by the percentage of cells in the panel which are lysed by the candidate's sera. This humoral immunity, which results in a high rate of hyperacute rejection of the graft, results from allogeneic sensitization to human HLA antigens through prior transplantation, pregnancy, or blood transfusion. Potential reci-pients with PRA >30% should undergo pro-spective cross-matching prior to heart transplantation. Although not a strict exclusion criterion, allosensitization can significantly pro-long the search for a suitable donor, and effec-tively render transplantation impossible. A desensitization protocol using intravenous gam-maglobulin (IVIG; 10% Gamimmune N®) may reduce the PRA and has allowed for the trans-plantation of a few highly sensitized indivi-duals.[41]

Pretransplant recipient management

'Routine' care

Ideally, 'routine' care of potential recipients should provide the continuity of care, detailed medical follow-up, education, and psychosocial support which has been shown to improve functional capacity and decrease the need for transplantation in this group of patients by as much as 30–50%.[42,43] The development of a dedicated heart failure and transplant evaluation clinic, or referral to an established one, can provide this framework.

The physician should ensure that aggressive medical therapy is uniformly offered to all patients and that it includes a regimen of diuretics, digitalis, vasodilators (angiotensin converting enzyme inhibitors in all those who tolerate them), and possibly beta blockers. A typical drug regimen is shown in Table 19.3. In addition, antiarrhythmic drugs such as amiodarone, implantable defibrillators, and conventional surgery should be considered before placing a patient on an active transplant waiting list.

It is a common mistake for health-care practitioners to underestimate the value of patient education and compliance with respect to sodium restriction, fluid restriction, and regular aerobic exercise. An advanced practice nurse can be especially important in helping patients comply with a complex medical regimen and

- ACE inhibitor, angiotensin II blocker if cough
- Hydralazine + nitrates for those intolerant of AT II blockers
- Loop diuretics
- Triamterene/hydrochlorathiazide
- Potassium supplements prn
- Digoxin (low dose)
- Enteric-coated aspirin if CAD
- HMG-CoA reductase inhibitor if CAD
- Warfarin sodium if atrial fibrillation, mural thrombus, ventricular aneurysm, or previous thromboembolic event
- Beta blocker trial

Table 19.3
Typical medical regimen for the treatment of advanced heart failure.

necessary behavior modification. Sodium intake should be limited to 2 g/day. This is nearly impossible to achieve without complete avoidance of processed food and great effort on the part of the patient to read labels carefully and calculate the sodium content of fresh ingredients. Written resource materials combined with frequent follow-up and encouragement by the physician or nurse are quite helpful. Fluid consumption should generally be restricted to 1.5–2 L/day, although greater amounts should be taken in the event of increased body fluid losses, such as diarrhea or especially hot weather. Patients should be advised to weigh themselves every day on a reliable and accurate scale, usually in the morning on rising and before dressing for the day. A weight gain or loss of more than 2 kg in a period of 1 week is probably due to body fluid shifts, and should be reported to the RN along with any changes in symptoms. In this way, close follow-up can be maintained over the telephone and clinic visits added when needed. The telephone consult for weight changes also serves as a good time for the nurse to reinforce good dietary and lifestyle practices and help the patients understand their own role in maintaining an optimal functional status for themselves. Weekly to monthly monitoring of electrolytes and renal function, as well as a history and physical exam, serve to detect changes in patient status before they become catastrophic.

Arrhythmia management

Sudden death from both tachyarrhythmias and bradyarrhythmias is the major cause of mortality in outpatients in stable condition awaiting cardiac transplantation. Placement of an automatic implantable cardiac defibrillator with a backup bradycardia pacing feature can reduce the incidence of sudden death in those patients at highest risk (patients with a history of sudden cardiac death).[44,45] Oral antiarrhythmics should be added to the regimen if frequent symptomatic arrhythmias or defibrillator firings occur.

Amiodarone has gained acceptance as part of a pretransplant treatment regimen because it is well tolerated compared with other agents and does not appear to increase mortality in patients with reduced left ventricular function. Whether low-dose amiodarone confers a survival benefit in heart failure patients who are in sinus rhythm and do not have a history of arrhythmia or sudden death remains unclear.[46,47] The incidence of serious side effects such as pulmonary fibrosis and thyroid dysfunction remains low with the use of doses in the 200–400 mg/day range, but less serious side effects such as symptomatic bradycardia and conduction abnormalities are common. If low-dose amiodarone is used empirically, it should be reserved for those patients without conduction abnormalities or a history of symptomatic bradycardia. At our institution, its use is generally reserved for those with documented life-threatening arrhythmias or a history of sudden death or syncope. Sotalol, a beta blocking agent with type III antiarrhythmic properties, is usually poorly tolerated in this patient population due to bradycardia and negative inotropy.

Inotropic therapy

Oral digitalis remains the only inotropic agent which has not been shown to increase overall mortality in patients with severe heart failure,[48] although clinical trials continue to investigate the use of newer agents. Recently, oral vesnarinone has been reported to increase mortality even at low dose and all survival trials have been stopped. The use of intermittent intravenous phosphodiesterase inhibitors such as milrinone is gaining acceptance for these patients, although the long-term effect on mortality remains to be seen.

Alternative therapies

The use of nonconventional surgeries remains of unproved efficacy. Cardiac myoplasty for end-stage heart disease is still an inferior treatment compared with transplantation due to the fairly high operative mortality rate (11–15% in one series),[49] modest improvements in ejection fraction, postoperative arrhythmias, and poorer survival than with transplantation beyond 24 months.[49–51] Recently, limited left ventricular resection has been touted to improve left ventricular mechanics and functional status, although the surgical mortality is high for this procedure as well. The efficacy of the procedure remains to be seen under the scrutiny of well-designed clinical trial.

Critical care

For the desperately ill, preterminal patients who can no longer maintain adequate blood pressure and/or end-organ function on maximal outpatient medical therapy, one must employ pharmacological or mechanical means to 'bridge' them to transplantation while awaiting a suitable donor organ.

This moves the patient to a higher priority status to receive a donor heart. In the USA, under United Network of Organ Sharing Guidelines, this is termed 'status I' while all other ambulatory patients are coded as 'status II'. Due to the ever-increasing number of patients awaiting transplants, approximately half of all recipients in the USA now deteriorate clinically to status I condition before receiving an organ.[52] This is an unfortunate occurrence, since the need for iv inotropic agents and/or mechanical ventilation prior to transplantation are risk factors for postoperative mortality.[53]

The usual choice of intravenous inotropic agents in these patients with decompensated class IV heart failure is a combination of alpha and beta-adrenergic agents such as dopamine and dobutamine. If adequate systemic perfusion pressures are maintained, dopamine should be used only at renal doses (<5 ug/kg/min) to enhance renal perfusion and promote diuresis. Patients with refractory hypoperfusion and hypotension despite moderate to high doses of dobutamine and dopamine can be supported with a combination of epinephrine, dobutamine, and inotropic agents which do not act at the beta receptor, such as amrinone or milrinone. This level of support usually indicates a grave prognosis. Patients with organ hypoperfusion despite an adequate arterial blood pressure and those with severe pulmonary hypertension can often benefit from a nitroprusside infusion when oral vasodilators have not proved sufficient.

The use of intravenous inotropic agents and/or vasodilators is usually more effectively managed with the help of a pulmonary artery catheter initially. In this way, therapy can be tailored to minimize the pulmonary capillary wedge and pulmonary artery pressures while maintaining adequate organ perfusion. Patients who require continued inotropic support beyond the initial stabilization period can be managed without further PA catheter monitoring. Every effort should be made to decrease the patient's risk of intravenous line infection, for example, low-dose inotropic agents can be infused via peripheral rather than central venous catheters as long as patency of the catheter can be demonstrated and the site is inspected closely and frequently for signs of subcutaneous tissue infiltration.

Mechanical bridges to transplantation

Intra-aortic balloon pumps (IABPs) augment cardiac output by approximately 20% under optimal conditions and can be used to stabilize a potential transplant recipient who cannot maintain end-organ function or who has unstable coronary ischemia. IABPs are attractive when immediate hemodynamic stabilization is required despite optimal medical therapy: they are widely available and relatively easy to place percutaneously via the femoral artery. However, there are several major drawbacks with these devices, including the risks of vascular injury and bleeding, occlusion of renal or mesenteric arteries with improper placement or sizing of the balloon, a high incidence of infection with prolonged use, forced bedrest for the patient, and insufficient augmentation of cardiac output.[54–56]

Mechanical ventricular assist device (VAD) technology has advanced steadily and left ventricular and biventricular devices are now available either commercially or through clinical research trials for patients who are in eminent danger of death from circulatory failure despite all other therapy. Some devices have wearable power generator systems which allow for patient ambulation and, under ideal conditions, discharge from the hospital.[57] Orthotopic cardiac replacement with a total artificial heart is again undergoing clinical trials, and appears to be comparable with implantable left ventricular assist devices in bridging patients to transplantation.[58]

The goal of mechanical circulatory support is to decrease cardiac work markedly and restore adequate organ perfusion pressure before irreversible ischemic damage occurs. Because most state-of-the-art devices can deliver up to $2.5 \text{ L/m}^2/\text{min}$ given an atrial pressure of 10–15 mmHg, they provide complete unloading of the assisted ventricle, but may increase the preload of the opposite ventricle. Despite encouraging results reported in a number of series,[59–62] the limitations preventing widespread implementation of such devices remain thromboembolism, bleeding complications, large pump sizes, infection, ineffective circulatory support in the setting of biventricular failure, and the lack of a compact and completely implantable power supply. Pediatric patients are generally too small to accommodate such devices but have been successfully 'bridged' to transplantation using centrifugal pump devices and extracorporeal membrane oxygenation.[63,64]

Donor selection

It is evident to physicians that the number of potential cardiac transplant recipients is immense and that the donor supply is limited. Organ donation rates remain low despite the efforts of local and national organ procurement organizations. Refusals by next of kin run at 30–40% in most European countries, irrespective of implied consent laws[65] and it is estimated that only 26–42% of eligible donors are utilized in the USA.[66] There has been a clear plateau in the number of heart transplant procedures, which remain between 3000 and 3500 worldwide annually (Figure 19.4). The clinical ramifications of this are evident from United Network of Organ Sharing (UNOS) statistics: the USA heart transplantation waiting list has nearly tripled between 1988 and 1994, but cadaveric donation rates have increased by only 25%.[53] Roughly 3500 people on the USA heart trans-

plant waiting list this year will face a median waiting time of 184 days, with an 11% chance of death before receiving an organ, and a 54% chance of requiring intravenous inotropic or mechanical support at the time they receive their donor heart.[52]

Successful heart transplantation depends upon a finite graft ischemia time (approximately 4 hours of cold ischemia), and so organs must be harvested from patients who meet established guidelines for irreversible brain death.[67] Criteria for heart donation vary somewhat between programs, but generally donors should be under the age of 40 years and free of cardiovascular disease, malignancy or acute infection. Patients with risk factors for cardiovascular disease should undergo sufficient screening tests to rule out pre-existing disease in the graft, including possible echocardiograms and cardiac catheterization with coronary angiography. All donors should be screened for HIV and hepatitis B and C infection before acceptance. Serologic screening for other latent infections such as cytomegalovirus (CMV), Epstein–Barr virus (EBV), and toxoplasmosis are performed by some programs because the information can be useful in the postoperative management of the recipient.

Physicians can play an important role by identifying potential donors and promptly con-

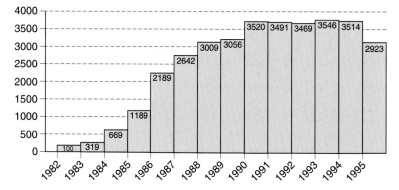

Figure 19.4
Heart transplantation procedures (1982–1995). The worldwide number of cardiac transplant procedures has remained stable since 1991 and is limited by donor availability. Reproduced from Hosenpud et al. (1996)[8] with permission from the International Society of Heart and Lung Transplantation.

tacting their local organ procurement organization (OPO). These organizations are frequently helpful both in obtaining consent for donation and in facilitating the proper medical management of the potential donor.

The operative procedure and perioperative period

Surgical technique

The surgical technique pioneered by Shumway and Lower is shown in Figure 19.5. Following cardiopulmonary bypass through cannulation of the ascending aorta near the takeoff of the innominate artery and bicaval cannulation via the right atrium, the recipient's native heart is removed by bilateral atriotomies and division of the great vessels just above the level of the annulus. The donor heart is then secured by bi-atrial anastamoses following repair of any patent foramen ovale noted in the donor heart, taking care to avoid the donor sinus node and coronary sinus. The pulmonary arteries and aortas are then anastamosed. This technique allows for the greatest simplicity and reduces ischemia time. Bicaval anastamosis has several theoretic advantages over this biatrial anastamosis technique, these being more normal right heart hemodynamics and more normal donor atrial conduction and pacemaker activity.[68] Recent reports suggest that the incidence of clinical events such as supraventricular arrhythmias, tricuspid regurgitation, and the need for permanent pacing may be lower with this technique.[69,70]

Heterotopic cardiac transplantations are rarely performed. The exceptions are a few patients who could not undergo the standard procedure due to irreversibly high pulmonary vascular resistance or donor–recipient size mismatch. Disadvantages of the surgery include compression atelectasis of the right lower lobe of the lung and emboli from the largely bypassed recipient ventricles. Mitral or tricuspid regurgitation is a contraindication to this procedure.

Complex congenital heart disease is a common indication for heart transplantation in the pediatric population. Some of the conditions which are surgically amenable to the procedure are corrected 'L' transposition of the great vessels, hypoplastic left heart syndrome, and patients who have undergone Fontan procedures for tricuspid atresia or univentricular hearts.[71–73] Even the difficult task of transplantation in a patient with situs inversus has been accomplished.[74] Preoperative MRI as well as angiography can be very helpful in defining the cardiopulmonary anatomy in these cases.

Perioperative course and potential complications

Aside from the institution of immunosuppressive drugs and careful monitoring for signs of rejection or infection, the immediate postoperative care of a transplant recipient is similar to that of patients undergoing other cardiac surgeries. At Stanford, the average length of stay for an uncomplicated heart transplantation is 7–10 days. This is accomplished by strict coordination of care between the transplant surgeons and a team of transplant specialists who provide frequent outpatient care in the first 12 weeks following surgery.

Several potential early complications deserve mention. Deaths occurring within the first 2 weeks after transplantation are principally related to donor preservation, right-sided heart failure, and hemorrhage.[75] The overall mortality rate for technical or primary cardiac failure is greater in the pediatric population,[75] probably due to the anatomic difficulties, previous surgeries, and secondary pulmonary hypertension encountered in patients with complex congenital heart disease.

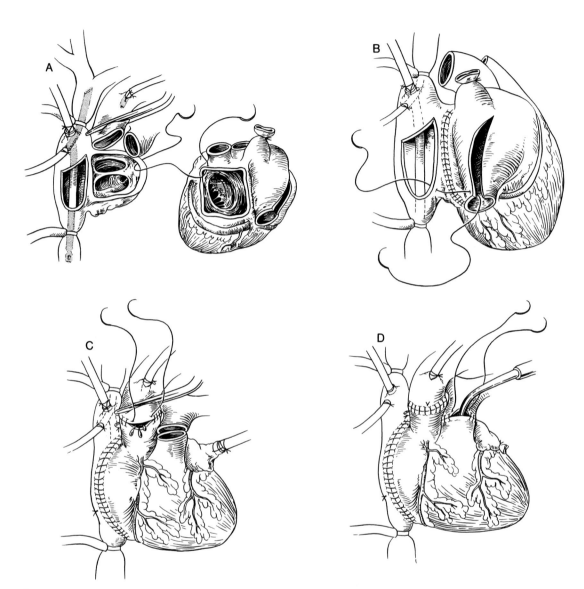

Figure 19.5
*Orthotopic cardiac transplantation technique: standard biatrial anastamosis. (A) The native heart has been excised by right and left atriotomies along the atrioventricular groove and by division of the great vessels just above the semilunar valves. The donor heart is positioned to begin the left atrial anastamosis.
(B) Following the left atrial anastamosis, the right atrial anastamosis proceeds. If a patent foramen ovale is present, it is closed prior to completion of the atrial anastamoses. (C) The aortic anastamosis is completed next, while cold saline or cold cardioplegia solution is dripped through the left atrial appendage. Decompression and de-airing of the ventricle occurs prior to release of the aortic cross clamp. (D) The procedure concludes with the pulmonary artery anastamosis and decompression of the right ventricle.*

Elevated right heart pressures are commonly encountered immediately after heart transplantation, for a variety of reasons including donor ischemia, tricuspid regurgitation, air embolus, and most importantly, recipient pulmonary hypertension.[76,77] This pulmonary hypertension typically resolves within the first 2 weeks if the recipient's preoperative pulmonary vascular resistance was normal.[78] Management of acute right ventricular failure in the perioperative period typically includes the use of vasodilators such as nitroprusside and nitroglycerin plus inotropic agents. Isoproterenol, a potent pulmonary vasodilator as well as a positive inotropic and chronotropic agent, can also be used for the first few days after transplantation.[79] Refractory cases have been managed successfully with prostaglandin E_1 and prostacyclin, and occasionally with right ventricular assist devices.[80–82]

Sinus node dysfunction is common (10–25%) in the early post-transplant period but usually resolves within the first week.[83,84] Epicardial pacing wires are typically placed at the time of surgery and are removed when the donor sinus node function recovers. Patients with persistent junctional rhythms or bradycardia should have a permanent pacemaker placed before discharge from the hospital due to the prohibitive cost of prolonged temporary pacing and the small but definable risk of symptomatic bradycardia and sudden death associated with rejection.[85]

Physiology and function

The physiologic function of the cardiac allograft differs from that of the native heart primarily due to denervation and the resultant alternations in autonomic control. Patients who undergo a bi-atrial anastamosis typically retain their sinus node on the residual posterior wall of the native right atrium. However the denervated donor sinus node controls the rate of the transplanted heart because the native impulse cannot cross the suture line. This dual sinus node activity can often be seen on the surface electrocardiogram. The donor sinus node typically maintains a resting rate of 90 to 110 beats per minute and is insensitive to innervation-dependent agents like atropine, but it can respond to catecholamines or other chronotropic agents which directly perfuse the sinus node. Afferent denervation results in an inability to perceive cardiac ischemic pain. A few long-term survivors will experience typical angina, an indicator that at least some reinnervation occurs in selected individuals.[86]

The ventricular response to exercise is slowed and proceeds in two phases. The early phase is dependent upon changes in ventricular volume and filling pressure and the second phase begins when circulating catecholamines begin to exert their inotropic and chronotropic effects. The transplanted heart has decreased heart rate reserve and a hemodynamic profile consistent with diastolic dysfunction. Nonetheless, a cardiac transplant recipient can expect to achieve a maximal cardiac output of 60–70% of predicted output for his or her age.[87,88]

Post-transplantation management

Immunosuppression

An ideal immunosuppressive regimen would be nontoxic and render the recipient tolerant of the donor organ without reducing the immune response to environmental pathogens. The reality is that our current methods of immunosuppression are both nonspecific and toxic, and the post-transplant physician must apply both knowledge and diligence to balance correctly between providing a patient with adequate immunosuppression and avoiding the adverse side effects of infection, malignancy, and direct organ toxicity. The risk of acute rejection is greatest at the time of the transplant and reduces gradually thereafter for reasons that remain only partially understood. Therefore, immunosuppression is greatest at the time of transplantation and in the first 2 weeks postoperatively, and is gradually reduced thereafter.

Standard therapy

Exact protocols differ between institutions, but a typical regimen is outlined in Table 19.4. The use of low-dose cyclosporin A, azathioprine, and corticosteriods minimizes the toxicity of the individual agents. Optimal adjustment of the cyclosporin dosage takes into account the frequently erratic gastrointestinal absorption of the drug, numerous possible drug interactions, and its renal toxicity. Cyclosporin preparations should be taken with food to optimize oral absorption. Twelve-hour trough blood levels and renal function should be monitored carefully, especially in the early postoperative period and when using any of the drugs known to interact with cyclosporin, as shown in Table 19.5. Therapeutic ranges for whole blood or serum levels of cyclosporin vary according to the assay performed, so physicians are advised to consult their laboratory for appropriate reference ranges. Increasing the maintenance dose of cyclosporin is not effective in the treatment of acute rejection, and the dosage is typically unchanged if the patient has serum trough levels in the therapeutic range.

Drug		Dosage	Route
cyclosporin A	preoperative	4–10 mg/kg once	oral
	postoperative	3–5 mg/kg every 12 h	oral or NG
		±	
		1–2 mg/hr continuous infusion for 3 days	intravenous
	maintenance	5–6 mg/kg/day adjust dose to therapeutic trough levels	oral
azathioprine	preoperative	2–3 mg/kg once	oral
	postoperative	1.5–2.5 mg/kg/day	oral
	maintenance	adjust to keep WBC count > 4500 cells/mm³	oral
methyl-prednisolone	intraoperative	500 mg once	intravenous
	perioperative	125 mg every 8 hours x 4 doses	intravenous
prednisone	begin on postoperative day 2	1 mg/kg/day every 12 hours, then taper by 10 mg every 3 days to a dose of 30 mg/day	oral
	maintenance	slow taper to 0.1–0.2 mg/kg/day by 6 months; adjust according to rejection grade on biopsy	oral

Table 19.4
Typical immunosuppressive regimen: triple drug therapy.

Drug class	Drugs increasing CSA levels	Drugs decreasing CSA levels	Drugs potentiating nephrotoxicity
antibiotics	erythromycin clarithromycin josamycin	rifampin nafcillin	erythromycin gentamicin tobramycin vancomycin trimethoprim- sulfamethoxazole
calcium channel blockers	diltiazem verapamil nicardipine		
antifungals	ketoconazole miconazole intraconazole		amphotericin B ketoconazole
glucocorticoids anticonvulsants	methylprednisolone phenytoin phenobarbital carbamazepine		
anti-inflammatory drugs			azapropazon diclofenac
gastrointestinal drugs	metoclopramide		cimetidine ranitidine
other drugs	allopurinol bromocriptine chloroquine danazol	octreotide ticlopidine	melphalan

Table 19.5
Cyclosporin drug interactions.

Azathioprine is adjusted to keep the white blood cell count >4500 cell/mm^3, and the dose of prednisone is tapered rapidly over 1 month to a dose of 30 mg/day. Prednisone is then tapered more slowly to a maintenance daily dose of 5–10 mg (0.1 mg/kg/day) over 3 to 6 months, depending upon whether there is evidence of rejection on the endomyocardial biopsy.

Deviations from this triple drug protocol have been developed in an effort to decrease early cyclosporin nephrotoxicity, early graft rejection, and chronic dependence on steroids. Some centers use potent anti-T cell induction therapy with antithymocyte globulins (ATG) or murine anti-CD3 antibodies (OKT3) during the first 2 weeks after surgery in combination with prednisone and azathioprine. Oral cyclosporin is added to the regimen 3–4 days before the completion of antibody therapy. Although this is a highly effective strategy for minimizing rejection and renal dysfunction in the early postoperative period, there are reports of more lymphoproliferative disorders and infectious complications with the use of these biological agents.[89,90] This may be the result of over-immunosuppression rather than toxicity of the immunoglobulins themselves. Corticosteriodsparing protocols aggressively attempt to discontinue corticosteriod mainenance within the first year and continue cyclosporin and azathioprine alone, often after antilymphocyte induction therapy. The advantages of minimizing steroid use are many, especially in the pediatric age group where growth retardation and the long-term side effects of these drugs can be especially devastating. Close monitoring for graft rejection using endomyocardial biopsy is necessary with this approach, and a significant number of patients will never be able to wean off steroids completely.

Adjuvant or alternative immunosuppressive agents

Adverse reactions and chronic or recurrent graft rejection sometimes necessitate the use of alternative or adjuvant immunosuppressive agents. For example, methotrexate has been used in addition to standard triple drug regimens for the treatment of recalcitrant rejection.[91–93] The immunomodulatory effect of methotrexate appears to be due to specific antiproliferative effects on locally activated lymphocytes. A second-line immunosuppressive is cyclophosphamide (Cytoxan®), which has been used as a substitute for azathioprine when pancreatitis or another form of intolerance precludes its use. However, it is a potent bone marrow depressant and can cause hemorrhagic cystitis. Total lymphoid irradiation has also been used as an adjuvant therapy in the treatment of persistent rejection, and it will be discussed in more detail later in the chapter.

More importantly, newer immunosuppressive agents have been developed which may prove superior to the current standard therapy. Two such agents which are now commercially available are tacrolimus (formerly FK506), and mycophenolate mofetil. Tacrolimus (Prograf®) is pharmacologically similar in action to cyclosporin but is more potent. Clinical trials, primarily in renal and liver transplant populations, have shown at least equivalent efficacy to cyclosporin in the prevention of allograft rejection and additional efficacy as a 'rescue' therapy for those with refractory rejection while on cyclosporin.[94–97] It has been used successfully in pediatric heart transplant recipients, and its use appears to reduce the incidence of moderate rejection, hypertension, and steroid-dependence compared with historical controls on a cyclosporin-based treatment regimen.[98] The major adverse effects are similar to CSA, the most common and significant being nephrotoxicity and neurotoxicity.

Mycophenolate mofetil (CellCept®), an inhibitor of purine synthesis, is another effective maintenance immunosuppressant which may also be effective in arresting acute graft rejection.[99,100] There is also hope that it may reduce the incidence of graft vascular disease; however, its major clinical advantage is that it causes less bone marrow suppression than azathioprine, and doses of 1000–4000 mg/day are being used as a substitute for azathioprine in those with leukopenia on standard therapy. The major adverse side effects include dose-dependent gastrointestinal intolerance, typically nausea and diarrhea.

Table 19.6 shows the currently available immunosuppressive agents and the major toxicities and side effects associated with the use of each. This table is not comprehensive, and the treating physician is advised to be acquainted thoroughly with full prescribing information before using these agents.

Surveillance and treatment of allograft rejection

Surveillance

Most patients will experience at least one episode of acute cellular rejection in the first year post-transplant.[101] It is the primary cause of

Drug	Toxicity	Side effects
cyclosporin A	renal dysfunction hypertension reversible hepatotoxicity neurotoxicity	hirsutism gingival hyperplasia renal magnesium wasting
azathioprine	bone marrow suppression hepatotoxicity; idiosyncratic pancreatitis	GI distress
corticosteriods	glucose intolerance hypertension osteoporosis avascular necrosis of bone truncal obesity peptic ulcer formation cataract formation	Cushingoid appearance acne mood disturbances
tacrolimus (FK506)	renal dysfunction neurotoxicity hypertension	insomnia tremors headache glucose intolerance
mycophenolate mofetil	bone marrow suppression	vomiting diarrhea
methotrexate	bone marrow suppression hepatic dysfunction abortifacient	ulcerative stomatitis gastrointestinal distress
cyclophosphamide	bone marrow suppression hemorrhagic cystitis infertility	reversible alopecia gastrointestinal distress

Table 19.6
Immunosuppressive agents: selected toxicities and side effects.

death in the first year, and remains a significant cause of late mortality.[8] Since the introduction of cyclosporin, there is no reliable means of detecting allograft rejection with physical examination or electrocardiographic criteria until it has reached an advanced state. A variety of noninvasive techniques have been investigated for the diagnosis of acute rejection, but none can approach the sensitivity and specificity of the endomyocardial biopsy. At our center, we routinely obtain a right ventricular biopsy and echocardiogram to screen for rejection at the time of discharge (7–10 days), and at weekly intervals for the first 4 to 6 weeks. The frequency of the endomyocardial biopsy can be reduced gradually to a frequency of every 3 months during the first year as long as the patient remains free of rejection. There is controversy over whether routine surveillance biopsies should be continued beyond the first year in stable patients.[102,103] However, many programs, including Stanford, continue to perform biopsies at least every 4 to 6 months because of the small but persistent risk of late rejection. In addition, endomyocardial biopsy and echocardiography should be performed to rule out rejection if the patient's clinical status suggests a decline in cardiac function, or if a new arrythmia occurs.

Endomyocardial biopsy is more difficult in neonates and small children. Therefore they are monitored for rejection noninvasively with echocardiography, the surface ECG, and frequent clinical examination. However, they should still undergo endomyocardial biopsy under general anesthesia in the first year while corticosteriods are being tapered. A typical schedule would include four biopsies within the first 6 months and another at 1 year in a clinically stable patient.

The endomyocardial biopsy procedure The most widely used technique utilizes a short, flexible bioptome to biopsy the right ventricular septum via cannulation of the right internal jugular vein. This can be accomplished on an outpatient basis in an angiography suite or procedure room. After introduction of a vascular sheath, the bioptome is advanced across the tricuspid valve and directed toward the ventricular septum under fluoroscopic or echocardiographic guidance and samples are obtained. There are now several bioptomes to choose from, including long instruments with an obligatory long sheath designed for a femoral approach. If a 9F bioptome is used, four tissue samples leads to an acceptable 2% false-negative rate. If a 7F bioptome is used, five or six specimens should be obtained to prevent sampling error.[104] The specimens should be immediately fixed in 10% formalin at room temperature. Additional samples may be snap frozen in liquid nitrogen or isopentane and dry ice if immunohistochemical studies for the diagnosis of humoral rejection are planned.

The possible complications of endomyocardial biopsy are many, including ventricular perforation, arrhythmias, coronary artery to right ventricle fistulae,[105] pneumothorax, arterial puncture, nerve paresis, hematoma, and injury to the tricuspid valvular apparatus.[106] The overall complication rate is reported to be 0.5–1.7% per procedure.[83,107] The development of right heart failure due to biopsy-induced tricuspid regurgitation is now being recognized in some patients. One group of investigators reported that the use of a 45 cm vascular sheath advanced into the right ventricle reduced the incidence of flail tricuspid regurgitation from 41% to 6% ($p < 0.0001$) and the average tricuspid regurgitation severity from 2^+ to 1^+ ($p < 0.0001$) in 72 patients over an average follow-up time of 2.5 years.[108]

Pathology Aside from antibody-mediated hyperacute rejection in the immediate post-transplant period, the vast majority of rejection is cell-mediated and is characterized by inflammatory infiltrates in the graft. In 1990, a standardized grading system for determining the severity of cellular rejection by endomyocardial biopsy was proposed and despite recent discussions regarding the elimination of the 'grade II' category,[109] it remains widely accepted today.[110] The pathologic features of rejection as they correlate with the grading system is illustrated in Table 19.7.

A common but apparently benign pathological finding in patients receiving cyclosporin are 'Quilty' lesions. These are endomyocardial lymphocytic infiltrates which are not associated with acute rejection or lymphoma.[111] They rarely cause a diagnostic dilemma to the trained cardiac pathologist unless there is extension of the infiltrate into the myocardium and there is rejection elsewhere in the biopsy. Their etiology is unknown.

Occasionally, patients will present with the clinical signs and symptoms of acute rejection, but will lack the cellular infiltrate typically associated with it. Several centers have reported this phenomenon, which has been termed 'humoral' or 'vascular' rejection.[112–115] The salient histological features are a scant cellular infiltrate

Grade	Description	Histopathologic findings
0	no rejection	No evidence of cellular rejection and no other histologic changes.
1A	focal, mild acute rejection	Focal, perivascular or interstitial infiltrates of large lymphocytes; no myoctye damage.
1B	diffuse, mild rejection	Diffuse, perivascular or interstitial infiltrate of large lymphocytes; no myocyte damage.
2	focal, moderate rejection	Only one focus of inflammatory infiltrate (large aggressive lymphocytes with or without eosinophils), which is sharply circumscribed. Architectural distortion with myocyte damage should be present within the solitary focus.
3A	mutifocal moderate rejection	Multifocal lymphocytic infiltrates with or without eosinophils; two or more foci causing myocyte necrosis or obvious myocyte replacement.
3B	diffuse, borderline severe acute rejection	Diffuse inflammatory process within several pieces of biopsy tissue. An aggressive inflammatory infiltrate of large lymphocytes and eosinophils, with an occasional neutrophil; associated with obvious myocyte damage. Hemorrhage is not usually seen in this grade.
4	severe acute rejection	The infiltrate may become polymorphous, including neutrophils and eosinophils. The process is diffuse; myocyte necrosis and damage is always seen. Edema, hemorrhage, and vasculitis are usually present.

Table 19.7
International Society of Heart and Lung Transplantation standardized grading system for cardiac allograft rejection.

scattered in an edematous interstitium and endothelial cell swelling of all vessels. Myocyte damage is typically minimal and hemorrhage may be present. Immunohistochemical staining reveals deposition of immunoglobulins, complement, and fibrinogen in linear staining patterns within the interstitium. The presence of immunoglobulin and complement deposits in the capillaries and vessels has no diagnostic value, as these changes can also be seen in association with ischemia and infection. Therefore, the diagnosis of humoral rejection should be made with caution and with knowledge of the clinical status of the patient.

Treatment of rejection
Graft rejection and its treatment can be subdivided into hyperacute rejection, acute cellular rejection, and humoral rejection. Antibody-mediated hyperacute rejection occurs in the immediate post-transplant period due to ABO incompatibility or preformed alloantibodies and is associated with a high mortality rate.[116,117] Antilymphocyte therapy with polyclonal antisera, plasmapheresis, and intravenous cyclosporin A and/or cyclophosphamide has been employed in the treatment of this condition.[118,119] However, graft failure often leads to the need for mechanical circulatory support

and emergency retransplantation. This scenario can be minimized by careful attention to ABO matching and checking for pre-existing circulating alloantibodies.

Acute cellular rejection is a common occurrence in the first 3 to 6 months following transplantation. In the early post-transplant period, mild to moderate rejection is usually treated with a pulse of 1 g methylprednisolone intravenously for 3 days, followed by a repeat endomyocardial biopsy in 7 days. After 3 months, grade 2 or 3A rejection episodes can be treated with an increase in prednisone to 50 mg twice daily for 3 days and a taper of 5 mg daily until the dose is reduced to 10 mg/day over the previous dose. A repeat biopsy should be obtained 1–2 weeks later to assess the response to therapy. Diffuse moderate (3B) rejection is still treated with an intravenous steroid pulse.

Severe rejection, regardless of the timing of occurrence, should be treated with initial hospitalization, intravenous corticosteriods, and antilymphocyte therapy such as ALG, ATG or the widely available monoclonal antibody preparation, OKT3. Despite a 90% efficacy of OKT3 in the treatment of rejection refractory to conventional therapy, there is a high incidence of recurrent rejection and sensitization to the antibody.[120–123] Monoclonal OKT3 antibody is directed against the CD3 glycoprotein that is present on the surface of all mature T cells and can effectively remove all circulating peripheral T lymphocytes within minutes of administration. The usual course of therapy is 5 mg/day intravenously for 10–14 days. Adverse reactions are usually most severe in the first 2 days of treatment, and include the development of antimouse antibodies in 14–41% of patients, and symptoms consistent with a cytokine-release syndrome — fever, chills, hypotension, diarrhea, and occasionally

pulmonary edema. For this reason, pretreatment with hydrocortisone, diphenlyhydramine, ranitidine, and acetaminophen is recommended. Patients who develop anti-OKT3 antibodies may be at higher risk of graft loss due to acute rejection.[122] Patients should be screened for the development of anti-OKT3 antibodies before repeat treatment with them for acute rejection.

Refractory cellular rejection has also been treated successfully with the addition of methotrexate to the regimen[91,92] and with total lymphoid irradiation.[124,125] Total lymphoid irradiation is fractionated over a 5-week period using the standard inverted-Y and mantel fields to a total dose of up to 2000 rad. Patients experience a period of generalized immunosuppression, usually necessitating a temporary discontinuation of azathioprine to minimize neutropenia. Tacrolimus has also been reported to reverse resistant rejection in renal transplant recipients[95] and in a small cohort of heart transplant recipients.[94] Therefore, it appears reasonable to substitute tacrolimus for cyclosporin in those with persistent rejection.

Vascular or humoral rejection has been associated with a poor prognosis and a higher incidence of irreversible fatal rejection.[113] The most efficacious method of treating this type of rejection remains unclear and the reported series are small. There are reports of response to conventional anti-rejection therapy plus plasmapheresis or extracorporeal immunoadsorption, and/or cyclophosphamide.[126–128] Although the utility of plasmapheresis and immunoadsorption remains unproved, these therapies appear to be beneficial in those patients with either unexplained graft dysfunction or vascular rejection on endomyocardial biopsy, suggesting that the dysfunction is mediated by soluble factors such as antibodies and complement.

Complications

Infections

The degree of immunosuppression required for the prevention of allograft rejection proportionally predisposes the post-transplant patient to infectious complications. Early postoperative infections are typically the same as those reported for other cardiothoracic surgeries, such as wound infections and pneumonia. Later, the most common sites of infection are the lungs, urinary tract, and central nervous system.[129] Surveillance is typically by chest radiograph and clinical examination. Aggressive attempts should be made to identify the organism responsible for any infection. An infectious disease consultant with experience in the care of immunocompromised patients can be very helpful, although physicians caring for transplant recipients should familiarize themselves with the more common opportunistic infections.

Several such infections deserve special attention because of the disproportionately great impact they have on the clinical outcome of patients. These are aspergillosis and CMV infections. Aspergillosis is the most common serious fungal infection in heart transplant recipients. The majority of cases occur within the first 3 months after transplantation and have a reported case fatality rate of 30% or more.[130] The most common site of infection is the lung, but it has a propensity to metastasize to other organs, including the central nervous system. The symptoms of CNS infection are usually neurological changes such as confusion, seizures, or focal neurological deficits rather than meningeal signs.[131] Asymptomatic pulmonary disease has a 50% chance of cure, whereas disseminated disease is nearly always fatal.[129] The treatment of choice is amphotericin B to a cumulative dose of 2-3 g, which must be administered with caution to avoid nephrotoxicity.

Cytomegalovirus (CMV) infection causes significant morbidity in heart transplant recipients. Reactivation of a latent infection in the recipient or transmission of the disease by the donor organ is common. One series reported viremia in 53% of recipients within the first 3 months after transplantation and subsequent symptomatic disease in 32%.[132] The severity of the disease can range from asymptomatic to life-threatening, and can affect multiple organ systems. A common intermediate syndrome is characterized by fever, leukopenia, thrombocytopenia, abnormal liver function tests, and diagnostic changes in CMV titers. Patients who are seronegative preoperatively and receive an organ from a seropositive donor have the highest rates and severest forms of the disease.[132,133] CMV infection is strongly associated with acute cellular rejection, bacterial superinfections, and the development of graft coronary artery disease. For this reason, prophylaxis is routinely given to patients at the highest risk for symptomatic illness with ganciclovir[134,135] and hyperimmune globulin (Cytogam®) early in the postoperative period.

Additional prophylactic measures to reduce infectious complications include the use of trimethoprim sulfamethoxizole three times weekly to prevent pneumocystis pneumonia, pyrimethamine if the donor was seropositive for toxoplasmosis, and standard endocarditis prophylaxis prior to gastointestinal or dental procedures.

Coronary artery disease

Progressive obliteration of the coronary arteries due to intimal proliferation and subsequent lipid deposition has become the main complication limiting long-term survival of heart transplant patients.[136] Based on yearly coronary angiographic studies at Stanford, there is evidence of graft vascular disease in 10% of survivors at 1 year and in 50% at 5 years post-transplantation. Characteristics of the disease include its diffuse nature, affecting distal vessels as well as proximal portions with frequent occlusion of distal branches (Figure 19.6). This diffuse nature has precluded traditional approaches to revascularization.

The diagnosis and detection of transplant coronary disease can be difficult since the heart remains denervated so that angina is usually not a presenting symptom. Sudden death or congestive heart failure may be the initial symptoms. In addition, noninvasive stress testing for transplant coronary artery disease is frequently not successful since the diffuse nature of the process does not allow for detection of differential abnormalities of

coronary flow or perfusion. Thus, most transplant centers continue to perform coronary arteriography every 1–2 years.

It had been hoped that the introduction of improved immunosuppression with cyclosporin in 1980 would lead to lessened vascular injury and graft disease. Comparison of our patients at Stanford pretreatment and posttreatment with cyclosporin demonstrated similar rates of angiographically detectable transplant CAD. In fact, although the 1-year survival of cyclosporin-treated patients was approximately 20% better than patients treated with prednisone and azathioprine, subsequent deterioration in survival was remarkably similar.[137]

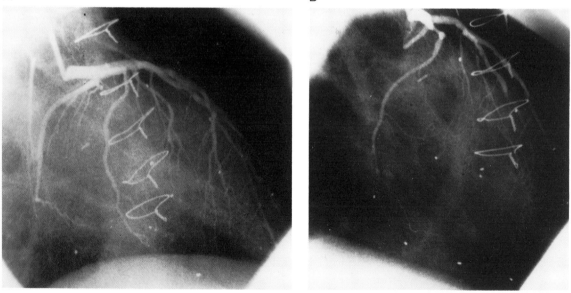

Figure 19.6

Cardiac allograft vasculopathy. (A) Right anterior oblique view of the left coronary artery showing essentially normal left coronary anatomy 1 year following cardiac transplantation. (B) Same view of the left coronary artery 5 years after transplantation, showing occlusion of the left circumflex artery and extensive distal pruning and diffuse irregularities of the first obtuse marginal branch of the left circumflex, the distal left anterior descending artery, and the diagonal branches.

C

D

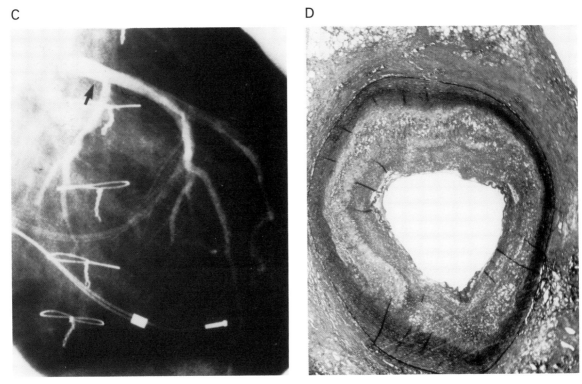

Figure 19.6 *(cont.)*
(C) Left coronary angiogram exhibiting essentially normal left main arteriographic anatomy (arrow)
4 days before the patient's death as a result of multiple myocardial infarcts secondary to severe coronary
artery disease. (D) Intracoronary ultrasound of the left main coronary artery showing concentric
atheromatous plaque, composed of a fibrous cap overlying a basal layer of extracellular and intracellular
lipid.

We have utilized intravascular ultrasound as a more sensitive method for detecting early coronary intimal proliferation post-transplantation. This approach can detect the proliferation process at a time when coronary arteriography appears to be entirely normal.[138,139] Currently, several new immunosuppressive agents in clinical trials are using intravascular ultrasound to detect the endpoint of transplant vascular disease.

Because the initial process of transplant coronary vascular disease appears to be intimal proliferation in response to chronic immune injury, several approaches have shown a pro-

phylactic effect when started early after transplantation. We have demonstrated in a randomized study of diltiazem versus no calcium antagonist that diltiazem started within a few days post-transplantation is not only an effective antihypertensive agent but also reduces intimal proliferation based on quantitative coronary arteriography.[140] In the no calcium antagonist group hypertension was controlled with antihypertensive agents other than calcium antagonist, primarily ACE inhibitors. Clinical events were also reduced (Figure 19.7). More recently, Kobashigawa reported on a randomized study of pravastatin versus placebo in

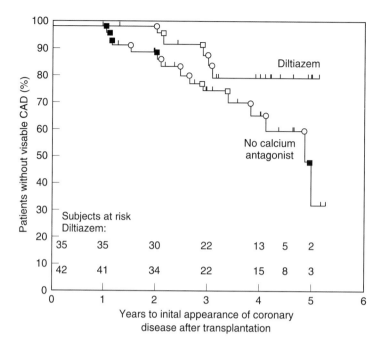

Figure 4.7
*The effect of calcium antagonists on the incidence of coronary artery disease after transplantation.
○ Initial CAD appearance without death, retransplantation* or ≥50% lesion; □ initial appearance with
≥50% lesion, but alive without retransplantation; ■ initial appearance ≥50% lesion, later death,
retransplantation*. *Death and retransplantation are included only if related to coronary disease.
(p = 0.082). The numbers at the bottom of the figure are the numbers of patients at risk in each group.*

97 transplant patients.[141] At 12 months the pravastatin group had less frequent cardiac rejection accompanied by hemodynamic compromise (three versus 14 patients; p = 0.005), better survival (94% versus 78%; p = 0.025) and a lower incidence of coronary vasculopathy by angiography and autopsy (three versus 10 patients; p = 0.049). Whether alterations in immune mechanisms and/or lipid lowering were responsible for these dramatic results remains to be established.

Based on the above findings, early initiation of a calcium antagonist such as diltiazem with adjustment in dosage to control cyclosporin-induced hypertension (usually 240–300 mg) and an HMG-CoA reductase inhibitor such as pravastatin appears wise in an effort to prevent this accelerated vascular coronary disease which defies treatment once it is established.

Malignancies
Chronic immunosuppression leads to an incidence of *de novo* malignant tumors which has been reported as 100 times that of the general population,[142] predominantly due to non-Hodgkin's lymphomas and carcinomas of the skin and the lips.[143] Interestingly enough, the incidence of some cancers commonly seen in the general population, such as cancer of the prostate, colon and rectum, female breast, uterine cervix and lung do not have an increased incidence in transplant recipients.[143] Malignancy accounts for 11.8% of deaths after transplantation according to the most recent

registry report.[8] For this reason, patients should be screened carefully for evidence of lymphoma and cutaneous malignancies on follow-up visits, be advised to wear sunscreen and avoid sun exposure, and undergo routine cancer screening tests appropriate for their age as well as serial chest radiographs.

Most post-transplantation non-Hodgkin's lymphomas are of the B-cell type and are believed to be related to primary or reactivated Epstein–Barr virus infection.[144,145] This entity is known as post-transplantation lymphoproliferative disease (PTLD); it affects 2–6% of cardiac transplant recipients and is correlated with the cumulative degree of immunosuppression an individual has received.[90,146,147] Patients at risk for primary EBV infection, that is EBV-negative recipients, are at an increased risk of developing PTLD. This may explain why, in at least one reported series, pediatric recipients had a three-times greater incidence of lymphomas than their adult cohorts.[148] At Stanford, the incidence of PTLD in the pediatric heart transplant population was 10% between the years of 1974 and 1992.[149] The clinical presentation is often atypical, tending to occur in extranodal sites and the central nervous system. The primary treatment consists of minimizing immunosuppression by withdrawing azathioprin and reducing the cyclosporin dosage while closely monitoring for graft rejection.[150] This is sometimes sufficient to cause complete regression of disease, but adjuvant therapy with interferon, antiviral agents, chemotherapy, and surgery or radiotherapy and surgery is employed if needed.[151]

Other complications

There are myriad effects of the post-transplant medical regimen, including hypertension, osteoporosis, renal dysfunction, dyslipidemia, and glucose intolerance. All these side effects take their eventual toll on end-organ function, but renal dysfunction and orthopedic complications account for a disproportionate degree of morbidity in recipients.

Cyclosporin-induced renal dysfunction is progressive and dose-dependent; therefore every effort should be made to use the lowest effective doses for a given individual and minimize the use of drugs which potentiate nephrotoxicity, as shown in Table 19.5. At Stanford, 3% of cyclosporin-treated survivors eventually progressed to renal failure between 1980 and 1993. Mid-term results for nine patients who have undergone renal transplantation for cyclosporin nephrotoxicity are excellent.[152]

Osteoporosis and its complications are common in heart transplant recipients. The most common complication is vertebral compression fracture, with a reported incidence of 15–35%.[153–155] Patients often have mild osteopenia prior to transplantation due to diuretic use, inactivity, previous tobacco smoking, and hypogonadism. Rapid bone dissolution occurs when therapy with corticosteriods and calcineurin phosphatase inhibitors such as cyclosporin or tacrolimus begins, and trabecular bone loss of 8.5–20% has been reported in the first year.[155,156] Avascular necrosis affecting the hips, knees, shoulders, and elbows occurs and may require joint replacement. This complication of steroid therapy does not appear to be dose dependent. Prevention of these disabling complications should involve identification of the osteopenic patient prior to transplantation, efforts to minimize corticosteriod use, the prophylactic use of calcium supplements post-transplant, and hormonal replacement when appropriate. Prophylactic vitamin D (alphacalcidiol) supplementation, and the use of newer bisphosphonates may also prove valuable in minimizing bone mineral density loss and reducing the incidence of fractures.

Graft failure

Retransplantation is the only viable option for patients with graft failure due to acute rejection, coronary vasculopathy, or severe constrictive disease. However, potential candidates for re-operation should be chosen carefully. The postoperative survival following retransplantation is significantly lower than for first transplants; the average survival in one registry is 52% at 1 year and 44% at 3 years.[8] Survival statistics following urgent retransplantation for acute rejection are even more dismal, with an approximate 33% 1-year survival.[157,158] At Stanford, the outcomes of 63 patients undergoing a total of 66 repeat heart transplants were reviewed to identify a subgroup of patients with good rehabilitation potential following retransplantation.[158] In this group, patients retransplanted for graft atherosclerosis had significantly better 1-year survival (69% versus 33%) and less infection and rejection than those retransplanted for acute rejection. However, there was equivalent survival between the groups at 5 years (34% versus 33%). Renal dysfunction (serum creatinine level >2.0 mg/dl) was a strong predictor of death following repeat transplantation; however, 3 patients who underwent simultaneous renal transplantation and cardiac retransplantation had good interim results. Based on these results, our institution is reluctant to offer retransplantation to candidates with intractable rejection, renal dysfunction, or other comorbid conditions which would limit their rehabilitative potential. For otherwise ideal candidates who have severe nephropathy, concomitant renal transplantation is favored.

Long-term follow-up and the role of the primary-care physician

Most transplant recipients will receive care from transplant specialists at their transplant center early after the operation, and then will return home for follow-up care with their primary cardiologist or internist if they are in a stable condition. A recommended follow-up schedule for examinations, endomyocardial biopsies, and routine screening tests is shown in Table 19.8. The primary-care physician should be vigilant for signs or symptoms of infection and rejection early on and for signs of graft dysfunction and malignancy thereafter. No new fever or clinical abnormality should be ignored or investigation delayed in these complex immunosuppressed patients. Encouragement and monitoring of medical compliance, the provision of psychological support, and physical and social rehabilitation are all important aspects of care.

A typical post-transplant drug regimen for the stable patient is outlined in Table 19.9. In addition to immunosuppressive agents, a variety of medications are employed as prophlyaxis against opportunistic infections and as treatments for the predictable adverse side effects of immunosuppressive therapy such as hypertension, mild fluid retension, hyperlipidemia, osteopenia, and gastric ulceration. Physicians caring for heart transplant patients must use the utmost care to check cyclosporin and other immunosuppressive drug interaction lists before starting any medication — even with something as simple as allopurinol. Some of these drug interactions are listed in Tables 19.5 and 19.9.

Approximately 85% of heart transplant survivors are physically and mentally able to return to their previous occupations at 1 year. The actual number who do return is much lower due to intercurrent complications post-transplantation, societal employing attitudes toward 'cardiac' patients and stringent rules for those patients receiving long-term disability allowance. Most programs require 'full disability' and so part-time work, which is ideally suited

Time post-transplant	Clinic visit frequency	Clinical evaluation and treatment plan	Heart biopsy frequency
0–1 month	biweekly	baseline ECG CBC with platelets chemistry panel with renal and hepatic indices chest X-ray CSA level monitor for infection and rejection CMV, toxoplasmosis prophylaxis prn	weekly
1–3 months	biweekly to weekly	same lab tests; no ECG monitor for infection or rejection reduce steroids if no rejection	monthly
3–6 months	every 2–3 weeks	same tests and examination continue to reduce steroids	monthly
6–12 months	every 4–6 weeks	same tests and examination attempt to wean off steroids	every 3 months
annual evaluation	yearly at transplant center	as above plus: 12-h creatinine clearance fasting lipid panel cardiac catheterization coronary angiography	include in evaluation
>12 months	reduce gradually to every 6–8 weeks	CBC with platelets chemistry panel and CSA level chest X-ray	every 3–6 months

Table 19.8
Outpatient care of the stable cardiac transplant patient.

to most transplant patients, is usually forbidden or jeopardizes disability payments.

If I had ...

If I had end-stage heart failure, I would first seek an experienced heart failure specialist at a high-volume transplant center for a definitive diagnosis and treatment plan, and I would enroll in their dedicated heart failure clinic. If I lived a long distance from the referral center, then I would identify a local physician who could provide close follow-up care and could execute the suggested treatment plan. I would definitely delay transplantation as long as possible, and would hope for stabilization or improvement in my condition considering our current knowledge of reversal of heart failure in some individuals. Such a course of action carries with it a risk of deteriorating to critical condition before receiving a donor organ. If I were on the verge of cardiovascular collapse despite intravenous inotropic therapy, I would want timely placement of an implantable VAD, so that I could be mobilized and avoid progressive multiorgan dysfunction, even though this carries a risk of stroke and infection.

Following transplantation, I would want my transplant physician to have a philosophy of minimizing immunosuppression whenever able and to be very attentive to clinical details

Drug	Dosage	Comments	Adverse drug interactions
prednisone	goal: taper to 0.1 mg/kg/day	usual discharge dose is 5–10 mg bid	see Table 19.5
cyclosporine	2–20 mg/kg/day	obtain level every 6 weeks; goal trough levels approximately: serum 70–200; whole blood 150–400	
azathioprine	25–200 mg QD	titrate to WBC >3500/ml; <5000/ml	ACE inhibitors or allopurinol; increased risk of leukopenia phenytoin, phenobarbital, rifampin: decreased blood levels ketoconazole, erythromycin: increased blood levels
diuretics: hydrochlorothiazide	25–50 mg/day	mild diuretic often used for sodium retention	
antihypertensives: diltiazem clonidine ACE inhibitors	180–240 mg/day TTS 1–TTS 3 patch weekly avoid high doses	watch renal function	increases cyclosporine level
ASA KCL	325 mg/day	prophylaxis against gastric ulcers needed most require	increased marrow suppression with azathioprine
antacids		Ca²⁺-containing antacids given early postoperation	tacrolimus may decrease or eliminate need for supplement
H₂-blockers: ranitidine mycostatin	150 mg bid swish or troches orally tid	watch renal function oral thrush prevention	potentiation CSA nephrotoxicity
sulfa/trimethoprim DS	prn		potentiation CSA nephrotoxicity
calcium, magnesium and Vit D supplements penicillin or erythromycin	standard doses prn	endocarditis prophylaxis prior to dental and GI procedures	

Table 19.9
Typical post-transplant drug regimen.

and meticulous in his or her attention to my complaints. I would prefer not to receive antilymphocyte antibodies as induction therapy if my preoperative renal function was normal, but rather save it for an acute rejection episode if needed. I would certainly want to know the serologic status of the donor with respect to cytomegalovirus, Epstein–Barr virus, and toxoplasmosis infections, and I would want appropriate prophylactic treatment. A comprehensive physical rehabilitation program would help me regain my sense of independence and well-being.

I would want the long-term treatment plan to include an attempt to wean me off steroids, and prudent but not aggressive invasive follow-up. By this, I mean endomyocardial biopsy every 6 to 12 months and cardiac catheterization with coronary angiography every 2 years, with non-invasive assessments more frequently.

References

1 Lower RR, Shumway NE, Studies in orthotopic homotransplantation of the canine heart, *Surg Forum* (1960)**11**:18–19.

2 Lower RR, Dong EJ, Shumway NE, Long-term survival of cardiac homografts, *Surgery* (1964)**58**:110–19.

3 Barnard CN, A human cardiac transplant: an interim report of the successful operation performed at the Groote Schuur Hospital, Cape Town, *South Africa Med J* (1967)**41**:1271–4.

4 Griepp RB, A decade of human heart transplantation, *Transplant Proc* (1979)**11**:285–92.

5 Griepp RB, Stinson EB, Dong EJ, Clark DA, Shumway NE, Determinants of operative risk in human heart transplantation, *Am J Surg* (1971)**122**:192–7.

6 Griepp RB, Stinson EB, Clark DA, Dong EJ, Shumway NE, The cardiac donor, *Surg Gynecol Obstet* (1971)**133**:792–8.

7 Oyer PE, Stinson EB, Jamieson SW, Hunt SA, Billingham M, Scott W, Cyclosporin A in cardiac allografting: a preliminary experience, *Transplant Proc* (1983)**15**:1247–52.

8 Hosenpud JD, Novak RJ, Bennet LE, Keck BM, Fiol B, Daily OP, The Registry of the International Society for Heart and Lung Transplantation: Thirteenth Offical Report-1996, *J Heart Lung Transplant* (1996)**15**:655–74.

9 Hosenpud JD, Novick RJ, Breen TJ, Keck B, Daily P, The Registry of the International Society for Heart and Lung Transplantation: Twelth Official Report — 1995, *J Heart Lung Transplant* (1995)**14**:805–15.

10 Hauptman PJ, Kartashov AI, Couper GS et al, Changing patterns in donor and recipient risk: a 10-year evolution in one heart transplant center, *J Heart Lung Transplant* (1995)**14**:654–8.

11 Rickenbacher PR, Trindade PT, Haywood GA et al, Transplant candidates with severe left ventricular dysfunction managed with medical treatment: characteristics and survival, *J Am Coll Cardiol* (1996)**27**:1192–7.

12 Kasper EK, Agema WR, Hutchins GM, Deckers JW, Hare JM, Baughman KL, The causes of dilated cardiomyopathy: a clinico-pathologic review of 673 consecutive patients, *J Am Coll Cardiol* (1994)**23**:586–90.

13 Costanzo MR, Augustine S, Bourge R et al, Selection and treatment of candidates for heart transplantation. A statement for health professionals from the Committee on Heart Failure and Cardiac Transplantation of the Council on Clinical Cardiology, American Heart Association, *Circulation* (1995)**92**:3593–612.

14 Kermani M, Stevenson LW, Chelimsky-Fallick C et al, Importance of serial excercise testing after evaluation for cardiac transplantation, *J Heart Lung Transplant* (1992)**11**:191.

15 Mancini DM, Eisen H, Kussmaul W, Mull R, Edmunds LH, Wilson JR, Value of peak excercise oxygen consumption for optimal timing of cardiac transplantation in ambulatory patients with heart failure, *Circulation* (1991)**83**:778–86.

16 Bourge RC, Naftel DC, Costanzo-Nordin MR et al, Pretransplantation risk factors for death after heart transplantation: a multiinstitutional study. The Transplant Cardiologists Research Database Group, *J Heart Lung Transplant* (1993)**12**:549–62.

17 Bull DA, Karwande SV, Hawkins JA et al, Long-term results of cardiac transplantation in patients older than sixty years. UTAH Cardiac Transplant Program, *J Thorac Cardiovasc Surg* (1996)**111**:423–7.

18 Drinkwater DC, Laks H, Blitz A et al, Outcomes of patients undergoing transplantation with older donor hearts, *J Heart and Lung Transplant* (1996)**15**:684–91.

19 Badellino MM, Cavarocchi B, Narins M et al, Cardiac transplantation in diabetic patients, *Transplant Proc* (1990)**22**:2384–8.

20 Ladowski JS, Kormos RL, Uretsky BP, Griffith BP, Armitage JM, Hardesty RL, Heart trans-

plantation in diabetic patients, *Transplantation* (1990)**49**:303–5.

21 Rhenman MJ, Rhenman B, Renogle T, Christensen R, Copeland J, Diabetes and heart transplantation, *J Heart Transplant* (1988)**7**: 356–8.

22 Disesa VJ, Sloss LJ, Cohn LH, Cardiac transplantation for intractable prosthetic valve endocarditis, *J Heart Transplant* (1990)**9**:142–3.

23 Kirklin JK, Naftel DC, McGiffin DC, McVay RF, Blackstone EH, Karp RB, Analysis of morbid events and risk factors for death after cardiac transplantation, *J Am Coll Cardiol* (1988)**11**:917–24.

24 Edwards BS, Hunt SA, Fowler MB, Valantine HA, Stinson EB, Schroeder JS, Cardiac transplantation in patients with pre-existing malignant disease, *Am J Cardiol* (1990)**65**:501–4.

25 Costard-Jackle A, Fowler MB, Influence of preoperative pulmonary artery pressure on mortality after heart transplantation: testing of potential reversibility of pulmonary hypertension with nitroprusside is useful in defining a high risk group, *J Am Coll Cardiol* (1992)**19**: 48–54.

26 Murali S, Uretsky BR, Armitage JM et al, Utility of prostaglandin E-1 in pretransplant evaluation of cardiac failure patients with significant pulmonary hypertension, *J Heart Lung Transplant* (1992)**11**:716–23.

27 Addonizio LJ, Cardiac transplantation in the pediatric patient, *Prog Cardiovasc Dis* (1990)**33**:19–34.

28 Bull DA, Hunter GC, Copeland JG et al, Peripheral vascular disease in heart transplant recipients, *J Vasc Surg* (1992)**16**:546–53.

29 Benvenisty AI, Todd GJ, Argenziano M et al, Management of peripheral vascular problems in recipients of cardiac allografts, *J Vasc Surg* (1992)**16**:895–901.

30 Baker AM, Levine TB, Goldberg AD, Levine AB, Natural history and predictors of obesity after orthotopic heart transplantation, *J Heart Lung Transplant* (1992)**11**:1156–9.

31 O'Connel J, Dec G, Goldenberg I et al, Results of heart transplantation for active lymphocytic myocarditis, *J Heart Transplant* (1990)**9**:351–6.

32 Cooper LTJ, Berry GJ, Rizeq M, Schroeder JS, Giant cell myocarditis, *J Heart Lung Transplant* (1995)**14**:394–401.

33 Gries W, Farkas D, Winters GL, Costanzo-Nordin MR, Giant cell myocarditis: first report of disease recurrence in the transplanted heart, *J Heart Lung Transplant* (1992)**11**:370–4.

34 Hosenpud JD, DeMarco T, Frazier OH et al, Progression of systemic disease and reduced long-term survival in patients with cardiac amyloidosis undergoing heart transplantation: follow-up results of a multicenter study, *Circulation* (1990)**82**(suppl III):713A.

35 Valantine HA, Tazelaar HD, Macoviak J et al, Cardiac sarcoidosis: response to steriods and transplantation, *J Heart Transplant* (1987)**6**: 244–50.

36 Rodriguez MD, Colon A, Santiago-Delphin EA, Psychosocial profile of noncompliant patients, *Transplant Proc* (1991)**23**:1807–9.

37 Rovelli M, Palmeri D, Vossler E, Bartus S, Hull D, Schweizer R, Noncompliance in organ transplant recipients, *Transplant Proc* (1989)**21**:833–4.

38 Kerman RH, Kimball P, Scheinen S et al, The relationship among donor-recipient HLA mismatches, rejection, and death from coronary artery disease in cardiac transplant recipients, *Transplantation* (1994)**57**:884–8.

39 Hosenpud JD, Edwards EB, Lin HM, Daily OP, Influence of HLA matching on thoracic transplant outcomes. An analysis from the UNOS/ISHLT Thoracic Registry, *Circulation* (1996)**94**:170–4.

40 De Mattos AM, Head MA, Everett J et al, HLA-DR mismatching correlates with early cardiac allograft rejection, incidence, and graft survival when high-confidence-level serological DR typing is used, *Transplantation* (1994)**57**(4):626–30.

41 Tyan DB, Li VA, Czer L, Trento A, Jordan SC, Intravenous immunoglobulin suppression of HLA alloantibody in highly sensitized transplant candidates and transplantation with a histoincompatible organ, *Transplantation* (1994)**57**:553–62.

42 Stevenson WG, Stevenson LW, Middlekauff HR et al, Improving survival for patients with advanced heart failure: a study of 737

consecutive patients, *J Am Coll Cardiol* (1995)**26**:1417–23.

43 Stevenson LW, Heart transplant centers: no longer the end of the road for heart failure, *J Am Coll Cardiol* (1996)**27**:1198–2000.

44 Grimm M, Wieselthaler G, Avanessian R et al, The impact of implantable cardioverter-defibrillators on mortality among patients on the waiting list for heart transplantation, *J Thorac Cardiovasc Surg* (1995)**110**:532–9.

45 Saxon LA, Wiener I, DeLurgio DB et al, Implantable defibrillators for high-risk patients with heart failure who are awaiting cardiac transplantation, *Am Heart J* (1995)**130**:501–6.

46 Singh SN, Fletcher RD, Fisher SG et al, Amiodarone in patients with congestive heart failure and asymptomatic ventricular arrhythmia. Survival Trial of Antiarrhythmic Therapy in Congestive Heart Failure, *N Engl J Med* (1995)**333**:77–82.

47 Doval HC, Nul DR, Grancelli HO, Perrone SV, Bortman GR, Curiel R, Randomised trial of low-dose amiodarone in severe congestive heart failure. Grupo de Estudio de la Sobrevida en la Insuficiencia Cardiaca en Argentina (GESICA), *Lancet* (1994)**344**:493–8.

48 Kelly RA, Smith TW, Digoxin in heart failure: implications of recent trials, *J Am Coll Cardiol* (1993)**22**:107A–112A.

49 Magovern GJS, Simpson KA, Clinical cardio-myoplasty: review of the ten-year United States experience, *Ann Thorac Surg* (1996)**61**:413–19.

50 Bocchi EA, Bellotti G, Moreira LF et al, Mid-term results of heart transplantation, cardio-myoplasty, and medical treatment of refractory heart failure caused by idiopathic dilated cardi-omyopathy, *J Heart Lung Transplant* (1996)**15**:736–45.

51 Moreira LF, Stolf NA, Bocchi EA et al, Clinical and left ventricular function outcomes up to five years after dynamic cardiomyoplasty, *J Thorac Cardiovasc Surg* (1995)**109**:353–62.

52 Bureau of Health Resources Development HRaSA, 1995 Annual Report of the US Scientific Registry for Transplant Recipients and the Organ Procurement and Transplantation Network — Transplant Data: 1988–1994. In:. Administrator of the National Organ Procurement and Transplantation Network and Scientific Registry of Organ Transplantation, Richmond, VA, and the Division of Transplantation, US Department of Health and Human Services, Rockville, MD, 1996.

53 UNOS Update. Administrator of the National Organ procurement and Transplantation Network and Scientific Registry of organ Transplantation, Richmond, VA, (1994)**10**:33–5.

54 Creswell L, Rosenbloom M, Cox JL, Fergusson TB, Kouchoukas NT, Spray TL, Intraaortic bal-loon counterpulsation: patterns of usage and outcome in cardiac surgery patients, *Ann Thorac Surg* (1992)**54**:11–20.

55 McEnany MT, Kay HR, Buckley MJ, Daggett WM, Endman AJ, Mundth ED, Clinical experi-ence with intra-aortic balloon pump support in 728 patients, *Circulation* (1978)**58**(suppl I):124–32.

56 Miller JF, Dodson TF, Salan AA, Smith RB, Vascular complications following intraaortic balloon pump insertion, *Am Surg* (1992)**58**:232–8.

57 Pristas JM, Winowich S, Nastala CJ et al, Protocol for releasing Novacor left ventricular assist system patients out-of-hospital, *Asaio J* (1995)**41**:M539–43.

58 Copeland JG, Pavie A, Duveau D et al, Bridge to transplantation with the CardioWest total artifical heart: the international experience 1993–1995, *J Heart Lung Transplant* (1996)**15**:94–9.

59 Frazier OH, Rose EA, McCarthy P et al, Improved mortality and rehabilitation of trans-plant candidates treated with a long-term implantable left ventricular assist system, *Ann Surg* (1995)**222**:327–36.

60 McCarthy PM, James KB, Savage RM et al, Implantable left ventricular assist device. Approaching an alternative for end-stage heart failure. Implantable LVAD Study Group, *Circulation* (1994)**90**:1183–6.

61 Pennington DG, McBride LR, Peigh PS, Miller LW, Swartz MT, Eight years' experience with bridging to cardiac transplantation, *J Thorac Cardiovasc Surg* (1994)**107**:472–80.

62 Vetter HO, Kaulbach HG, Schmitz C et al, Experience with the Novacor left ventricular assist system as a bridge to cardiac transplanta-

tion, including the new wearable system, *J Thorac Cardiovasc Surg* (1995)**109**:74–80.

63 Ashton RJ, Oz MC, Michler RE et al, Left ventricular assist device options in pediatric patients, *Asaio J* (1995)**41**:M277–80.

64 del Nido PJ, Extracorporeal membrane oxygenation for cardiac support in children, *Ann Thorac Surg* (1996)**61**:336–9.

65 Cohen B, Wright C, The shortage of donor organs: the European experience, *Xenobiotica* (1993)**1**:21–2.

66 O'Connel JB, Gunnar RM, Evens RW, Fricker FJ, Hunt SA, Kirklin JK, Task Force 1: organization of heart transplantation in the US; 24th Bethesda Conference, Cardiac Transplantation, *J Am Coll Cardiol* (1993)**22**:8–14.

67 Report of the Medical Consultants on the Diagnosis of Death to the President's Commission for the Study of Ethical Problems in Medicine and Biomedical and Behavioral Research, Guidelines for the determination of death, *JAMA* (1981)**246**:2184–6.

68 Dreyfus G, Jebara V, Mihaileanu MD, Carpentier A, Total orthotopic heart transplantation: an alternative to the standard technique, *Ann Thorac Surg* (1991)**52**:1181–4.

69 Deleuze PH, Benvenuti C, Mazzucotelli MD et al, Orthotopic cardiac transplantation with direct caval anastamosis: is it the optimal procedure? *J Thorac Cardiovasc Surg* (1995)**109**: 731–7.

70 El Gamel A, Yonan NA, Grant S et al, Orthotopic cardiac transplantation: a comparison of standard and bicaval Wythenshawe techniques, *J Thorac Cardiovasc Surg* (1995)**109**:721–30.

71 Bailey L, Concepcion W, Shattuck H, Huang L, Method of heart transplantation for treatment of hypoplastic left heart syndrome, *J Thorac Cardiovasc Surg* (1986)**92**:1–5.

72 Pearl JM, Laks H, Drinkwater DC, Case reports: cardiac transplantation following the modified Fontan procedure, *Transplant Sci* (1992)**2**:1–3.

73 Reitz BA, Jamieson SW, Gaudiani VA, Oyer PE, Stinson EB, Method for cardiac transplantation in corrected transposition of the great arteries, *J Cardiovasc Surg* (1982)**23**:293–6.

74 Doty DB, Renlund DG, Caputo GR, Burton NA, Jones KW, Cardiac transplantation in situs inversus, *J Thorac Cardiovasc Surg* (1990)**99**:493–9.

75 Kriett JM, Kaye MP, The registry of the International Society for Heart and Lung transplantation: eighth official report — 1991, *J Heart Lung Transplant* (1991)**10**:491–8.

76 Erickson KW, Constanzo-Nordin MR, O'Sullivan EJ et al, Influence of preoperative transpulmonary gradient on late mortality after orthotopic heart transplantation, *J Heart Transplant* (1990)**9**:526–37.

77 Young JB, Leon CA, Short HDI et al, Evolution of hemodynamics after orthotopic heart and heart-lung transplantation: early restrictive patterns persisting in occult fashion, *J Heart Transplant* (1987)**6**:34–43.

78 Bhatia SJ, Kirschenbaum JM, Shemin JR et al, Time course of resolution of pulmonary hypertension and right ventricular remodeling after orthotopic cardiac transplantation, *Circulation* (1987)**76**:819–26.

79 Stinson EB, Caves PK, Griepp RB, Oyer PE, Rider AK, Shumway NE, Hemodynamic observations in the early period after human heart transplantation, *J Thorac Cardiovasc Surg* (1975)**69**:264–70.

80 Armitage JM, Hardesty RL, Griffith BP, Prostaglandin E1: an effective treatment of right ventricular heart failure after orthotopic heart transplantation, *J Heart Transplant* (1987)**6**:348–51.

81 Fonger JD, Borken AM, Baumgartner WA, Achuff SC, Augustine S, Reitz B, Acute right ventricular failure following heart transplantation: improvement with prostaglandin E and right ventricular assist, *J Heart Transplant* (1986)**5**:317–21.

82 Pascual JM, Fiorelli AI, Bellotti GM, Stolf NA, Jatene AD, Prostacyclin in the management of pulmonary hypertension after heart transplantation, *J Heart Transplant* (1990)**9**:644–51.

83 Frist WH, Management of complications. In: Shumway SJ, Shumway NE, eds. *Thoracic transplantation* (Blackwell Scientific: Cambridge, 1995) 226–51.

84 Miyamoto Y, Curtiss EI, Kormos RL, Armitage JM, Hardesty RL, Griffith BP, Bradyarrhythmia after heart transplantation. Incidence, time course, and outcome, *Circulation* (1990)**82**(suppl IV):313–17.

85 Schroeder JS, Berke DK, Graham AF, Rider AK, Harrison DC, Arrhythmias after cardiac transplantation, *Am J Cardiol* (1974)**33**:604–7.

86 Stark RP, McGinn AL, Wilson RF, Chest pain in cardiac transplant recipients. Evidence of sensory reinnervation after cardiac transplantation, *N Engl J Med* (1991)**324**:1791–4.

87 Kao AC, Van Trigt Pr, Shaeffer-McCall GS et al, Allograft diastolic dysfunction and chronotropic incompetence limit cardiac output response to exercise two to six years after heart transplantation, *J Heart Lung Transplant* (1995)**14(1 Pt 1)**:11–22.

88 Nixon PA, Fricker FJ, Noyes BE, Webber SA, Orenstein DM, Armitage JM, Exercise testing in pediatric heart, heart-lung, and lung transplant recipients, *Chest* (1995)**107**:1328–35.

89 Miller LW, Naftel DC, Bourge RC et al, Infection after heart transplantation: a multiinstitutional study. Cardiac Transplant Research Database Group, *J Heart Lung Transplant* (1994)**13**:381–92.

90 Swinnen LJ, Costanzo-Nordin MR, Fisher SG et al, Increased incidence of lymphoproliferative disorders after immunosuppression with monoclonal antibody OKT3 in cardiac transplant recipients, *N Engl J Med* (1990)**323**:1723–8.

91 Bouchart F, Gundry SR, Van Schaack-Gonzales J et al, Methotrexate as rescue/adjunctive immunotherapy in infant and adult heart transplantation, *J Heart Lung Transplant* (1993)**12**:427–33.

92 Costanzo-Nordin MR, Grusk BB, Silver MA, Reversal of recalcitrant cardiac allograft rejection with methotrexate, *Circulation* (1988)**78** (**suppl III**):47–57.

93 Hosenpud JD, Hershberger RE, Ratkovec RR et al, Methotrexate for the treatment of patients with multiple episodes of acute cardiac allograft rejection, *J Heart Lung Transplant* (1992)**11**:739–45.

94 Armitage JM, Kormos RL, Morita S et al, Clinical trial of FK 506 immunosuppression in adult cardiac transplantation, *Ann Thorac Surg* (1992)**54**:205–10.

95 Jordan ML, Shapiro R, Vivas CA et al, FK506 'rescue' for resistant rejection of renal allograft under primary cyclosporin immunosuppression, *Transplantation* (1994)**57**:860–5.

96 Pham SM, Kormaos RL, Hattler BG et al, A prospective trial of tacrolimus (FK506) in clinical heart transplantation: intermediate term results, *J Thorac Cardiovasc Surg* (1996)**111**: 1–9.

97 Todo S, Fund JJ, Tzakis A et al, One hundred and ten consecutive primary orthotopic liver transplants under FK506 in adults, *Transplant Proc* (1991)**23**:1397–402.

98 Armitage JM, Fricker FJ, del Nido P, Starzl TE, Hardesty RL, Griffith BP, A decade (1982 to 1992) of pediatric cardiac transplantation and the impact of FK 506 immunosuppression, *J Thorac Cardiovasc Surg* (1993)**105**:464–72.

99 Rescue therapy with mycophenolate mofetil. The Mycophenolate Mofetil Renal Refractory Rejection Study Group, *Clin Transplant* (1996)**10**:131–5.

100 Renlund DG, Gopinathan SK, Kfoury AG, Taylor DO, Mycophenolate mofetil (MMF) in heart transplantation: rejection, prevention and treatment, *Clin Transplant* (1996)**10**:136–9.

101 Kobashigawa JA, Naftel DC, Bourge RC et al, Pretransplantation risk factors for acute rejection after heart transplantation: a multiinstitutional study. The Transplant Cardiologists Research Database Group, *J Heart Lung Transplant* (1993)**12**:355–66.

102 Sethi GK, Kosaraju S, Arabia FA, Rosado LJ, McCarthy MS, Copeland JG, Is it necessary to perform surveillance endomyocardial biopsies in heart transplant recipients? *J Heart Lung Transplant* (1995)**14**:1047–51.

103 White JA, Guiraudon C, Pflugfelder PW, Kostuk WJ, Routine surveillance myocardial biopsies are unnecessary beyond one year after heart transplantation, *J Heart Lung Transplant* (1995)**14**:1052–6.

104 Spiegelhalter DJ, Stovin PGI, Analysis of repeated biopsies following cardiac transplantation, *Stat Med* (1983)**2**:33–40.

105 Henslova MJ, Nath H, Bucy RB, Bourge RC, Kirlin JK, Rogers WJ, Coronary artery to right ventricle fistula in heart transplant recipients: a complication of endomyocardial biopsy, *J Am Coll Cardiol* (1989)**14**:258–61.

106 Braverman AC, Coplen SE, Mudge GH, Lee RT, Ruptured chordae tendinae of the tricuspid valve as a complication of endomyocardial

biopsy in heart transplant patients, *Am J Cardiol* (1990)**66**:111–13.

107 Deckers JW, Hare JM, Baughman KL, Complications of transvenous right ventricular endomyocardial biopsy in patients with cardiomyopathy: a seven year survey of 546 consecutive diagnostic procedures in a tertiary referral center, *J Am Coll Cardiol* (1992)**19**:43–7.

108 Williams MJ, Lee MY, DiSalvo TG et al, Biopsy-induced flail tricuspid leaflet and tricuspid regurgitation following orthotopic cardiac transplantation, *Am J Cardiol* (1996)**77**:1339–44.

109 Winters GL, McManus BM, Consistencies and controversies in the application of the International Society for Heart and Lung Transplantation working formulation for heart transplant biopsy specimens, *J Heart Lung Transplant* (1996)**15**:728–35.

110 Billingham ME, Cary NRB, Hammond ME et al, A working formulation for the standardization of nomenclature in the diagnosis of heart and lung rejection: heart rejection study group, *J Heart Transplant* (1990)**9**:587–92.

111 Joshi A, Masek MA, Brown BWJ, Weiss LM, Billingham ME, 'Quilty' revisited: a 10-year perspective, *Hum Pathol* (1995)**26**:547–57.

112 Ensley RD, Hammond EH, Renlund DG et al, Clinical manifestations of vascular rejection in cardiac transplantation, *Transplant Proc* (1991)**23**(suppl 1):1130–2.

113 Hammond EH, Yowell RL, Nunosa S et al, Vascular (humoral) rejection in heart transplantation: pathologic observations and clinical implications, *J Heart Transplant* (1989)**8**:430–43.

114 Hammond EH, Ensley RD, Yowell RL et al, Vascular rejection of human cardiac allografts and the role of humoral immunity in chronic allograft rejection, *Transplant Proc* (1991)**23** (suppl 2):26–30.

115 Schuurman HJ, Jambroes G, Borleffs J, Slootweg P, Meyling FH, de Gast GC, Acute humoral rejection after heart transplantation, *Transplantation* (1988)**46**:603–5.

116 Trento A, Hardesty RL, Griffith BP, Zerbe T, Kormos RL, Bahnson HT, Role of antibody to vascular endothelial cells in hyperacute rejection in patients undergoing cardiac transplantation, *J Thorac Cardiovasc Surg* (1988) **95**:37–41.

117 Weil R, Clarke DR, Iwaki Y et al, Hyperacute rejection of a transplanted human heart, *Transplantation* (1981)**32**:71–2.

118 Ippoliti G, Martinelli L, Minzioni G et al, Emergency retransplantation with a positive donor cross-match, *J Heart Transplant* (1989)**8**:184–8.

119 Pikul FJ, Bolman RM, Saffitz JE, Chaplin H, Anti-B-mediated rejection of an ABO-incompatible cardiac allograft despite aggressive plasma exchange transfusions, *Transplant Proc* (1987)**19**:4601–4.

120 Costanzo-Nordin MR, Silver MA, O'Connell JB et al, Successful reversal of acute cardiac allograft rejection with OKT3 monoclonal antibody, *Circulation* (1987)**76**(suppl 5):71–9.

121 Costanzo-Nordin MR, O'Sullivan EJ, Hubbell EA et al, Long-term follow-up of heart transplant recipients treated with murine antihuman mature T-cell monoclonal antibody (OKT3): the Loyola experience, *J Heart Transplant* (1989)**8**:288–95.

122 O'Connel JB, Renlund DG, Hammond EH et al, Sensitization to OKT3 monoclonal antibody in heart transplantation: correlation with early graft loss, *J Heart Lung Transplant* (1991)**10**:217–22.

123 Macris MP, Frazier OH, Lammermeier D, Radovancevic B, Duncan MJ, Clinical experience with muromonoab-CD3 monoclonal antibody (OKT3) in heart transplantation, *J Heart Transplant* (1989)**8**:281–7.

124 Hunt SA, Strober S, Hoppe RT, Stinson EB, Total lymphoid irradiation for the treatment of intractable cardiac allograft rejection, *J Heart Lung Transplant* (1991)**10**:211–16.

125 Levin B, Bohannan L, Warvariv V, Bry W, Collins G, Total lymphoid irradiation (TLI) in the cyclosporin era — use of TLI in resistant cardiac allograft rejection, *Transplant Proc* (1989)**21**:1793–5.

126 Ballester M, Obrador D, Carrio I et al, Reversal of rejection-induced coronary vasculitis detected early after heart transplantation with increased immunosuppression, *J Heart Transplant* (1989)**8**:413–17.

127 Olivari MT, May CB, Johnson NA, Ring WS, Stephens MK, Treatment of acute vascular

rejection with immunoadsorption, *Circulation* (1994)**90**:1170–3.

128 Partanen J, Nieminen MS, Krogerus L, Harjula ALJ, Mattila S, Heart transplant rejection treated with plasmapheresis, *J Heart Lung Transplant* (1992)**11**:301–5.

129 Stinson EB, Oyer PE, Infectious complications in thoracic transplantation. In: Shumway SJ, Shumway NE, eds. *Thoracic transplantation* (Blackwell Scientific: Cambridge, 1995) 252–72.

130 Paya CV, Fungal infections in solid-organ transplantation, *Clin Infect Dis* (1993)**16**:677–88.

131 Torre-Cisneros J, Lopez OL, Kusne S et al, CNS aspergillosis in organ transplantation: a clinico-pathological study, *J Neurol Neurosurg Psychiatry* (1993)**56**:188–93.

132 Grossi P, Minoli L, Percivalle E, Irish W, Vigano M, Gerna G, Clinical and virological monitoring of human cytomegalovirus infection in 294 heart transplant recipients, *Transplantation* (1995)**59**:847–51.

133 Boland GJ, Hene RJ, Ververs C, de Haan MA, de Gast GC, Factors influencing the occurrence of active cytomegalovirus (CMV) infections after organ transplantation, *Clin Exper Immunol* (1993)**94**:306–12.

134 Merigan TC, Renlund DG, Keay S et al, A controlled trial of ganciclovir to prevent cytomegalovirus disease after heart transplantation, *N Engl J Med* (1992)**326**:1182–6.

135 Wagner JA, Ross H, Hunt S et al, Prophylactic ganciclovir treatment reduces fungal as well as cytomegalovirus infections after heart transplantation, *Transplantation* (1995)**60**:1473–7.

136 Gao SZ, Schroeder JS, Alderman EL et al, Clinical and laboratory correlates of accelerated coronary artery disease in the cardiac transplant patient, *Circulation* (1987)**76** (**suppl V**):56–61.

137 Gao SZ, Schroeder JS, Alderman EL et al, Prevalence of acclerated coronary artery disease in heart transplant survivors: comparison of cyclosporin and azathioprine regimens, *Circulation* (1989)**80**(**suppl III**):100–05.

138 Heroux AL, Silverman P, Costanzo MR et al, Intracoronary ultrasound assessment of morphological and functional abnormalities associated with cardiac allograft vasculopathy, *Circulation* (1994)**89**:272–7.

139 St. Goar FG, Pinto FJ, Alderman EL, Intracoronary ultrasound in cardiac transplant recipients: *in vivo* evidence of 'angiographically silent' intimal thickening, *Circulation* (1992)**85**:979–87.

140 Schroeder JS, Gao SZ, Alderman EL et al, A preliminary study of diltiazem in the prevention of coronary artery disease in heart transplant recipients, *N Engl J Med* (1993)**328**:164–70.

141 Kobashigawa JA, Katznelson S, Laks H et al, Effect of pravastatin on outcomes after cardiac transplantation, *N Engl J Med* (1995)**333**:621–7.

142 Penn I, Neoplastic consequences of immunosuppression. In: Dean JH, Luster MI, Munson AE, Amos H, eds. *Immunotoxicology and immunopharmacology* (Raven Press: New York, 1985) 78–89.

143 Penn I, Malignant neoplasia in the immunocompromised patient. In: Cooper DKC, Novitsky E, eds. *The transplantation and replacement of thoracic organs* (Kluwer Academic: Boston, 1990) 183–90.

144 Hanto DW, Frizzera G, Gaul-Peczalska J et al, The Epstein-Barr virus (EBV) in the pathogenesis of post-transplant lymphoma, *Transplant Proc* (1981)**8**:756–60.

145 Young I, Alfieri C, Hennessy K et al, Expression of the Epstein-Barr virus transformation-associated genes in the tissue of patients with EBV lymphoproliferative disease, *N Engl J Med* (1989)**321**:1080–5.

146 Brumbaugh J, Baldwin JC, Stinson EB et al, Quantitative analysis of immunosuppression in cyclosporin-treated heart transplant patients with lymphoma, *Heart Transplant* (1985)**4**:307–11.

147 Penn I, Cancers after cyclosporin therapy, *Transplant Proc* (1988)**20**:276–9.

148 Amitage JM, Kormaos RL, Stuart RS et al, Posttransplant lymphoproliferative disease in thoracic organ transplant patients: ten years of cyclosporin-based immunosuppression, *J Heart Lung Transplant* (1991)**10**:877–87.

149 Bernstein D, Baum D, Berry G et al, Neoplastic disorders after pediatric heart transplantation, *Circulation* (1993)**88**:II230–7.

150 Starzl TE, Porter FA, Iwatsuki S et al, Reversibility of lymphoma and lymphoproliferative lesions developing under cyclosporin-steriod therapy, *Lancet* (1984)**1**:583–7.

151 Swinnen LJ, Mullen GM, Carr TJ, Costanzo MR, Fisher RI, Aggressive treatment for post-cardiac transplant lymphoproliferation, *Blood* (1995)**86**:3333–40.

152 Kuo PC, Luikart H, Busse-Henry S et al, Clinical outcome of interval cadaveric renal transplantation in cardiac allograft recipients, *Clin Transplant* (1995)**9**:92–7.

153 Lee AH, Mull RL, Keenan GF et al, Osteoporosis and bone morbidity in cardiac transplant recipients, *Am J Med* (1994)**96**:35–41.

154 Shane E, Rivas MC, Silverberg SJ, Kim TS, Staron RB, Bilezikian JP, Osteoporosis after cardiac transplantation, *Am J Med* (1993)**94**:257–64.

155 Van Cleemput J, Daenen W, Nijs J, Geusens P, Dequeker J, Vanhaecke J, Timing and quantification of bone loss in cardiac transplant recipients, *Transplant Int* (1995)**8**:196–200.

156 Blockman RS, Weinerman SA, Steriod-induced osteoporosis, *Orthop Clin North Am* (1990)**21**:97–107.

157 Ubel PA, Arnold RM, Caplan AL, Rationing failure. The ethical lessons of the retransplantation of scarce vital organs, *JAMA* (1993)**270**:2469–74.

158 Smith JA, Ribakove GH, Hunt SA et al, Heart retransplantation: the 25-year experience at a single institution, *J Heart Lung Transplant* (1995)**14**:832–9.

Index

Note: page numbers in *italics* refer to figures and tables

    cardiovascular risk intervention 18
    echocardiography 307
    lack 1
    redistribution thallium imaging 130
exercise testing in women 71–2
    coronary artery disease 74
exhaustion
    cardiovascular conditions 215–16
    hyperventilation 220

F18-fluorodeoxyglucose (FDG) single-photon imaging
        150, 151, 152
familial hypercholesterolaemia 334, 335, 344–5
familial hyperhomocysteinemia 12
fatty acids, myocardial metabolism 149
FDG-PET 150
FDG-SPECT 150
fetus, hypertension in pregnancy 49
fibrates, diabetes 36
fibroblast growth factor 1 (FGF1) 345
fibroblast growth factor
    secreted (FGF-5) 350, 352
    see also basic fibroblast growth factor (bFGF)
fight–flight reaction 219
fish
    consumption 15
    oils 14–15
FK506 see tacrolimus
flecainide 198
    atrial fibrillation 245
folic acid 12
Framingham study 3
    coronary artery disease in women 63–4
    Offspring Study 19
    type A behaviour pattern 213
French paradox 13

β-galactosidase 337
    genes encoding 347, 350
    reporter gene 352
ganciclovir 383
gemfibrozil 7
    diabetes 36
gene
    expression duration 335
    marker 333, 354
gene therapy 333–54
    antisense oligonucleotides 343–4
    arterial for peripheral vascular disease 348–9

delivery devices
    diffusion 341–3
    mechanical 343
    pressure-driven 343
    mRNA formation 343–4
    single gene disorders 334
    vectors 335–6, 337, 338, 339, 340
    viral conjugates 340–38
gene transfer 333
    angioplasty restenosis 345
    bioprostheses 347–8
    cell proliferation inhibition 345–6
    DNA 334–5
    endothelial function restoration 347
    ischaemic heart disease 349–50
    myocardium 350, 351
    principles 334–5
    therapeutic targets 350, 352–3
    thrombosis prevention 346–7
    vector 334
    vein grafts 347–8
    see also familial hypercholesterolaemia
genetic counselling 334
glucocorticoids 290
glucose, myocardial metabolism 150
glucose tolerance
    coronary heart disease 34
    impaired 31, 34
Goldman index 303, 304, 308
graft failure, retransplantation 388
graft rejection 375–6
    acute cellular 382
    endomyocardial biopsy 379–80
    grading system 381
    humoral 380–1, 382–3
    refractory cellular 382
    surveillance in heart transplantation 378–83
    treatment 381–3
    vascular 380–1, 382–3
    see also heart transplantation; immunosuppression

haemagglutinating virus of Japan 340, 346
haemorheological indices
    abnormalities with oral contraceptives 50
    hypertension 47
heart failure
    aspirin 197
    aspirin/ACE inhibitor interaction 202–3
    diabetes 30
    emotional stress 222